MITOCHONDRIAL DISEASES

Edited by **Eylem Taskin, Celal Guven**
and **Yusuf Sevgiler**

Mitochondrial Diseases
http://dx.doi.org/10.5772/67963
Edited by Eylem Taskin, Celal Guven and Yusuf Sevgiler

Contributors

Srinivasa R. Sripathi, Weilue He, Johnpaul Offor, Diana R. Gutsaeva, Wan Jin Jahng, Rodrigo Quintanilla, Cheril Tapia-Rojas, María José Pérez, Claudia Jara, Erick H Vergara, Janka Vašková, Ladislav Vaško, Jozef Firment, Danielle R. Bruns, Lori A. Walker, Grazyna Nowak, Namik Kaya, Zuhair Al-Hassnan, Dilek Colak, Mazhor Aldosary, Maha Abdurrahim, Jiann Ruey Hong, Lateef Reshi, Hao -Ven Wang, Anibal E Vercesi, Estela Busanello, Ana Carolina Marques, Estela Lorza-Gil, Helena Oliveira, Fumiaki Uchiumi, Sei-Ichi Tanuma, Jun Arakawa, Yutaka Takihara, Motohiro Akui, Hiroshi Hamada, Yusuf Sevgiler, Eylem Taskin, Celal Guven, Hongyu Qiu, Shaunrick Stoll, Christiana Leimena, Nahum Rosenberg, Nasra Yassin, Leo Veenman, Orit Rosenberg, Abraham Weizman, Moshe Gavish, Kiyoshi Kita, Madhavi Priyanka Paranagama, Sandra Cardoso, Ana Esteves, Diana F Silva, Daniel Santos, Emanuel Candeias, Filipa Filipe, C. Roger White, Samantha Giordano, Ved Mooga, Xiaowen Bai, Danielle Twaroski, Yasheng Yan, Congshan Jiang, Sarah Logan, Zeljko J Bosnjak, Zuzana Tatarkova, Martin Kolisek, Ivana Pilchova, Peter Racay, Peter Kaplan

First published in London, United Kingdom, 2018 by IntechOpen
IntechOpen is the global imprint of INTECHOPEN LIMITED, registered in England and Wales, registration number: 11086078, The Shard, 25th floor, 32 London Bridge Street
London, SE19SG – United Kingdom
Printed in Croatia

British Library Cataloguing-in-Publication Data
A catalogue record for this book is available from the British Library

Additional hard copies can be obtained from orders@intechopen.com

Mitochondrial Diseases, Edited by Eylem Taskin, Celal Guven and Yusuf Sevgiler
p. cm.
Print ISBN 978-1-78923-674-3
Online ISBN 978-1-78923-675-0

For EU product safety concerns:
IN TECH d.o.o., Prolaz Marije Krucifikse Kozulić 3, 51000 Rijeka, Croatia,
info@intechopen.com or visit our website at intechopen.com.

Meet the editors

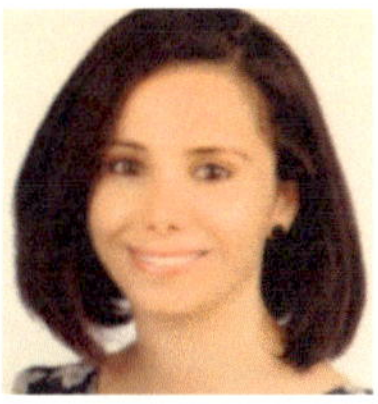

Eylem Taskin is a physiologist. She worked as a postdoctoral researcher at New York University for two years. She has published more than twenty articles and four international book chapters. She has also edited a book. She has worked on the editorial board for several scientific journals.

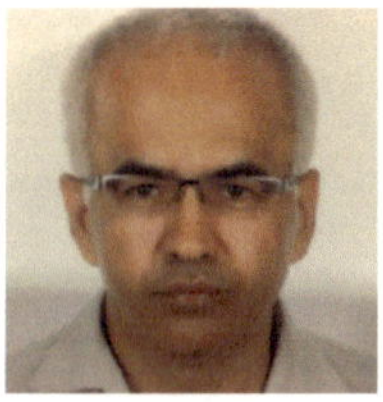

Celal Guven graduated from the Department of Biophysics, Istanbul University. He has been working on protein-chemical interactions. He has published almost ten articles and four international book chapters. He has also edited a book. Dr. Guven has worked on an editorial board for a national journal.

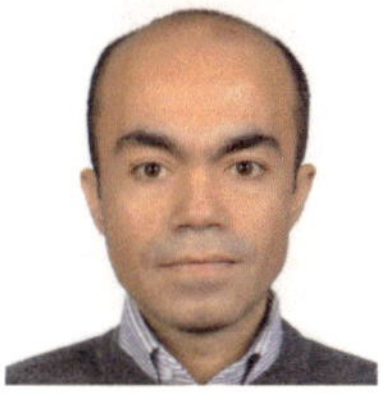

Yusuf Sevgiler graduated from the Department of Biology, Çukurova University. He has published twenty articles about oxidative and neurotoxic potentials of xenobiotics and reviewed many. Dr Sevgiler has also published two international book chapters and has edited a book as well.

Contents

Preface

The cell has a dynamic and complex architecture; therefore, it is not in equilibrium with its environment. The environment constantly disrupts this dynamic and complex harmony. For cell maintenance, cells must absorb different types of energy from their environment and convert this energy into usable chemical forms. The mitochondrion plays a major role in supporting cellular homeostasis and formalizes the physiology of a cell as the most significant energy producer in aerobes. It also participates in cell death mechanisms. Therefore, mitochondrial dysfunction is implicated in the mode of action of many harmful factors for cells such as drugs and environmental contaminants, dysfunction of the oxygen transport system, malnutrition, intense exercise, and genetic variations.

Multicellular organisms need oxygen to execute chemical transformations for ATP utilization and production as an energy transducer, and they need a pump for oxygen transport to the cells in hypoxic environments of their bodies. Heart function depends on continuous energy supply, and therefore a complex mitochondrial network. Any factor affecting the mitochondrial network will produce heart-related diseases and heart failure. Dr Stoll et al. tried to explain the role and the mechanism of mitochondria in the development of heart disease, and the progress in clinical diagnosis and treatments on a mitochondrial basis in recent studies. They proposed that further studies are required to confirm the effectiveness and toxicity of metabolic-modulating drugs and mitochondria-targeting antioxidants. As explained in this chapter, changes in substrate utilization mechanisms should be solved for further understanding in developing effective treatment strategies against heart failure. Drs Bruns and Walker focused on the mechanism of right ventricular failure, which is less common than the left ventricle failure. Both are mitochondria-related pathologies. A detailed explanation of the embryological, physiological, and pathophysiological differences between left and right ventricles is presented in their chapter in the view of recent studies. They reported that there is no right ventricle failure-targeted therapy and the current approach is extrapolating the therapeutic interventions for the left ventricular failure to the right one. However, there are some recent considerations to develop an effective therapy for right ventricle failure with further evaluations. Mitochondria accumulate the damaged and/or modified proteins and mitochondrial DNA (mtDNA) during their life cycles. Mitophagy is an important physiological component for mitochondrial turnover to eliminate damaged or dysfunctional mitochondria to prevent further risk to the cell, especially to avoid unregulated reactive oxygen formation. The healthy heart needs a fine balance between mitophagy and mitochondriogenesis; however, accumulation of damaged proteins and altered proteostasis in mitochondria is an important factor in age-related diseases of the heart. Dr Tatarkova et al. have detailed the current knowledge on the physiological and biochemical changes in the mitochondrial functioning of the aging heart. They proposed that the development of restoration strategies against changed protein machinery should be beneficial against age-related disorders, especially heart-related disorders.

Mitochondrial dysfunction can also be seen in many pathophysiological situations, for example, tumor progression. Therefore, there are recent studies to control cancer cells via mitochondrial component targeting. Drs Paranagama and Kita presented their recent study that defines the complex II of electron transport chain targeted therapy against cancer cells. According to their results, Atpenin A5, a complex II Q site inhibitor, elevates the reactive oxygen formation at this site in cancer cells while there is no effect in healthy cells. They hypothesized that there is a difference at this site via post-translational modification between healthy and cancer cells. Although cancer is known to be a genetic disorder, it has recently and predominantly been accepted as a metabolic disease. Moreover, Dr Uchiumi et al. have explained cancer as a transcriptional disease. They described the general scheme of mitochondrial dysfunction and the characteristic properties of the genes that have a role in this process. The relationship between the metabolic status, specially designated as NAD^+/NADH ratio, and the transcriptional profile of these genes has been explained in detail in the progression of cancer and aging. Finally, a list of possible genes to be targeted to improve mitochondrial functions and then to convert the cancer cells into the normal ones is provided.

Because of its ancestral bacterial origin, damage-associated molecular patterns are sequestered within the mitochondrion, and their releases trigger the sterile innate immune responses. This type of pathology is significant especially in age-related neurodegenerative disorders such as Alzheimer's and Parkinson's diseases. Dr Esteves et al. described innate immune responses observed in these neurodegenerative diseases and the interplay between innate immunity and mitochondria. They concluded that a better understanding of the contribution of mitochondria in neuroinflammatory processes and the exploration of markers would be useful to prevent and treat these disorders.

A mitochondrion contains different components in a delicate balance to produce energy from substrates and to decide the fate of a cell. While most of the proteins of the mitochondrion are encoded in the nuclear DNA, mtDNA encodes 13 genes participating in the electron transfer chain (ETC). The ETC is localized in the inner membrane, while inner and outer mitochondrial membranes contain many proteins to transport ATP, substrates, Ca^{2+}, reactive oxygen, etc. from the other parts of a cell. The proper functioning of ETC and trafficking proteins is vital and their deficiency or failure causes inadequate energy production, abnormal production of reactive oxygen, and then cell death. Dr Nowak reported that 354 mitochondrial proteins are phosphoproteins, and their phosphorylation leads to the progression of mitochondrial damage depending on their phosphorylation site and the kinase as a catalyzer in the context of ischemia/reperfusion injury. She carefully reviewed and grouped the phosphoproteins according to their function in a mitochondrion. Therefore, mitochondrial-related kinases may be a potential therapeutic target for the treatment of ischemic injury. There is a dynamic relationship between the cytoskeleton and mitochondrial proteins for effective energy production, and compensating the damaged parts of mitochondrial structures, they reunite, which is named fusion. On the other hand, denser mitochondrial damage causes the splitting of mitochondria called fission. In all these situations, the mitochondrial morphology is changed. Pathophysiological conditions such as cardiovascular, neurodegenerative, metabolic, tumor progression, etc. cause the change in mitochondrial dynamics and therefore morphology. Dr Sripathi et al. presented their recent work on the pathophysiologic dynamics of mitochondria in age-related macular degeneration via interaction mapping of mitochondrial trafficking proteins. They proposed that the adequate description of the modulation of the mitochondrial network will be useful to develop effective strategies against neurodegenerative diseases. However, this explanation will also be used for the treatment of all the mitochondrial-related diseases. In the other two chapters of the book, authors focused on the mitochondrial transport proteins and their roles in the pathogenesis of mitochondrial diseases. Dr Rosenberg et al. defined the role of the 18 kDa translocator protein (TSPO) in mitochondrial pathologies exemplified by the traumatic brain injury model. Nuclear-encoded proteins located on/in the inner and outer mitochondrial membranes have an interactive role in the proper functioning of the mitochondrion to balance the required amounts of intermediates between two sides of the mitochondrial membranes. Their interaction can also be useful to determine the fate of a cell. Therefore, their contribution in mitochondrial physiology and pathophysiology is discussed in the chapter by Dr Vaskova et al. They concluded that the definition of mitochondrial transport mechanisms could contribute to better diagnosis and treatment of metabolic disorders. In another chapter, Dr Kaya et al. focused on the iron-sulfur cluster assembly proteins that have a role in the assembly of some of the inner membrane localized ETC and some of the cytosolic and matricial proteins. Their inheritance is carried out by nuclear DNA, and some recessive inheritance modes are inhibited with multiple mitochondrial dysfunctions syndrome characterized by various symptoms. Authors listed the case studies related to the inheritance of iron-sulfur clustering assembly proteins.

The mitochondrion is also a key player in the mode of action of drugs and environmental toxicants. These chemicals interfere with the mitochondrial function via interaction with mitochondrial structures that play a role in different layers of mitochondrial homeostasis. Dr Guven et al. discussed the adverse effects of pyrethroids on mitochondrial mechanism as an example of environmental toxicants and doxorubicin as an example of therapeutic agents. They concluded that the most pronounced effects of these agents on mitochondria are the excessive production of reactive oxygen and the disruption of calcium homeostasis via direct and/or indirect pathways. Dr Twaroski et al. introduced their recent studies related to the role of the neurodegenerative potential of ketamine in developing neurons derived from human embryonic stem cells. Ketamine can induce the neuroapoptosis and can alter the mitochondrial ultrastructure through the dysregulated intracellular calcium/microRNA pathway. Collectively, their results put forward the safety of anesthesia, especially in pediatric patients. Dr Busanello et al. presented a well-defined scheme about the toxicity of statins, which are the most prevalent cholesterol-lowering agents. After the presentation of mitochondrial toxicity of these agents, they proposed the coadministration of antioxidants specifically the coenzyme Q10 against the statins' toxicity. As a widespread legal drug, ethanol also targets mitochondrial function and the general mechanism of ethanol toxicity where the mitochondrion is the central mediator is discussed with different consumption scenarios in the chapter by Dr Tapia-Rojas et al. They concluded that the neuronal sites related to the ethanol dependence, learning, and memory are particularly vulnerable toward ethanol toxicity; therefore, knowing all the events that induce mitochondrial dysfunction leads to the development of effective strategies against the toxicity observed in different patterns of ethanol consumption.

An entirely different role of mitochondria can be seen in virus infections. Because the fate of a cell is generally imposed by mitochondrial events, viruses target the mitochondria to increase their survival in their host cells. Interestingly, inheritance materials of these pathogens encode different mitochondrion-resident proteins to control the cell functions. However, some viral proteins act as pro-apoptotic depending on the cellular environment according to Dr Reshi et al. The most vulnerable parameter in a virus infection is the loss of mitochondrial membrane potential, for which the exact mechanism is not currently understood. They concluded that more information on the virus-host cell interaction is needed to treat challenging virus infections.

Dr Mooga et al. discussed the role of estrogen-a pleiotropic hormone-and its receptors in inflammation, cardiovascular diseases, neurodegeneration, aging, and cancer in the view of mitochondrial regulation. Gender-specific differences and age-related challenges in females are well-explained in this chapter. Several cytoprotective mechanisms of estrogen and its receptors support mitochondrial function such as mitochondrial respiration and ATP production, attenuation of reactive oxygen formation, and inhibition of mitochondrial cell death pathways essential in the normal physiological and pathophysiological conditions. On the contrary, these events are also crucial in the estrogen-related promotion of normal and neoplastic breast cancer cells.

Collectively, as the powerhouse of a cell, the mitochondrion is one of the targets of therapeutic interventions because of its role in normal physiologic and pathophysiologic conditions. Different layers of mitochondrial mechanisms become an essential part of a specific pathophysiologic condition. However, reactive oxygen formation, altered calcium homeostasis, and mitochondrial morphology are the most common indicators of mitochondrial dysfunction. There are still many unknowns in inner mitochondrial mechanisms and their interplay and dependence with other components of the cell such as endoplasmic reticulum, cytosol, plasma membrane, and nuclear DNA. Therefore, research on mitochondrial diseases, determination of specific markers, and development of effective treatments will be a competing area in the medical and biological fields.

Eylem Taskin
Nigde Omer Halisdemir University
Medical Faculty
Physiology Department
Nigde, Turkey

Celal Guven
Nigde Omer Halisdemir University
Medical Faculty
Biophysics Department
Nigde, Turkey

Yusuf Sevgiler
Adiyaman University
Faculty of Science and Letters
Department of Biology
Adiyaman, Turkey

Section 1

Mitochondrial Dysfunction and Cardiovascular Diseases

Chapter 1

Mitochondria and Metabolism in Right Heart Failure

Danielle R. Bruns and Lori A. Walker

Additional information is available at the end of the chapter

http://dx.doi.org/10.5772/intechopen.70450

Abstract

Heart failure (HF) is a clinically complex and heterogenous disease characterized by an inability of the heart to pump sufficient blood to the periphery. As such, it has historically been thought of and studied as a disease of the left ventricle (LV). While LV failure is the most common form of HF, it is the ability of the right heart to function that predicts survival in many clinical settings. Extrapolation of mechanisms of left HF to the right ventricle (RV) has yet to prove fruitful in identification of therapeutic approaches, in large part due to a lack of basic mechanistic understanding of the RV which is embryologically, anatomically, and physiologically distinct from the LV. The failing LV is characterized by mitochondrial dysfunction and a metabolic switch, both of which contribute to an energetically starved heart with poor contractile ability. These mechanisms, however, are far less described in the failing RV. The purpose of this chapter is to present the current literature examining the role of mitochondria and metabolism in the healthy right heart, treatments to target deficits in the failing RV, and to identify knowledge gaps for future research in this clinically important area.

Keywords: heart failure, right ventricle, mitochondria, metabolism, ventricular dysfunction, pulmonary hypertension

1. Introduction

Cardiovascular disease is the leading cause of death worldwide, of which heart failure (HF) constitutes a growing public health concern. In the United States alone, close to 6 million individuals currently suffer from HF, accounting for nearly one of out every nine deaths [1]. Morbidity and mortality from HF are high, with 50% mortality within the first 5 years of diagnosis. HF is also a financial burden on the healthcare system, with direct costs estimated at $32 billion per year in the United States [2], roughly 2–3% of total global healthcare spending.

While HF constitutes a complex syndrome of diseases, it generally refers to the inability of the heart to pump sufficient blood to the periphery. As such, historically HF has been studied as a disease of the left ventricle (LV), and most treatments for HF are designed to improve function of the failing LV. Hallmarks of current HF therapies include neurohormonal targets, vasodilators, and/or reducing heart rate- all of which should reduce myocardial oxygen consumption and workload and rebalance energy supply and demand in the heart. However, these therapeutic approaches are largely based on symptom management and have not significantly changed the clinical course of the disease, as the staggering HF morbidity and mortality statistics have remained largely the same over the past 15 years [3]. These data suggest new therapeutic strategies are needed for successful HF therapy, and targeting the bioenergetic deficit through restoration of mitochondrial abnormalities has recently emerged as a promising strategy [4].

While LV-centered pathology constitutes the largest number of HF cases, it is ability of the right ventricle (RV) to function that predicts survival in many cardiovascular disease contexts including pulmonary hypertension [5], (which will be reviewed in much greater detail below), heart failure with preserved ejection fraction [6], and dilated cardiomyopathy [7]. However, no RV-directed therapies exist, and far less is known about the pathophysiology of the failing right heart than the LV. So, while considerable progress has been made to elucidate the metabolic and mitochondrial derangements that underlie LV failure, basic understanding of mitochondrial and metabolic derangements in RV dysfunction continues to be ill-defined. Here, we will present what is known about RV failure and the role of mitochondria and metabolism in models of experimental RV failure and in human populations with right HF. We believe successful HF therapies must target the failing RV for significant improvement in clinical and therapeutic outcomes.

2. The healthy right and left ventricles

Although many similarities exist between the ventricles, and they work in concerted effort to efficiently contract and relax for sufficient blood delivery, important embryological, physiological, and pathophysiological differences exist between the right and left ventricles [8]. We will briefly discuss a few of these differences, with a specific focus on mitochondria and metabolism.

2.1. Embryology, anatomy, and physiology

The RV and LV have different embryological origins and diverge early in development. The RV derives from the anterior (secondary) heart field, while the LV derives from the early heart tube (primary heart field) [9]. This early divergence is transcriptionally regulated, and several transcription factors have been identified which are responsible for the chamber-specific development including Hand2 and Tbx20 [10]. During gestation, the RV functions as the systemic pump. After birth, the RV becomes coupled to the low-pressure pulmonary circulation. As the ductus arteriosus and foramen ovale close, peripheral vascular resistance (PVR) decreases, leading to an increase in RV compliance, regression of muscle mass, and shifting of the interventricular septum toward the RV, resulting in a concave shape of the ventricle in adulthood. Consequently, right sided pressures are significantly lower than the systemically-coupled left sided pressures. Due to its coupling to a low-pressure circuit, the RV is approximately 1/3 the thickness of the LV. As a result of lower pressures and wall stress, the RV has a lower O_2 requirement both at rest and during exercise. Consistent with a lower workload, coronary blood flow and O_2 delivery to the RV are comparatively lower than the LV [11]. At rest, the LV extracts 75% of O_2 and the RV ~50% of the available coronary O_2. These basal differences in oxygen uptake are important under periods of physiological or pathological stress, particularly those in which oxygen availability changes. Further, the ventricles can adapt to changes in oxygen availability through different mechanisms, with the RV meeting O_2 demands by either increasing coronary flow or by increased O_2 extraction [12], whereas the LV primarily increases coronary flow to match demand [13]. These data are consistent with the response of the ventricles to pathological insult, which will be discussed in greater detail below.

2.2. Mitochondrial function and metabolism in the healthy heart

2.2.1. Cardiac metabolism

In healthy states, the heart derives energy from multiple sources to match the demand of contractile function, and can serve as an energetic omnivore based on substrate availability. When given a choice, however, the heart prefers lipid, based on significantly higher ATP production per carbon molecule compared to glycolysis. The first report of the heart's preference for lipid was published in 1953 [14], with subsequent studies confirming that fatty acids constitute 60–90% of cardiac ATP sources with carbohydrates supplying the remaining 10–40% [15]. Fatty acids are transported into cardiomyocytes through fatty acid transporters and subsequently into the mitochondria by carnitine palmitoyltransferase-1 into the matrix where they undergo β-oxidation. The successive oxidation of fatty acid chains provides acetyl CoA that enters the Kreb's Cycle to produce energy to supply the demand of contraction. Glucose is transported into cardiomyocytes by facilitated diffusion mediated by glucose transporters GLUT1 and GLUT4 (insulin-dependent). Once inside the cell, glucose is phosphorylated by hexokinase as the first step in glycolysis. Nine steps later, pyruvate is either decarboxylated by pyruvate dehydrogenase (PDH) to form acetyl CoA to be transported into the mitochondria to begin Kreb's Cycle, or reduced to form lactate and subsequent anaerobic metabolism.

Assuming similar metabolism and mechanisms of control of these pathways between the ventricles might be overly simplistic. As discussed above, the RV is thinner and has a different shape than the LV, which contributes to differential responses to pathological load (discussed below). Transcriptional profiles, including those which regulate metabolism, differ between ventricles, as a comparative gene expression of mRNA and microRNA between control RV and LV samples identified numerous genes with differential expression between the ventricles [16]. These genes spanned a wide variety of biological processes including metabolism, with carbohydrate metabolism (three differentially expressed genes), lipid, fatty acid and steroid metabolism (11 genes), nucleic acid (30 genes) and protein metabolism (22 genes), as well as other metabolic genes (11 genes) significantly varying between ventricles [16].

2.2.2. Mitochondrial content, dynamics, and function

The heart is an extremely energetically active organ. Despite accounting for less than 1% of body weight, it consumes roughly 8% of total ATP [4]. The process of energy production and consumption is incredibly dynamic, as the heart only stores enough energy to supply a few beats and turns over the entire metabolite pool every 10 seconds [17]. To meet this costly energy demand, the heart is the most mitochondrially-dense tissue, with mitochondria comprising 25–30% of cardiac myocyte cell volume [18]. Mitochondria are responsible for the majority of ATP production in the healthy heart, with some estimates suggesting that close to 95% of cardiac ATP production occurs through mitochondrial oxidative phosphorylation [19]. Mitochondria are double membrane-bound organelles which are tightly regulated within the myocardium to facilitate efficient energy production. ATP is produced through oxidation of metabolic fuel to provide reducing equivalents (NADH and $FADH_2$) that are coordinately used to generate a proton motive force across the inner mitochondrial membrane to drive ATP synthesis. Successive electron transfer through complexes I through IV of the electron transport chain culminates in ATP synthesis through complex V (ATP Synthase) in an oxygen-dependent manner.

It has been recognized for quite some time that mitochondria exist in a dynamic reticulum and not as isolate organelles [20]. This network not only allows for efficient ATP production, but also facilitates mitochondrial quality control. The maintenance of this network occurs through continuous mitochondrial fusion and fission, a process mediated by both inner and outer mitochondrial membrane proteins. Fusion, the elongation of the mitochondrial network, increases mitochondrial mass and is regulated mainly by mitofusin-1 and mitofusin-2 (Mfn1 and Mfn2) of the outer mitochondrial membrane and optic atrophy-1 (Opa1) of the inner membrane. Fission, the fragmentation of the mitochondrial network, results in a greater number of smaller mitochondria, and is mediated in part by dynamin-related protein-1 (DRP-1) and fission protein 1 homolog (Fis1) [21]. Fusion and fission are critically necessary for cardiac development as loss of any of these proteins is embryonically lethal [22–24]. Substantial evidence suggests they are also important in the adult heart, as genetic manipulation of these proteins has profound impact on cardiac function.

In addition to regulating mitochondrial shape and size, mitochondrial fission and fusion proteins also regulate mitochondrial quality control through mediating mitophagy, the cellular process of removing damaged mitochondria through autophagy [25]. Autophagy, a highly conserved lysosomal-dependent process of removing damaged cargo and recycling long-lived proteins and organelles, plays a pivotal role in a number of disease states, including cardiovascular diseases [26]. Though the exact mechanisms of mitophagy are far from resolved, it is generally believed that too much mitophagy results in cardiomyocyte death and can contribute to cardiac dysfunction [27] while too little may impair the removal of damaged mitochondria, causing the accumulation of damaged mitochondria which lose mitochondrial membrane potential, produce excess reactive oxygen species, and impart cellular damage [28]. Microtubule associated protein light chain 3 (LC3) is often used as a marker of autophagy; LC3-I (the cytosolic isoform) is converted to LC3-II during the formation of autophagosomes. Additional mitochondrial specific regulators of this process include PINK1 and Parkin [28]. In addition to these protein markers of mitophagy, the process can also be visualized by electron microscopy (EM).

In addition to dynamically undergoing fission and fusion to regulate the mitochondrial network, mitochondrial turnover or biogenesis, creates new mitochondria. Mitochondria have their own DNA (mtDNA) and genetic code that is distinct from nuclear genetics. The biogenesis of mitochondria is a cooperative effort between mitochondrial and nuclear-encoded genes to synthesize all proteins which comprise the five electron transport chain complexes. Biogenesis is transcriptionally regulated by peroxisome proliferator-activated receptor-gamma coactivator 1-α (PGC-1α), the "master regulator" of biogenesis [29], transcription factor of mitochondria (TFAM), and nuclear respiratory factor 1 (NRF1) [30]. Biogenesis of mitochondria also requires the synthesis of cardiolipin, a mitochondrial-specific phospholipid located on the inner mitochondrial membrane which regulates respiratory enzyme super complex assembly [31]. The transcriptional assessments of TFAM, PGC-1α and NRF1 or markers of mitochondrial content are often used as surrogates of biogenesis, a cumulative process which is truly represented by net synthesis of mitochondrial proteins and/or lipids into functioning organelles [32].

Mitochondrial biology and physiology are further complicated when we consider the arrangement of mitochondrial populations within the adult heart. Three distinct cardiac populations have been identified: the subsarcolemmal mitochondria (SSM), located along the perimeter of the cell, interfibrillar mitochondria (IFM), located between the myofibrils [33], and perinuclear mitochondria which are arranged in clusters surrounding nuclei and are presumably involved with transcriptional activity. Although never directly tested, SSM are hypothesized to provide ATP for basic cell functions, whereas IFM provide energy for the contractile apparatus. The original description of IFM and SSM populations identified differences in biochemical and respiratory properties, as well as ultrastructural differences [33]. Following years of debate as to whether these two populations were different and discrepancy over the causal role of isolation procedures in obscuring differences, consensus seems to have been reached regarding important physiological differences in IFM and SSM. It should be noted that these differences have only been identified in LV mitochondria, and to our knowledge, subpopulations of SSM and IFM have never been described in the RV.

Indeed, most of what we know about mitochondrial structure and function in the healthy heart derives from studies of the LV, and only a few studies have compared healthy right and left ventricles. However, a small report suggests differential expression of autophagy and mitophagy regulators in the RV compared to LV [34]. A proteomic analysis of healthy rabbit and porcine LV and RV free walls demonstrated similar cellular aerobic capacity, mitochondrial volume, mitochondrial electron transport chain content (complexes I, III, IV, and V), as well as mitochondrial enzyme activity [35]. Our group assessed mitochondrial content and electron transport chain activity, as well as protein markers of mitochondrial dynamics in the RV and LV from healthy 2-week old cows (**Figure 1**). While we generally found similar mitochondrial profiles between the ventricles, there were some subtle differences including higher relative copy number of COXI (mt/nDNA) and higher expression of Mfn1 in the RV compared to the LV. Together, the few published papers comparing the LV and RV and the data from our group suggest that though small or subtle, differences exist in mitochondrial physiology in the RV and LV, consistent with the different energetic and functional capacities of the ventricles. A more careful description of interventricular differences will aid in understanding pathological adaptations that occur within these organelles, and the contribution they play in development of cardiac disease.

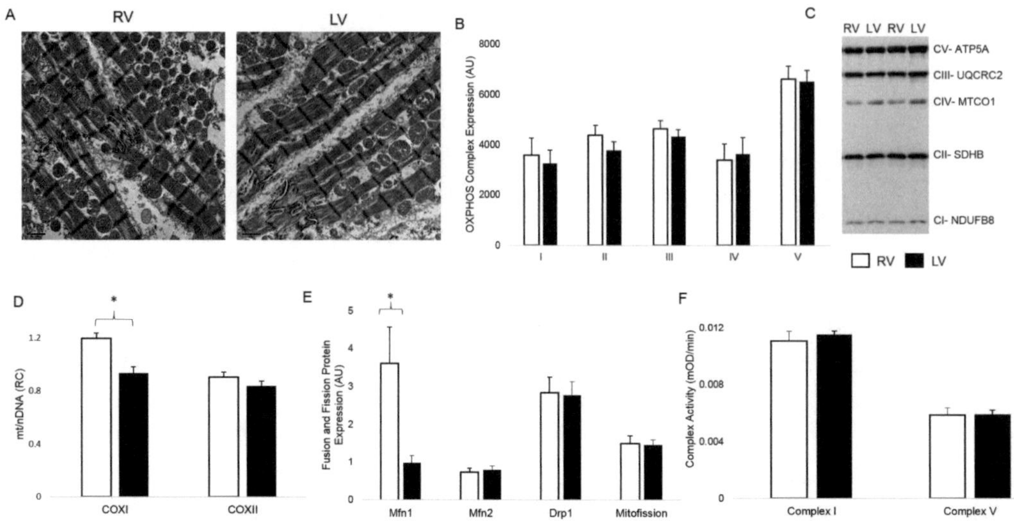

Figure 1. Mitochondrial content, dynamics, and activity in healthy right ventricle (RV) and left ventricle (LV) from neonatal cows. (A) Representative electron micrographs of the mid-RV and LV of control cows. (B) Expression of electron transport chain complexes does not differ in the healthy ventricles. OXPHOS complex expression was assessed by immunoblotting using an antibody against one subunit of each complex. (C) Representative image. (D) Mitochondrial content, as assessed by mt/nDNA copy number, is slightly different between ventricles, as COX1 copy number is higher in the RV than the LV. (E) Mitofusin-1 (Mfn1) expression is significantly higher in the RV than the LV, with no differences in other mitochondrial dynamics markers. (F) Complex I and V activity do not differ between healthy RV and LV, as assessed by spectrophotometric assay. All comparisons were assessed by Student's t-test. *$p < 0.05$, n = 10 in each ventricle. White bars: RV; black bars: LV. Adapted from Bruns, DR et al. AJP-lung, 2014.

2.2.3. Non-energy producing roles for mitochondria in the healthy heart

Mitochondria are a major source of cardiac reactive oxygen species (ROS), and the largest producer of ROS within the cell [36]. Several labs have identified superoxide ($O_2^{\bullet-}$) as the primary mitochondrial source of ROS. Superoxide formation occurs on the outer mitochondrial membrane, in the matrix, and on both sides of the inner membrane. The relative contribution of each site to total $O_2^{\bullet-}$ varies from tissue to tissue and depends on respiration state of the mitochondria. In heart mitochondria, complex III appears to be most responsible for $O_2^{\bullet-}$ formation [37]. When mitochondria are functioning normally, ROS production is low. Although a physiological amount of ROS are produced for oxidant-sensitive cell signaling, these ROS are balanced by both mitochondrial and cytosolic scavenging systems to prevent oxidative damage. The matrix contains a specific form of superoxide dismutase (SOD) with manganese in the active site (MnSOD, or SOD2) [38]. SOD2 dismutates $O_2^{\bullet-}$ into hydrogen peroxide (H_2O_2), which is catalyzed to water and molecular oxygen by catalase, a major detoxifying enzyme present in heart mitochondria [39]. In addition to these enzymes, other enzymes including glutathione peroxidases, as well as non-enzymatic molecules like vitamins C and E, help to attenuate excess ROS production. However, if ROS production exceeds the ability to remove them, oxidant damage occurs in the form of lipid peroxidation (including oxidation of both inner and outer membranes, and cardiolipin), mitochondrial protein oxidation, and oxidant damage to mtDNA.

In addition to damaging macromolecules, excess ROS can trigger apoptosis. The observation that mitochondria trigger cardiomyocyte apoptosis was first described in 1999 [40]. This study demonstrated that when cardiomyocytes are exposed to hydrogen peroxide, Bad, a pro-apoptotic family member of Bcl-2 family, translocates to the mitochondria, resulting in the release of cytochrome c into cytoplasm which leads to the activation of caspase 3 and programmed cell death. Furthermore, both pro-apoptotic proteins Bax and Bak co-localize with Mfn2 on the outer mitochondrial membrane [41]. Drp1 is also recruited by Bax in response to apoptotic stimuli, and colocalizes with Bax at the outer mitochondrial membrane [41]. Conversely, OPA1 is strongly anti-apoptotic by preventing cytochrome c release independent from modulation of fusion [42]. Taken together, these findings suggest that in addition to their roles as primary energy producers, the mitochondria are key contributors to redox homeostasis and regulation of programmed cell death, both of which contribute to healthy and pathological cardiac function.

While little is known regarding basal differences in ROS production, antioxidant defenses, and apoptotic signaling between the healthy LV and RV, two recent studies suggest differences may exist between the ventricles in healthy hearts and in response to cardiac stress. Schreckenberg and colleagues [43] used a model of systemic nitric oxide (NO) depletion in rats by administration of the pharmacological nitric oxide synthase inhibitor L-NAME. They evaluated cardiac antioxidant capacity in response to L-NAME and in a control (untreated) group. Chronic NO deficiency is associated with oxidant stress, however it appears to do so in a ventricle-specific manner. Dihydroethidium staining, used to detect ROS, showed elevated free radical load in untreated RV control samples compared with the LV, as well as elevated peroxynitrite, both of which were further increased during L-NAME treatment. To identify mechanisms underlying the differential formation of ROS in the LV and RV, the authors examined expression of antioxidant enzymes and found that L-NAME treatment induced SOD2 expression in the LV by 51%, but depressed SOD2 by 30% in the RV. The authors concluded that while the LV increases SOD2 to compensate for increased oxidant load with NO deficiency, the RV does not. Importantly, these biochemical differences in redox status were correlated with changes in RV geometry and function indicative of cardiac dysfunction. A second small study of ischemia–reperfusion injury in a bi-ventricular isolated working heart preparation suggests that mechanisms of myocardial apoptosis also differ between the ventricles. While both ventricles saw similar upregulation of apoptosis in response to ischemia as assessed by cleaved caspase-3 expression, the RV downregulated anti-apoptotic regulator Bcl, while the LV did not [34]. Though this study was small, and performed no follow-up of additional apoptotic regulators or ROS signaling in the healthy heart, it does suggest that different mechanisms may underlie the ability of the two ventricles to regulate ROS production, antioxidant defenses, and apoptosis. Together, this work suggests that inherent differences between the ventricles with respect to these signaling pathways may be especially relevant in response to stresses which promote redox dys-homeostasis including ischemia, reperfusion, and hypoxia.

3. Cardiac remodeling and heart failure

In response to pathological stress, the heart remodels, resulting in changes in structure, shape, or physiology of the heart and its cellular components. While remodeling can occur physiologically such as in response to exercise or pregnancy, pathophysiologic remodeling is a maladaptive process that occurs with stress such as myocardial infarction or hypertension (chronic pressure overload). Adaptations evidenced at the organ level can occur at the level of myocyte, as well as within other cardiac cell types including fibroblasts and endothelial cells. Typically, remodeling is not an acute event, but rather occurs as a continuum of changes both adaptive and maladaptive, first evidenced by ventricular hypertrophy, dysfunction and abnormalities in filling and contraction. In the continued face of stress and/or adverse signaling modalities the heart continues to remodel resulting in overt failure - the inability of the heart to supply sufficient circulation for the needs of the body. The response of the RV or LV to pathological stress is complex and is likely a cumulation of the nature, severity, and chronicity (acute versus chronic) of the insult. In addition, the timing of the insult (newborn, juvenile, adult, or aged) likely has a large impact on cardiac remodeling. Insults that are initiated early in life tend to be better tolerated than those in adulthood [44]. Though cardiac aging research and RV aging are understudied, the aged heart has been suggested to perform even poorer in response to pathological stress, an area which warrants future research efforts.

It should come as no surprise given the physiological differences between ventricles, that the ability to adapt to pathological load greatly varies between the left and right heart. While it is generally accepted that the RV is able to tolerate volume overload well [45], it poorly tolerates pressure overload (afterload). Experimentally, an increase in pulmonary artery pressure of 20 mmHg compared to a similar increase in systolic afterload resulted in a 30% decline in RV stroke volume, compared to only a 10% reduction in LV stroke volume [46]. Mechanistically, the thin wall of the RV along with reduced elastance is thought to reflect this poor tolerance for increases in afterload. This observation is clinically highly relevant, as patients with systemic hypertension compensate for the increased load for many years before diagnosis or treatment of cardiac disease, but patients with pulmonary hypertension (PH, which will be discussed in greater detail below), often rapidly progress to right heart failure.

3.1. Right heart failure

Right heart failure (RHF) is a syndrome reflecting the inability of the RV to fill or eject properly. Clinically, it manifests as fluid retention (peripheral edema) and decreased systolic reserve or cardiac output, which often presents as exercise intolerance [47]. In the case of RV geometry, the ventricle becomes more concentric, and the interventricular septum flattens. In humans, right heart failure is diagnosed through a combination of clinical findings, laboratory tests and imaging. Similarly, in larger animal models of RV failure (below), it can be measured by echocardiography, whereas in mouse models it is generally demonstrated by morphometric changes including RV/LV ratios and myocyte size.

3.2. Models of right heart failure

Understanding RV failure requires the use of animal models that are primarily or predominantly right-sided. Therefore, although the most common cause of RV failure in humans is left-sided heart failure, it is more helpful to study the RV in diseases and models in which it is primary. For reasons including methodological constraints, clinical relevance, and the sensitivity of the RV to increased afterload (compared to the insensitivity of the RV to volume overload), most groups use models of RV pressure overload. However, we should mention that other causes of RV failure include valvular insufficiency, congenital disease including tetralogy of fallot, pulmonary atresia, truncus arteriosus, and hypoplastic left heart syndrome, RV ischemia/infarct, and amyloid and sarcoid [44]. Below, we'll briefly overview common animal models of RV failure and how they recapitulate human disease, which are summarized in **Table 1**.

Pulmonary artery banding (PAB) involves surgical constriction of the pulmonary artery, in a manner equivalent to the commonly used transaortic constriction (TAC) model of LV pressure overload. Administration of a band around the pulmonary artery results in pulmonary constriction, increased afterload, RV hypertrophy, and eventually failure. While similar methodologically and conceptually to TAC, an RNA-seq experiment comparing the RV and LV in isolated TAC or PAB suggests that the two ventricles do not respond in an entirely similar manner [48]. Of the nearly 3600 genes identified, only 192 were commonly expressed in both ventricles, 565 were unique to the RV, and 327 were unique to the LV. Canonical pathway enrichment only revealed oxidative phosphorylation as similar between the two ventricles [48]. Therefore, despite being methodologically and conceptually equivalent models of isolated pressure overload, TAC and PAB do not elicit identical molecular signatures, again suggesting that important differences between the ventricles may explain disease trajectory and prognosis.

A more clinically relevant model of RV afterload is pulmonary hypertension (PH). The World Health Organization classifies five distinct groups of PH based on etiology, prognosis, and therapy. However, they're all linked by an increase in mean pulmonary artery pressure of >25 mmHg at rest [49]. The increased pulmonary pressures cause pressure overload in the RV, isolated RV

Human RHF	Experimental RHF
LV failure	Pulmonary artery banding (PAB)
Pulmonary hypertension	Pulmonary hypertension: chronic hypoxia, MCT, SuHx, BMP2R
Congenital disease: hypoplastic left heart syndrome, tetralogy of fallot, pulmonary atresia	Not available
Amyloid sarcoid	Microbial infection, genetic knockout
RV Ischemia/infarct	Right coronary ligation (sheep)
Valvular disease	Not available

Legend: LV failure is the most common cause of RHF in humans. Pulmonary hypertension is a heterogenous disease, classified into five groups by the World Health Organization, but generally refers to an increase in pulmonary arterial pressure, causing increased RV afterload. Congenital diseases, amyloid, sarcoid, RV ischemia and infarct, and valvular disease (tricuspid, pulmonic) also contribute to RHF. In experimental RHF, pulmonary artery banding/constriction causes an isolated increased RV afterload, similar to transaortic banding in left heart failure. Animal models of PH (rats, mice, cows) are also frequently used to cause predominant RHF. MCT: monocrotaline, SuHx: Sugen hypoxia, BMP2R: bone morphogenetic peptide receptor models (BMP2R plays a critical role in the pathogenesis of familiar idiopathic PH).

Table 1. Selected causes of clinical right heart failure (RHF) and the corresponding experimental model.

hypertrophy, dysfunction, and eventual failure. PH can be modeled in animals by different approaches including chronic exposure to hypoxia, pharmaceuticals which accelerate pulmonary dysfunction, or their combination. Here, we will briefly discuss the most common laboratory approaches to PH, but refer readers to an extensive review of animal models of PH [50].

Exposure to chronic hypoxia while causing systemic reduction in oxygen supply, selectively induces pressure overload on the RV. Animal models of chronic hypoxia are often driven by normobaric hypoxia, accomplished by nitrogen replacement to reduce partial pressure of oxygen, or by hypobaric hypoxia (simulated ~14,000–17,000 feet), reducing overall atmospheric pressure and thus reducing oxygen partial pressure in the inhaled air. Animal models of hypoxia-driven PH have been used at least since the early 1960s [51] and can be used to elicit predictable and reproducible PH within many animal strains. However, there are some unique differences between species worth noting. Bovine models produce robust responses to simulated altitude and hypoxia, and were among the most common model used in early research [52]. Neonatal calves exposed to chronic hypobaric hypoxia develop severe PH with striking remodeling of the pulmonary vasculature [52]. Rodent models of hypoxia are also common in the literature, with certain strains of rats developing more severe PH, and mice developing the least severe perivascular remodeling [50].

In addition to hypoxia exposure, other models of PH include monocrotaline (MCT) injection, a pyrrolizidine alkaloid oxidized in the liver to a bioactive molecule which selectively injures the lung vascular endothelium, causing PH [53]. MCT as a model of PH has been in use for almost 50 years, and can be produced by a single subcutaneous or intraperitoneal injection of the drug. Within hours of injection, pulmonary damage occurs, by 2 weeks PVR has increased, and by 3 weeks, increased RV mass is often reported [54]. Some reports also describe liver and kidney damage [55], as well as myocarditis of both the RV and LV [56], limiting the use of MCT to study isolated RV hypertrophy and failure. A relatively recent model to the PH literature is a model of severe PH that combines chronic hypoxia plus a pharmaceutical vascular endothelial growth factor (VEGF) receptor inhibitor. This model, coined the Sugen hypoxia (SuHx) model after the VEGF receptor inhibitor Sugen 5416, has been modified for both mice and rats, and is characterized by persistent pulmonary vasculature disease and right heart failure [57]. Alternative animal models of PH worth mentioning include bleomycin injury and single gene mutations. Bleomycin, an antibiotic, is a common model for pulmonary fibrosis in mice. A single intratracheal dose results in PH after 2–5 weeks, a doubling of right ventricular systolic pressure, and a drop in cardiac output [58]. Lastly, several human mutations have been linked to elevated pulmonary pressures and PH, with the bulk of experimental PH studies using models with mutations of bone morphogenetic protein receptor type II [59].

4. Molecular mechanisms of left heart failure

All cell types within the heart respond to stress, including in response to chronic pressure overload [60]. However, the majority of research has focused on changes within the myocytes as they are the primary cell type responsible for contraction and heart failure is a disease of impaired cardiac function. The hallmark molecular change of myocyte remodeling is hypertrophy. In response to pathological load such as pressure overload, myocyte size increases via synthesis of new sarcomeres. Myocytes also reactivate a fetal program of gene expression, now often referred to as the hypertrophic gene program [61]. While initially characterized in the failing left heart, the fetal (hypertrophic) gene program has now been shown to also occur in RV failure [62]. While believed to be compensatory at first, over time this is maladaptive, and likely contributes to the energy deficit of the failing heart.

4.1. Metabolic remodeling and mitochondrial dysfunction in left heart failure

Mitochondrial and metabolic abnormalities are well-established in left-sided HF. Since this topic will be more extensively covered elsewhere, we will just briefly discuss mitochondrial dysfunction and the metabolic switch in the failing left heart. Considerable evidence exists for an energetic deficit in HF, both in pre-clinical animal models of disease, and in studies from explanted human hearts (reviewed in [4]). One of the hallmarks of the hypertrophied or failing heart is a metabolic switch [63]. As the heart remodels, it undergoes a switch from fatty acid oxidation (FAO) to glycolytic carbohydrate metabolism. Although it is still a matter of debate whether this switch is causal, associative or compensatory, it is clear that the energy starved heart no longer produces the majority of its ATP from lipid sources. It has been suggested that this switch is designed to allow more efficient energy production with respect to oxygen since under states of low oxygen availability carbohydrate metabolism produces more ATP per mole of oxygen [64].

Due to their primary role as ATP generators, mitochondrial dysfunction has been mechanistically linked to the energy starved failing heart. Mitochondrial dysfunction is well described in the failing LV across many different pre-clinical models including guinea pigs [65], rats [66], rabbits [67], and dogs [68] with dilated, ischemic, and diabetic heart failure. Similarly, decreased respiration and respiratory control ratios, associated with an overall loss of oxidative capacity [69], have been observed in human explanted hearts from patients with ischemic and dilated cardiomyopathy. In addition to depressed oxidative phosphorylation, mitochondrial biogenic signaling is depressed in HF, with PGC-1α downregulated in different models of HF [70, 71]. Together, substantial data links mitochondrial respiratory deficits with the failing LV and suggests interventions aimed at preservation of mitochondrial function may have therapeutic potential. Observations of changes in the shape of mitochondria in HF spurred the idea that the major proteins regulating mitochondrial dynamic could be causally involved in development of the disease [72–74].

As discussed above, ROS production in the healthy heart is countered by enzymatic and non-enzymatic scavenging of ROS to prevent cellular damage. However, increased ROS and oxidant stress have been reported in many types have cardiovascular disease, including early in the development of pressure overload-induced left HF [75]. In addition to damaging cellular macromolecules, increased ROS can activate several cell-signaling processes including apoptosis and opening of the mitochondrial transition pore (mPTP) which are known to correlate with adverse health outcomes. Opening of this pore is associated with oxidant stress and mitochondrial dysfunction, and increased opening is observed in HF [75]. Although apoptosis of cardiomyocytes is rare in the healthy heart, it is well-established that apoptosis increases in human HF [76]. As adult cardiac myocytes have limited regenerative capacity, the loss of these cells is often counteracted by replacement with non-myocytes, promoting fibrosis and cardiac dysfunction.

5. Molecular mechanisms of right heart failure

The bulk of the research thus far in the field of RV failure and mitochondrial function has focused on PH-associated changes within the pulmonary vasculature (pulmonary artery smooth muscle cells, endothelial cells, and fibroblasts [77]) and metabolic changes that underlie activated inflammatory cells (reviewed in [78, 79]). In addition, a systemic metabolic and mitochondrial hypothesis has been put forward, based on similar changes in mitochondrial function observed in skeletal muscle in models of PH [80]. However, a few RV-specific investigations of changes in metabolism and mitochondrial function exist, and we'll review this evidence below.

5.1. Metabolic remodeling in right heart failure

Although the data are less extensive than in the LV, the metabolic switch that occurs during LV hypertrophy and dysfunction also occurs in models of RV dysfunction [81, 82]. Several groups have reported upregulated glycolysis with suppression of FAO, and associated global changes in gene expression favoring glucose oxidation and downregulation of PPARα target genes [62]. Mechanistically, pyruvate dehydrogenase kinase (PDK) has been linked to the metabolic switch. PDK, an inhibitor of pyruvate dehydrogenase, is upregulated in RV hypertrophy. This PDK-mediated metabolic switch is associated with decreased RV myocyte contractility and cardiac output [81]. The shift to aerobic glycolysis has several consequences for the heart. First, greater amounts of lactate are produced, shifting redox status and other homeostatic outcomes, and second, fewer ATP molecules/glucose molecule are produced (32 during glucose oxidation, and 2 during glycolysis). To compensate for increased glycolysis, glucose uptake is accelerated, and can be assessed by positron emission tomography, both in experimental PH and RV dysfunction [83, 84], and in patients with pulmonary arterial hypertension [85].

As in left heart failure, researchers have attempted to explain the metabolic switch based on energy production relative to oxygen availability. The pressure overloaded RV is oxygen deprived. In the setting of an oxygen limited hypertrophic RV, energy production which favors a high ATP/O_2 ratio would benefit the working heart, and FAO uses 12% more oxygen than glucose oxidation to generate the same amount of ATP [86]. Some experimental data support this hypothesis, with reports of systolic perfusion gradients limiting coronary artery flow [87], coupled with increased metabolic demands in the hypertrophied heart, which result in a localized RV ischemia. However, the question of oxygen supply in RV hypertrophy is insufficiently answered. While it may be true that angiogenic potential in the failing RV is attenuated, resulting in ischemia [88], methodological difficulties have precluded accurate assessment of RV oxygen supply. Further, other groups have argued that reliance on carbohydrate metabolism predisposes the hypertrophied myocardium to contractile dysfunction, and maintaining the inherent metabolic profile of fatty acid fuel preference may be a more beneficial approach [89].

5.2. Mitochondrial dysfunction in right heart failure

Similar to the LV, mitochondrial dysfunction is also implicated in RHF, albeit with less literature supporting the mechanistic link, and more conflicting reports depending on the model. MCT and SuHx models of RHF tend to demonstrate more severe mitochondrial dysfunction and depression of mitochondrial biogenesis. Decreased PGC-1α expression and a net loss of mitochondrial protein and oxidative capacity have been reported in SuHx rats, alongside abnormal mitochondrial shape and size by electron microscopy [90]. On the other hand, changes in mitochondrial function in chronic hypoxia models have been particularly discordant and warrant further discussion. Chronic hypoxia decreased ATP synthesis and measurements of mitochondrial number in a rat model of chronic hypoxia in both ventricles, however, the effect was slightly delayed in the right compared to LV [91]. Data from our lab in the neonatal calf model of PH-induced RV dysfunction also demonstrated similar changes to mitochondrial function in both ventricles, with no additional impact of pressure overload on the RV [92]. In these models of PH and RV dysfunction, the hypoxic stimulus is administered systemically using a hypobaric chamber. Thus, the LV experiences similar degrees of hypoxia as the RV, yet does not show signs of contractile or relaxation deficits until much later in disease progression. It's possible that interventricular differences in oxygen supply and demand explain the similar findings in both ventricles, and support the need for better mechanistic understanding of the similarities and differences in oxygen delivery and metabolism in the RV exposed to pathological load.

Mitochondrial dynamics are not well-described in the failing right heart. However, in a study by Marsboom et al., administration of the Drp1 inhibitor Mdivi-1 regressed PH in rodents by arresting proliferation of pulmonary artery smooth muscle cells, resulting in improved exercise capacity and RV function. Therefore, while not described in the RV, modulation of mitochondrial dynamics may be therapeutically viable for right heart failure [93]. Even less has been described on the role of mitophagy in the setting of right heart failure. However, one group has attempted to elucidate the impact of autophagy on remodeling following PAB. p62 and LC3 II/I were both increased in the hypertrophied RV [94]. These data support similar findings in MCT-induced RV dysfunction, with increased autophagy signaling and autophagosome formation by EM [95]. Expression of these markers temporally increased post MCT injection, which the authors suggest indicates a causal role for autophagy during the progression from hypertrophy to failure. Future work is needed to elucidate the changes that occur with mitochondrial dynamics and mitophagy in the failing right heart, and future investigations should test myocyte-specific deletion of Mfn1, Mfn2, and Drp1 in experimental RV failure.

Our understanding of mitochondrial abnormalities in human RV failure is equally as understudied. Although availability of human samples is methodologically limiting, the use of pediatric congenital heart explants has shed some light on changes which underlie human RHF. One study of RV samples obtained from 31 pediatric patients undergoing cardiac surgery for congenital heart disease classified patients based on compensated RV function or failure based on echocardiography, right heart catheterization and MRI. Citrate synthase activity was maintained during hypertrophy, but decreased at failure, while mtDNA content progressively decreased with worsening clinical disease [96]. In addition, adult RV samples of various etiologies demonstrate increased mitochondrial membrane potential which positively correlates with the degree of hypertrophy [97]. A complete understanding of mitochondrial function in human right heart failure is limited by methodological constraints of assessing comprehensive ETC function.

5.3. Non-energy producing mitochondrial mechanisms of right heart failure

Studies of non-energy producing roles of mitochondria are in their infancy in the RV. However, some evidence supports a causative role of ROS, as increased lipid peroxidation is observed in the RV 6 weeks following MCT injection [98]. NADPH oxidase is significant source of ROS in LV hypertrophy, and its expression increases during MCT-induced RV hypertrophy alongside decreased SOD1 and SOD2 expression [99]. Increased expression of pro-apoptotic proteins Bax and capase-3 have also been noted in the RV after PAB, with concomitant increased RV myocyte cell death [100]. Together, the limited investigations of the metabolic and non-metabolic roles of mitochondria in right heart failure highlight the need for additional work to elucidate similarly and differentially regulated pathways in left and right HF.

6. Therapeutic intervention

To date, no RV-directed therapies exist. Right-sided heart failure is typically treated with the goal of improving LV function or lowering pulmonary pressures. Extrapolation of LV pathophysiology and pharmacology to the failing RV has not yet proven fruitful, and in some cases, has accelerated disease progression [101]. Interestingly, lowering of pulmonary pressures (either by pharmaceutical approaches or by lung transplant) does not consistently improve RV function [102], suggesting a cardiac-specific irreversible effect of long-term pressure overload, or contribution of circulating systemic factors. Whatever the reason for insufficient return of RV function despite reduction in afterload, we and others believe that identification of new, or repurposing of old therapies requires an RV-centric approach.

6.1. Metabolic therapeutic interventions

Enhancing glucose oxidation at the expense of FAO as emerged as a therapeutic strategy in RV dysfunction, based on the reciprocal relationship between these two energy sources. In large part, enhancing glucose oxidation has gained attention as a strategy because of the higher ATP production per oxygen molecule provided by carbohydrate compared to lipid sources. Partial inhibitors of FAO are approved for a few human cardiovascular indications including refractory ischemia [103]. These drugs (trimetazidine) have also been experimentally tested in RV dysfunction [86]. Rats with PAB-induced RV dysfunction treated with partial FAO inhibitors had elevated RV glucose oxidation alongside increased exercise capacity and cardiac output. The beneficial effect of this drug has also been demonstrated in MCT-induced RV dysfunction, where trimetazidine enhanced cardiac mitochondrial function and increased oxygen consumption while reducing ROS formation [104].

The metabolic switch that occurs in the hypertrophied RV is suggested to be mediated in part through PDK4 [81]. Dichloroacetate (DCA), a small molecule inhibitor of pyruvate dehydrogenase, improves glucose oxidation and has reported improvements in RV stroke volume, cardiac output, and exercise capacity [81, 105]. It is also associated with restoration of RV mitochondrial function and mitochondrial-dependent apoptosis [106]. Though a Phase I clinical trial has been completed in subjects with advanced PH (Clinical Trial Identifier NCT01083524), study results have not been published, and the therapeutic potential of DCA in human RV failure remains unknown. As discussed above, the therapeutic strategy of FAO and improved glucose oxidation lacks consensus [89], and in part is predicated on the balance between ATP production and oxygen availability. While continued efforts to test metabolic mediators in RHF are warranted, a mechanistic understanding of energy production, relative RV ischemia, and the molecular regulators of these processes are necessary for development of targeted metabolic therapy.

6.2. Mitochondrial therapeutic interventions

The causal role of ROS in cardiac dysfunction led to the early belief that antioxidants would attenuate cardiovascular disease. In experimental models, treatments with antioxidants have somewhat inconsistently tended to improve cardiac function [107]. However, clinical trials have largely failed to show benefit of antioxidants in treatment of chronic disease [108]. In light of these disappointing results, many groups have taken fundamentally different approaches to improving redox status. Induction of endogenous antioxidants by a phytochemical supplement preserved RV function and prevented RV fibrosis and capillary loss [109], suggesting activation of cytoprotective transcription factors may more robustly attenuate oxidant stress than traditional vitamin supplements. Other groups use mitochondrially-directed peptides to scavenge free radicals. One such peptide, SS31, accumulates more than 1000-fold in mitochondria [110]. This peptide prevented LV hypertrophy, fibrosis, and diastolic dysfunction [111], and reduced mitochondrial oxidant damage [112]. To date, however, targeted mitochondrial peptides have not been tested in models of RV failure.

Interventions which boost mitochondrial function and/or biogenesis have large therapeutic potential in many types of cardiovascular disease, including RV failure. Phytochemical compounds which elicit mitochondrial biogenic properties have received attention lately, such as resveratrol. Resveratrol, the primary polyphenol in red wine, stimulates mitochondrial content, ATP production, and FAO, while inhibiting mitochondrial ROS production in several tissue types and disease contexts [113, 114]. In addition, it is currently in testing as a therapy for chronic obstructive pulmonary disorder (NCT02245932) and non-ischemic heart failure (NCT01914081). Identification of other plant-based or pharmaceutical approaches which stimulate the synthesis of new mitochondria to increase energy production while decreasing oxidant damage may have profound impact on the failing right heart.

6.3. Exercise as right heart therapy

Exercise-induced cardiac hypertrophy has been known to be cardioprotective for decades [115], though the exact mechanisms underlying physiological hypertrophy have remained somewhat elusive. RV-specific adaptations to exercise, however, have lagged, in large part due to clinical concerns. Even in healthy individuals with normal pulmonary vascular function, the hemodynamic load on the RV increases with a relatively greater proportion during exercise than LV hemodynamic load. This disproportionate increase in load is accentuated in patients with PH. Exercise-induced increases in pulmonary artery pressures may exceed RV contractile reserve, resulting in attenuated cardiac output and exercise intolerance. Thus only recently have clinical and preclinical studies begun looking at the cardioprotective role of exercise specifically on the RV.

The primary goal of most of the recent studies of exercise in PH patients was to evaluate safety of low-level exercise training and changes in systolic pulmonary artery pressure. A recent meta-analysis assessing safety outcomes in low intensity aerobic exercise in the form of walking, cycling, and light resistance training found improvement of non-invasive measurements of cardiac performance and exercise capacity, as well as improvement of PH functional class and quality of life [116]. Preclinical studies in rodents with MCT-induced PH also support the benefit of aerobic exercise training. Several animal studies show improvement of mean pulmonary arterial pressure, measured by right heart catheterization following 3–5 weeks of exercise training consisting of 30–60 min of 50–60% maximal aerobic capacity [117]. Subsequent work to investigate the timing of exercise for therapeutic benefit in experimental PH induced by MCT found that exercise initiated early, before MCT injection, was markedly more successful at improving disease outcomes such as survival, diastolic RV function, cardiac output and exercise tolerance, although some benefit was also observed in the cohort who began exercise training 2 weeks after MCT injection [118].

Though exercise stimulates a multitude of cardioprotective mechanisms, endurance exercise is a well-known stimulator of mitochondrial biogenesis, first reported by measuring mitochondrial mass in the myocardium in 1967 [119]. Subsequent mechanistic studies have shown lower mPTP opening rates and apoptosis resistance in endurance trained animals [120], decreased mitochondrial ROS production in exercise trained rats [121], and increased oxidative capacity and mitochondrial volume [122], and increased mitochondrial biogenesis [123]. To our knowledge, no groups have investigated these mechanisms in RV failure and exercise, and virtually nothing is known about the molecular adaptations within the RV that occur in response to exercise therapy.

7. Conclusions and future investigations

Understanding of RV metabolism and mitochondrial function has lagged that of the left heart, and arguably even less is known about how RV mitochondria adapt to pathological stress. What little is known about the role of mitochondrial function and metabolism in the dysfunctional or failing RV (summarized in **Table 2**) has largely been extrapolated from studies of LV dysfunction, and there is a large need for more mechanistic studies of the failing RV to more successfully target therapies. In addition to a need for both pre-clinical and clinical investigations of the right heart, a reductionist approach may be needed to make significant strides in RV therapy. The heart (and the RV) is comprised of multiple different cell types. Due to the fact that cardiac myocytes are the work horses of the heart, heart failure studies have historically been myocyte-centric. However, emerging data from our group and others suggests that

Mitochondrial phenotype	Regulators/assessment	LV failure	RV failure
Content: % of cell occupied by mitochondria	mt/nDNA, EM, citrate synthase activity	↓ [68, 71, 77]	↓ [98, 99, 104]
Function: electron transport chain activity	Complex I-V activity respiration (Ouroboros, Seahorse)	↓ [68–75]	NC [98–100, 112]
Fusion: elongation of mitochondrial network	Mfn1, Mfn2, OPA1 mitochondrial volume	↓ [21, 68]	NC [99, 100]
Fission: fragmentation of mitochondrial network	Fis1, Drp1 mitochondrial size	↑ [21, 79]	↑ [99–101]
Biogenesis: turnover and synthesis of new mitochondria	PGC-1α, NRF1, TFAM mitochondrial protein synthesis	↓ [76, 77]	NC [98, 104]
Mitophagy: removal of damaged mitochondria	LC3 II/I, Pink/Parkin, EM	NC [28, 80, 81]	NC [102, 103]
Apoptosis	Pro: Bax, caspase 3 Anti: Bcl-2	↑ [34, 69, 70, 84]	↑ [34, 108, 114]
ROS and oxidant damage	Protein, lipid, DNA oxidation, ROS production ($O_2^{\bullet -}$, H_2O_2)	↑ [68–70, 74, 82]	↑ [106, 107]
Antioxidant defenses	Antioxidant enzyme expression (SOD2, catalase) and non-enzymatic antioxidants	↓ [68]	↓ [43, 106, 117]

Legend: Mitochondrial alterations in left and right heart failure. Assessment of mitochondrial content, function, dynamics, biogenesis, quality control, and non-energy production roles of mitochondria and changes in HF are summarized. Arrows indicate directional change with heart failure. NC: no consensus.

Table 2. Mitochondrial changes in left and right HF.

other cell types within the heart and within the dysfunctional RV may be causally involved in disease progression. Specifically, the cardiac fibroblast is emerging as a vital cell type in regulating cardiac function and pathophysiology [124]. Not only do these cells primarily regulate the extracellular matrix (and thus fibrosis, electrical remodeling, and inflammation), but it is becoming increasingly apparent that they communicate with other cell types such as myocytes to regulate cardiac function. Virtually nothing is known about RV fibroblast mitochondrial metabolism or biology, or how these cell types respond to cardiac stress. In conclusion, the RV is not a thinner, lower pressure LV. Significant physiological and pathophysiological differences separate the two ventricles, and RV-centric approaches are necessary for the identification, repurposing, or development of therapies for RHF.

Author details

Danielle R. Bruns* and Lori A. Walker

*Address all correspondence to: danielle.bruns@ucdenver.edu

Division of Cardiology, Department of Medicine, University of Colorado-Denver, Aurora, CO, USA

References

[1] Go AS, Mozaffarian D, Roger VL, Benjamin EJ, Berry JD, Borden WB, et al. Heart disease and stroke statistics—2013 update: A report from the American Heart Association. Circulation. 2013;**127**(1):e6-e245

[2] Braunschweig F, Cowie MR, Auricchio A. What are the costs of heart failure? Europace. 2011;**13**(Suppl 2 ii):13-17

[3] Yancy CW, Jessup M, Bozkurt B, Butler J, Casey DE Jr, Drazner MH, et al. 2013 ACCF/AHA guideline for the management of heart failure: A report of the American College of Cardiology Foundation/American Heart Association task force on practice guidelines. Journal of the American College of Cardiology. 2013;**62**(16):e147-e239

[4] Brown DA, Perry JB, Allen ME, Sabbah HN, Stauffer BL, Shaikh SR, et al. Expert consensus document: Mitochondrial function as a therapeutic target in heart failure. Nature Reviews. Cardiology. 2017;**14**(4):238-250

[5] Voelkel NF, Quaife RA, Leinwand LA, Barst RJ, McGoon MD, Meldrum DR, et al. Right ventricular function and failure: Report of a National Heart, Lung, and Blood Institute working group on cellular and molecular mechanisms of right heart failure. Circulation. 2006;**114**(17):1883-1891

[6] Melenovsky V, Hwang SJ, Lin G, Redfield MM, Borlaug BA. Right heart dysfunction in heart failure with preserved ejection fraction. European Heart Journal. 2014;**35**(48):3452-3462

[7] Gulati A, Ismail TF, Jabbour A, Alpendurada F, Guha K, Ismail NA, et al. The prevalence and prognostic significance of right ventricular systolic dysfunction in nonischemic dilated cardiomyopathy. Circulation. 2013;**128**(15):1623-1633

[8] Walker LA, Buttrick PM. The right ventricle: Biologic insights and response to disease. Current Cardiology Reviews. 2009;**5**(1):22-28

[9] Zaffran S, Kelly RG, Meilhac SM, Buckingham ME, Brown NA. Right ventricular myocardium derives from the anterior heart field. Circulation Research. 2004;**95**(3):261-268

[10] Srivastava D, Olson EN. A genetic blueprint for cardiac development. Nature. 2000;**407**(6801):221-226

[11] Kusachi S, Nishiyama O, Yasuhara K, Saito D, Haraoka S, Nagashima H. Right and left ventricular oxygen metabolism in open-chest dogs. The American Journal of Physiology. 1982;**243**(5):H761-H766

[12] Zong P, Tune JD, Downey HF. Mechanisms of oxygen demand/supply balance in the right ventricle. Experimental Biology and Medicine (Maywood, N.J.). 2005;**230**(8):507-519

[13] Tune JD, Gorman MW, Feigl EO. Matching coronary blood flow to myocardial oxygen consumption. Journal of Applied Physiology (1985). 2004;**97**(1):404-415

[14] Bing RJ, Siegel A, Vitale A, Balboni F, Sparks E, Taeschler M, et al. Metabolic studies on the human heart in vivo. I. Studies on carbohydrate metabolism of the human heart. The American Journal of Medicine. 1953;**15**(3):284-296

[15] van der Vusse GJ, van Bilsen M, Glatz JF. Cardiac fatty acid uptake and transport in health and disease. Cardiovascular Research. 2000;**45**(2):279-293

[16] Drake JI, Bogaard HJ, Mizuno S, Clifton B, Xie B, Gao Y, et al. Molecular signature of a right heart failure program in chronic severe pulmonary hypertension. American Journal of Respiratory Cell and Molecular Biology. 2011;**45**(6):1239-1247

[17] Balaban RS. Cardiac energy metabolism homeostasis: Role of cytosolic calcium. Journal of Molecular and Cellular Cardiology. 2002;**34**(10):1259-1271

[18] Barth E, Stammler G, Speiser B, Schaper J. Ultrastructural quantitation of mitochondria and myofilaments in cardiac muscle from 10 different animal species including man. Journal of Molecular and Cellular Cardiology. 1992;**24**(7):669-681

[19] Neely JR, Morgan HE. Relationship between carbohydrate and lipid metabolism and the energy balance of heart muscle. Annual Review of Physiology. 1974;**36**:413-459

[20] Lewis MR, Lewis WH. Mitochondria in tissue culture. Science. 1914;**39**(1000):330-333

[21] Ong SB, Hall AR, Hausenloy DJ. Mitochondrial dynamics in cardiovascular health and disease. Antioxidants & Redox Signaling. 2013;**19**(4):400-414

[22] Chen H, Detmer SA, Ewald AJ, Griffin EE, Fraser SE, Chan DC. Mitofusins Mfn1 and Mfn2 coordinately regulate mitochondrial fusion and are essential for embryonic development. The Journal of Cell Biology. 2003;**160**(2):189-200

[23] Davies VJ, Hollins AJ, Piechota MJ, Yip W, Davies JR, White KE, et al. Opa1 deficiency in a mouse model of autosomal dominant optic atrophy impairs mitochondrial morphology, optic nerve structure and visual function. Human Molecular Genetics. 2007;**16**(11):1307-1318

[24] Manczak M, Sesaki H, Kageyama Y, Reddy PH. Dynamin-related protein 1 heterozygote knockout mice do not have synaptic and mitochondrial deficiencies. Biochimica et Biophysica Acta. 2012;**1822**(6):862-874

[25] Zhao T, Huang X, Han L, Wang X, Cheng H, Zhao Y, et al. Central role of mitofusin 2 in autophagosome-lysosome fusion in cardiomyocytes. The Journal of Biological Chemistry. 2012;**287**(28):23615-23625

[26] Nishida K, Otsu K. Autophagy during cardiac remodeling. Journal of Molecular and Cellular Cardiology. 2016;**95**:11-18

[27] Zhang X, Li ZL, Crane JA, Jordan KL, Pawar AS, Textor SC, et al. Valsartan regulates myocardial autophagy and mitochondrial turnover in experimental hypertension. Hypertension. 2014;**64**(1):87-93

[28] Palikaras K, Daskalaki I, Markaki M, Tavernarakis N. Mitophagy and age-related pathologies: Development of new therapeutics by targeting mitochondrial turnover. Pharmacology & Therapeutics. 2017

[29] Steinberg GR, Kemp BE. AMPK in health and disease. Physiological Reviews. 2009;**89**(3):1025-1078

[30] Fernandez-Marcos PJ, Auwerx J. Regulation of PGC-1alpha, a nodal regulator of mitochondrial biogenesis. The American Journal of Clinical Nutrition. 2011;**93**(4):884S-8890

[31] Chicco AJ, Sparagna GC. Role of cardiolipin alterations in mitochondrial dysfunction and disease. American Journal of Physiology. Cell Physiology. 2007;**292**(1):C33-C44

[32] Miller BF, Hamilton KL. A perspective on the determination of mitochondrial biogenesis. American Journal of Physiology. Endocrinology and Metabolism. 2012;**302**(5):E496-E499

[33] Palmer JW, Tandler B, Hoppel CL. Biochemical properties of subsarcolemmal and interfibrillar mitochondria isolated from rat cardiac muscle. The Journal of Biological Chemistry. 1977;**252**(23):8731-8739

[34] Zungu-Edmondson M, Suzuki YJ. Differential stress response mechanisms in right and left ventricles. Journal of Rare Diseases Research & Treatment. 2016;**1**(2):39-45

[35] Phillips D, Aponte AM, Covian R, Neufeld E, ZX Y, Balaban RS. Homogenous protein programming in the mammalian left and right ventricle free walls. Physiological Genomics. 2011;**43**(21):1198-1206

[36] Turrens JF. Mitochondrial formation of reactive oxygen species. The Journal of Physiology. 2003;**552**(Pt 2):335-344

[37] Turrens JF, Boveris A. Generation of superoxide anion by the NADH dehydrogenase of bovine heart mitochondria. The Biochemical Journal. 1980;**191**(2):421-427

[38] Fridovich I. Superoxide radical and superoxide dismutases. Annual Review of Biochemistry. 1995;**64**:97-112

[39] Radi R, Turrens JF, Chang LY, Bush KM, Crapo JD, Freeman BA. Detection of catalase in rat heart mitochondria. The Journal of Biological Chemistry. 1991;**266**(32):22028-22034

[40] Cook SA, Sugden PH, Clerk A. Regulation of bcl-2 family proteins during development and in response to oxidative stress in cardiac myocytes: Association with changes in mitochondrial membrane potential. Circulation Research. 1999;**85**(10):940-949

[41] Karbowski M, Lee YJ, Gaume B, Jeong SY, Frank S, Nechushtan A, et al. Spatial and temporal association of Bax with mitochondrial fission sites, Drp1, and Mfn2 during apoptosis. The Journal of Cell Biology. 2002;**159**(6):931-938

[42] Frezza C, Cipolat S, Martins de Brito O, Micaroni M, Beznoussenko GV, Rudka T, et al. OPA1 controls apoptotic cristae remodeling independently from mitochondrial fusion. Cell. 2006;**126**(1):177-189

[43] Schreckenberg R, Rebelo M, Deten A, Weber M, Rohrbach S, Pipicz M, et al. Specific mechanisms underlying right heart failure: The missing upregulation of superoxide

dismutase-2 and its decisive role in antioxidative defense. Antioxidants & Redox Signaling. 2015;**23**(15):1220-1232

[44] Walker LA, Buttrick PM. The right ventricle: Biologic insights and response to disease: Updated. Current Cardiology Reviews. 2013;**9**(1):73-81

[45] Webb G, Gatzoulis MA. Atrial septal defects in the adult: Recent progress and overview. Circulation. 2006;**114**(15):1645-1653

[46] MacNee W. Right ventricular function in cor pulmonale. Cardiology. 1988;**75**(Suppl 1):30-40

[47] Haddad F, Doyle R, Murphy DJ, Hunt SA. Right ventricular function in cardiovascular disease, part II: Pathophysiology, clinical importance, and management of right ventricular failure. Circulation. 2008;**117**(13):1717-1731

[48] Friehs I, Cowan DB, Choi YH, Black KM, Barnett R, Bhasin MK, et al. Pressure-overload hypertrophy of the developing heart reveals activation of divergent gene and protein pathways in the left and right ventricular myocardium. American Journal of Physiology. Heart and Circulatory Physiology. 2013;**304**(5):H697-H708

[49] McLaughlin VV, Archer SL, Badesch DB, Barst RJ, Farber HW, Lindner JR, et al. ACCF/AHA 2009 expert consensus document on pulmonary hypertension: A report of the American College of Cardiology Foundation task force on expert consensus documents and the American Heart Association: Developed in collaboration with the American College of Chest Physicians, American Thoracic Society, Inc., and the Pulmonary Hypertension Association. Circulation. 2009;**119**(16):2250-2294

[50] Stenmark KR, Meyrick B, Galie N, Mooi WJ, McMurtry IF. Animal models of pulmonary arterial hypertension: The hope for etiological discovery and pharmacological cure. American Journal of Physiology. Lung Cellular and Molecular Physiology. 2009;**297**(6):L1013-L1032

[51] Alexander AF, Will DH, Grover RF, Reeves JT. Pulmonary hypertention and right ventricular hypertrophy in catle at high altitude. American Journal of Veterinary Research. 1960;**21**:199-204

[52] Orton EC, Reeves JT, Stenmark KR. Pulmonary vasodilation with structurally altered pulmonary vessels and pulmonary hypertension. Journal of Applied Physiology (1985). 1988;**65**(6):2459-2467

[53] Wilson DW, Segall HJ, Pan LC, Lame MW, Estep JE, Morin D. Mechanisms and pathology of monocrotaline pulmonary toxicity. Critical Reviews in Toxicology. 1992;**22**(5-6):307-325

[54] Werchan PM, Summer WR, Gerdes AM, McDonough KH. Right ventricular performance after monocrotaline-induced pulmonary hypertension. The American Journal of Physiology. 1989;**256**(5 Pt 2):H1328-H1336

[55] Roth RA, Dotzlaf LA, Baranyi B, Kuo CH, Hook JB. Effect of monocrotaline ingestion on liver, kidney, and lung of rats. Toxicology and Applied Pharmacology. 1981;**60**(2):193-203

[56] Miyauchi T, Yorikane R, Sakai S, Sakurai T, Okada M, Nishikibe M, et al. Contribution of endogenous endothelin-1 to the progression of cardiopulmonary alterations in rats with monocrotaline-induced pulmonary hypertension. Circulation Research. 1993;**73**(5):887-897

[57] Vitali SH, Hansmann G, Rose C, Fernandez-Gonzalez A, Scheid A, Mitsialis SA, et al. The Sugen 5416/hypoxia mouse model of pulmonary hypertension revisited: Long-term follow-up. Pulmonary Circulation. 2014;**4**(4):619-629

[58] Hemnes AR, Zaiman A, Champion HC. PDE5A inhibition attenuates bleomycin-induced pulmonary fibrosis and pulmonary hypertension through inhibition of ROS generation and RhoA/rho kinase activation. American Journal of Physiology. Lung Cellular and Molecular Physiology. 2008;**294**(1):L24-L33

[59] Best DH, Austin ED, Chung WK, Elliott CG. Genetics of pulmonary hypertension. Current Opinion in Cardiology. 2014;**29**(6):520-527

[60] Frieler RA, Mortensen RM. Immune cell and other noncardiomyocyte regulation of cardiac hypertrophy and remodeling. Circulation. 2015;**131**(11):1019-1030

[61] Parker TG, Packer SE, Schneider MD. Peptide growth factors can provoke "fetal" contractile protein gene expression in rat cardiac myocytes. The Journal of Clinical Investigation. 1990;**85**(2):507-514

[62] Adrogue JV, Sharma S, Ngumbela K, Essop MF, Taegtmeyer H. Acclimatization to chronic hypobaric hypoxia is associated with a differential transcriptional profile between the right and left ventricle. Molecular and Cellular Biochemistry. 2005;**278**(1-2):71-78

[63] Lehman JJ, Kelly DP. Transcriptional activation of energy metabolic switches in the developing and hypertrophied heart. Clinical and Experimental Pharmacology & Physiology. 2002;**29**(4):339-345

[64] Abozguia K, Clarke K, Lee L, Frenneaux M. Modification of myocardial substrate use as a therapy for heart failure. Nature Clinical Practice. Cardiovascular Medicine. 2006;**3**(9):490-498

[65] Goh KY, Qu J, Hong H, Liu T, Dell'Italia LJ, Wu Y, et al. Impaired mitochondrial network excitability in failing guinea-pig cardiomyocytes. Cardiovascular Research. 2016;**109**(1):79-89

[66] Ahmed LA, El-Maraghy SA. Nicorandil ameliorates mitochondrial dysfunction in doxorubicin-induced heart failure in rats: Possible mechanism of cardioprotection. Biochemical Pharmacology. 2013;**86**(9):1301-1310

[67] Kawai K, Qin F, Shite J, Mao W, Fukuoka S, Liang CS. Importance of antioxidant and antiapoptotic effects of beta-receptor blockers in heart failure therapy. American Journal of Physiology. Heart and Circulatory Physiology. 2004;**287**(3):H1003-H1012

[68] Sabbah HN, Gupta RC, Kohli S, Wang M, Hachem S, Zhang K. Chronic therapy with elamipretide (MTP-131), a novel mitochondria-targeting peptide, improves left

ventricular and mitochondrial function in dogs with advanced heart failure. Circulation. Heart Failure. 2016;**9**(2):e002206

[69] Sharov VG, Todor AV, Silverman N, Goldstein S, Sabbah HN. Abnormal mitochondrial respiration in failed human myocardium. Journal of Molecular and Cellular Cardiology. 2000;**32**(12):2361-2367

[70] Sun CK, Chang LT, Sheu JJ, Wang CY, Youssef AA, Wu CJ, et al. Losartan preserves integrity of cardiac gap junctions and PGC-1 alpha gene expression and prevents cellular apoptosis in remote area of left ventricular myocardium following acute myocardial infarction. International Heart Journal. 2007;**48**(4):533-546

[71] Garnier A, Fortin D, Delomenie C, Momken I, Veksler V, Ventura-Clapier R. Depressed mitochondrial transcription factors and oxidative capacity in rat failing cardiac and skeletal muscles. The Journal of Physiology. 2003;**551**(Pt 2):491-501

[72] Papanicolaou KN, Khairallah RJ, Ngoh GA, Chikando A, Luptak I, O'Shea KM, et al. Mitofusin-2 maintains mitochondrial structure and contributes to stress-induced permeability transition in cardiac myocytes. Molecular and Cellular Biology. 2011;**31**(6): 1309-1328

[73] Ikeda Y, Shirakabe A, Maejima Y, Zhai P, Sciarretta S, Toli J, et al. Endogenous Drp1 mediates mitochondrial autophagy and protects the heart against energy stress. Circulation Research. 2015;**116**(2):264-278

[74] Billia F, Hauck L, Konecny F, Rao V, Shen J, Mak TW. PTEN-inducible kinase 1 (PINK1)/ Park6 is indispensable for normal heart function. Proceedings of the National Academy of Sciences of the United States of America. 2011;**108**(23):9572-9577

[75] Schwarzer M, Osterholt M, Lunkenbein A, Schrepper A, Amorim P, Doenst T. Mitochondrial reactive oxygen species production and respiratory complex activity in rats with pressure overload-induced heart failure. The Journal of Physiology. 2014;**592**(17): 3767-3782

[76] Hein S, Arnon E, Kostin S, Schonburg M, Elsasser A, Polyakova V, et al. Progression from compensated hypertrophy to failure in the pressure-overloaded human heart: Structural deterioration and compensatory mechanisms. Circulation. 2003;**107**(7):984-991

[77] Plecita-Hlavata L, Tauber J, Li M, Zhang H, Flockton AR, Pullamsetti SS, et al. Constitutive reprogramming of fibroblast mitochondrial metabolism in pulmonary hypertension. American Journal of Respiratory Cell and Molecular Biology. 2016;**55**(1):47-57

[78] Paulin R, Michelakis ED. The metabolic theory of pulmonary arterial hypertension. Circulation Research. 2014;**115**(1):148-164

[79] Ryan J, Dasgupta A, Huston J, Chen KH, Archer SL. Mitochondrial dynamics in pulmonary arterial hypertension. Journal of Molecular Medicine (Berlin). 2015;**93**(3):229-242

[80] Enache I, Charles AL, Bouitbir J, Favret F, Zoll J, Metzger D, et al. Skeletal muscle mitochondrial dysfunction precedes right ventricular impairment in experimental pulmonary hypertension. Molecular and Cellular Biochemistry. 2013;**373**(1-2):161-170

[81] Piao L, Sidhu VK, Fang YH, Ryan JJ, Parikh KS, Hong Z, et al. FOXO1-mediated upregulation of pyruvate dehydrogenase kinase-4 (PDK4) decreases glucose oxidation and impairs right ventricular function in pulmonary hypertension: Therapeutic benefits of dichloroacetate. Journal of Molecular Medicine (Berlin). 2013;**91**(3):333-346

[82] Do E, Baudet S, Verdys M, Touzeau C, Bailly F, Lucas-Heron B, et al. Energy metabolism in normal and hypertrophied right ventricle of the ferret heart. Journal of Molecular and Cellular Cardiology. 1997;**29**(7):1903-1913

[83] Sutendra G, Dromparis P, Paulin R, Zervopoulos S, Haromy A, Nagendran J, et al. A metabolic remodeling in right ventricular hypertrophy is associated with decreased angiogenesis and a transition from a compensated to a decompensated state in pulmonary hypertension. Journal of Molecular Medicine (Berlin). 2013;**91**(11):1315-1327

[84] Takeyama D, Kagaya Y, Yamane Y, Shiba N, Chida M, Takahashi T, et al. Effects of chronic right ventricular pressure overload on myocardial glucose and free fatty acid metabolism in the conscious rat. Cardiovascular Research. 1995;**29**(6):763-767

[85] Lundgrin EL, Park MM, Sharp J, Tang WH, Thomas JD, Asosingh K, et al. Fasting 2-deoxy-2-[18F]fluoro-D-glucose positron emission tomography to detect metabolic changes in pulmonary arterial hypertension hearts over 1 year. Annals of the American Thoracic Society. 2013;**10**(1):1-9

[86] Fang YH, Piao L, Hong Z, Toth PT, Marsboom G, Bache-Wiig P, et al. Therapeutic inhibition of fatty acid oxidation in right ventricular hypertrophy: Exploiting Randle's cycle. Journal of Molecular Medicine (Berlin). 2012;**90**(1):31-43

[87] van Wolferen SA, Marcus JT, Westerhof N, Spreeuwenberg MD, Marques KM, Bronzwaer JG, et al. Right coronary artery flow impairment in patients with pulmonary hypertension. European Heart Journal. 2008;**29**(1):120-127

[88] Reddy S, Bernstein D. Molecular mechanisms of right ventricular failure. Circulation. 2015;**132**(18):1734-1742

[89] Chambers KT, Leone TC, Sambandam N, Kovacs A, Wagg CS, Lopaschuk GD, et al. Chronic inhibition of pyruvate dehydrogenase in heart triggers an adaptive metabolic response. The Journal of Biological Chemistry. 2011;**286**(13):11155-11162

[90] Gomez-Arroyo J, Mizuno S, Szczepanek K, Van Tassell B, Natarajan R, dos Remedios CG, et al. Metabolic gene remodeling and mitochondrial dysfunction in failing right ventricular hypertrophy secondary to pulmonary arterial hypertension. Circulation. Heart Failure. 2013;**6**(1):136-144

[91] Nouette-Gaulain K, Malgat M, Rocher C, Savineau JP, Marthan R, Mazat JP, et al. Time course of differential mitochondrial energy metabolism adaptation to chronic hypoxia in right and left ventricles. Cardiovascular Research. 2005;**66**(1):132-140

[92] Bruns DR, Brown RD, Stenmark KR, Buttrick PM, Walker LA. Mitochondrial integrity in a neonatal bovine model of right ventricular dysfunction. American Journal of Physiology. Lung Cellular and Molecular Physiology. 2015;**308**(2):L158-L167

[93] Marsboom G, Toth PT, Ryan JJ, Hong Z, Wu X, Fang YH, et al. Dynamin-related protein 1-mediated mitochondrial mitotic fission permits hyperproliferation of vascular smooth muscle cells and offers a novel therapeutic target in pulmonary hypertension. Circulation Research. 2012;**110**(11):1484-1497

[94] Qipshidze N, Tyagi N, Metreveli N, Lominadze D, Tyagi SC. Autophagy mechanism of right ventricular remodeling in murine model of pulmonary artery constriction. American Journal of Physiology. Heart and Circulatory Physiology. 2012;**302**(3):H688-H696

[95] Deng Y, Wu W, Guo S, Chen Y, Liu C, Gao X, et al. Altered mTOR and Beclin-1 mediated autophagic activation during right ventricular remodeling in monocrotaline-induced pulmonary hypertension. Respiratory Research. 2017;**18**(1):53

[96] Karamanlidis G, Bautista-Hernandez V, Fynn-Thompson F, Del Nido P, Tian R. Impaired mitochondrial biogenesis precedes heart failure in right ventricular hypertrophy in congenital heart disease. Circulation. Heart Failure. 2011;**4**(6):707-713

[97] Nagendran J, Gurtu V, Fu DZ, Dyck JR, Haromy A, Ross DB, et al. A dynamic and chamber-specific mitochondrial remodeling in right ventricular hypertrophy can be therapeutically targeted. The Journal of Thoracic and Cardiovascular Surgery. 2008;**136**(1):168-178 e1-e3

[98] Farahmand F, Hill MF, Singal PK. Antioxidant and oxidative stress changes in experimental cor pulmonale. Molecular and Cellular Biochemistry. 2004;**260**(1-2):21-29

[99] Redout EM, Wagner MJ, Zuidwijk MJ, Boer C, Musters RJ, van Hardeveld C, et al. Right-ventricular failure is associated with increased mitochondrial complex II activity and production of reactive oxygen species. Cardiovascular Research. 2007;**75**(4):770-781

[100] Braun MU, Szalai P, Strasser RH, Borst MM. Right ventricular hypertrophy and apoptosis after pulmonary artery banding: Regulation of PKC isozymes. Cardiovascular Research. 2003;**59**(3):658-667

[101] Vaidya B, Gupta V. Novel therapeutic approaches for pulmonary arterial hypertension: Unique molecular targets to site-specific drug delivery. Journal of Controlled Release. 2015;**211**:118-133

[102] van de Veerdonk MC, Kind T, Marcus JT, Mauritz GJ, Heymans MW, Bogaard HJ, et al. Progressive right ventricular dysfunction in patients with pulmonary arterial hypertension responding to therapy. Journal of the American College of Cardiology. 2011;**58**(24):2511-2519

[103] Bhandari B, Subramanian L. Ranolazine, a partial fatty acid oxidation inhibitor, its potential benefit in angina and other cardiovascular disorders. Recent Patents on Cardiovascular Drug Discovery. 2007;**2**(1):35-39

[104] Guarnieri C, Muscari C. Beneficial effects of trimetazidine on mitochondrial function and superoxide production in the cardiac muscle of monocrotaline-treated rats. Biochemical Pharmacology. 1988;**37**(24):4685-4688

[105] Michelakis ED, McMurtry MS, XC W, Dyck JR, Moudgil R, Hopkins TA, et al. Dichloroacetate, a metabolic modulator, prevents and reverses chronic hypoxic pulmonary hypertension in rats: Role of increased expression and activity of voltage-gated potassium channels. Circulation. 2002;**105**(2):244-250

[106] Sun XQ, Zhang R, Zhang HD, Yuan P, Wang XJ, Zhao QH, et al. Reversal of right ventricular remodeling by dichloroacetate is related to inhibition of mitochondria-dependent apoptosis. Hypertension Research. 2016;**39**(5):302-311

[107] Dhalla AK, Hill MF, Singal PK. Role of oxidative stress in transition of hypertrophy to heart failure. Journal of the American College of Cardiology. 1996;**28**(2):506-514

[108] Bjelakovic G, Nikolova D, Gluud LL, Simonetti RG, Gluud C. Mortality in randomized trials of antioxidant supplements for primary and secondary prevention: Systematic review and meta-analysis. Journal of the American Medical Association. 2007;**297**(8):842-857

[109] Bogaard HJ, Natarajan R, Henderson SC, Long CS, Kraskauskas D, Smithson L, et al. Chronic pulmonary artery pressure elevation is insufficient to explain right heart failure. Circulation. 2009;**120**(20):1951-1960

[110] Zhao K, Zhao GM, Wu D, Soong Y, Birk AV, Schiller PW, et al. Cell-permeable peptide antioxidants targeted to inner mitochondrial membrane inhibit mitochondrial swelling, oxidative cell death, and reperfusion injury. The Journal of Biological Chemistry. 2004;**279**(33):34682-34690

[111] Dai DF, Chen T, Szeto H, Nieves-Cintron M, Kutyavin V, Santana LF, et al. Mitochondrial targeted antioxidant peptide ameliorates hypertensive cardiomyopathy. Journal of the American College of Cardiology. 2011;**58**(1):73-82

[112] Dai DF, Hsieh EJ, Chen T, Menendez LG, Basisty NB, Tsai L, et al. Global proteomics and pathway analysis of pressure-overload-induced heart failure and its attenuation by mitochondrial-targeted peptides. Circulation. Heart Failure. 2013;**6**(5):1067-1076

[113] Zhang H, Li Y, Su W, Ying Z, Zhou L, Zhang L, et al. Resveratrol attenuates mitochondrial dysfunction in the liver of intrauterine growth retarded suckling piglets by improving mitochondrial biogenesis and redox status. Molecular Nutrition & Food Research. 2017;**61**(5)

[114] Csiszar A, Labinskyy N, Pinto JT, Ballabh P, Zhang H, Losonczy G, et al. Resveratrol induces mitochondrial biogenesis in endothelial cells. American Journal of Physiology. Heart and Circulatory Physiology. 2009;**297**(1):H13-H20

[115] Abrahams A. Exercise and cardiac hypertrophy. Lancet. 1946;**2**(6425):565

[116] Babu AS, Padmakumar R, Maiya AG, Mohapatra AK, Kamath RL. Effects of exercise training on exercise capacity in pulmonary arterial hypertension: A systematic review of clinical trials. Heart, Lung & Circulation. 2016;**25**(4):333-341

[117] Colombo R, Siqueira R, Becker CU, Fernandes TG, Pires KM, Valenca SS, et al. Effects of exercise on monocrotaline-induced changes in right heart function and pulmonary artery remodeling in rats. Canadian Journal of Physiology and Pharmacology. 2013;**91**(1):38-44

[118] Moreira-Goncalves D, Ferreira R, Fonseca H, Padrao AI, Moreno N, Silva AF, et al. Cardioprotective effects of early and late aerobic exercise training in experimental pulmonary arterial hypertension. Basic Research in Cardiology. 2015;**110**(6):57

[119] Laguens RP, Gomez-Dumm CL. Fine structure of myocardial mitochondria in rats after exercise for one-half to two hours. Circulation Research. 1967;**21**(3):271-279

[120] Kavazis AN, McClung JM, Hood DA, Powers SK. Exercise induces a cardiac mitochondrial phenotype that resists apoptotic stimuli. American Journal of Physiology. Heart and Circulatory Physiology. 2008;**294**(2):H928-H935

[121] Judge S, Jang YM, Smith A, Selman C, Phillips T, Speakman JR, et al. Exercise by lifelong voluntary wheel running reduces subsarcolemmal and interfibrillar mitochondrial hydrogen peroxide production in the heart. American Journal of Physiology. Regulatory, Integrative and Comparative Physiology. 2005;**289**(6):R1564-R1572

[122] Eisele JC, Schaefer IM, Randel Nyengaard J, Post H, Liebetanz D, Bruel A, et al. Effect of voluntary exercise on number and volume of cardiomyocytes and their mitochondria in the mouse left ventricle. Basic Research in Cardiology. 2008;**103**(1):12-21

[123] Tao L, Bei Y, Lin S, Zhang H, Zhou Y, Jiang J, et al. Exercise training protects against acute myocardial infarction via improving myocardial energy metabolism and mitochondrial biogenesis. Cellular Physiology and Biochemistry. 2015;**37**(1):162-175

[124] Gourdie RG, Dimmeler S, Kohl P. Novel therapeutic strategies targeting fibroblasts and fibrosis in heart disease. Nature Reviews. Drug Discovery. 2016;**15**(9):620-638

Chapter 2

Mitochondria and Heart Disease

Shaunrick Stoll, Christiana Leimena and Hongyu Qiu

Additional information is available at the end of the chapter

http://dx.doi.org/10.5772/intechopen.72611

Abstract

Mitochondria play a key role in the normal functioning of the heart and in the pathogenesis and development of various types of heart disease. In addition, specific mitochondrial cardiomyopathies due to mutations in mitochondrial DNA have been identified. Increasing studies demonstrate that mitochondrial function has emerged as a therapeutic target in heart disease. This chapter addresses the recent studies of the role and the mechanism of mitochondria in the development of heart disease, and the progress in clinical diagnosis and treatments on a mitochondrial basis. Consequently, the aim of this chapter is to outline current knowledge about mitochondria in the heart disease.

Keywords: mitochondria, heart, heart failure, cardiac hypertrophy, heart disease

1. Introduction

The heart is the most metabolically active organ in the body and highly depends on oxidative energy generation in mitochondria to supply the large amount of adenosine triphosphate (ATP) required for its continuous contractile activity. In addition, cardiac mitochondria also serve other cellular functions such as generating and regulating reactive oxygen species (ROS), buffering cytosolic calcium ions (Ca^{2+}), and regulating cellular apoptosis through the mitochondrial permeability transition pore (mPTP).

Heart disease is the leading cause of mortality worldwide. Although the study of mitochondrial function in the human heart faces many obstacles, the role of mitochondria in cardiac diseases has been elucidated from the studies with animal models. Increasing evidences have shown that abnormalities in the mitochondrial structure and function are tightly associated with development of various cardiovascular diseases, which prompted new therapies to treat and prevent heart disease by aiming at metabolic modulation.

Mitochondrial abnormalities include impaired mitochondrial electron transport chain (ETC) activity, increased formation of ROS, shifted metabolic substrate utilization, aberrant mitochondrial dynamics, and altered ion homeostasis. Some of the mitochondrial abnormalities may have a genetic basis due to the changes of mitochondrial DNA (mtDNA) or the mutation of specific nuclear DNA (nDNA), while other abnormalities are due to environmental cardiotoxic insult or uncharacterized reasons. Although many specific mitochondrial targets have proven to be promising therapeutic strategies in experimental studies, most of them are pending for validation through clinical trials. Better understanding the molecular mechanism of mitochondria in cardiac pathology is important to provide diagnosis and treatment of mitochondrial-based cardiac diseases.

In order to better understand the role that the mitochondrion plays in the heart, we provide in this chapter a brief background describing the regulation and function of mitochondria during normal cardiac development and aging as well as the pathological mechanisms involved in cardiac diseases. We also address the mitochondrial abnormalities–based diagnosis and therapeutic options available in heart disease.

2. The role of mitochondria in the normal heart

Mitochondria have long been described as the powerhouses of the cell. They are responsible for the generation of ATP, the main energy currency of the cell, while playing important roles in intracellular signaling, activation of apoptosis, and other mechanisms. Little information is currently available on mitochondrial function in the normal human heart as most of the studies on the role of mitochondria have relied on animal models, which may not be representative of the human. However, the development of new methods to study mitochondrial function provides an opportunity to use the small amount of tissue available from surgeries to understand mitochondrial function. In the near future, we expect more studies to be developed utilizing these techniques.

2.1. Basis of the regulation of cardiac mitochondrial function

2.1.1. Cardiac energy production and metabolism

The heart relies mainly on mitochondrial metabolism to provide most of its energy. The heart has the largest demand for energy among all organs, since it beats continuously from its formation in the fetus until death, and thus cardiomyocytes contain the highest concentration of mitochondria in the body in order to meet its energy requirements [1]. Several interacting bioenergetic pathways contribute to energy metabolism of cardiac muscle including pyruvate oxidation, the tricarboxylic acid (TCA) cycle, the mitochondrial fatty acids oxidation (FAO), and oxidative phosphorylation (OXPHOS), which generates 80–90% of cellular ATP [2]. While the oxidation of pyruvate takes place in the cytosol, the other procedures occur in the mitochondria.

In the normal heart tissue, the supply of ATP from glycolytic mechanism is limited [2]. Fatty acids are the primary energy substrates used to produce ATP in cardiac muscle by OXPHOS, utilizing the carnitine shuttle to transport the fatty acids into the mitochondria. The heart also maintains stored high-energy phosphates, such as creatine phosphate (CP), that are produced from creatine by mitochondrial creatine kinase (mitoCK) using ATP from the closely associated adenine nucleotide translocase (ANT) and mitochondrial ATP synthase [2].

Additionally, the heart is a well vascularized organ, allowing for delivery of freshly oxygenated blood and quick removal of the waste products of metabolism. This constant supply of oxygen is important for OXPHOS to take place, as oxygen serves as the final electron acceptor in the ETC. Understanding the factors involved in the development and function of mitochondrial energy production pathways is increasingly important due to the many diseases associated with defects in this machinery.

Energy production within the cardiomyocytes of the heart is influenced by genetic factors as well as environmental factors. nDNA and mtDNA affect the enzymes and their cofactors as well as the availability of substrates to the mitochondria from their surroundings, which further influence OXPHOS. Cardiac tissue has specific gene regulations to meet its physiological and developmental needs. For example, the ATP synthase β-subunit is expressed at higher levels in cardiomyocyte-differentiated cells compared to control cells [3], and some isoforms of enzymes, e.g., cardiac specific isoforms of cytochrome c oxidase subunits VIa, VIIa, and VIII, are differentially expressed across tissues [4].

Besides the expression and function of the main proteins associated with the OXPHOS, the component of the ETC complexes I-IV and ATP synthase (complex V), many other molecules have been found to be involved in the regulation of the mitochondrial energy production through posttranslational modification. For example, proteins within the mitochondrial complexes can be nitrosylated (the addition of an NO group) or *O*-GlcNAcylated (the addition of *O*-linked β-*N*-acetylglucosamine (*O*-GlcNAc)) [5, 6]. These protein modifications modulate the activity of the complexes and hence change the efficiency of the mitochondria to meet the physiological function of the heart. In addition, our recent studies have also found a specific cell survival-promoting signaling that plays an important regulatory role in promoting ETC efficiency in cardiomyocytes, remarkably under the cardiac stress [7–9]. In particular, we found that this signaling pathway, which includes the heat shock protein 22(Hsp22), AKT, and valosin-containing protein (VCP), promotes ETC efficiency in cardiomyocyte through the increase of mitochondrial inducible nitric oxide synthase (iNOS) [7–9].

2.1.2. Modulation of calcium signaling

Ca^{2+} concentration is highly regulated in the myocardium and is responsible for the induction and intensity of contraction in the myocytes [10]. Mitochondria are able to modulate the Ca^{2+} concentration in the cardiomyocyte, which plays an important role in the cardiac function [11].

Mitochondria can directly decrease the Ca^{2+} concentration in the cytosol of the cell by importing Ca^{2+} via the mitochondrial Ca^{2+} uniporter. Reciprocally, they can also increase the Ca^{2+} concentration in the cytosol by expelling calcium stored within the mitochondria through Na^+/Ca^{2+} or H^+/Ca^{2+} exchangers [12]. This elaborate system of channels and transporters allows for physiological responses to cytosolic calcium signals and the loading of Ca^{2+} in the mitochondrial matrix. Mitochondria partake in the cardiac excitation-contraction coupling (ECC) by storing Ca^{2+}, responding to cytosolic calcium signals and generating the ATP required for cardiac contraction. Ca^{2+} influx via L-type Ca^{2+} channels triggers further release of Ca^{2+} from the sarcoplasmic reticulum (SR), which binds to troponin C, and allows for the myosin and actin filaments to interact [10]. During diastole, the Ca^{2+} either goes back into the SR or is exported out of the cell via the Na^{+}/Ca^{2+} exchanger [13]. An increase in workload, as triggered by β-adrenergic stimulation, increases the number of Ca^{2+} transients as well as the size of the transients, leading to stronger cardiac contractions [14]. Additionally, mitochondria can also indirectly contribute to Ca^{2+} regulation by inducing changes in the concentration of ATP, NAD(P)H, pyruvate, and ROS, which in turn regulate other Ca^{2+} signaling machinery components [15]. This associated Ca^{2+} signaling is involved in the Ca^{2+} buffering, the Ca^{2+} release from internal stores and the influx from the extracellular solution, the Ca^{2+} uptake into cellular organelles, and the extrusion by plasma membrane Ca^{2+} pumps [16].

Calcium signaling in the mitochondria also contributes to the regulation of cellular energy metabolism. ATP is hydrolyzed to ADP in order to power energy-requiring processes and is shuttled into the mitochondria to be reconverted into ATP as a final step in respiration. This enhances the electron flux within the ETC, resulting in the oxidation of NADH to NAD^{+}. Concurrently, Ca^{2+} is transferred into the mitochondria through the mitochondrial Ca^{2+} uniporter (MCU), activating the enzymes of the Krebs cycle to adjust NADH regeneration to match its oxidation [14]. In addition, excessive mitochondrial Ca^{2+} uptake and Ca^{2+} accumulation, irreversible $\Delta\Psi$ collapse, ATP depletion, and oxidative stress contribute to the opening of the mPTP [17].

Type 2 ryanodine receptors (RyR2s) and type 2 inositol 1,4,5-trisphosphate receptors (IP3R2s) are Ca^{2+} release channels found on cardiac SR. Recent studies have demonstrated that leaky RyR2 channels, but not IP3R2, contribute to mitochondrial Ca^{2+} overload and dysfunction in heart failure (HF) [11]. NO signaling and its downstream effectors such as *S*-nitrosylation have also been shown to be key processes in regulating calcium signaling. The neuronal nitric oxide synthase (nNOS or NOS1) has been linked to the reduction of calcium influx through the L-type Ca^{2+} channel [5, 18]. This decrease in Ca^{2+} influx may be responsible for the cardioprotection induced by NO. Furthermore, decreased *S*-nitrosylation of key SR Ca^{2+} handling proteins such as the RyR2s due to impaired NOS1 can result in increased Ca^{2+}-mediated ventricular arrhythmia in the setting of elevated myocardia $[Ca^{2+}]_i$ [19]. Inhibition of *S*-nitrosylation of the SR Ca^{2+} ATPase (SERCA) has been associated with lower Ca^{2+} uptake in the SR and impaired myocardial relaxation [20].

While substantial efforts were undertaken to characterize the kinetic properties of mitochondrial calcium cycling, the experimental approaches and techniques have not been able to reach explicit conclusions on cardiac mitochondrial responses to cytosolic Ca^{2+} oscillations during each heartbeat. However, it is widely accepted that Ca^{2+} is a second messenger for the regulation of mitochondrial tasks and represents a crucial link for the role of mitochondria for excitation-metabolism and excitation-contraction coupling in the heart.

2.1.3. Generation of ROS

Mitochondria are also a large cellular source of ROS. ROS includes the superoxide anion radical ($O_2^{\cdot-}$) and hydroxyl radical ($^{\cdot}OH$), as well as nonradical oxidants, such as hydrogen peroxide (H_2O_2) and singlet oxygen ($^{1}O_2$) [21]. They can be converted from one to the other by enzymatic and nonenzymatic mechanisms. The most abundant form of ROS in the body is $O_2^{\cdot-}$, which is enzymatically or spontaneously dismutated to H_2O_2. In the human body, there are three superoxide dismutase (SOD) isoforms with precise subcellular compartmentalization: the Cu,Zn-dependent isoform (Cu,Zn SOD, SOD1) is found in the cytosol; the Mn-dependent isoform (Mn SOD, SOD2) is located in the mitochondrial matrix; and Cu,Zn SOD is located in the extracellular space (ecSOD, SOD3) [22]. Mitochondrial ROS have emerged as an important mechanism of disease and redox signaling in the cardiovascular system.

O_2^- is the proximal mitochondrial ROS and is produced by the one-electron reduction of oxygen [23]. Mitochondrial O_2^- production takes place at redox-active prosthetic groups within proteins where the kinetic factors are key to the production of O_2^- formation [23]. Under physiological conditions, the balance between ROS generation and ROS scavenging is highly controlled. ROS generation can initiate diverse cellular responses, which include triggering signaling pathways involved in cell protection, initiating coordinated activation of mitochondrial fission and autophagy to optimize removal of abnormal mitochondria and cells, and ensuring that the damage does not spread to neighboring mitochondria and cells [21]. Both high levels of ROS (oxidative stress) and excessively low levels of ROS (reductive stress) are harmful and may play causative roles in the pathologies related to the dramatic change of redox environment [21]. Excess ROS production in the heart under pathophysiological conditions leads to mitochondrial dysfunction and bioenergetic decline and contributes to a number of cell pathologies in the heart. For example, ROS is favored by high membrane potential, low ATP formation, and hampering the flow of electrons through the complexes in cardiomyocytes. In addition, ROS formation is the result of the uncoupling of respiration as seen during the opening of the mPTP [21]. Although many studies have detected O_2^- produced in isolated mitochondria, there are few reliable methods that can be used to measure the mitochondrial ROS production *in vivo* [24].

The molecular mechanisms of ROS generation in the cardiac mitochondrion remain unclear. It has been showed that complex I (NADH-ubiquinone oxidoreductase) is the main source of ROS in the mitochondrion. However, the ROS production at complex I is high under pathological conditions, not physiological condition [21]. Further mechanistic studies suggest that the major site of ROS production in complex I is either upstream of a rotenone-binding site or tightly coupled to the increased level of NAD(P)H after rotenone supplementation [21]. ROS production at complex II is low at physiological concentrations of succinate, suggesting that complex II is not a key contributor to the mitochondrial ROS. ROS production at complex III only occurs after the binding of antimycin A, suggesting that conformational changes that occur on antimycin A binding may be responsible for the production of ROS [21].

2.1.4. mPTP opening

Mitochondria can mediate cell death through the opening or activation of the mPTP [25]. The mPTP is a high conductance channel that generates a sudden increase in inner mitochondrial membrane (IMM) permeability to ions and small solutes when opened [26, 27]. The pore is regulated by the concentration of Ca^{2+}, ADP, NADH, and ROS. Regulation of the mPTP opening is a key essential mechanism for cardiomyocyte survival and function.

Intense research efforts have been focused on elucidating the molecular components of the mPTP. The original mPTP model hypothesized that the channel comprised these principal proteins: cyclophilin D (CyPD), located in the mitochondrial matrix; the ANT, found in the inner membrane; the voltage-dependent anion channel (VDAC) in the outer membrane [28];

and other interacting mitochondrial molecules such as the phosphate carrier, BH3 proteins, and p53 [29]. However, genetic ablation of the proposed components revealed that only the deletion of the CyPD gene resulted in impaired opening of the mPTP, suggesting that the other proposed components are not a necessary part of the pore [30, 31].

Recent studies indicated that the ATP synthase is a major component of the mPTP [32]. There are two working proposals about the mechanism for ATP synthase in the mPTP formation. The first one suggests that the pore forms at the interface of two dimers of ATP synthase [33]. It has been showed that the current that was observed from reconstituted lipid bilayers with purified dimers of the ATP synthase was electrophysiologically equivalent to that of the mPTP. Additionally, genetic ablation of two specific subunits of the F0 subcomplex that are necessary for dimerization did not result in opening of the pore, which further underscores the importance of dimerization for the formation of the mPTP [34]. The second hypothesis focuses on the c-subunit ring of the F0 subcomplex [35]. In purified ATP synthase extracts in yeast, the ring structure produced by the c-subunits exhibited a current that was equivalent to that of the mPTP [34], and the currents were inhibited by regulators of the mPTP, suggesting that the ring and the mPTP are the same. While debate continues about the precise components and mechanism of the mPTP, its importance in physiology and pathology is clear and its regulation is paramount to cell survival.

While a short-term opening of the mPTP appears to act as a normal calcium-release mechanism that is required for proper metabolic regulation [29, 36–38], irreversible formation and consequent opening of the mPTP are key factors in mitochondrial dysfunction and mitochondria-driven cell death [32, 39, 40]. When the mitochondria are exposed to high concentrations of calcium, they undergo a massive and permanent swelling that leads to an abrupt increase in permeability to small solutes of the IMM, abolishing the chemiosmotic gradient across the IMM [29], which subsequently uncouples OXPHOS, leading to a decrease in ATP production and an increase in ROS formation [25]. Further rupture of the outer mitochondrial membrane results in the extrusion of cytochrome c, a key step in the initiation of apoptosis [41]. The mPTP may also play a role in the regulation of energy production due to the dual role of the ATP synthase in both ATP production and mPTP formation [25].

Interestingly, small increases in *O*-GlcNAcylation were correlated with improved ability of cardiac mitochondria to sequester Ca^{2+} as well as resistance to mPTP opening. Key regulatory proteins in the mPTP, the VDAC and ANT, were also found to be able to be *O*-GlcNAcylated. The ATP synthase, the key molecule that forms the mPTP, has also been shown to be able to be *O*-GlcNAcylated [6]. Since mPTP opening is influenced by the loss of the mitochondrial potential as well as calcium overload, any change in mitochondrial potential or calcium dynamics may have adverse effects in the mitochondria. Key calcium signaling participants of mPTP regulation include the pore of the outer membrane, VDAC, the pore of the IMM calcium uniporter, and a key regulator of the mPTP, cyclophilin D [42]. Our most recent study also showed that overexpression of VCP protects against stress-induced mPTP opening in cardiomyocyte through an iNOS-dependent mechanism [9].

2.2. Cardiac mitochondrial changes during cardiac development

There are significant differences in mitochondrial metabolism and function during the cardiac development through the fetus, neonatal, and adult heart.

One of the major changes during the cardiac development is the use of energy fuels to generate ATP in cardiomyocyte. In the fetal heart, glucose and lactate are the predominant substrates used in the generation of ATP [43, 44]. The fetal heart boasts of a large endogenous glycogen supply, which is a significant source of the glucose on which the heart relies. Glycogenolysis is also particularly important in conditions of oxygen deprivation, allowing the fetal heart to resist the effects of hypoxia and ischemia better than the adult heart [43]. Fetal hearts have less mitochondria and therefore lower levels of respiratory and TCA cycle activities [2]. Notably, circulating levels of fatty acids are low, reducing the role of FAO in the generation of ATP. FAO is further inhibited by the high lactate levels present in the fetal heart [2]. Postnatally, an important switch occurs as fatty acids replace glucose and lactate as the primary energy substrates in the developing heart [43]. Consequently, the activity of the proteins of the carnitine shuttle, particularly the M isoform of the mitochondrial carnitine palmitoyltransferase I (CPT I) and mitochondrial carnitine palmitoyltransferase II (CPT II), is markedly increased during the early postnatal period [45]. Other key proteins that have been associated with the uptake of fatty acids into cardiac muscle cells also exhibit increased mRNA expression during maturation of the heart, reflecting increased fatty acid uptake and metabolism [46].

In addition, there is a change in the transfer and use of the energy currency in the mitochondria during the cardiac development. MitoCK is responsible for the production of high-energy phosphates in adult heart. In the fetal heart, mitoCK levels are undetectable, with its expression starting between weeks 1 and 2 in the Wistar rat pup and rising to adult levels after 6 weeks [47]. MitoCK expression was associated with creatine-activated respiration and the affinity of OXPHOS to ADP. Importantly, there is a change in the organization of the cardiac mitochondria from a random arrangement from day 1 in a rat to a fine network of myofibrils by week 3, as mitoCK allows maximal activation of the processes of OXPHOS [47].

2.3. Cardiac mitochondria during aging

Aging is a major risk factor for cardiovascular diseases. During aging, mitochondrial oxidative stress responses, mitochondrial damage, and biogenesis as well as the cross-talk between mitochondria and cellular signaling are changed.

Aging may induce changes to the shape and size of mitochondria in the heart [48]. In aged mice, mitochondria appeared more rounded and less spherical [49]. It was further noted that aged mitochondria exhibit a lower total area of inner membrane per mitochondria, suggesting a reduced capacity for OXPHOS [50]. Reciprocally, increased levels of large-scale deletions and point mutations in cardiac mtDNA, as well as reduced levels of mitochondrial enzymatic activities, may occur with aging.

Additionally, the multiple metabolic changes that occur in cardiac muscle with advancing age include increasing levels of saturated fatty acids and reduced levels of polyunsaturated fatty acids and cardiolipin [51]. Cardiolipin is a key cellular phospholipid and an important constituent of the mitochondrial inner membrane. Reduced cardiolipin influences cardiac mitochondrial membrane transport function, fluidity, and stability of the membrane and facilitates optimal energy generation [51]. Significant reduction in carnitine and acetyl carnitine levels has also been reported in older subjects, suggesting lowered ability to transfer fatty acids into the mitochondria to be metabolized [52]. In addition, the effect of aging on cardiac OXPHOS enzymatic function has been reported. Within cardiomyocytes, the interfibrillar mitochondria consume less oxygen and show a decrease in the ETC enzyme activity, particularly complexes III and IV during aging [53, 54]. This decrease in enzyme activity may lead to the lowered ability to meet the energy demands of the heart as aging ensues.

Furthermore, mitochondrial abnormalities have been proposed due to the increased mitochondrial production of ROS during aging. The rate of oxidative phosphorylation decreases with aging, allowing for increased leakage of electrons [48], these electrons are then able to interact with oxygen, generating superoxide anions and other forms of ROS. Excessive ROS formation has harmful consequences, including cellular dysfunction and cell death [48]. This high level of ROS is also able to oxidize mtDNA. Moreover, opening of the mPTP has been found to be changed in the heart during aging [55]. Increased opening of the mPTP may be linked to higher ROS levels and thus may be facilitating the aging process.

3. Mitochondria in heart diseases

Although the pathophysiology of heart diseases is divergent, mitochondrial dysfunction appears to be a common mechanism that determines cardiac survival and function. Cardiac mitochondrial abnormalities include shifted metabolic substrate utilization, impaired mitochondrial ETC activity, increased formation of ROS, altered calcium homeostasis, and increased mPTP opening. Defects in mitochondrial structure and function have been found in association with cardiovascular diseases such as dilated and hypertrophic cardiomyopathy (DCM and HCM, respectively), cardiac conduction defects and sudden death, ischemic and alcoholic cardiomyopathy, and myocarditis. This section focuses on the changes of mitochondrial bioenergetics that are associated with cardiac survival and growth in heart diseases, including heart failure (HF), ischemia/reperfusion (I/R), pressure overload–induced cardiac hypertrophy and the cardiomyopathies in diabetes, and genetic mitochondrial diseases (MD).

3.1. Mitochondrial dysfunction in HF

HF is an end stage of many heart disorders and a complex chronic clinical syndrome. Although the causes of HF are variable, HF is viewed as an energy-mismatched disease [1, 56]. The first link between HF and mitochondrial dysfunction was described in 1962 in a guinea pig model with HF induced by an aortic restriction [57]. Since this observation, there has been growing interest in the investigation of mitochondrial function in failing hearts [58], and emerging evidence supports the concept that dysregulation of myocardial energetics is tightly associated with the development and progression of HF [1, 56, 59, 60].

The heart requires large amounts of energy to facilitate its continuous contraction and relaxation cycles. HF occurs when the energy demand outweighs the energy supply. Any contributor that leads to HF is accompanied with a gradual but progressive decline in the activity of mitochondrial respiration, leading to diminished capacity for ATP production and subsequent progression of the heart to fail. Reciprocally, a failed heart reduces the blood and oxygen supply to the peripheral tissues and to the heart itself, further exacerbating the decline in cardiac energy production. On the other hand, the amount of ATP required from the mitochondria is increased to meet the abnormally enlarged myocardium size and failing function, augmenting

http://dx.doi.org/10.5772/intechopen.72611

the imbalance between the requirement and supplement of oxygen in the cardiac muscle during the contraction and relaxation cycle. Consequently, the bioenergetic requirements of the heart are beyond what the mitochondria can cope with, and the heart begins to progress to HF. Thus, energy deficiency can be a cause and effect of HF. There are considerable evidences of links between HF and impairment of the energetics of myocardial mitochondria, such as declined mitochondrial synthesis/resynthesis of ATP, shifted fuel selection, impaired mitochondrial biogenesis, and abnormal calcium transport.

3.1.1. Reduction of ATP synthesis

Like all the other cells, there are three energy systems that contribute to the production of ATP in cardiac muscles: phosphagen system (ATP-creatine phosphate cycling; high power, short duration), glycolysis (moderate power/short duration), and FAO (low power/long duration). Three energy systems can be selectively recruited, depending on the amount of oxygen available, as part of the cellular respiration process to generate the ATP for the cardiac muscles. Since the heart has a limited capacity for substrate storage, energy is required to rebuild or resynthesize it. The energy released from any of these three series of reactions is coupled with the energy requirements of the reaction that resynthesizes ATP.

ATP-CP system is the quickest way to resynthesize ATP. CP, like ATP, is stored in cardiac muscle cells and serves as the main energy store in myocardium. If oxygen is unavailable, the ATP-CP system does not use oxygen and does not produce lactic acid. This is the primary system behind the very short, powerful movements of the cardiac contraction and relaxation cycle. When CP is broken down, a large amount of energy is released. This energy released is coupled to the energy requirement necessary for the resynthesis of ATP. CP can easily diffuse through the inner mitochondrial membrane to the cytosol to generate ATP from ADP catalyzed by the cytosolic CK (cytoCK). Normal beating cardiomyocytes, even under variations of workload, maintain a constant level of ATP and CP in the cytosolic and mitochondrial compartments [58]. The CP/ATP ratio of 1.7–2.1 reflects normal mitochondrial ATP production and CK efficiency. This ratio has become a powerful index of the bioenergetics of the heart and its decrease has been reported in both the human and animal models of HF [61–65]. In HF patients and animal models, the total CK, as well as both the cytoCK and mitoCK, positively correlates with ejection fraction and can decrease as much as 50% [66–68]. It is observed that the decrease in CK activity, rather than the level of hypertrophy itself, is a hallmark of the transition from severe hypertrophy to HF [62, 69]. Interestingly, healthy myocardial cell size, myofibrillar and cytoskeletal organization, and positioning of the mitochondria near the SR allow for the ATP production in both mitochondrial and cytosolic regions and work concurrently to meet the energy demand [69]. However, in the failing hearts, the increase in myocardial cell size, the shrinkage of mitochondrial content, the alterations in microtubules, and the disorganization of cytoskeletal protein and their reduced expression contribute to decrease the efficiency of mitoCK and cytoCK for the energy transfer between the mitochondria and the cytosol [70–73].

The glycolysis system is the second-fastest way to resynthesize ATP. In the normal heart, pyruvate is converted into a metabolic intermediary molecule called acetyl coenzyme A (acetyl-CoA), which enters the mitochondria for oxidation and the production of more ATP. In the failing heart, the conversion to lactate occurs due to the greater demand for oxygen than the available supply. Although the catabolism of sugar supplies the necessary energy from which

ATP is manufactured, it is only partially broken down when sugar is metabolized anaerobically. Only a few moles of ATP can be resynthesized from the breakdown of sugar as compared to the yield possible when oxygen is present. In addition, there is an increase in hydrogen ions due to the formation of lactic acid, causing the muscle pH to decrease. This leads to acidosis and the accumulation of other metabolites such as ADP, P_i, and potassium ions that may further induce the inhibition of specific enzymes involved in metabolism and muscle contraction.

The aerobic system includes the Krebs cycle and the ETC. Mitochondria are crucial for the working of the cardiomyocytes as these powerhouses provide the aerobic metabolism for the cardiomyocyte function. Reduced mitochondrial oxidative capacity has been observed in rodent HF models. The onset of HF is not an overnight process but a progression of continual abnormalities in the bioenergetics due to the disruption of metabolic regulatory signaling pathway or the lack of oxygen supply, which leads to failure in mitochondrial dysfunction and decline in ATP production.

3.1.2. The shift of fuel selection of mitochondrial bioenergetics

Numerous studies have demonstrated that cardiac substrate preference is altered in the failing heart. Fatty acids are the preferential energy substrates of the heart and contribute to 60–90% of cardiac ATP production [74]. At the early phase of HF, there is a decline in FAO. An adaptive mechanism is to switch from fatty acid to glucose via the glycolytic pathway. The decrease in the capacity for the mitochondria to oxidize fatty acids is linked to the reduced expression of the master regulator of energy metabolism in mitochondria, PGC-1α (transcriptional co-activator peroxisome proliferator–activated receptor-γ coactivator-1α) [75–77]. In mouse model, PGC-1α is shown to be crucial for the functional efficiency of mitochondrial FAO, lipid regulation, and ATP synthesis, particularly in instances of increased cardiac demand [78]. The overexpression of PGC-1α in transgenic mice induces enhancement of mitochondrial respiration and an increase in mitochondrial numbers [79]. The downregulation of PGC-1α leads to reduction of its downstream targets, e.g., nuclear respiratory factor (NRFs), estrogen receptor–related receptor (ERRα/γ), peroxisome proliferator–activated receptors (PPARs), and subsequently regulates FAO, glucose utilization, and mitochondrial biogenesis [1, 69]. PPARα, as a transcription factor that enables fatty acids to be transported into the mitochondria and peroxisomes, is downregulated in failing hearts of animals and humans [80, 81]. In human HF patients (both ischemic and idiopathic DCM), ERRα and its target genes were downregulated, which may contribute to the reduction of mitochondrial metabolic capacity [81].

It is yet unclear whether the myocardial substrate shifts serve as adaptive functions or cause deleterious effects on the failing heart, but the evidences from reports in animal models and in rare genetic human diseases provide some light. In mice studies, the rapid decline in the cardiac mitochondrial FAO capacity induces cardio-lipotoxic effects due to the accumulation of lipids [82, 83]. Furthermore, when FAO enzymes such as the very-long-chain acyl-CoA dehydrogenase (VLCAD) or the long-chain acyl-CoA dehydrogenase (LCAD) are disrupted in mice, cardiomyopathic profiles similar to human cases are observed [84, 85]. Likewise, with cardiac-specific deletion of the PPARβ gene, which is involved in the oxidation of the FA, the mice developed cardiomyopathy with cardiomyocyte apoptosis and death [86]. Moreover, in human cases, reports of deficiencies in children of enzymes that are part of the mitochondrial long-chain FAO have caused a stress-induced cardiomyopathy due to accumulation of myocardial lipids [87]. Despite these evidences of the cardiac pathologies that come from reduced mitochondrial FAO, the shift from FAO to glucose in the hypertrophied heart may be beneficial and adaptive for the short term. PPARα-null mice, for example, have reduced FAO efficiency, but the hearts showed no ventricular dysfunction. However, in a rat pressure overload model, when FAO was reactivated, the hearts developed ventricular dysfunction [88]. In addition, the degree and duration of the pathophysiological stimulus as well as the systemic metabolic state (e.g., levels of circulating lipids) may contribute to the consequence of alterations of FAO capacity in the pathogenesis of HF.

3.1.3. Dysregulation of Ca^{2+} homeostasis

The reduction of energy production rate in dysfunctional mitochondria is also attributed by the dysregulation of Ca^{2+} homeostasis within the cardiomyocyte. Mitochondria act as a calcium sensor detecting the increase and decrease of the cytosolic Ca^{2+} to meet the needs of the cardiomyocyte. Ca^{2+} is transported into the mitochondria via MCU and out of the mitochondria via the sodium-calcium exchanger (NCX). Both the MCU and mitochondrial NCX are localized to the IMM. In normal physiological conditions, in the event of increased workload, the cytosolic Ca^{2+} is increased, triggering the opening of the MCU to transport Ca^{2+} into the mitochondrial matrix. The influx of the mitochondrial Ca^{2+} in the matrix increases the ATP synthase and the dehydrogenase activity of the citric acid cycle to generate more ATP [58]. Another transporter of Ca^{2+} into the mitochondria is the mPTP, which requires oxidative stress, elevated phosphate, and adenine nucleotide depletion to be opened. Increased uptake of Ca^{2+} into the mitochondria has been linked to cellular dysfunction and energy reduction [89, 90]. Also, the accumulation of Ca^{2+} in the mitochondria induces activation of the apoptotic and necrotic pathways [91]. In addition, in postmyocardial infarction HF mouse model, diastolic SR Ca^{2+} leak induces mitochondrial Ca^{2+} overload and dysfunction [92]. In HF, Ca/calmodulin-dependent protein kinase II (CamKII) has been involved in increasing mitochondrial Ca^{2+} uptake through the MCU and promotes mPTP opening and myocardial cell death [93].

3.1.4. Impaired mitochondrial biogenesis

Efficient mitochondrial capacity to meet the heart's workload also involves maintaining and protecting its biogenesis. It has been shown that the mitochondrial biogenesis was declined in failing heart, which is associated with the downregulation of the transcription factors such as NRF and ERRα [94].

3.1.5. Excess generation of ROS

The respiratory chain regularly generates ROS in the form of O_2^-, which can initiate the formation of other ROS such as OH, peroxynitrite, and H_2O_2. These O_2^- are not able to easily permeate outside the mitochondria and become trapped within. Since mtDNA has no protective histones and a poor DNA repair system, mtDNA is more susceptible to damage and has a high mutation rate [58]. Presence of ROS generates oxidative stress and damage not only to DNA, but also to proteins of the cell, which include those in signaling of the mechanical and structural roles. In a canine model of HF and HF patient blood samples, O_2^- production by the mitochondria is increased [95, 96]. The reduction of PGC-1α in HF has also been found to promote oxidative stress and mitochondrial damage [97]. Another source of ROS is one of the isoforms of NADP oxidase (Nox). Nox 4 is abundant in cardiomyocytes and is localized primarily in the mitochondria. Nox 4 has been reported to enhance ROS production in aging and in pressure overload–HF models [98–100] and also is highly active in failing human hearts [101]. Moreover, ROS plays a part in regulating cardiac hypertrophic pathways: Ras, protein kinase C, Jun N-terminal kinase, and mitogen-activated protein kinase [94, 102].

In summary, HF is characterized by bioenergetic imbalance between the energy production from mitochondria and demands from the myocardial performance. There are many complex simultaneous interplays between: the maintenance of ratio of CP/ATP, the level of total CK as a catalyst, the cycling of Ca^{2+} between the cytosol and the mitochondrial matrix, the major regulatory role of PGC-1α for mitochondrial biogenesis, FAO and glucose metabolism, and even the volume of cardiomyocyte in affecting mitochondria positioning that influences efficiency of ATP production in cardiac mitochondria.

3.2. Mitochondria and ischemia/reperfusion (I/R)

The normal function of the mitochondria maintains the endurance of the cardiomyocyte in the events of stress and increased workload. However, as soon as the series of biochemical alterations and damage in the mitochondria occur, the cell viability declines and regresses to cell death. Mitochondrial dysfunction contributes to cell damage during I/R. Myocardial ischemia is the result of the narrowing or blockage of the coronary artery, thereby depriving the cardiomyocytes from oxygen leading to hypoxia and damage to the heart region and disabling the heart to efficiently pump. The effects of hypoxia induce sudden biochemical and metabolic changes in the cardiomyocytes. These alterations induce mitochondrial membrane depolarization, reduction of ATP synthesis, and damage to the contractile function. With the cardiomyocytes being devoid of O_2, the cell metabolism changes to anaerobic respiration, inducing lactate accumulation and pH reduction. The increase in proton drives the Na^+-H^+ ion exchanger to expel H^+ from the cell in exchange for entry of Na^+ ions [103]. Furthermore, due to the lack of ATP, $3Na^+$-2 K^+ATPase fail to function causing more accumulation of Na^+ and inducing the reverse function of the NCX pump to extrude Na^+ and accumulate Ca^{2+} ions, promoting Ca^{2+} overload [104]. However, with prolonged ischemia, the increase in mitochondrial Ca^{2+}, ROS, and decline of ATP level, the mPTP is triggered to be opened. These changes further result in mPTP opening, mediating both the necrotic and apoptotic cell death.

Although reperfusion restores the region of ischemia with new influx of O_2, and the necessary substrates for aerobic ATP synthesis are delivered and extracellular pH has been restored, reperfusion has been proven to deliver damage at the same time. As blood flow reintroduces molecular oxygen to the damaged areas, ROS is generated. While the mitochondria generate ROS in normal physiology, the reperfusion of the ischemic region induces bursts of ROS production that overwhelms the ability of the cells to normally scavenge the reactive species [105]. It has been reported that upon reperfusion, while O_2 supply is suddenly restored, the rapid normalization of the pH and the existing Ca^{2+} overload and oxidative stress triggers the mPTP to be opened [106, 107]. If the duration of the ischemia is relatively short, the biochemical changes would not be as severe, mPTP remains closed, and the cell will recover [58]. The activation of mPTP occurs in two stages [107]. In the first stage, during ischemia, due to the accumulation of fatty acids, loss of cytochrome c and antioxidants, the dissipation of the electrical potential across the membrane establishes the 'priming' formation of the mPTP. When reperfusion is introduced, the opening of the mPTP is triggered by multiple factors such as Ca^{2+} overload, increased free phosphate, ROS, and acidosis [107]. In addition, as the mitochondrial membrane potential continues to decline, mitochondrial and cytosolic Ca^{2+} levels continue to increase, leading to cell necrosis and apoptosis.

3.3. Mitochondria and pressure overload–induced cardiac remodeling

Under physiological or pathological cardiac workload, the heart adapts through structural remodeling to meet the requirements. Remodeling at the cellular level induces alterations in organelle structure, intercellular protein, and gene expression [108]. At the early stages of cardiac hypertrophy, there are enhancement and preservation of the mitochondrial oxidative capacity, but as hypertrophy progresses to HF, mitochondrial function is gradually impaired [109]. Mitochondrial alterations and dysfunction have been linked to cardiac remodeling including morphology, FAO, ATP synthesis, biogenesis, ROS, and mitophagy.

It has been widely accepted that pressure overload–induced cardiac remodeling alters the mitochondrial morphology in size, volume, and numbers. For example, the mitochondria were found to be swollen, with degraded mtDNA and altered cristae structures in HCM model in pigs [110]. There were distorted cristae and reduced mitochondrial density and volume in a pressure overload–induced cardiac hypertrophic mouse model without difference in mitochondrial numbers between the hypertrophic hearts and the sham control [111]. Despite these evidence from animal models, observations from electron microscopy show remarkable variabilities in HF patients of cardiomyopathy in terms of the mitochondrial numbers, size, and matrix density [112].

In addition, in the pressure overloaded heart, the fuel that drives mitochondria to synthesize ATP switches from FA to glucose, which causes lesser ATP production and depletion in cellular energy. In normal physiology, the uptake of FAs involves the conjugation of FA to acetyl CoA (FA-CoA). FA-CoA enters the mitochondrial matrix and is metabolized by the beta oxidation process through the carnitine shuttle, CPT-1 and CPT-2 [113]. In the pressure overload heart, FAO rate is reduced, along with the decrease in mRNA expression of CPT-1 [114–116]; however, some report it to be unchanged [113]. The variable data might be due to the varying degrees of hypertrophy in different animals [113].

Furthermore, pressure overload–induced cardiac remodeling also affects mitochondrial biogenesis. In response to metabolic status of the cell, the mitochondria undergo controlled cycles of biogenesis with fusion and fission. The processes of the fusion and fission are well regulated by PGC-1α, which then regulates ERRα to act on the group of guanosine triphosphatases (GTPases). Fusion involves mitofusin proteins (MFN 1 and 2) in the outer mitochondrial membrane and optical atrophy protein 1 (OPA1) in the IMM. The fusion process is switched on to balance the mitochondrial membrane potential and allows for the exchange of matrix components, as well as damaged mtDNA [117]. Fission, on the other hand, allows for more mitochondria to be distributed further to release cytochrome c during apoptosis and mitochondrial degradation by mitophagy. Fission occurs through dynamin-1-like protein (DRP1), mitochondrial fission factor (MFF), and adapter protein mitochondrial fission 1 (FIS1). In physiological hypertrophy, PGC-1α activates biogenesis to meet the demands of the heart [77]. At early stages of pathological hypertrophy, mitochondrial biogenesis increases, and mitochondrial numbers increase, but as hypertrophy worsens to HF, PGC-1α expression is downregulated and biogenesis activity is impaired [79, 118]. In addition, as hypertrophy transits to HF, the expression of OPA1 is reduced and mitochondria become small and fragmented. Furthermore, in decompensated hypertrophy and HF, the mitochondrial biogenesis also declines due to depletion of ATP synthesis, which then halts the increase in new mitochondria in the cardiomyocyte [109].

Moreover, cardiac hypertrophy also affects the energetic cross-talk between mitochondria and other organelles to transfer ATP. There is direct communication between the mitochondria and the ATPases of the myofibrils and the SR [119]. Muscle mitochondria in its ordered bundled organization around the myofibrils and the SR are highly clustered at regions of high-energy demand where there is a tightly regulated ATP/ADP ratio [69]. In the pressure overload–induced hypertrophic heart, the direct channeling of ATP within the high-energy demand sites becomes weakened due to the decrease in mitochondrial content and numbers [69, 119]. In addition, mitophagy is activated in pressure overloaded cardiomyocytes due to the increased cellular damage from mitochondrial dysfunction. The causative factors of autophagy in cardiac hypertrophy are complex. Although low baseline autophagy allows the cardiomyocytes to adapt to hypertrophic demands, exacerbation of autophagy promotes hypertrophic contractile dysfunction [120].

In summary, pressure overload causes cardiac remodeling through disruption of the cell signaling pathway, altering the mitochondrial morphology in size, volume, and numbers, regulating the mitochondrial biogenesis and affecting the energetic cross-talk between mitochondria and other organelles to transfer ATP for utilization by the cardiomyocyte or mitophagy. These changes further lead to the failing of the myocardium.

3.4. Mitochondria and diabetic cardiomyopathy

Although coronary artery disease remains as the top cause of mortality and morbidity in western countries, the link between HF and diabetes is growing with the rising incidence of diabetes and prediabetes [121]. Based on epidemiological studies, diabetic individuals are likely to develop HF compared to those who have no diabetic history [122]. This link describes the term diabetic cardiomyopathy, which is due to the myocardium of chronic diabetes patients showing diastolic dysfunction and left ventricular hypertrophy, followed by later onset systolic dysfunction that regresses to decompensated HF [123]. Approximately 60% of type 2 diabetic patients have diabetic cardiomyopathy [124]. The causes of diabetic cardiomyopathy are multifactorial and complex. Cardiac mitochondrial abnormalities were found in both diabetic mouse models and human diabetic hearts. Diabetic cardiomyopathy has been linked to the increased myocardial oxygen consumption and increased oxidative stress. Mouse models of type 2 diabetes (*db/db* and *ob/ob*) showed dysfunctional mitochondrial state 3 respiration and decline in ATP production [125, 126]. In right atrial myofibers of diabetic patients, defects in respiratory complex were observed with the reduction of state 3 respiration on impairment in complex I alone [127]. Another respiration deficiency was detected in myofibers from diabetic patients that showed deficiency in respiration with substrate palmitoyl-L-carnitine [127].

Interestingly, opposite to the reduction of FAO in failing heart, diabetic hearts had more FAO and a reduction in glucose oxidation. The increase in FAO is attributed to the increased expression of PPARα, which increases the genes that are involved with cardiac FA utilization [128]. Additionally, in type 2 diabetes, reduction of cardiac efficiency is also caused by an increase in mitochondrial uncoupling that in turn increases O_2 consumption. The series of events begins with the increased availability and delivery of FA that forces the mitochondria to increase FA uptake. This stimulates the increase in ROS production [129]. ROS generation activates the uncoupling proteins (UCs) and promotes proton leak via ANT. The increase in mitochondrial uncoupling propagates the increase of mitochondrial O_2 consumption, which promotes the activation of FAO. As mitochondrial uncoupling causes the rise in O_2 consumption, the ATP production will not be increased. This reduces the cardiac efficiency of the cell in the generation and usage of energy, which subsequently reduces the provision of ATP for the cell and leads to contractile dysfunction. Thus, this is the link between the type 2 diabetes mechanism merging with contractile dysfunction and development of muscle pathology, with diastolic dysfunction and left ventricular hypertrophy.

3.5. Genetic mitochondrial heart disease

Genetic MD can be caused by a mutation in either the mtDNA or the nDNA [130, 131]. MDs arising from mtDNA are more prevalent in adults, whereas diseases arising from nDNA tend to be more prevalent in infants and children [132]. MDs can also be classified by the function of the proteins involved in the disease. For example, MDs have been found to be associated with the mutations in genes that encode subunits of the ETC complexes [130] and ATP synthase [133, 134], ancillary proteins that participate in the assembly, transport, and function of the ETC complexes, or the regulatory proteins that control activities of the mitochondria [130, 131]. In addition, mutations have been described in gene-encoding proteins that synthesize cardiolipin, an integral part of the inner mitochondrial membrane [135, 136]. The most frequently identified biochemical abnormalities are deficiencies in NADH-coenzyme Q (CoQ) reductase (complex I) and cytochrome-c oxidase (complex IV) [135, 136].

The mitochondrion is a unique organelle as it possesses its own DNA system. While mutated DNA can affect any organ, the presence of the mtDNA mutations in highly metabolic tissues, such as brain, heart, skeletal muscle, and eyes, exhibits a more severe and progressive prognosis. Patients with the known mitochondrial mutation of m.3243A > G develop early death, whereas if this mutation has a cardiac cause, sudden deaths would occur [137]. A healthy individual may possess mutated DNA, but the onset of the disease will not be obvious until a certain mutation threshold of ~60–90% is present [138]. Inheritance of mtDNA occurs only through the maternal line with single, large-scale deletions being rare and the point mutations frequently transmitted [139].

Cross-sectional studies have shown that specific mitochondrial mutations have been presented with a certain cardiac phenotype, and cardiac disorders could inherit different mtDNA mutations [140]. For example, there are inherited familial cardiomyopathies (in both children and adult) linked to mutations in the mtDNA [139, 141]. Mutation m.1555A > G mt-rRNA has only been associated with restrictive cardiomyopathy [142]. Conversely, up to 40% of MD patients have HCM [143]; atrioventricular (AV) block is one of the manifestations of Kearns-Sayre syndrome (KSS) that is due to the large-scale deletions in the mtDNA [143]. The symptoms of HCM patients who have sarcomeric protein gene mutations differ from the those of MD patients who developed HCM. Generally, these MD patients who develop HCM have left ventricular dysfunction but no left ventricular outflow tract obstruction [144, 145]. Another cardiomyopathy-presenting phenotype that is less common in the MD patients is DCM. The echocardiographic findings showed slow progression of disease [146, 147].

Cardiac phenotype association with genetic MD is more common than realized; however, the mechanism of association of some mutations with specific cardiac phenotypes is not clearly understood. Since myocardial cells depend heavily upon mitochondria for its energy requirements, it is no wonder that specific MD involves specific cardiac pathology phenotype.

4. Clinical applications

4.1. Diagnosis of mitochondrial dysfunction in heart disease

Although it has been widely accepted that mitochondria play a key role in cardiac pathological conditions, effectively diagnosing mitochondrial dysfunction in the clinical setting has been challenging. MDs often affect multiple organ systems in the body and clinical presentation varies; however, there are a few "tell-tale" signs and combinations that may enable clinicians to better identify MDs [148]. For example, patients with KSS, which is typically associated with single deletion mutations, may present with ptosis, retinal pigmentary abnormalities, ataxia, and cardiac conduction abnormalities [148]. In patients with myoclonic epilepsy with ragged-red fibers (MERRF), myoclonus, cerebellar ataxia, and elevated blood lactate are key symptoms in their presentations [149]. A high suspicion is important when considering a diagnosis of MD. Cardiologists who evaluate patients for hypertrophy, conduction abnormalities, and DCM should be aware of the spectrum of MD so that they can collaborate with MD specialists to make accurate diagnoses.

Since there are variabilities in the MD symptom presentations, in addition to the clinical diagnosis, a multiple-parametric approach that involves histological, biochemical, and genetic testing is required to identify abnormalities of blood, urine, or cerebrospinal fluid (CSF) analyte values, microscopic irregularities, biochemical deviations on polarographic assays, or a diagnostic genetic finding [150].

4.1.1. Genetic tests

It is crucial to understand that not all persons with mtDNA mutations will manifest the symptoms. Nuclear DNA and mtDNA mutation screening can be performed in the consented family, but the challenge remains that only a small proportion of these nDNA mutations have been identified. The presence of family history of maternal inheritance or multisystemic diseases will be important to note. Furthermore, mitochondrial genome screening can also be performed on the muscle sample [132].

4.1.2. Laboratory tests

Muscle biopsy in conjunction with molecular genetic testing is required for effective diagnosis of MD [151]. A major feature of the histological result of the biopsy using the Gomori Trichrome stain shows >2% ragged red fibers that come from the sub-sarcolemmal mitochondrial accumulation. However, these ragged red fibers are present only in the late stage of the disease and commonly absent in children [132]. The key diagnostic feature is the presence of fibers that are deficient for cytochrome c oxidase (COX) activity [with >2% of COX negative fibers], reflecting low activity of complex IV of the respiratory chain, in patients less than 50 years [148, 151]. COX activity may be decreased in healthy older patients, so its use in diagnosis is limited to younger patients. Laboratory tests for the levels of creatine phosphokinase, pyruvate, albumin, lactate, transaminases, and blood count are also recommended [152]. An elevated postprandial lactate:pyruvate ratio (>20) is commonly found in MD patients; however, some MD patients may show normal ratio and thus other tests are required to confirm the disease [146]. Next-generation sequencing is also proposed for screening of the multiple mutations associated with MDs [152]. Additionally, fibroblast growth factor-21 (FGF-21) has been recently identified as a serum biomarker of MDs associated with both mtDNA and nDNA mutations [148], potentially simplifying the clinical diagnosis of MD.

4.1.3. Cardiac imaging

The cardiac presentation of MD patients varies; however, progressive cardiac conduction defects may develop into a complete heart block in KSS, while Wolff-Parkinson-White (WPW) syndrome can develop in patients with mitochondrial encephalomyopathy, lactic acidosis, and stroke-like episodes (MELAS) syndrome owing to the m.3243A > G mutation [153, 154]. There is no characteristic manifestation of cardiomyopathy that differentiates MD, although HCM is common [150]. Cardiac imaging using cardiovascular magnetic resonance (CMR) with late gadolinium enhancement (LGE) can be used to effectively evaluate the heterogeneous presentation of HCM, offering a more reliable measurement of all segments of the heart than echocardiography [155].

4.1.4. Electrocardiogram

In the early stage of the diagnosis process of MD, 12-lead electrocardiogram results are useful to add to the diagnostic criteria [146]. ECG results will be variable depending on the kinds of syndrome the mitochondrial myopathy is associated with [156]. Ocular myopathy patients may in general show normal ECG profile, but two out of the six patients were presented with ST depression and inverted T wave [156]. Patients with MELAS/MERRF may show atrial or ventricular premature contraction (APC or VPC) with T-wave abnormalities such as inverted T wave, as well as ST depression [156]. These abnormalities can be present even without the presentation of left ventricular hypertrophy [146]. A profile of short PR, or WPW, was also found for a MELAS patient [146, 156]. Patients with KSS presented cardiac conduction abnormalities with a variation of ECG profile of AV blocks, complete right bundle branch block with inverted T, or left axis deviation (LAD) and prolonged His ventricular (HV) interval [156]. Though some patients may show normal ECG profile at diagnosis, performing another ECG every 1–3 years may be important to detect uprise of cardiac abnormalities or complications [151].

4.2. Mitochondria as a drug target in heart disease

Most standard-of-care pharmacological approaches to HF, such as β-blockers, ivabradine, a cyclic nucleotide-gated channel blocker, and antagonism of the renin-angiotensin-aldosterone system, focus on the reduction of the energy requirements of cardiac muscle, including modulation of neurohormonal abnormalities, unloading the heart (vasodilatation), and/or reducing the heart rate, which subsequently reduces myocardial oxygen consumption. Although these therapies have improved survival in patients over the past 2–3 decades, death and poor quality of life continue to adversely affect this ever-increasing patient population [94]. The search for more effective and complementary therapy for these patients must be focused on improving the intrinsic function of the cardiomyocytes [157, 158], such as finding ways to increase/restore the energy supply, in addition to reducing the energy demand of the heart [1].

Since disruption of metabolic signaling pathways such as in FAO, glucose utilization, or ATP generation contributes to the development of heart dysfunction, proteins in these metabolic pathways have become attractive targets of novel therapeutic strategies for the prevention or early treatment of HF [159]. Selective agonists for each of the PPARs have been established and are currently used to treat hyperlipidemia (fibrates) and diabetes (thiazolidinediones). It must be noted that stimulation of the PPAR pathway in the heart or extra cardiac tissues, e.g., adipose or hepatic tissue, potentially diminishes cardiac lipotoxicity by reducing lipid delivery or increasing mitochondrial oxidation. However, chronic activation of PPARα could lead to deleterious effects, particularly in the context of diabetes, hyperlipidemic states, or the ischemic heart [159].

Additionally, although the molecular mechanisms responsible for mitochondria-mediated disease processes are not yet clear, oxidative stress seems to play an important role. Accordingly, strategies for the targeted delivery of antioxidants to mitochondria are being developed. A typical "mitochondrial cocktail," which may include coenzyme Q10 (CoQ10), creatine, L-carnitine, thiamine, riboflavin, folate, as well as other antioxidants such as vitamins C and E, has been reported to partially improve clinical manifestations, though others have disputed its effectiveness [160]. Although, L-carnitine supplementation may be highly effective in patients diagnosed with DCM secondary to primary systemic carnitine deficiency, supplementation has little effect on other types of mitochondrial cardiomyopathy [132]. Recent developments in mitochondrial-targeted antioxidants that concentrate on the matrix-facing surface of the IMM protect against mitochondrial oxidative damage and hold therapeutic potential for future treatment of cardiovascular diseases (CVDs) [161].

Because a cure for mitochondrial genetic defects is still not available, the management of genetic MD with presentation of cardiac pathology, β-blockers, ACE inhibitors, or angiotensin receptor blockers should be administered [146]. Providing rudimentary nutritional education along with nutritional assessment and exercise will be important for the patients to take preventative measures from further lifestyle disease complications [146, 162]. Should there be advanced second- and third-degree AV block coupled with neuromuscular disorders, a permanent pacemaker is highly recommended [163]. Depending on the severity of the mitochondrial cardiomyopathy, cardiac transplantation could be recommended depending on the presence of neuromuscular weakness as it can complicate anesthesia administration [164].

5. Future direction

Because diagnosing MD can be challenging for clinicians, research is needed to better understand the complex bioenergetic arrangements and redox networks of the mitochondrion in cardiac cell. Improved understanding of mitochondrial mechanism in the pathophysiology in the heart will help the discovery of novel biomarkers and clinical diagnostic standards for the heart disease. In addition, current pharmacologic strategies are incompletely effective, and large randomized controlled trials are warranted to direct future therapy. Since HF is recognized as a state of myocyte energy starvation, greater evidence, in the form of large randomized, controlled trials, is required to confirm the role of metabolic-modulating drugs in the treatment of HF, which will be expected to be an area of great advances in the future. Additionally, more preclinical and clinical studies are necessary to evaluate the effectiveness and toxicity of mitochondrial-targeted antioxidants. Furthermore, the identification of the mechanisms by which alterations in substrate utilization cause cardiomyopathy is also a necessary area of intense research.

Author details

Shaunrick Stoll, Christiana Leimena and Hongyu Qiu*

*Address all correspondence to: hqiu@llu.edu

Division of Physiology, Department of Basic Sciences, School of Medicine, Loma Linda University, Loma Linda, CA, USA

References

[1] Brown DA et al. Expert consensus document: Mitochondrial function as a therapeutic target in heart failure. Nature Reviews. Cardiology. 2017;**14**(4):238-250

[2] Marín-García J, Goldenthal MJ. The mitochondrial organelle and the heart. Revista Española de Cardiología. 2002;**55**(12):1293-1310

[3] Bisetto E et al. Proteomic analysis of F1F0-ATP synthase super-assembly in mitochondria of cardiomyoblasts undergoing differentiation to the cardiac lineage. Biochimica et Biophysica Acta. 2013;**1827**(7):807-816

[4] Grossman LI, Lomax MI. Nuclear genes for cytochrome c oxidase. Biochimica et Biophysica Acta. 1997;**1352**(2):174-192

[5] Zhang YH. Nitric oxide signalling and neuronal nitric oxide synthase in the heart under stress. F1000Research. 2017;**6**:742

[6] Ma J et al. *O*-GlcNAcomic profiling identifies widespread *O*-linked beta-N-acetylglucosamine modification (*O*-GlcNAcylation) in oxidative phosphorylation system regulating cardiac mitochondrial function. The Journal of Biological Chemistry. 2015;**290**(49):29141-29153

[7] Qiu H et al. H11 kinase/heat shock protein 22 deletion impairs both nuclear and mitochondrial functions of STAT3 and accelerates the transition into heart failure on cardiac overload. Circulation. 2011;**124**(4):406-415

[8] Rashed E et al. Heat shock protein 22 (Hsp22) regulates oxidative phosphorylation upon its mitochondrial translocation with the inducible nitric oxide synthase in mammalian heart. PLoS One. 2015;**10**(3):e0119537

[9] Lizano P et al. The valosin-containing protein is a novel mediator of mitochondrial respiration and cell survival in the heart in vivo. Scientific Reports. 2017;**7**:46324

[10] Eisner D. Calcium in the heart: From physiology to disease. Experimental Physiology. 2014;**99**(10):1273-1282

[11] Santulli G et al. Mitochondrial calcium overload is a key determinant in heart failure. Proceedings of the National Academy of Sciences of the United States of America. 2015;**12**(36):11389-11394

[12] Finkel T et al. The ins and outs of mitochondrial calcium. Circulation Research. 2015; **116**:1810-1819

[13] Bers DM. Altered cardiac myocyte Ca regulation in heart failure. Physiology. 2006; **21**(6):380-387

[14] Kohlhaas M et al. Mitochondrial energetics and calcium coupling in the heart. The Journal of Physiology. 2017;**595**(12):3753-3763

[15] Walsh C et al. Modulation of calcium signalling by mitochondria. Biochimica et Biophysica Acta. 2009;**1787**(11):1374-1382

[16] Clapham DE. Calcium signaling. Cell. 2007;**131**(6):1047-1058

[17] Bhosale G et al. Calcium signaling as a mediator of cell energy demand and a trigger to cell death. Annals of the New York Academy of Sciences. 2015;**1350**:107-116

[18] Sears CE et al. Cardiac neuronal nitric oxide synthase isoform regulates myocardial contraction and calcium handling. Circulation Research. 2003;**92**(5):e52-e59

[19] Cutler MJ et al. Aberrant S-nitrosylation mediates calcium-triggered ventricular arrhythmia in the intact heart. Proceedings of the National Academy of Sciences of the United States of America. 2012;**109**(44):18186-18191

[20] Bencsik P et al. Cardiac capsaicin-sensitive sensory nerves regulate myocardial relaxation via S-nitrosylation of SERCA: Role of peroxynitrite. British Journal of Pharmacology. 2008;**153**(3):488-496

[21] Zorov DB et al. Mitochondrial reactive oxygen species (ROS) and ROS-induced ROS release. Physiological Reviews. 2014;**94**(3):909-950

[22] Zelko IN et al. Superoxide dismutase multigene family: A comparison of the CuZn-SOD (SOD1), Mn-SOD (SOD2), and EC-SOD (SOD3) gene structures, evolution, and expression. Free Radical Biology & Medicine. 2002;**33**(3):337-349

[23] Murphy MP. How mitochondria produce reactive oxygen species. The Biochemical Journal. 2009;**417**(1):1-13

[24] Chance B, Sies H, Boveris A. Hydroperoxide metabolism in mammalian organs. Physiological Reviews. 1979;**59**(3):527-605

[25] Pérez MJ, Quintanilla RA. Development or disease: Duality of the mitochondrial permeability transition pore. Developmental Biology;**426**(1):1-7

[26] Hunter DR, Haworth RA. The Ca^{2+}-induced membrane transition in mitochondria. Archives of Biochemistry and Biophysics. 1979;**195**(2):468-477

[27] Haworth RA, Hunter DR. The Ca^{2+}-induced membrane transition in mitochondria. Archives of Biochemistry and Biophysics. 1979;**195**(2):460-467

[28] Rao VK, Carlson EA, Yan SS. Mitochondrial permeability transition pore is a potential drug target for neurodegeneration. Biochimica et Biophysica Acta (BBA) – Molecular Basis of Disease. 2014;**1842**(8):1267-1272

[29] Elrod JW, Molkentin JD. Physiologic functions of cyclophilin D and the mitochondrial permeability transition pore. Circulation Journal. 2013;**77**(5):1111-1122

[30] Kokoszka JE et al. The ADP/ATP translocator is not essential for the mitochondrial permeability transition pore. Nature. 2004;**427**(6973):461-465

[31] Baines CP et al. Voltage-dependent anion channels are dispensable for mitochondrial-dependent cell death. Nature Cell Biology. 2007;**9**(5):550-555

[32] Jonas EA et al. Cell death disguised: The mitochondrial permeability transition pore as the c-subunit of the F1FO ATP synthase. Pharmacological Research. 2015;**99**:382-392

[33] Giorgio V et al. Dimers of mitochondrial ATP synthase form the permeability transition pore. Proceedings of the National Academy of Sciences of the United States of America. 2013;**110**(15):5887-5892

[34] Carraro M et al. Channel formation by yeast F-ATP synthase and the role of dimerization in the mitochondrial permeability transition. The Journal of Biological Chemistry. 2014;**289**(23):15980-15985

[35] Alavian KN et al. An uncoupling channel within the c-subunit ring of the F1FO ATP synthase is the mitochondrial permeability transition pore. Proceedings of the National Academy of Sciences of the United States of America. 2014;**111**(29):10580-10585

[36] Hausenloy D et al. Transient mitochondrial permeability transition pore opening mediates preconditioning-induced protection. Circulation. 2004;**109**(14):1714-1717

[37] Lu X et al. Individual cardiac mitochondria undergo rare transient permeability transition pore openings. Circulation Research. 2016;**118**(5):834-841

[38] Saotome M et al. Transient opening of mitochondrial permeability transition pore by reactive oxygen species protects myocardium from ischemia-reperfusion injury. American Journal of Physiology. Heart and Circulatory Physiology. 2009;**296**(4):H1125-H1132

[39] Bernardi P et al. From ATP to PTP and back: A dual function for the mitochondrial ATP synthase. Circulation Research. 2015;**116**(11):1850-1862

[40] Bernardi P et al. The mitochondrial permeability transition pore: Channel formation by F-ATP synthase, integration in signal transduction, and role in pathophysiology. Physiological Reviews. 2015;**95**(4):1111-1155

[41] Kroemer G, Galluzzi JD, Brenner C. Mitochondrial membrane permeabilization in cell death. Physiological Reviews. 2007;**87**(1):99-163

[42] Williams GS, Boyman L, Lederer WJ. Mitochondrial calcium and the regulation of metabolism in the heart. Journal of Molecular and Cellular Cardiology. 2015;**78**:35-45

[43] Lopaschuk GD, Collins-Nakai RL, Itoi T. Developmental changes in energy substrate use by the heart. Cardiovascular Research. 1992;**26**(12):1172-1180

[44] Marin-Garcia J, Ananthakrishnan R, Goldenthal MJ. Human mitochondrial function during cardiac growth and development. Molecular and Cellular Biochemistry. 1998; **179**(1-2):21-26

[45] Brown NF et al. Mitochondrial carnitine palmitoyltransferase I isoform switching in the developing rat heart. The Journal of Biological Chemistry. 1995;**270**(15):8952-8957

[46] Van Nieuwenhoven FA et al. Co-expression in rat heart and skeletal muscle of four genes coding for proteins implicated in long-chain fatty acid uptake. The International Journal of Biochemistry & Cell Biology. 1999;**31**(3-4):489-498

[47] Tiivel T et al. Developmental changes in regulation of mitochondrial respiration by ADP and creatine in rat heart in vivo. Molecular and Cellular Biochemistry. 2000;**208**(1-2):119-128

[48] Boengler K et al. Mitochondria and ageing: Role in heart, skeletal muscle and adipose tissue. Journal of Cachexia, Sarcopenia and Muscle. 2017;**8**(3):349-369

[49] Cheng Z et al. Characteristics of cardiac aging in C57BL/6 mice. Experimental Gerontology. 2013;**48**(3):341-348

[50] El'darov CM et al. Morphometric examination of mitochondrial ultrastructure in aging cardiomyocytes. Biochemistry (Mosc). 2015;**80**(5):604-609

[51] Lesnefsky EJ, Chen Q, Hoppel CL. Mitochondrial metabolism in aging heart. Circulation Research. 2016;**118**(10):1593-1611

[52] Costell M, O'Connor JE, Grisolia S. Age-dependent decrease of carnitine content in muscle of mice and humans. Biochemical and Biophysical Research Communications. 1989;**161**(3):1135-1143

[53] Lesnefsky EJ et al. Aging decreases electron transport complex III activity in heart interfibrillar mitochondria by alteration of the cytochrome c binding site. Journal of Molecular and Cellular Cardiology. 2001;**33**(1):37-47

[54] Suh JH, Heath S-H, Hagen TM. Two subpopulations of mitochondria in the aging rat heart display heterogenous levels of oxidative stress. Free Radical Biology & Medicine. 2003;**35**(9):1064-1072

[55] Picard M et al. Mitochondrial function in permeabilized cardiomyocytes is largely preserved in the senescent rat myocardium. PLoS One. 2012;**7**(8):e43003

[56] Rosca MG, Hoppel CL. Mitochondrial dysfunction in heart failure. Heart Failure Reviews. 2013;**18**(5):607-622

[57] Schwartz A, Lee KS. Study of heart mitochondria and glycolytic metabolism in experimentally induced cardiac failure. Circulation Research. 1962;**10**(3):321-332

[58] Griffiths EJ. Mitochondria and heart disease. Advances in Experimental Medicine and Biology. 2012;**942**:249-267

[59] Rosca MG, Hoppel CL. New aspects of impaired mitochondrial function in heart failure. Journal of Bioenergetics and Biomembranes. 2009;**41**(2):107-112

[60] Scolletta S, Biagioli B. Energetic myocardial metabolism and oxidative stress: let's make them our friends in the fight against heart failure. Biomedicine & Pharmacotherapy. 2010;**64**(3):203-207

[61] Neubauer S et al. Impairment of energy metabolism in intact residual myocardium of rat hearts with chronic myocardial infarction. The Journal of Clinical Investigation. 1995;**95**(3):1092-1100

[62] Ye Y et al. High-energy phosphate metabolism and creatine kinase in failing hearts: A new porcine model. Circulation. 2001;**103**(11):1570-1576

[63] Ye Y et al. Myocardial creatine kinase kinetics and isoform expression in hearts with severe LV hypertrophy. American Journal of Physiology. Heart and Circulatory Physiology. 2001;**281**(1):H376-H386

[64] Hardy CJ et al. Altered myocardial high-energy phosphate metabolites in patients with dilated cardiomyopathy. American Heart Journal. 1991;**122**(3 Pt 1):795-801

[65] Zhang J et al. Bioenergetic abnormalities associated with severe left ventricular hypertrophy. The Journal of Clinical Investigation. 1993;**92**(2):993-1003

[66] Nascimben L et al. Creatine kinase system in failing and nonfailing human myocardium. Circulation. 1996;**94**(8):1894-1901

[67] SylvÉN C et al. Dynamics of creatine kinase shuttle enzymes in the human heart. European Journal of Clinical Investigation. 1991;**21**(3):350-354

[68] De Sousa E et al. Subcellular creatine kinase alterations. Implications in heart failure. Circulation Research. 1999;**85**(1):68-76

[69] Ventura-Clapier R et al. Bioenergetics of the failing heart. Biochimica et Biophysica Acta (BBA) – Molecular Cell Research. 2011;**1813**(7):1360-1372

[70] Sabbah HN et al. Mitochondrial abnormalities in myocardium of dogs with chronic heart failure. Journal of Molecular and Cellular Cardiology. 1992;**24**(11):1333-1347

[71] Gupta A et al. Impairment of ultrastructure and cytoskeleton during progression of cardiac hypertrophy to heart failure. Laboratory Investigation. 2010;**90**(4):520-530

[72] Hein S et al. The role of the cytoskeleton in heart failure. Cardiovascular Research. 2000; **45**(2):273-278

[73] Cooper 4th G. Cytoskeletal networks and the regulation of cardiac contractility: Microtubules, hypertrophy, and cardiac dysfunction. American Journal of Physiology. Heart and Circulatory Physiology. 2006;**291**(3):H1003-H1014

[74] Stanley WC, Recchia FA, Lopaschuk GD. Myocardial substrate metabolism in the normal and failing heart. Physiological Reviews. 2005;**85**(3):1093-1129

[75] Garnier A et al. Depressed mitochondrial transcription factors and oxidative capacity in rat failing cardiac and skeletal muscles. The Journal of Physiology. 2003;**551**(Pt 2):491-501

[76] Sun C-K et al. Losartan preserves integrity of cardiac gap junctions and PGC-1 α gene expression and prevents cellular apoptosis in remote area of left ventricular myocardium following acute myocardial infarction. International Heart Journal. 2007;**48**(4):533-546

[77] Watson PA et al. Restoration of CREB function is linked to completion and stabilization of adaptive cardiac hypertrophy in response to exercise. American Journal of Physiology. Heart and Circulatory Physiology. 2007;**293**(1):H246-H259

[78] Wu Z et al. Mechanisms controlling mitochondrial biogenesis and respiration through the thermogenic coactivator PGC-1. Cell. 1999;**98**(1):115-124

[79] Lehman JJ et al. The transcriptional coactivator PGC-1alpha is essential for maximal and efficient cardiac mitochondrial fatty acid oxidation and lipid homeostasis. American Journal of Physiology. Heart and Circulatory Physiology. 2008;**295**(1):H185-H196

[80] Sack MN et al. Fatty acid oxidation enzyme gene expression is downregulated in the failing heart. Circulation. 1996;**94**(11):2837-2842

[81] Sihag S et al. PGC-1alpha and ERRalpha target gene downregulation is a signature of the failing human heart. Journal of Molecular and Cellular Cardiology. 2009;**46**(2):201-212

[82] Chiu HC et al. A novel mouse model of lipotoxic cardiomyopathy. The Journal of Clinical Investigation. 2001;**107**(7):813-822

[83] Yagyu H et al. Lipoprotein lipase (LpL) on the surface of cardiomyocytes increases lipid uptake and produces a cardiomyopathy. The Journal of Clinical Investigation. 2003;**111**(3):419-426

[84] Exil VJ et al. Very-long-chain acyl-coenzyme a dehydrogenase deficiency in mice. Circulation Research. 2003;**93**(5):448-455

[85] Kurtz DM et al. Targeted disruption of mouse long-chain acyl-CoA dehydrogenase gene reveals crucial roles for fatty acid oxidation. Proceedings of the National Academy of Sciences of the United States of America. 1998;**95**(26):15592-15597

[86] Cheng L et al. Cardiomyocyte-restricted peroxisome proliferator-activated receptor-delta deletion perturbs myocardial fatty acid oxidation and leads to cardiomyopathy. Nature Medicine. 2004;**10**(11):1245-1250

[87] Kelly DP, Strauss AW. Inherited cardiomyopathies. The New England Journal of Medicine. 1994;**330**(13):913-919

[88] Young ME et al. Reactivation of peroxisome proliferator-activated receptor alpha is associated with contractile dysfunction in hypertrophied rat heart. The Journal of Biological Chemistry. 2001;**276**(48):44390-44395

[89] Odagiri K et al. Local control of mitochondrial membrane potential, permeability transition pore and reactive oxygen species by calcium and calmodulin in rat ventricular myocytes. Journal of Molecular and Cellular Cardiology;**46**(6):989-997

[90] Balaban RS et al. Role of calcium in metabolic signaling between cardiac sarcoplasmic reticulum and mitochondria in vitro. American Journal of Physiology. Heart and Circulatory Physiology. 2003;**284**(2):C285-C293

[91] Nakayama H et al. Ca(2+)- and mitochondrial-dependent cardiomyocyte necrosis as a primary mediator of heart failure. The Journal of Clinical Investigation. 2007;**117**(9):2431-2444

[92] Santulli G et al. Mitochondrial calcium overload is a key determinant in heart failure. Proceedings of the National Academy of Sciences of the United States of America. 2015; **112**(36):11389-11394

[93] Joiner ML et al. CaMKII determines mitochondrial stress responses in heart. Nature. 2012;**491**(7423):269-273

[94] Bayeva M, Gheorghiade M, Ardehali H. Mitochondria as a therapeutic target in heart failure. Journal of the American College of Cardiology. 2013;**61**(6):599

[95] Chen Y et al. Increased superoxide production causes coronary endothelial dysfunction and depressed oxygen consumption in the failing heart. American Journal of Physiology. Heart and Circulatory Physiology. 2005;**288**(1):H133-H141

[96] Ijsselmuiden AJ et al. Circulating white blood cells and platelets amplify oxidative stress in heart failure. Nature Clinical Practice. Cardiovascular Medicine. 2008;**5**(12):811-820

[97] Lu Z et al. PGC-1 alpha regulates expression of myocardial mitochondrial antioxidants and myocardial oxidative stress after chronic systolic overload. Antioxidants & Redox Signaling. 2010;**13**(7):1011-1022

[98] Lambeth JD. NOX enzymes and the biology of reactive oxygen. Nature Reviews. Immunology. 2004;**4**(3):181-189

[99] Ago T et al. Upregulation of Nox4 by hypertrophic stimuli promotes apoptosis and mitochondrial dysfunction in cardiac myocytes. Circulation Research. 2010;**106**(7):1253-1264

[100] Kuroda J et al. NADPH oxidase 4 (Nox4) is a major source of oxidative stress in the failing heart. Proceedings of the National Academy of Sciences of the United States of America. 2010;**107**(35):15565-15570

[101] Heymes C et al. Increased myocardial NADPH oxidase activity in human heart failure. Journal of the American College of Cardiology. 2003;**41**(12):2164-2171

[102] Kwon SH et al. H(2)O(2) regulates cardiac myocyte phenotype via concentration-dependent activation of distinct kinase pathways. Journal of Molecular and Cellular Cardiology. 2003;**35**(6):615-621

[103] Jurkowitz MS, Brierley GP. H^+-dependent efflux of Ca^{2+} from heart mitochondria. Journal of Bioenergetics and Biomembranes. 1982;**14**(5-6):435-449

[104] Haigney MC et al. Sodium channel blockade reduces hypoxic sodium loading and sodium-dependent calcium loading. Circulation. 1994;**90**(1):391-399

[105] Granger DN, Kvietys PR. Reperfusion injury and reactive oxygen species: The evolution of a concept. Redox Biology. 2015;**6**:524-551

[106] Turer AT, Hill JA. Pathogenesis of myocardial ischemia-reperfusion injury and rationale for therapy. The American Journal of Cardiology. 2010;**106**(3):360-368

[107] Honda HM, Korge P, Weiss JN. Mitochondria and ischemia/reperfusion injury. Annals of the New York Academy of Sciences. 2005;**1047**(1):248-258

[108] Verdejo HE et al. Mitochondria, myocardial remodeling, and cardiovascular disease. Current Hypertension Reports. 2012;**14**(6):532-539

[109] Rosca MG, Tandler B, Hoppel CL. Mitochondria in cardiac hypertrophy and heart failure. Journal of Molecular and Cellular Cardiology. 2013;**55**:31-41

[110] Lin CS, Sun YL, Liu CY. Structural and biochemical evidence of mitochondrial depletion in pigs with hypertrophic cardiomyopathy. Research in Veterinary Science. 2003; **74**(3):219-226

[111] Bugger H et al. Proteomic remodelling of mitochondrial oxidative pathways in pressure overload-induced heart failure. Cardiovascular Research. 2010;**85**(2):376-384

[112] Baandrup U et al. Electron microscopic investigation of endomyocardial biopsy samples in hypertrophy and cardiomyopathy. A semiquantitative study in 48 patients. Circulation. 1981;**63**(6):1289-1298

[113] Abel ED, Doenst T. Mitochondrial adaptations to physiological vs. pathological cardiac hypertrophy. Cardiovascular Research. 2011;**90**(2):234-242

[114] Akki A, Smith K, Seymour AM. Compensated cardiac hypertrophy is characterised by a decline in palmitate oxidation. Molecular and Cellular Biochemistry. 2008; **311**(1-2):215-224

[115] Barger PM et al. Deactivation of peroxisome proliferator-activated receptor-α during cardiac hypertrophic growth. The Journal of Clinical Investigation. 2000;**105**(12):1723-1730

[116] Rimbaud S et al. Stimulus specific changes of energy metabolism in hypertrophied heart. Journal of Molecular and Cellular Cardiology. 2009;**46**(6):952-959

[117] Neely JR, Morgan HE. Relationship between carbohydrate and lipid metabolism and the energy balance of heart muscle. Annual Review of Physiology. 1974;**36**:413-459

[118] Asayama K et al. Lipid peroxidation and free radical scavengers in thyroid dysfunction in the rat: A possible mechanism of injury to heart and skeletal muscle in hyperthyroidism. Endocrinology. 1987;**121**(6):2112-2118

[119] Kaasik A et al. Energetic crosstalk between organelles: Architectural integration of energy production and utilization. Circulation Research. 2001;**89**(2):153-159

[120] Delbridge LMD et al. Myocardial stress and autophagy: Mechanisms and potential therapies. Nature Reviews. Cardiology. 2017;**7**:412-425

[121] Calton EK et al. Certain dietary patterns are beneficial for the metabolic syndrome: Reviewing the evidence. Nutrition Research. 2014;**34**(7):559-568

[122] Stamler J et al. Diabetes, other risk factors, and 12-yr cardiovascular mortality for men screened in the multiple risk factor intervention trial. Diabetes Care. 1993;**16**(2):434-444

[123] Ernande L, Derumeaux G. Diabetic cardiomyopathy: Myth or reality? Archives of Cardiovascular Diseases. 2012;**105**(4):218-225

[124] Bell DSH. Diabetic cardiomyopathy. Diabetes Care. 2003;**26**(10):2949-2951

[125] Kuo TH et al. Defective oxidative metabolism of heart mitochondria from genetically diabetic mice. Diabetes. 1983;**32**(9):781-787

[126] Boudina S et al. Reduced mitochondrial oxidative capacity and increased mitochondrial uncoupling impair myocardial energetics in obesity. Circulation. 2005;**112**(17):2686-2695

[127] Anderson EJ et al. Substrate-specific derangements in mitochondrial metabolism and redox balance in atrium of type 2 diabetic human heart. Journal of the American College of Cardiology. 2009;**54**(20):1891-1898

[128] Aoyama T et al. Altered constitutive expression of fatty acid-metabolizing enzymes in mice lacking the peroxisome proliferator-activated receptor alpha (PPARalpha). The Journal of Biological Chemistry. 1998;**273**(10):5678-5684

[129] Bugger H, Abel ED. Mitochondria in the diabetic heart. Cardiovascular Research. 2010; **88**(2):229-240

[130] Alston CL et al. The genetics and pathology of mitochondrial disease. The Journal of Pathology. 2017;**241**(2):236-250

[131] Spinazzola A. Mitochondrial DNA mutations and depletion in pediatric medicine. Seminars in Fetal & Neonatal Medicine. 2011;**16**(4):190-196

[132] Meyers DE, Basha HI, Koenig MK. Mitochondrial cardiomyopathy: Pathophysiology, diagnosis, and management. Texas Heart Institute Journal. 2013;**40**(4):385-394

[133] Xu T, Pagadala V, Mueller DM. Understanding structure, function, and mutations in the mitochondrial ATP synthase. Microbial Cell. 2015;**2**(4):105-125

[134] Mayr JA et al. Mitochondrial ATP synthase deficiency due to a mutation in the ATP5E gene for the F1 epsilon subunit. Human Molecular Genetics. 2010;**19**(17):3430-3439

[135] DiMauro S. Mitochondrial myopathies. Current Opinion in Rheumatology. 2006;**18**(6): 636-641

[136] DiMauro S, Hirano M. Mitochondrial encephalomyopathies: An update. Neuromuscular Disorders. 2005;**15**(4):276-286

[137] Majamaa-Voltti K et al. Causes of death in pedigrees with the 3243A>G mutation in mitochondrial DNA. Journal of Neurology, Neurosurgery, and Psychiatry. 2008;**79**(2):209-211

[138] Bates MG et al. Cardiac involvement in mitochondrial DNA disease: Clinical spectrum, diagnosis, and management. European Heart Journal. 2012;**33**(24):3023-3033

[139] Greaves LC et al. Mitochondrial DNA and disease. The Journal of Pathology. 2012; **226**(2):274-286

[140] Wahbi K et al. Cardiac involvement is frequent in patients with the m.8344A>G mutation of mitochondrial DNA. Neurology. 2010;**74**(8):674-677

[141] Taylor RW, Turnbull DM. Mitochondrial DNA mutations in human disease. Nature Reviews. Genetics. 2005;**6**(5):389-402

[142] Santorelli FM et al. Maternally inherited cardiomyopathy: An atypical presentation of the mtDNA 12S rRNA gene A1555G mutation. American Journal of Human Genetics. 1999;**64**(1):295-300

[143] Limongelli G et al. Prevalence and natural history of heart disease in adults with primary mitochondrial respiratory chain disease. European Journal of Heart Failure. 2010;**12**(2):114-121

[144] Montaigne D, Pentiah AD. Mitochondrial cardiomyopathy and related arrhythmias. Cardiac Electrophysiology Clinics. 2015;**7**(2):293-301

[145] Stalder N et al. Mitochondrial A3243G mutation with manifestation of acute dilated cardiomyopathy. Circulation. Heart Failure. 2012;**5**(1):e1-e3

[146] Limongelli G, Masarone D, Pacileo G. Mitochondrial disease and the heart. Heart. 2017;**103**(5):390-398

[147] Weisz SH et al. Left ventricular non compaction in children. Congenital Heart Disease. 2010;**5**(5):384-397

[148] Liang C, Ahmad K, Sue CM. The broadening spectrum of mitochondrial disease: Shifts in the diagnostic paradigm. Biochimica et Biophysica Acta. 2014;**1840**(4):1360-1367

[149] Lorenzoni PJ et al. When should MERRF (myoclonus epilepsy associated with ragged-red fibers) be the diagnosis? Arquivos de Neuro-Psiquiatria. 2014;**72**:803-811

[150] Cohen BH. Neuromuscular and systemic presentations in adults: Diagnoses beyond MERRF and MELAS. Neurotherapeutics. 2013;**10**(2):227-242

[151] Pfeffer G, Chinnery PF. Diagnosis and treatment of mitochondrial myopathies. Annals of Medicine. 2013;**45**(1):4-16

[152] Parikh S et al. Diagnosis and management of mitochondrial disease: A consensus statement from the mitochondrial medicine society. Genetics in Medicine. 2015;**17**(9):689-701

[153] Vydt TC et al. Cardiac involvement in adults with m.3243A > G MELAS gene mutation. American Journal of Cardiology. 2007;**99**(2):264-269

[154] Kenny D, Wetherbee J. Kearns-Sayre syndrome in the elderly: Mitochondrial myopathy with advanced heart block. American Heart Journal. 1990;**120**(2):440-443

[155] Karamitsos TD et al. The role of cardiovascular magnetic resonance imaging in heart failure. Journal of the American College of Cardiology. 2009;**54**(15):1407-1424

[156] Anan R et al. Cardiac involvement in mitochondrial diseases. A study on 17 patients with documented mitochondrial DNA defects. Circulation. 1995;**91**(4):955-961

[157] Wilcox JE et al. "targeting the heart" in heart failure: Myocardial recovery in heart failure with reduced ejection fraction. JACC: Heart Failure. 2015;**3**(9):661-669

[158] Gheorghiade M et al. Developing new treatments for heart failure: Focus on the heart. Circulation: Heart Failure. 2016;**9**(5)

[159] Huss JM, Kelly DP. Mitochondrial energy metabolism in heart failure: A question of balance. Journal of Clinical Investigation. 2005;**115**(3):547-555

[160] Chinnery P et al. Treatment for mitochondrial disorders. Cochrane Database of Systematic Reviews. 2006;**1**:CD004426

[161] Milagros Rocha M, Victor VM. Targeting antioxidants to mitochondria and cardiovascular diseases: The effects of mitoquinone. Medical Science Monitor. 2007;**13**(7): RA132-RA145

[162] Taivassalo T, Haller RG. Exercise and training in mitochondrial myopathies. Medicine and Science in Sports and Exercise. 2005;**37**(12):2094-2101

[163] Page RL et al. 2015 ACC/AHA/HRS guideline for the management of adult patients with supraventricular tachycardia: A report of the American College of Cardiology/American Heart Association Task Force on Clinical Practice Guidelines and the Heart Rhythm Society. Circulation. 2015;**134**(11):e234-e2345

[164] Schmauss D et al. Cardiac transplantation in a 14-yr-old patient with mitochondrial encephalomyopathy. Pediatric Transplantation. 2007;**11**(5):560-562

Interplay Between Mitochondrial Proteins and Age-Associated Risk of Cardiovascular Diseases

Zuzana Tatarkova, Martin Kolisek, Ivana Pilchova,
Peter Racay and Peter Kaplan

Additional information is available at the end of the chapter

http://dx.doi.org/10.5772/intechopen.71789

Abstract

Normal functioning of mitochondria is crucial for cardiac performance. Mitochondria undergo mitophagy (mitochondrial autophagy) and biogenesis, and mitochondrial proteins are subject to extensive post-translational modifications (PTMs). The state of mitochondrial homeostasis reflects overall cellular fitness and longevity. Perturbed mitochondria produce less adenosine triphosphate (ATP), release greater amounts of reactive molecules, and are more prone to apoptosis. Therefore mitochondrial turnover is an integral aspect of quality control in which dysfunctional mitochondria are selectively eliminated through mitophagy. Currently, the progressive deterioration of physiological functions is seen as accumulation of modified/damaged proteins with limiting regenerative ability throughout aging in myocardial cells. Mitochondrial stress response to reactive species was evaluated as electron transport chain (ETC) complexes, redox-active molecules, and their possible communication. Protein-protein interactions revealed a strong linkage between age and ETC protein subunits. Redox state was strongly affected in senescent mitochondria with shift in favor of more pro-oxidizing condition within cardiomyocytes. Assume all together, dysfunctional proteostasis can play a causative role in aging and restoration of protein homeostasis machinery is protective against aging and possibly age-related disorders.

Keywords: aging, heart, mitochondria, protein-protein interactions, redox homeostasis

1. Introduction

The world population ages rapidly, mostly because of increasing longevity and declining fertility [1]. The average lifespan of the human populations is increasing worldwide and it is predicted that in 2035, nearly every fourth individual will be 65 years or older [2]. Aging is a complex phenomenon with a large impact on society. Aging is recently an emerging topic since the life expectancy is rising and because aging itself is the basis for the development of age-related diseases such as cardiovascular disease (CVD), cancer, neurodegenerative diseases and degenerative metabolic diseases (e.g. *diabetes mellitus* type 2) [3]. Since age is the largest risk factor for CVD, the prevalence of these ailments increases dramatically with increasing age. Over 80% of all cases of coronary artery disease and more than 75% of those of congestive heart failure are observed in elderly patients [4]. In order to improve prevention and care for patients, it is important to analyze processes linked with cardiac aging. Prevalence of high blood pressure, obesity and metabolic syndrome correlate with age, and all these conditions facilitate the development of cardiomyopathies that are the major cause of chronic disability, morbidity and mortality in the elderly. Although the long-term exposure to cardiovascular risk factors plays a major role in the etiopathogenesis of CVD and neurodegeneration, intrinsic alterations in the heart and the vascular system occur during lifespan and render the cardiovascular system more vulnerable during senescence. The possible link between aging and senescence was first described in 1961 [5] and it based on the inability of telomeres to sustain their lengths. In addition to this, other events and signals were identified including non-telomeric/genotoxic stress generated by various signals, such as mitochondrial deterioration, oxidative stress, DNA-replication "stress" or activated oncogenes [6]. Several lines of evidence indicate mitochondrial dysfunction to be a major contributor to cardiovascular senescence. Damaged mitochondria are bioenergetically less efficient and they are producing excessive amounts of reactive oxygen species (ROS) with detrimental structural and functional consequences [7]. The ROS impair excitation-contraction coupling, cause arrhythmias, and contribute to cardiac remodeling by inducing cardiac hypertrophy, apoptosis, necrosis, and fibrosis [8]. However, antioxidant interventions in patients with CVD yielded only disappointing results so far [9].

The accumulation of abnormal/dysfunctional mitochondria is usually a consequence of impaired clearance of damaged organelles by autophagy and inadequate replenishment of the cellular mitochondrial pool by mitochondriogenesis [7]. Autophagic flux is generally decreased in aging hearts. Murine loss-of-function models for autophagy develop exacerbated cardiac dysfunction that is accompanied by accumulation of misfolded proteins and dysfunctional organelles. On the other hand, stimulation of autophagy in mouse models improves cardiac function and enables to study a protein aggregation by removing accumulated misfolded proteins, dysfunctional mitochondria, and damaged DNA, thereby alleviating aging-associated pathology in the heart. Multiple lines of evidence suggest that autophagy is required for many mechanisms that mediate lifespan extension, such as caloric restriction. These results are pointing out the possibility that autophagy may play an important role in combating the adverse effects of aging in the heart [10]. At the molecular level, the aging process is associated with accumulation of damaged proteins and organelles, partially due to defects in protein quality control systems. Since most cellular functions are performed by proteins, aging may be, in part, the consequence of a deregulation or malfunction of the cellular proteome [11]. Modern techniques enabled the investigation of the internal structure and morphology of mitochondria and revealed a highly complex compartmentalization [12] with the challenge to dissect the communication and maintenance of the individual compartments. Part of this is to ensure proteostasis (folding, unfolding and degradation) to generate a homeostasis of the functional proteome and to clear mistargeted/damaged proteins. It is not easy, because every submitochondrial compartment needs to control its redox milieu, which is interestingly highly different, e.g. the inner membrane separates the reducing matrix from the more oxidizing intermembrane space [13]. The complexity of the proteome supersedes that of the genome due to alternative splicing events and post-translational modifications (PTMs). Specific position has the mitochondrial intermembrane space (MIMS) with its role in protein and lipid transport, regulation and assembly of the respiratory transport system, regulation of redox processes, coordination of apoptosis and metal ion homeostasis [14]. One of the big challenges of future research will be to investigate how the mitochondrion communicates with the cytosol and the nucleus. The MIMS exhibits specific redox environment and controlled porine-facilitated leakiness through the outer membrane allowing the free diffusion of small molecules (less than 5 kDa) that might harbor candidates mediating the communication from signaling pathways occurring inside the mitochondria toward other organelles [15].

Mitochondrial homeostasis is associated with overall cellular fitness and cellular longevity. Therefore, it determines also normal physiology of organ systems and performance of the body. Recent studies suggest that restoration of mitochondrial dynamics and mitophagy could delay organ senescence and prevent age-associated cardiac diseases. Here, we discuss the current understanding of mitochondria with particular focus on the heart, specifically the close relationship between mitochondrial dynamics or mitophagy suggesting a possible link to the regulation of redox metabolism, and intercellular protein communication.

2. Cellular senescence and mitochondria

Cells undergo widespread changes and develop specific characteristics during senescence that are considered as senescence markers. However, no individual marker has been so far identified as entirely selective parameter for cellular senescence. Nevertheless, a combination of several markers might be evaluated and can help to define the current stage of senescence. Phenotypically, the increase in size and protein content was reported in senescent cells [16, 17] which is in agreement with our results. The data in **Table 1** show that the total protein concentration was elevated in senescent (27 months old) rat mitochondria by 40% ($p < 0.01$).

Protein concentration (mg/ml)	Age (months)		
	6	14	27
Homogenate	20.87 ± 2.50	23.96 ± 1.46	19.19 ± 2.96
Mitochondria	5.69 ± 0.61	5.38 ± 0.49	9.56 ± 0.05**

Values are expressed as Mean ± SEM of 5 individual experiments, **p<0.01; significantly different in comparison to 6 months old rats.

Table 1. Protein concentration in homogenate and mitochondria during aging in heart (yet unpublished data).

However, the protein content in homogenates as well as in isolated mitochondrial fraction was maintained during overall aging process comparing the samples from old (14 months old) and adult (6 months old) rat hearts.

Further, senescent cells exhibit enlarged nuclei and lysosomes, which possess elevated senescence-associated β-galactosidase activity (SA-β-Gal), the most widely used marker [17]. They also enter a proliferative arrest state, detected by cell cycle inhibitor levels such as p53/p21, tumor suppressor $p16^{INK4a}$ [18, 19] and markers of proliferation like Ki-67 and 5-bromodeoxyuridine [20]. Other factors secreted during senescence are cytokines, chemokines, growth factors, proteases, fibronectin as well as ROS and reactive nitrogen species (RNS). Additionally, proteostatic changes during senescence accompanied by an increase in modified proteins, accumulation of protein aggregates and reduced functionality of the proteasomal and autophagy systems [3] will be discussed in following chapters. Only two parameters currently correlate with species longevity in the right sense: the mitochondrial rate of ROS production and the degree of fatty acid unsaturation of tissue membranes. Their basal level is in both cases low in long-lived animals. In addition, the best-known manipulation that extends longevity, dietary restriction, also decreases the rate of mitochondrial ROS production and oxidative damage to mtDNA [21]. The available information supports a mitochondrial free radical theory of aging focused on low generation of endogenous damage and low sensitivity of membranes to oxidation in long-lived animals.

2.1. Mitochondrion – organelle with two faces

According to mitochondrial theory of aging, mitochondria are both the main source and targets of detrimental reactions initiated in association with age-dependent deterioration of the cellular functions. Reactions leading to increased ROS generation, mtDNA mutations, oxidation of mitochondrial proteins and lipids result in subsequent induction of apoptotic events, impaired oxidative phosphorylation capacity, mitochondrial dynamics, and autophagy [22]. In addition, mitochondrial function may be affected by subject parameters like physical activity history [23], caloric restriction [21], drugs [24] and various comorbidities including obesity [25], insulin resistance and hypertension [26]. The primary function of mitochondria is to produce adenosine triphosphate (ATP) by the process of oxidative phosphorylation. In fact, about 90–95% of cellular oxygen is used up in oxidative phosphorylation and 3% from that pool can be converted to superoxide anion radical ($O_2^{\bullet-}$). This is a very strong argument to mitochondria as a main source of this oxygen radical [27]. Among the most relevant ROS sources in heart belong NADPH oxidases (NOX) and mitochondria [28]. Recent studies demonstrate that mitochondrial ROS play a critical role in mediating the cellular effects of angiotensin II in the cardiovascular system [29]. Angiotensin II binds to angiotensin receptor 1, thereby activating NOX isoform 2 and 4 leading to increased mitochondrial ROS production in vascular endothelial cells as well as in cardiac myocytes [30].

Two principal scenarios can be envisioned that favor increased mitochondrial ROS-formation: increased formation of $O_2^{\bullet-}$ at the electron transport chain (ETC) and decreased elimination of $O_2^{\bullet-}$ or hydrogen peroxide (H_2O_2) in the mitochondrial matrix. In heart failure, the first scenario occurs when modifications of ETC complexes like disturbed stoichiometry and

PTMs hamper electron flux along the ETC to provoke excessive $O_2^{\bullet -}$ formation [31] mostly by NADH dehydrogenase (complex I) and Cytochrome c reductase (complex III) causing functional uncoupling of the respiratory chain. The extent and way of individual ETC complexes inhibition is different. According to **Figure 1**, the decline in activity of complex I and cytochrome c oxidase (complex IV) was more obvious during aging when compared to the succinate dehydrogenase (complex II) and complex III activities. Literature data are inconsistent among the studies, mainly due to differences in the experimental age groups and animal models, isolation/purity of mitochondria or enzyme substrate/inhibitor used for study. Complex I is considered to be the most important player in the game of ROS production and/or proton-motive cascade. Loss of its activity has been attributed to the mutations in mitochondrial DNA (mtDNA) in aging animals and recently was linked to the apoptotic cell death pathway [32].

Reduced complex I activity was seen in the rat heart [33], brain synaptic mitochondria [34] as well as continual decrease in the frontal cortex of Parkinson disease patients [35]. It is important to note that the activity and stability of this respiratory complex are determined by its abundance, PTMs and/or specific protein–protein interactions. In contrary, other studies have reported no age-related decrease in complex I activity [36]. Most of the inconsistencies are related to the complexes II, III and IV, where activities of respiratory complexes have been also shown to decline [37], remain unchanged or increased during aging [38]. Our data show age-dependent decrease in all ETC enzyme activities, although the extent of inhibition is different (**Figure 1**). Among them, complex IV was most affected throughout aging and reached 63.4% of adult respiring mitochondria. While complexes I, II and III maintained activities in 14 months old rat mitochondria, cytochrome c oxidase showed deprivation by

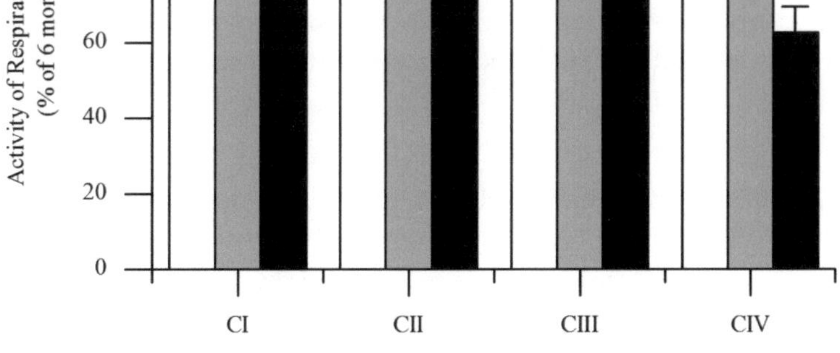

Figure 1. Activities of ETC complexes in heart mitochondria during aging (yet unpublished data). Values are expressed as Mean ± SEM of 5 individual experiments, $^{**}p < 0.01$, $^{***}p < 0.001$; significantly different in comparison to 6 months old rats.

21.6% ($p < 0.01$) when compared to the adults. Unique role in both, Krebs cycle and ETC, has in inner mitochondrial membrane (IMM) embedded complex II. Its function is cardiolipin-independent and is not taking part in respiratory supercomplexes but has been identified as an isolated entity in mildly solubilized mitochondrial membranes [39]. This confirms the least damage by 13.6% in senescent mitochondria when compared to the other respiratory complexes. Interestingly, recent works described the direct connection of the $O_2^{\bullet-}$ formation and respiratory chain complex II [40] when lack of succinate was present. At saturated succinate concentration and high membrane potential complex II is tightly bound with reverse transfer of electrons to $O_2^{\bullet-}$ -producing complex I [41].

Several factors have impact on ETC with specific role of mtDNA. ETC complexes are composed of both nuclear DNA-encoded (more than 80 proteins subunits) and 13 mtDNA-encoded subunits proteins. Respiratory chain and F_1F_0-ATPase deficits are adverse effects on a variety of cellular and tissue functions, causing a wide range of complex clinical phenotypes. The incidence of inherited mitochondrial diseases is estimated to be about 1 in 5000 but a much larger population may be affected when somatic genetic defects, such as mtDNA mutation and deletions accompanying normal aging, are considered. The frequency of the common 4977-bp mtDNA deletion, a typical consequence of oxidative stress [42], increases with age in the human heart and is estimated to be 5- to 15-fold higher in people over 40 years of age relative to younger individuals [43]. This deletion affects genes encoding 7 polypeptide components of the mitochondrial ETC. Bioenergetic consequences of 4977-bp deletions will be reflected when the proportion of deleted mtDNA exceeds 50–55% of total mtDNA. The involvement of mtDNA mutations in cardiac aging is supported by findings in mice that express a proof reading deficient version of mtDNA polymerase (PolG) [44]. A high load of mtDNA mutations and deletions accumulate in the heart of these mice, in conjunction with the early onset of several age-associated changes including cardiac enlargement, fibrosis, impairment of systolic and diastolic function [30], and reduced activity of ETC complexes [44].

To maintain proton-motive force and electron transfer through ETC, reduced equivalents are required. In mitochondria, the Krebs cycle generates NADH, which delivers electrons to the ETC inducing translocation of protons across the inner mitochondrial membrane. This establishes a membrane potential that fuels the F_1F_0-ATPase to generate ATP. At the ETC, electrons can leak to produce $O_2^{\bullet}$ which is dismutated to H_2O_2 by Mn-dependent superoxide dismutase (Mn-SOD) and, in turn, is detoxified by enzymes that require NADPH. Accordingly, equilibrium exists between reduced and oxidized forms of equivalents NADH/NAD^+ and NADPH/$NADP^+$ [45].

In experiments, citrate synthase is frequently used as basal mitochondrial activity marker to avoid possible effects of different yield of mitochondria. Increase in its activity shown in **Figure 2** led to more pronounced activity changes in ETC complexes with age. Starting from citrate synthase, some of the Krebs cycle enzymes play inevitable role in reduced equivalents machinery, such as $NAD(P)^+$-isocitrate dehydrogenase (ICDH) and α-ketoglutarate dehydrogenase (KGDH). Both of the enzymes share some common features as NADH production and they are regulated by calcium (Ca^{2+}). Calcium uptake dynamically controls the redox state of NAD(P)H in working cardiac myocytes [28] and availability of NADPH together with reduced glutathione is required for H_2O_2 removal by glutathione peroxidase/glutathione reductase

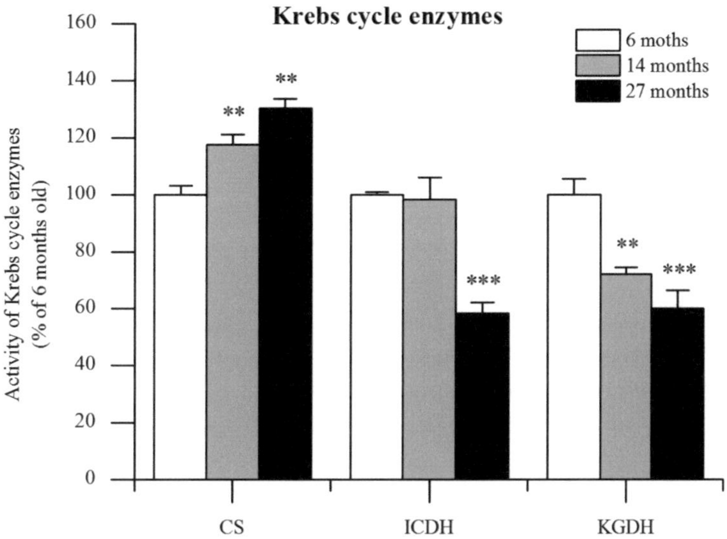

Figure 2. Activities of Krebs cycle enzymes in heart mitochondria during aging (yet unpublished data). Values are expressed as Mean ± SEM of 5 individual experiments, $^{**}p < 0.01$, $^{***}p < 0.001$; significantly different in comparison to 6 months old rats.

cycling. Therefore regeneration of NADPH is very important and depends on Krebs cycle enzymes, especially ICDH [46]. Interestingly, the activity of ICDH was affected only in senescent mitochondria but by a significant 42.5% decrease (from 246.52 ± 1.90 to 144.04 ± 5.58) μmol/min/mg protein. Almost equivalent to ICDH activity in senescent hearts was drop in KGDH activity but this enzyme has shown gradual decline during whole aging process (**Figure 2**). In heart failure, elevated intracellular Na^+ promotes ROS-formation by reducing mitochondrial Ca^{2+} uptake. Therefore, mitochondrial Ca^{2+} uptake critically regulates mitochondrial ROS production/removal [28] in cooperation with Krebs cycle enzymes and other ions to maintain mitochondrial homeostasis. Activation of ion channels in the IMM such as mitochondrial permeability transition pore (MPTP), the inner membrane anion channel (IMAC) and ATP-dependent K^+-channel causes depolarization of IMM. This is accompanied by an increase in electron flux required to maintain ATP production. Opening of these channels might promote ROS production, but interestingly they can be activated by ROS themselves. Moreover, $O_2^{\bullet-}$ can be released from mitochondria via MPTP and IMAC. ROS in such a situation trigger oscillations of membrane potential leading to higher incidence of arrhythmias during reperfusion in the heart [47]. It seems that oxidative stress is one of the key events in myocardial senescence progression and development; however, during evolution cells were equipped with antioxidant defense mechanisms that can prevent/recover cells from an oxidative to a reductive state.

3. Redox homeostasis in mitochondria

Mitochondria play important role in generation of ROS and RNS but they are themselves players in different signaling pathways, in which the mitochondrial oxidative defense system contributes to maintain redox homeostasis. Cellular redox state is determined by the reduction potentials and reducing capacities of the redox couples, such as GSH/GSSG, NAD(P)H/NAD(P)$^+$, thioredoxin (reduced/oxidized), glutaredoxin (reduced/oxidized) and cysteine/cystine, From these the GSH/GSSG system is considered to be the most abundant among endogenous antioxidants with 2 to 4-fold higher abundance than other redox systems.

3.1. Thiol–disulfide redox state of mitochondria

Reduced form of GSH (γ-L-glutamyl-L-cysteinyl glycine) is two electron donating molecule and in humans is almost uniquely present in a quite high concentration (1–10 mmol/L). This allows GSH to scavenge ROS either directly or indirectly. As an antioxidant, it reacts with reactive forms and radicals produced in association with electron transport, xenobiotic metabolism and inflammatory responses [48]. GSH homeostasis is not only regulated by its *de novo* synthesis, but also by other factors such as utilization, recycling and cellular export. Cooperation with other antioxidant, redox-related enzymes is important for recycling and maintenance of the optimal redox environment. It was reported that GSH level decreases over time in heart mitochondria [49] and several brain regions [50]. This phenomenon was confirmed by GSH measurement in three age groups (**Table 2**). Rapid decline of GSH level was accompanied by increase in oxidized GSSG form in senescent rat hearts. Interestingly, 14 months old hearts were able to maintain basal concentrations of that present in adult ones. The relative GSH/GSSG ratio indicates a decrease in GSH levels leading to more oxidized environment in senescent cardiomyocytes and experimentally dilated cardiomyopathy in mice [51]. The total content of thiol-containing compounds (R-SH), in contrary to GSH, decreases very slowly (by 19.2% in senescent) during aging process.

(μmol/g of tissue)	Age (months)		
	6	14	27
R-SH content	8.66 ± 0.46	7.12 ± 0.26	7.00 ± 0.09*
GSH content	3.00 ± 0.25	3.74 ± 0.39	1.68 ± 0.19**
GSSG content	1.77 ± 0.21	1.61 ± 0.25	3.81 ± 0.31**
GSH/GSSG ratio	1.64	2.10	0.51
Enzyme activity (μmol/min/mg protein)			
GPx activity	9.033 ± 0.860	8.239 ± 0.081***	6.489 ± 0.112***
GR activity	4.790 ± 0.093	4.194 ± 0.306**	3.960 ± 0.124***
TrxR activity	0.085 ± 0.018	0.050 ± 0.008**	0.052 ± 0.013**

Values are expressed as means ± SEM of 5 individual experiments. *p < 0.05, **p < 0.01, ***p < 0.001; significantly different in comparison to 6 months old rats.

Table 2. The content and activities of GSH cycle-related molecules in heart during aging (yet unpublished data).

Aerobic respiration may result in an increase of H_2O_2, which is metabolized by glutathione peroxidase (GPx), while GSH is recycled by the action of glutathione reductase (GR). Since both of the enzymes were affected in old as well as senescent rat hearts, overproduction of H_2O_2 or lack of reduced NADPH was present. Moreover, peroxidase-mediated elimination of H_2O_2 will also augment the level of GSSG. This in turn, may not only lower the glutathione redox potential, but also increase in amount of protein mixed disulfides. Addition of GSH to protein cysteine residues results to post-translational modification known as S-glutathionylation. It is a reversible process with potential to activate or inactivate protein function by modulating different cellular pathways. It is able to influence gene expression by affecting different transcription factors such as Nrf2 (nuclear factor erythroid 2-related factor 2) or NF-κB (nuclear factor kappa-light-chain-enhancer of activated B cells) [52]. The Nrf2-Keap1 (Kelch-like ECH-associated protein 1) pathway is the major regulator of cytoprotective responses to oxidative and electrophilic stress. In the presence of ROS, critical cysteine residues in Keap1 become oxidized leading to a conformational change, which prevents its binding to Nrf2. As a consequence, Nrf2 degradation is stopped and its nuclear translocation promoted [53]. Recently was shown that S-glutathionylation of endothelial NO synthase (eNOS) at Cys^{689} and Cys^{908} leads to eNOS uncoupling, diminished NO production and enhanced oxidative stress linked with superoxide overproduction [54]. S-glutathionylation as well as GSH alone interacts with earlier mentioned nuclear factor Nrf2. This factor is key transcription factor of 4-hydroxy-2-nonenal (HNE). HNE is highly reactive aldehyde product of lipid peroxidation with potential to modulate function of proteins and lipids. The Nrf2 under stress conditions activates HNE-mediated antioxidant protection, when at a sub-lethal concentration 5 μmol/l HNE stimulates biosynthesis of GSH in cardiomyocytes. In contrary, glutathione after oxidation to the glutathione radical ($GS^•$) has deleterious effects. It is able to take H^+ from lipid side chains and polyunsaturated fatty acids or to induce lipid peroxidation [55]. Altogether, S-glutathionylation may be a double-edged sword in the sense that it promotes antioxidant or pro-oxidant responses.

Peroxidase activity is found in GPx and in the thiol-specific proteins called peroxiredoxins (Prx). They react with H_2O_2 at a very high rate and their activity depends on cysteine residue in the active site. Peroxiredoxins can also reduce and detoxify peroxynitrite anion and a wide range of organic hydroperoxides. The highest reaction rate and abundance has Prx2 which traps almost all H_2O_2 *in vivo* [56]. The level of this powerful thiol-specific protein was maintained until the age of 14 months, but senescent mitochondria lost 35.1% of Prx2 amount (**Figure 3**). Oxidized cysteine residues of Prx are specifically reduced by Trx. Oxidized Trx as well as other oxidized cellular proteins can be reversibly reduced by TrxR in a NADPH-dependent manner. The Trx/TrxR system appears to have a protective function against oxidative stress, e.g. supports the activity of ribonucleotide reductase and inhibits apoptosis signal-regulated kinase-1 [57]. Thioredoxin reductase has been severely affected during aging process by 41.9% in group of 14 months old hearts with an extension until the age of 27 months (**Table 2**). The same scenario was observed in Trx protein level where the amount of protein has decreased to 62.4% in 14 months old as well as 27 months

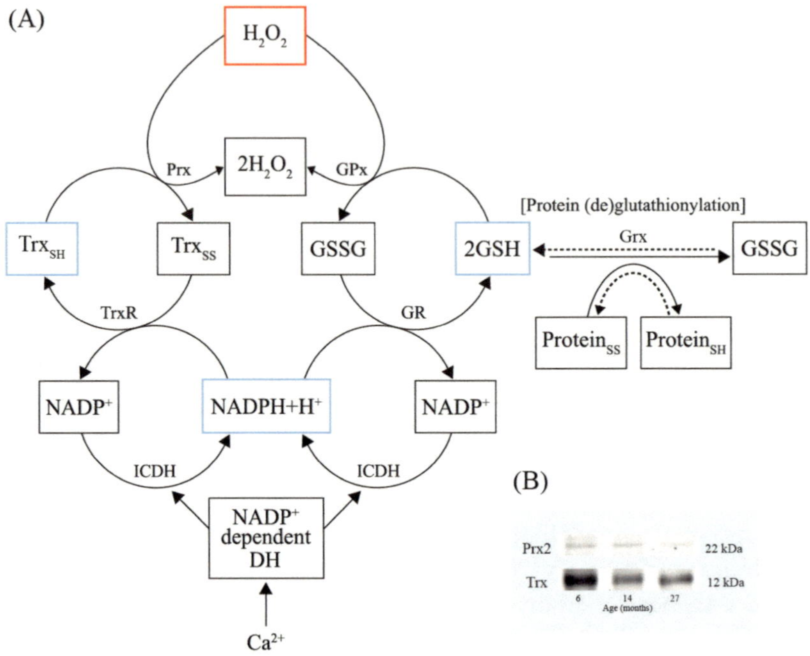

Figure 3. Scheme of (A) Thiol-disulfide network and (B) protein level for Prx2, Trx (yet unpublished data). GSH-reduced glutathione, GSSG-oxidized glutathione, GPx-Glutathione peroxidase, GR-Glutathione reductase, Grx-Glutaredoxin, Prx-Peroxiredoxin, Trx-Thioredoxin, TrxR-Thioredoxin reductase, SH-reduced and SS-oxidized form of Protein, ICDH-isocitrate dehydrogenase.

old rat hearts (**Figure 3**). Low Trx level is probably result of TrxR malfunctioning due to lack of NADPH, overproduction of ROS and/or RNS. Thioredoxin also plays a role in the reversible S-nitrosylation of cysteine residues in target proteins, and thereby contributes to the response of intracellular nitric oxide (NO). In addition, Trx is able to block caspase-3 activity through nitrosylation of the active cysteine site in response to NO. Therefore, Trx protein deficiency may contribute to the stimulation of caspase-dependent apoptosis. The most studied enzyme in the process of protein S-glutathionylation is glutaredoxin (Grx). The high specificity of Grx to S-glutathionylated proteins is used as a tool for studying and identifying them. In general, it is stated that the main task of Grx is to remove GSH from S-glutathionylated proteins. Thus, reduced thiol-containing protein is restored, which was confirmed in experiments with siRNA (small interfering RNA). The suppression of Grx genes with siRNA is an approach to study not only the "antioxidant" properties of Grx but also the role of protein S-glutathionylation [58]. Grx2 catalyzes S-glutathionylation of IMM proteins in a relatively reduced GSH/GSSG ratio equal to 6. The fact that thiol-disulfide oxidoreductases can catalyze both oxidizing and reducing reactions is not exclusive to Grx. Thioredoxin can act as an oxidant in oxidizing environment. Currently, the biggest challenge of researchers is to identify which enzymes are responsible for (de)glutathionylation, and if it is spontaneous process or catalyzed by enzymes. Existing information suggests that the mechanisms involved in resistance to various types of stress together with maintenance of bioenergetic capacity and redox homeostasis may be critical in the evolution of longevity.

3.2. Mitochondrial protein-protein network

One of the major goals of gerontology is to understand the comprehensive mechanisms involved in aging at different levels and hopefully to help understand age-related diseases. The complexity of the proteome supersedes that of the genome, due to alternative splicing events and PTMs of proteins. Proteomes are expected to be two to three orders of magnitude more complex than would be predicted from numbers of protein-encoding genes present in the respective genomes [59]. It is widely recognized that cellular aging causes changes in the proteome. However, the nature and targets of these changes and their consequences have not yet been completely identified. In recent years, mass spectrometry (MS) has been recognized as a golden standard tool for the identification and analysis of individual proteins. For further understanding of the molecular changes during heart aging, we have identified several proteins and compared the differences in the mitochondrial protein expression profiles among two age groups.

Precipitated proteins from mitochondria of 6 and 27 months old rat hearts were separated with two-dimensional electrophoresis (2-DE) to provide a protein profile (**Figure 4**). Interestingly, the change in protein level was statistically significant (1.5-fold change, 95% confidence interval) in only 12 proteins (marked with red circles) from the total protein pool of mitochondria. All the proteins were down-regulated in senescent mitochondria in comparison to the adult ones. Despite the small number of quantitatively modified proteins, these create an interesting protein-protein network. The strength of data support represents line thickness of protein-protein interaction network generated by String

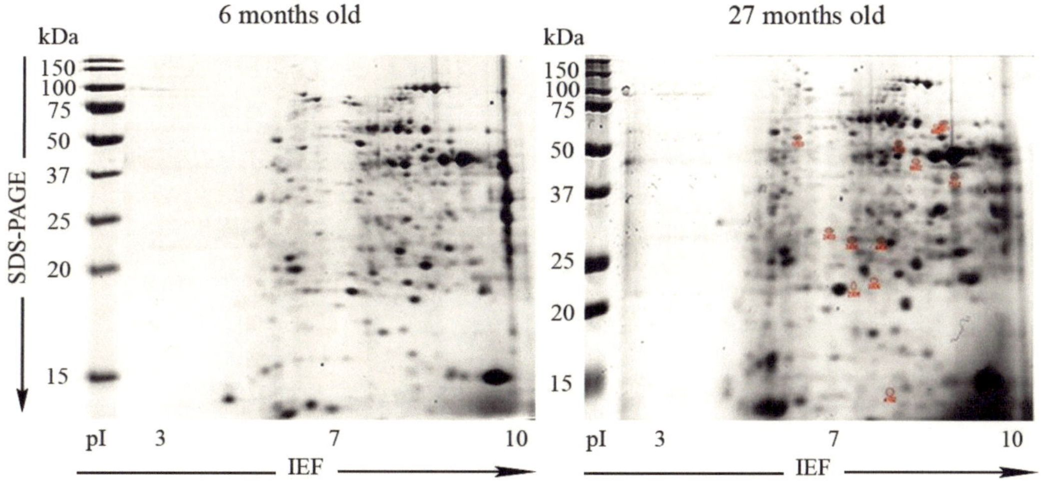

Figure 4. Representative 2-DE analysis of mitochondrial proteins in aging rat heart (yet unpublished data).

software and using *gene IDs* (**Figure 5**). Two proteins, methylmalonate-semialdehyde dehydrogenase [acylating] (Gene ID: *Aldh6a1*) and carnitine O-palmitoyltransferase 2 (*Cpt2*) did not fit to the protein-protein interaction map. However, their role in fatty acid metabolism is very important in connection to the heart muscle work and energy production. The rest of the proteins participate in various metabolic pathways of mitochondria. Three take part in Krebs cycle – malate dehydrogenase (*Mdh1*), dihydrolipoyl dehydrogenase (*Dld*) and aconitate hydratase (*Aco2*). Post-translational cysteine-related modification of aconitase was reported to be a key in linkage between Krebs cycle, redox signaling and metabolism of ROS [60]. Next five down-regulated proteins were directly connected with cardiac muscle contraction and the risk of developing age-related neuronal disorders - Huntington, Parkinson and Alzheimer disease. All of them are subunits of ETC, thus regulate production of energy in mitochondria: NADH dehydrogenase 1 alpha subcomplex subunit 5 (*Ndufa5*), cytochrome bc1 complex subunit 1 (*Uqcrc1*) and cytochrome bc1 complex subunit Rieske (*Uqcrsf2*), cytochrome c oxidase subunit 5B (*Cox5b*), electron transfer flavoprotein subunit beta (*Etfb*). Combined defects in oxidative phosphorylation and fatty acid beta oxidation were detected in mitochondrial diseases [61]. Creatine kinase M-type (*Ckm*) was only one cytoplasmic enzyme interacting with mitochondria through transfer of phosphate and the last one is voltage-dependent anion-selective channel protein 1 (*Vdac1*),

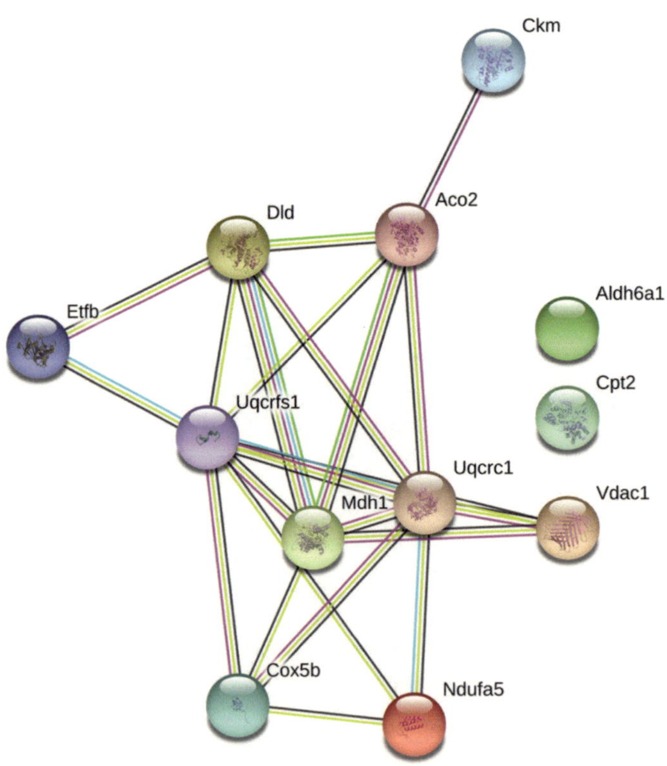

Figure 5. Functional protein-protein interactions during aging in rat mitochondria (yet unpublished data).

which plays a role in outer mitochondrial membrane permeabilization and cellular death. This outer mitochondrial membrane protein is tightly bound with Alzheimer disease, where mediates amyloid β toxicity and represents a potential target for Alzheimer disease therapy [62].

Currently available evidence indicates that the steady-state amounts of structural damage to proteins accumulated during life are relatively small, and are often present only in trace amounts. On the other hand, the pro-oxidizing changes in the redox state reflected by the decline in redox potential, increases in production of H_2O_2 and level of protein modifications are significant and ubiquitous. However, the oxidative PTMs are relevant only if these are connected to functional consequences. It is important to consider that a slight modification in low abundance proteins may be of physiological importance. Distinguishing between inconsequential modifications and functionally significant ones requires careful biochemical/biophysical analysis of target proteins [63]. Thus, proteomic approaches represent powerful tools to address these questions by identifying the targeted proteins and the extent of their modifications.

3.3. Post-translational modifications of proteins during aging

The detailed examination of enzyme molecules by mass spectrometry and other techniques continues to identify hundreds of distinct PTMs. Global analyses of enzymes using proteomics revealed widespread distribution of PTMs on many key enzymes located in all cellular compartments. Multiple PTMs within a single enzyme molecule and their mutual interplays are critical for the regulation of catalytic activity. Enzymatic PTMs can be detected in ever increasing amounts and they appear to be critical for folding and assembly (e.g. glycosylation), function as key regulators of catalytic activity of enzymes (e.g. binding of prosthetic groups, phosphorylation), or mark enzyme molecules for targeted destruction (e.g. ubiquitylation). In parallel with these processes there are non-enzymatic PTMs caused by ROS and RNS continuously interacting with individual enzyme molecules. These PTMs contribute to molecular aging and may also be involved in regulation of enzymes' catalytic activity [64]. There are two groups of PTMs observed during oxidative stress mediated aging, reversible and irreversible. The major types of *irreversible PTMs* are carbonylation and 3-nitrotyrosilation.

- *Carbonylation* is covalent adduction of lipid aldehyde to the side chains of lysine, histidine or cysteine residues. Extensive amount of information about this modification can be found in the recently published book [65].
- *3-nitrotyrosilation*, frequently called tyrosine nitration is formed between RNS (peroxynitrite anion) and a tyrosine residue of target protein. Extensive research was done during last years in failing human [66] and rat hearts [67].

Second group of *reversible PTMs* which are related to the aging process are sulfur-mediated S-Sulfenylation, S-nitrosylation, S-glutathionylation and lipid peroxidation pathway-related HNE modification.

- Protein *S-Sulfenylation* leads to the production of sulfur-hydroxylation product (P-SOH), disulfide bond and sulfenyl-amide bond formation. It may be a precursor to the process of S-sulfinylation and S-sulfonylation. This type of modification is believed to be a fleeting molecular switch that regulates non-enzymatic oxidative folding [68].
- *S-nitrosylation* occurs when NO is covalently incorporated into the Cysteine thiol group forming S-nitrosothiol (SNO). It plays important role in redox metabolism through GSH interaction in failing heart in rats [67] and human heart disease [69]. This PTM has been progressively implicated in virtually every NO-regulated process within the cardiovascular system. The current, widely-held paradigm is that S-nitrosylation plays an equivalent role as phosphorylation, providing a stable and controllable PTM [70].
- *S-glutathionylation* is covalent attachment of GSH to protein thiol groups. The function of protein S-glutathionylation reactions in metabolism is a rapid and reversible redox signaling mechanism that involves the conjugation and removal of glutathione from cysteine switches. Several observations have shown that unlike other redox modifications S-glutathionylation reactions fulfill the requisite criteria to serve as an effective PTM that controls protein function, links energy metabolism to redox signaling in mitochondria. Because of its role in modulation of ROS production in myocardial mitochondria, currently the usage of mitochondria penetrating antioxidants is discussed in context of the heart disease treatment [71].
- During last decade *HNE modification* was under extensive research because of its dual role as pro- and anti-oxidant. This most abundant reactive aldehyde attacks predominantly nitrogen of histidine, lysine (less commonly arginine) or cysteine, and it is related to wide range of metabolic diseases [72].

Above mentioned PTMs occur the most frequently during oxidative stress-related aging process. However, there are virtually hundreds of additional PTMs that may occur in enzymes. To support results from protein profiling of mitochondria is important to focus on deep protein analyzes of individual selected proteins, their interactions within the individual compartments, between different organelles or the intercellular communication. For this purpose, proteomics is now integrated with molecular genetics, transcriptomics, and other areas leading to systems biology strategies.

3.4. Turnover of mitochondrial proteins - role of mitophagy in cardiomyocytes

Proper functioning of mitochondria is crucial for cardiac function. Damaged mitochondria produce less ATP, release greater amounts of ROS, and have a lower threshold for cytochrome c release resulting in apoptosis, undergo mitochondrial permeability transition pore opening resulting in necrosis or may release mitochondrial components into cytosol where are recognized by receptors for removal. Mitochondrial turnover is therefore an integral aspect of quality control in which dysfunctional mitochondria are selectively eliminated through autophagy or mitochondrial autophagy (mitophagy) and replaced through expansion of preexisting mitochondria (biogenesis). In the heart mitochondria turnover is with a half life of 14 days. Rat cardiomyocytes have roughly 1000 mitochondria per cell, suggesting that under basal resting conditions, one mitochondrion per cell is replaced every 40 minutes [73]. In order to facilitate and initiate mitophagy, mitochondrial fusion and fission play a critical role in mitochondrial turnover. Fission of mitochondria into smaller fragments is a crucial requirement for mitophagy to occur. The key regulator of this process is dynamin-related protein 1 (Drp1), which in concert with proteins fission 1 (Fis1), mitochondrial fission factor (Mff), mitochondrial dynamics proteins of 49 kDa (MiD49) and 51 kDa (MiD51) is responsible for mitochondrial fragmentation. The role of last three proteins appears essential. Mff assists in the assembly of Drp1. MiD49 and MiD51 may play a regulatory role by recruiting Drp1 and maintaining it in inactive state until fission is required [74]. Proteins that promote outer mitochondrial membrane (OMM) fusion such as Mitofusin 1 and 2 (Mfn1 and 2) are ubiquitinated and eliminated by the ubiquitin proteasome system. E3 ubiquitin ligase Parkin (also known as Park2) and PTEN-induced putative kinase 1 (PINK1) have been shown to play an important role in mitophagy. PINK1 targets to the mitochondria but is normally degraded by presenilin associated rhomboid-like protease (PARL). In response to loss of mitochondrial membrane potential, PARL is inactivated; PINK1 is stabilized and recruits Parkin. Parkin ubiquitinates several mitochondrial associated proteins and they are then recognized by p62 and bring mitochondria to the autophagosomes. Thus mitochondria with membrane potential loss can be selectively degraded. Parkin substrates include e.g. voltage-dependent anion-selective channel protein (VDAC), translocase of the outer membrane (TOM), mitochondrial fission 1 (FIS1), hexokinase, mitochondrial Rho-GTPase (MIRO) 1 and 2, although whether ubiquitination of these proteins is required or sufficient for mitophagy is unclear and highly dependent on the specific cellular context [75].

The importance of mitophagy for the preservation of cardiovascular homeostasis, the cardiomyocyte-specific deletion of Parkin and the expression of a mutant Mfn2 (mitofusin 2) at birth prevented the switch from fetal to adult mitochondria in the mice heart [76]. Another example, mice bearing a heart-specific deletion of Mfn2 prematurely succumbed to a progressive cardiomyopathy characterized by impaired contractile function [77]. Such a detrimental phenotype could be reversed, at least partially by Mfn2 to prevent the targeted mitochondria from rejoining the mitochondrial network through fusion. Under basal conditions Mfn2 functions in mitochondrial fusion events and links endoplasmic reticulum to mitochondria. Also acts as Parkin receptor during mitophagy following phosphorylation by PINK1 and recruiting Parkin to the mitochondria. So even in case of Parkin-dependent mitophagy, some outer mitochondrial membrane proteins are recycled through transfer to the endoplasmic reticulum. Most studies have relied on the systemic modulation of autophagy with nutritional or pharmacological interventions or the homozygous/heterozygous deletion of a relevant gene. Nutritional and pharmacological interventions commonly used to modulate autophagy in the cardiovascular system *in vivo*, including caloric restriction or caloric restriction mimetics, rapamycin, 3-methyladenine, and lysosomal inhibitors, are rather nonspecific. Genetic interventions offer increased specificity, but are not devoid of potential problems that should be kept under attentive consideration. Linking mitophagy with cardiomyocytes is the field of interest in many publications [78]. While mitophagy is responsible for bulk degradation of mitochondria, turnover of individual components may proceed at asynchronous rates through redistribution of components via fusion events, selective degradation of proteins by mitochondrial proteases, and proteasomal elimination of some outer mitochondrial membrane proteins. Some studies suggest that inner mitochondrial membrane proteins, especially oxidative phosphorylation constituents, may be primarily cleared via mitophagy. There is more to discuss, especially communication between intracellular organelles (mitochondria and endoplasmic reticulum) and oxidative phosphorylation events in mitochondria in relation to redox network, apoptosis/necrosis or mitophagy. These appear to be key players in cardiomyocytes survival during aging.

4. Conclusions

Maintenance of mitochondrial function and energy/redox homeostasis requires both generation of newly synthesized and elimination of dysfunctional mitochondria. Taken together, age-dependent decline of mitophagy inhibits removal of dysfunctional or redundant mitochondria as well as impairs mitochondrial biogenesis. It results to progressive mitochondrial accretion and consequently, deterioration of cardiomyocytes function. At present it is pointed out that the steady-state amounts of structural damage accumulated during life are relatively small. However, changes in the redox state reflected by the decline in redox potential, increases in production of H_2O_2 and level of protein modifications are significant and ubiquitous. Activities of ETC complexes revealed that the most affected throughout aging was complex IV, in contrast to relatively small age-related changes in complex II. These non-uniform changes in ETC enzyme complexes may lead to altered electron transfer through the chain, leading to impairment of ATP synthesis and overall functionality of cardiomyocytes during aging. The ability of the main regulatory Krebs cycle enzymes to supplement NADH to ETC was altered in senescent mitochondria. ICDH and KGDH had only half activity in senescent mitochondria; however ICDH was not affected in group of 14 months old. This might support promotion of H_2O_2 in senescent cardiac myocytes where peroxiredoxin 2 ability to trap H_2O_2 was also significantly affected. Decrease in GSH levels indicates low GSH/GSSG ratio leading to more oxidized environment in senescent cardiomyocytes but 14-month old hearts were able to maintain basal levels of adult mitochondria. Despite the variations in enzyme activities, the overall proteomic analyses revealed only 12 significantly affected proteins during aging. All these were more or less deprived but question is what is responsible for such a changes. Are these proteins really relevant? Is change in protein amount important? These and other questions are waiting for us and other researchers to be answered.

Specific marker of senescence was yet not identified, but evaluating a series of markers can help to define the senescent state. Senescent cells have greater proportion of protein content, which might be modulated by several PTMs. If these protein modifications are connected to functional consequences and protein-protein interactions are revealed, link may lead to the solution. Unfortunately, the proteome is much more complicated than the genome. To fit all the proteins together with their different characteristics in various pathways and cellular compartments is almost infeasible. At present, various nutritional, pharmacological and genetic interventions have higher or lower specificity, but are not devoid of potential problems that should be kept under attentive consideration. Collectively, these studies suggest that dysfunctional proteostasis has a causative role in aging and that restoration of protein homeostasis is protective against age-related diseases. New window is opened and hopefully with help of bioinformatics collecting huge amounts of data from proteomics, genomics and other scientific approaches will lead to personalized therapeutic procedures for individual patient and age-related disorder(s).

Acknowledgements

This work was supported by the project APVV-15-0107 and the project "Competence Center for Research and Development in the field of Diagnostics and Therapy of Oncological diseases", ITMS: 26220220153, co-financed from EU sources. We thank Mrs. Zdena Cetlova for technical assistance.

Author details

Zuzana Tatarkova[1*], Martin Kolisek[2], Ivana Pilchova[2], Peter Racay[1,2] and Peter Kaplan[1,2]

*Address all correspondence to: tatarkova@jfmed.uniba.sk

1 Department of Medical Biochemistry, Jessenius Faculty of Medicine in Martin, Comenius University in Bratislava, Martin, Slovakia

2 Biomedical Center Martin, Jessenius Faculty of Medicine in Martin, Comenius University in Bratislava, Martin, Slovakia

References

[1] Steenman M, Lande G. Cardiac aging and heart disease in humans. Biophysical Reviews. 2017;**9**(2):131-137. DOI: 10.1007/s12551-017-0255-9

[2] Lakatta EG, Sollott SJ. Perspectives on mammalian cardiovascular aging: Humans to molecules. Comparative Biochemistry and Physiology. Part A, Molecular & Integrative Physiology. 2002;**132**(4):699-721. DOI: 10.1016/S1095-6433(02)00124-1

[3] Höhn A, Weber D, Jung T, Ott C, Hugo M, Kochlik B, et al. Happily (n)ever after: Aging in the context of oxidative stress, proteostasis loss and cellular senescence. Redox Biology. 2017;**11**:482-501. DOI: 10.1016/j.redox.2016.12.001

[4] Lopez-Lluch G, Hunt N, Jones B, Zhu M, Jamieson H, Hilmer S, et al. Calorie restriction induces mitochondrial biogenesis and bioenergetic efficiency. Proceedings of the National Academy of Sciences of the United States of America. 2006;**103**:1768-1773. DOI: 10.1073/pnas.0510452103

[5] Hayflick L, Moorhead PS. The serial cultivation of human diploid cell strains. Experimental Cell Research. 1961;**25**:585-621

[6] Kuilman T, Michaloglou C, Mooi WJ, Peeper DS. The essence of senescence. Genes & Development. 2010;**24**(22):2463-2479. DOI: 10.1101/gad.1971610

[7] Marzetti E, Csiszar A, Dutta D, Balagopal G, Calvani R, Leeuwenburgh C. Role of mitochondrial dysfunction and altered autophagy in cardiovascular aging and disease: From mechanisms to therapeutics. American Journal of Physiology. Heart and Circulatory Physiology. 2013;**305**:H459-H476. DOI: 10.1152/ajpheart.00936.2012

[8] Ago T, Matsushima S, Kuroda J, Zablocki D, Kitazono T, Sadoshima J. The NADPH oxidase Nox4 and aging in the heart. Aging (Albany NY). 2010;**2**:1012-1016. DOI: 10.18632/aging.100261

[9] Barger JL, Kayo T, Vann JM, Arias EB, Wang J, Hacker TA, et al. A low dose of dietary resveratrol partially mimics caloric restriction and retards aging parameters in mice. PLoS One. 2008;**3**(6):e264. DOI: 10.1371/journal.pone.0002264

[10] Shirakabe A, Ikeda Y, Sciarretta S, Zablocki DK, Sadoshima J. Aging and autophagy in the heart. Circulation Research. 2016;**118**:1563-1576. DOI: 10.1161/CIRCRESAHA.116.307474

[11] Flatt T. A new definition of aging? Frontiers in Genetics. 2012;**23**(3):148. DOI: 10.3389/fgene.2012.00148

[12] Scorrano L. Keeping mitochondria in shape: A matter of life and death. European Journal of Clinical Investigation. 2013;**43**(8):886-893. DOI: 10.1111/eci.12135

[13] Hu J, Dong L, Outten CE. The redox environment in the mitochondrial intermembrane space is maintained separately from the cytosol and matrix. The Journal of Biological Chemistry. 2008;**283**(43):29126-29134. DOI: 10.1074/jbc.M803028200

[14] Herrmann JM, Riemer J. The intermembrane space of mitochondria. Antioxidants & Redox Signaling. 2010;**13**(9):1323-1326. DOI: 10.1089/ars.2010.3270

[15] Nuebel E, Manganas P, Tokatlidis K. Orphan proteins of unknown function in the mitochondrial intermembrane space proteome: New pathways and metabolic cross-talk. Biochimica et Biophysica Acta. 2016;**1863**(11):2613-2623. DOI: 10.1016/j.bbamcr.2016.07.004

[16] Young AR, Narita M, Ferreira M, Kirschner K, Sadaie M, Darot JF, et al. Autophagy mediates the mitotic senescence transition. Genes & Development. 2009;**23**(7):798-803. DOI: 10.1101/gad.519709

[17] Lee BY, Han JA, Im JS, Morrone A, Johung K, Goodwin EC, et al. Senescence-associated beta-galactosidase is lysosomal beta-galactosidase. Aging Cell. 2006;**5**(2):187-195. DOI: 10.1111/j.1474-9726.2006.00199.x

[18] Beauséjour CM, Krtolica A, Galimi F, Narita M, Lowe SW, Yaswen P, et al. Reversal of human cellular senescence: Roles of the p53 and p16 pathways. The EMBO Journal. 2003;**22**(16):4212-4222. DOI: 10.1093/emboj/cdg417

[19] Helman A, Klochendler A, Azazmeh N, Gabai Y, Horwitz E, Anzi S, et al. p16(Ink4a)-induced senescence of pancreatic beta cells enhances insulin secretion. Nature Medicine. 2016;**22**(4):412-420. DOI: 10.1038/nm.4054

[20] Muñoz-Espín D, Cañamero M, Maraver A, Gómez-López G, Contreras J, Murillo-Cuesta S, et al. Programmed cell senescence during mammalian embryonic development. Cell. 2013;**55**(5):1104-1118. DOI: 10.1016/j.cell.2013.10.019

[21] Barja G. The mitochondrial free radical theory of aging. Progress in Molecular Biology and Translational Science. 2014;**127**:1-27. DOI: 10.1016/B978-0-12-394625-6.00001-5

[22] Cedikova M, Pitule P, Kripnerova M, Markova M, Kuncova J. Multiple roles of mitochondria in aging processes. Physiological Research. 2016;**65**(5):5519-5531

[23] Gnaiger E. Capacity of oxidative phosphorylation in human skeletal muscle: New perspectives of mitochondrial physiology. The International Journal of Biochemistry & Cell Biology. 2009;**41**(10):1837-1845. DOI: 10.1016/j.biocel.2009.03.013

[24] Milane L, Trivedi M, Singh A, Talekar M, Amiji M. Mitochondrial biology, targets, and drug delivery. Journal of Controlled Release. 2015;**207**:40-58. DOI: 10.1016/j.jconrel.2015.03.036

[25] Boudina S, Graham TE. Mitochondrial function/dysfunction in white adipose tissue. Experimental Physiology. 2014;**99**(9):1168-1178. DOI: 10.1113/expphysiol.2014.081414

[26] Bonomini F, Rodella LF, Rezzani R. Metabolic syndrome, aging and involvement of oxidative stress. Aging and Disease. 2015;**6**(2):109-120. DOI: 10.14336/AD.2014.0305

[27] Maurel A, Hernandez C, Kunduzova O, Bompart G, Cambon C, Parini A, et al. Age-dependent increase in hydrogen peroxide production by cardiac monoamine oxidase A in rats. American Journal of Physiology. Heart and Circulatory Physiology. 2003;**284**(4): H1460-H1467. DOI: 10.1152/ajpheart.00700.2002

[28] Kohlhaas M, Liu T, Knopp A, Zeller T, Ong MF, Böhm M, et al. Elevated cytosolic Na^+ increases mitochondrial formation of reactive oxygen species in failing cardiac myocytes. Circulation. 2010;**121**(14):1606-1613. DOI: 10.1161/CIRCULATIONAHA.109.914911

[29] Dai DF, Chen T, Wanagat J, Laflamme M, Marcinek DJ, Emond MJ, et al. Age-dependent cardiomyopathy in mitochondrial mutator mice is attenuated by overexpression of catalase targeted to mitochondria. Aging Cell. 2010;**9**(4):536-544. DOI: 10.1111/j.1474-9726.2010.00581.x

[30] Dai DF, Rabinovitch PS, Ungvari Z. Mitochondria and cardiovascular aging. Circulation Research. 2012;**110**(8):1109-1124. DOI: 10.1161/CIRCRESAHA.111.246140

[31] Balaban RS, Nemoto S, Finkel T. Mitochondria, oxidants, and aging. Cell. 2005;**120**(4):483-495. DOI: 10.1016/j.cell.2005.02.001

[32] Shulga N, Pastorino JG. GRIM-19-mediated translocation of STAT3 to mitochondria is necessary for TNF-induced necroptosis. Journal of Cell Science. 2012;**125**:2995-3003

[33] Preston CC, Oberlin AS, Holmuhamedov EL, Gupta A, Sagar S, Syed RH, et al. Aging-induced alterations in gene transcripts and functional activity of mitochondrial oxidative phosphorylation complexes in the heart. Mechanisms of Ageing and Development. 2008;**129**(6):304-312. DOI: 10.1016/j.mad.2008.02.010

[34] Petrosillo G, Matera M, Casanova G, Ruggiero FM, Paradies G. Mitochondrial dysfunction in rat brain with aging Involvement of complex I, reactive oxygen species and cardiolipin. Neurochemistry International. 2008;**53**(5):126-131. DOI: 10.1016/j.neuint.2008.07.001

[35] Navarro A, Boveris A. Brain mitochondrial dysfunction in aging, neurodegeneration, and Parkinson's disease. Frontiers in Aging Neuroscience. 2010;**2**:34. DOI: 10.3389/fnagi.2010.00034

[36] Cocco T, Sgobbo P, Clemente M, Lopriore B, Grattagliano I, Di Paola M, et al. Tissue-specific changes of mitochondrial functions in aged rats: Effect of a long-term dietary treatment with N-acetylcysteine. Free Radical Biology & Medicine. 2005;**38**(6):796-805. DOI: 10.1016/j.freeradbiomed.2004.11.034

[37] Kumaran S, Subathra M, Balu M, Panneerselvam C. Age-associated decreased activities of mitochondrial electron transport chain complexes in heart and skeletal muscle: Role of L-carnitine. Chemico-Biological Interactions. 2004;**30**(148):11-18. DOI: 10.1016/j.cbi.2003.10.010

[38] Choksi KB, Papaconstantinou J. Age-related alterations in oxidatively damaged proteins of mouse heart mitochondrial electron transport chain complexes. Free Radical Biology & Medicine. 2008;**44**(10):1795-1805. DOI: 10.1016/j.freeradbiomed.2008.01.032

[39] Lenaz G, Genova ML. Supramolecular organisation of the mitochondrial respiratory chain: A new challenge for the mechanism and control of oxidative phosphorylation. Advances in Experimental Medicine and Biology. 2012;**748**:107-144. DOI: 10.1007/978-1-4614-3573-0_5

[40] Dröse S. Differential effects of complex II on mitochondrial ROS production and their relation to cardioprotective pre- and postconditioning. Biochimica et Biophysica Acta. 2013;**1827**(5):578-587. DOI: 10.1016/j.bbabio.2013.01.004

[41] Quinlan CL, Orr AL, Perevoshchikova IV, Treberg JR, Ackrell BA, Brand MD. Mitochondrial complex II can generate reactive oxygen species at high rates in both the forward and reverse reactions. The Journal of Biological Chemistry. 2012;**287**(32):27255-27264. DOI: 10.1074/jbc.M112.374629

[42] Puche JE, García-Fernández M, Muntané J, Rioja J, González-Barón S, Castilla Cortazar I. Low doses of insulin-like growth factor-I induce mitochondrial protection in aging rats. Endocrinology. 2008;**149**(5):2620-2627. DOI: 10.1210/en.2007-1563

[43] Mohamed SA, Hanke T, Erasmi AW, Bechtel MJ, Scharfschwerdt M, Meissner C, et al. Mitochondrial DNA deletions and the aging heart. Experimental Gerontology. 2006;**41**(5):508-517. DOI: 10.1016/j.exger.2006.03.014

[44] Trifunovic A, Wredenberg A, Falkenberg M, Spelbrink JN, Rovio AT, Bruder CE, et al. Premature ageing in mice expressing defective mitochondrial DNA polymerase. Nature. 2004;**429**(6990):417-423. DOI: 10.1038/nature02517

[45] Aon MA, Cortassa S, O'Rourke B. Redox-optimized ROS balance: A unifying hypothesis. Biochimica et Biophysica Acta. 2010;**1797**(6-7):865-877. DOI: 10.1016/j.bbabio.2010.02.016

[46] Moreno-Sánchez R, Gallardo-Pérez JC, Rodríguez-Enríquez S, Saavedra E, Marín-Hernández Á. Control of the NADPH supply for oxidative stress handling in cancer cells. Free Radical Biology & Medicine. 2017;**112**:149-161. DOI: 10.1016/j.freeradbiomed.2017.07.018

[47] Akar FG, Aon MA, Tomaselli GF, O'Rourke B. The mitochondrial origin of postischemic arrhythmias. The Journal of Clinical Investigation. 2005;**115**:3527-3535. DOI: 10.1172/JCI25371

[48] Ray PD, Huang BW, Tsuji Y. Reactive oxygen species (ROS) homeostasis and redox regulation in cellular signaling. Cellular Signalling. 2012;**24**(5):981-990. DOI: 10.1016/j.cellsig.2012.01.008

[49] van der Vlies D, Woudenberg J, Post JA. Protein oxidation in aging: Endoplasmic reticulum as a target. Amino Acids. 2003;**25**(3-4):397-407. DOI: 10.1007/s00726-003-0025-9

[50] Tong J, Fitzmaurice PS, Moszczynska A, Mattina K, Ang LC, Boileau I, et al. Do glutathione levels decline in aging human brain? Free Radical Biology & Medicine. 2016;**93**:110-117. DOI: 10.1016/j.freeradbiomed.2016.01.029

[51] Rajasekaran NS, Connell P, Christians ES, Yan LJ, Taylor RP, Orosz A, et al. Human alpha B-crystallin mutation causes oxido-reductive stress and protein aggregation cardiomyopathy in mice. Cell. 2007;**130**(3):427-439. DOI: 10.1016/j.cell.2007.06.044

[52] Pastore A, Piemonte F. S-S-glutathionyation signaling in cell biology: Progress and prospects. European Journal of Pharmaceutical Sciences. 2012;**46**(5):279-292. DOI: 10.1016/j.ejps.2012.03.010

[53] Ungvari Z, Bailey-Downs L, Sosnowska D, Gautam T, Koncz P, Losonczy G, et al. Vascular oxidative stress in aging: A homeostatic failure due to dysregulation of nrf2-mediated antioxidant response. The American Journal of Physiology. 2011;**301**:H363-H372. DOI: 10.1152/ajpheart.01134.2010

[54] De Pascali F, Hemann C, Samons K, Chen CA, Zweier JL. Hypoxia and reoxygenation induce endothelial nitric oxide synthase uncoupling in endothelial cells through tetrahydrobiopterin depletion and S-glutathionyation. Biochemistry. 2014;**53**(22):3679-3688. DOI: 10.1021/bi500076r

[55] Zhang Y, Sano M, Shinmura K, Tamaki K, Katsumata Y, Matsuhashi T, et al. 4-hydroxy-2-nonenal protects against cardiac ischemia-reperfusion injury via the Nrf2-dependent pathway. Journal of Molecular and Cellular Cardiology. 2010;**49**(4):576-586. DOI: 10.1016/j.yjmcc.2010.05.011

[56] Sies H. Hydrogen peroxide as a central redox signaling molecule in physiological oxidative stress. Redox Biology. 2017;**11**(6):613-619. DOI: 10.1016/j.redox.2016.12.035

[57] Go YM, Jones DP. Redox control systems in the nucleus: Mechanisms and functions. Antioxidants & Redox Signaling. 2010;**13**(4):489-509. DOI: 10.1089/ars.2009.3021

[58] Qanungo S, Starke DW, Pai HV, Mieyal JJ, Nieminen AL. Glutathione supplementation potentiates hypoxic apoptosis by S-glutathionylation of p65-NFkappaB. The Journal of Biological Chemistry. 2007;**282**(25):18427-18436

[59] Černý M, Skalák J, Cerna H, Brzobohatý B. Advances in purification and separation of posttranslationally modified proteins. Journal of Proteomics. 2013;**9**:2-27. DOI: 10.1016/j.jprot.2013.05.040

[60] Lushchak OV, Piroddi M, Galli F, Lushchak VI. Aconitase post-translational modification as a key in linkage between Krebs cycle, iron homeostasis, redox signaling, and metabolism of reactive oxygen species. Redox Report. 2014;**19**(1):8-15. DOI: 10.1179/1351000213Y.0000000073

[61] Nsiah-Sefaa A, McKenzie M. Combined defects in oxidative phosphorylation and fatty acid β-oxidation in mitochondrial disease. Bioscience Reports. 2016;**36**(2):e00313. DOI: 10.1042/BSR20150295

[62] Smilansky A, Dangoor L, Nakdimon I, Ben-Hail D, Mizrachi D, Shoshan-Barmatz V. The voltage-dependent anion channel 1 mediates amyloid β toxicity and represents a potential target for Alzheimer disease therapy. The Journal of Biological Chemistry. 2015;**290**(52): 30670-30683. DOI: 10.1074/jbc.M115.691493

[63] Ortuño-Sahagún D, Pallàs M, Rojas-Mayorquín AE. Oxidative stress in aging: Advances in proteomic approaches. Oxidative Medicine and Cellular Longevity. 2014;**2014**:573208. DOI: 10.1155/2014/573208

[64] Ryšlavá H, Doubnerová V, Kavan D, Vaněk O. Effect of posttranslational modifications on enzyme function and assembly. Journal of Proteomics. 2013;**92**:80-109. DOI: 10.1016/j.jprot.2013.03.0252

[65] Ros J, editor. Protein Carbonylation: Principles, Analysis, and Biological Implications. 1st ed. Hoboken, New Jersey, USA: John Wiley & Sons; 2017. 416 p

[66] Sheeran FL, Pepe S. Posttranslational modifications and dysfunction of mitochondrial enzymes in human heart failure. American Journal of Physiology. Endocrinology and Metabolism. 2016;**311**(2):E449-E460. DOI: 10.1152/ajpendo.00127.2016

[67] Wang X, Shults NV, Suzuki YJ. Oxidative profiling of the failing right heart in rats with pulmonary hypertension. PLoS One. 2017;**12**(5):e0176887. DOI: 10.1371/journal.pone.0176887

[68] Beedle AE, Lynham S, Garcia-Manyes S. Protein S-sulfenylation is a fleeting molecular switch that regulates non-enzymatic oxidative folding. Nature Communications. 2016;**7**:12490. DOI: 10.1038/ncomms12490

[69] Zhang YH. Nitric oxide signalling and neuronal nitric oxide synthase in the heart under stress. F1000Res. 2017;**6**:742. DOI: 10.12688/f1000research.10128.1

[70] Wolhuter K, Eaton P. How widespread is stable protein S-nitrosylation as an end-effector of protein regulation? Free Radical Biology & Medicine. 2017;**109**:156-166. DOI: 10.1016/j.freeradbiomed.2017.02.013

[71] Mailloux RJ, Treberg JR. Protein S-glutathionlyation links energy metabolism to redox signaling in mitochondria. Redox Biology. 2016;**8**:110-118. DOI: 10.1016/j.redox.2015.12.010

[72] Castro JP, Jung T, Grune T, Siems W. 4-Hydroxynonenal (HNE) modified proteins in metabolic diseases. Free Radical Biology & Medicine. 2017;**111**:309-315. DOI: 10.1016/j.freeradbiomed.2016.10.497

[73] Carreira RS, Lee Y, Ghochani M, Gustafsson ÅB, Gottlieb RA. Cyclophilin D is required for mitochondrial removal by autophagy in cardiac cells. Autophagy. 2010;**6**(5):462-472. DOI: 10.4161/auto.6.4.11553

[74] Losón OC, Song Z, Chen H, Chan DC. Fis1, Mff, MiD49, and MiD51 mediate Drp1 recruitment in mitochondrial fission. Molecular Biology of the Cell. 2013;**24**(5):659-667. DOI: 10.1091/mbc.E12-10-0721

[75] Zhang J. Teaching the basics of autophagy and mitophagy to redox biologists—Mechanisms and experimental approaches. Redox Biology. 2015;**4**:242-259. DOI: 10.1016/j.redox.2015.01.003

[76] Gong G, Song M, Csordas G, Kelly DP, Matkovich SJ, Dorn GW II. Parkin-mediated mitophagy directs perinatal cardiac metabolic maturation in mice. Science. 2015;**350**:aad2459. DOI: 10.1126/science.aad2459

[77] Chen Y, Dorn GW II. PINK1-phosphorylated mitofusin 2 is a Parkin receptor for culling damaged mitochondria. Science. 2013;**340**:471-475. DOI: 10.1126/science.1231031

[78] Bravo-San Pedro JM, Kroemer G, Galluzzi L. Autophagy and mitophagy in cardiovascular disease. Circulation Research. 2017;**120**(11):1812-1824. DOI: 10.1161/CIRCRESAHA.117.311082

Section 2

Mitochondrial Dysfunction and Anticancer Drug Development

Chapter 4

Differential Effect of Atpenin A5 on ROS Production from Wild-Type Mitochondrial Complex II in Human Cancer Cells and Normal Cells

Madhavi P. Paranagama and Kiyoshi Kita

Additional information is available at the end of the chapter

http://dx.doi.org/10.5772/intechopen.71638

Abstract

Human mitochondrial complex II is an intriguing enzyme, which has been the focus of medical research during the past few decades since it contributes to pathogenesis of mitochondrial diseases as well as a target for chemotherapy. Reactive oxygen species (ROS) produced by this enzyme has been implicated in both these conditions. While ROS produced from mutated mitochondrial complex II has been implicated in pathogenesis of mitochondrial diseases, ROS produced from pharmacologically inhibited mitochondrial complex II has been implicated in cancer cell death. In this chapter, we show that inhibition of mitochondrial complex II in human cancer cells with atpenin A5 produces detectable levels of ROS while normal cells do not. Thus, this enzyme may be used as a potential target for developing new anticancer drugs to trigger ROS-mediated selective death of cancer cells.

Keywords: mitochondrion complex II, ROS, anticancer agents, atpenin A5

1. Introduction

Human mitochondrial complex II (succinate:ubiquinone oxidoreductase; succinate dehydrogenase (SDH)) is an intriguing enzyme, which has been the focus of medical research during the past few decades since it contributes to pathogenesis of mitochondrial diseases (for recent reviews, see [1, 2]) and also a target for chemotherapy [3–5].

1.1. Structure of mitochondrial complex II

Mitochondrial complex II is a heterotetrameric protein embedded in the inner mitochondrial membrane. Its four subunits are referred as flavoprotein subunit (Fp), iron-sulfur subunit

(Ip), cytochrome *b* large subunit (CybL), and cytochrome *b* small subunit (CybS). The Fp and Ip subunits comprise the catalytic domain of the enzyme. The Fp subunit has a flavin adenine dinucleotide (FAD) as a prosthetic group and contains the dicarboxylate-binding site, which serves as the binding site for succinate and fumarate. The Ip subunit generally contains three iron-sulfur clusters $[2Fe\text{-}2S]^{2+,1+}$, $[4Fe\text{-}4S]^{2+,1+}$, and $[3Fe\text{-}4S]^{1+,0}$ as prosthetic groups. Subunits CybL and CybS, with heme *b* as the prosthetic group, form the anchor domain of the enzyme. This anchors the catalytic domain to the inner mitochondrial membrane and also forms the quinone (Q)-binding site, together with the Ip subunit [6, 7] (**Figure 1**).

In 2003, our laboratory revealed that human mitochondrial complex II exists in two isoforms, which differ in the Fp subunit. These two human Fp subunits, which are referred as Fp I and Fp II, differ only in two amino acids in the C-terminal of the protein-Tyr629Phe and Val657Ile [8, 9]. The majority of human tissues have shown expression of both isoforms of complex II with predominant expression of type I Fp. However, some cancer cell lines and fetal tissues have shown predominant expression of type II Fp also [4]. Furthermore, type II Fp expression has been found to increase in cultured cells under ischemic conditions [10]. Moreover, our laboratory has revealed that Fp subunit of human complex II undergoes posttranslational modifications by phosphorylation of its tyrosine, threonine, and serine residues under tumor mimicking microenvironments (hypoxic and hypoglycemic conditions), which affects its enzymatic activity [11].

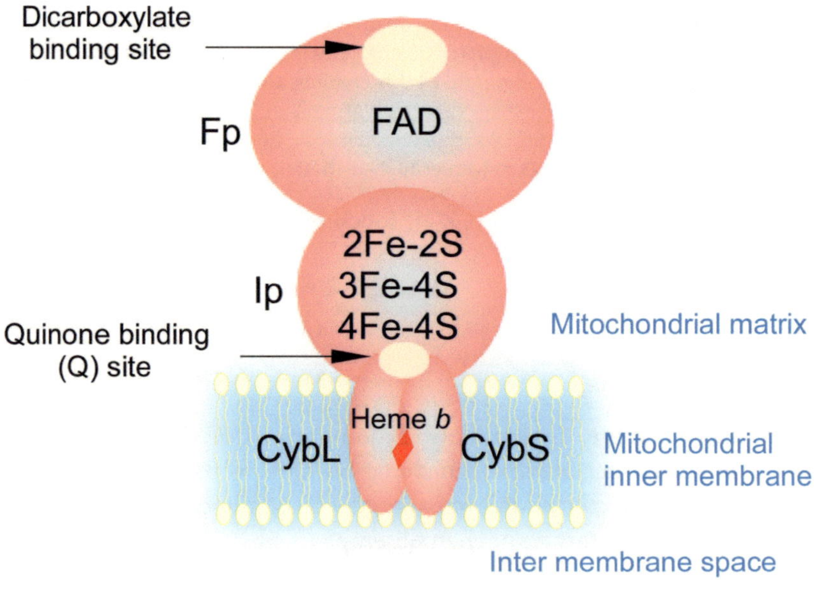

Figure 1. Schematic representation of the mitochondrial complex II. The four subunits of the complex II, namely the flavoprotein subunit, iron sulfur subunit, cytochrome *b* large subunit, and cytochrome *b* small subunit are labeled as Fp, Ip, CybL, and CybS, respectively. The prosthetic groups that participate in the electron transfer are the flavin adenine dinucleotide (FAD), three iron sulfur clusters 2Fe-2S, 3Fe-4S, 4Fe-4S, and heme *b*. Dicarboxylate-binding site in the Fp subunit serves as the catalytic site for succinate oxidation/fumarate reduction. Quinone-binding site comprised of Ip, CybL, and CybS subunits serves as the catalytic site for quinone reduction/quinol oxidation.

1.2. Function of mitochondrial complex II

In human cells, this enzyme plays dual roles as an indispensable enzyme in the TCA cycle as well as in the aerobic respiratory chain (**Figure 2**). It oxidizes succinate to fumarate in the TCA cycle and reduces quinone to quinol in the aerobic respiratory chain [6, 12]. This is in contrast to the function of the mitochondrial complex II of the anaerobic organisms such as *Ascaris suum,* which oxidizes quinol into quinone that is coupled with reduction of fumarate to succinate (**Figure 3**) [13]. However, our laboratory has revealed distinct fumarate reductase (FRD) activity in the human cancer cells, which have significantly increased upon exposure to hypoxia and hypoglycemia. In these cells, mitochondrial complex II is reported to acquire FRD activity through phosphorylation of its Fp subunit [11]. This finding is further supported

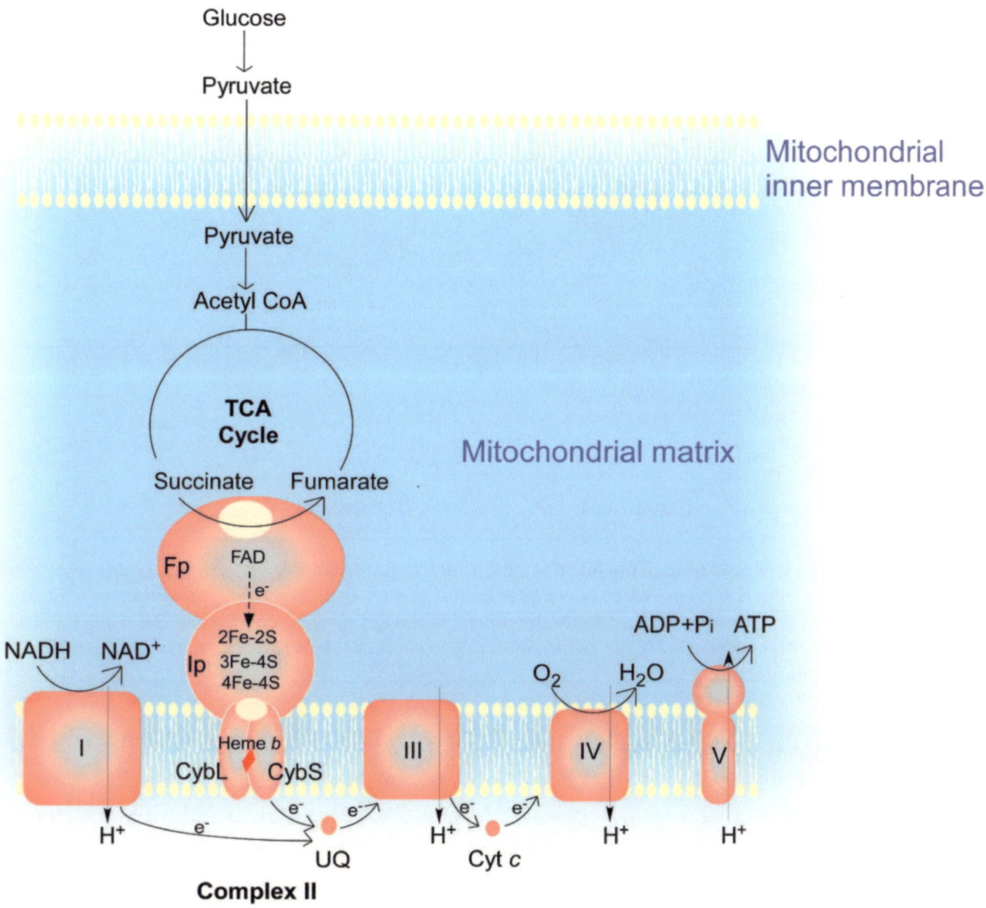

Figure 2. Schematic representation of the function of the mitochondrial complex II in the aerobic respiratory chain and the TCA cycle. Functioning as a component of the TCA cycle, mitochondrial complex II catalyzes the oxidation of succinate to fumarate with transfer of electrons to FAD. Functioning as a component of the aerobic respiratory chain, the electrons on FAD are transferred through Fe-S clusters and heme *b* to reduce the ubiquinone. For simplicity of the representation, the subunit composition of the respiratory chain complexes I, III, IV, and V is not shown.

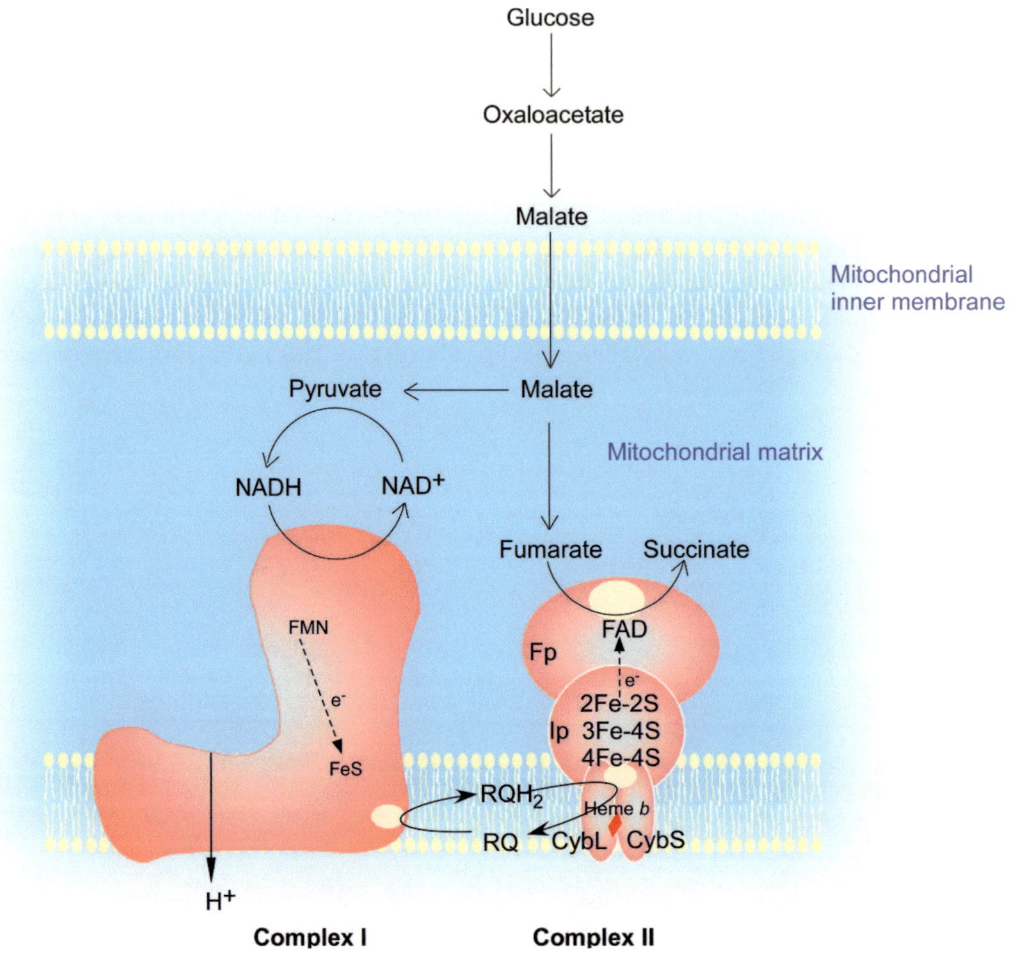

Figure 3. A schematic representation of the function of the mitochondrial complex II in the anaerobic respiratory chain. Electrons originating from NADH oxidation in complex I reduce the rhodoquinone (RQ) to rhodoquinol (RQH2) at its Q site. Rhodoquinol is subsequently oxidized to rhodoquinone at the Q site of the complex II. The resulting electrons are transferred via the Fe-S clusters and FAD to reduce fumarate to succinate. Fumarate is the terminal electron acceptor of the anaerobic respiratory chain.

by recent metabolic profiling studies also on gastric and colon carcinomas [14]. In addition to its role in energy metabolism, mitochondrial complex II has been identified to have a novel function as a tumor suppressor in certain tissues. Mutations in its subunits are reported to cause cancers such as pheochromocytoma (tumors of the chromaffin cells in the adrenal medulla) and paraganglioma (extra adrenal tumors of sympathetic or parasympathetic origin). Moreover, breast, thyroid, and renal carcinomas are also known to be associated with complex II mutations. More recently, mutations in the complex II assembly factors, succinate dehydrogenase assembly factor 1 (SDHAF1) and succinate dehydrogenase assembly factor 2 (SDHAF2), are also reported to be linked with infantile leukoencephalopathy and paraganglioma (for a recent review, see [2]).

1.3. ROS production from mitochondrial complex II

Reactive oxygen species (ROS) are inevitable byproducts of the aerobic respiratory chain. Major ROS produced by the respiratory chain is superoxide (O_2^-). It is subsequently dismutated into hydrogen peroxide (H_2O_2) by superoxide dismutase (**Figure 4**). Both O_2^- and H_2O_2 are known to contribute to physiological and pathological redox signaling [15, 16].

However, conventionally, mitochondrial complex II is not identified as a significant source of ROS. But, two potential ROS-producing sites can be identified in mitochondrial complex II when its sequence of electron transport is considered together with the spatial arrangement of its redox centers. When one molecule of succinate is oxidized by complex II, FAD is reduced with two electrons, but subsequent transfer of electrons through Fe-S clusters occurs one at a time. Hence, when one electron is delivered to the proximal Fe-S cluster from FAD, a flavin radical is formed until the second electron is delivered. Similarly, after sequential transfer of single electrons through Fe-S clusters, quinone is reduced with two electrons. Hence, when one electron arrives at the Q site, until another electron arrives from Fe-S clusters, a quinone radical is formed. These two radicals have the potential to generate ROS, if there is accessibility to oxygen (**Figure 5**).

During the past two decades, complex II has emerged as an important source of ROS. On the one hand, ROS produced from mutated complex II has been proposed to be the underlying cause of complex II–associated human diseases. Thus, numerous studies have been conducted to understand ROS production from human complex II. Most of these studies have been conducted on model organisms such as *Escherichia coli, Saccharomyces cerevisiae, and Caenorhabditis elegans* [17–20]. A hallmark in these studies is the finding that the *mev-1* mutation in the mitochondrial complex II of *C. elegans* results in enhanced O_2^- production and oxygen hypersensitivity [19, 20]. Later on, this finding was further reinforced by a study using a transgenic mouse cell line with the equivalent mutation in the *CybL* gene as the *mev-1* mutation demonstrating O_2^- overproduction from mitochondria that leads to tumorigenesis [21]. More recently, mutations in the Ip subunit in the *C. elegans* have also been found to display enhanced ROS production [22]. Site-directed mutagenesis of CybS subunit in *E. coli* [23] and the Ip and CybS subunits in *S. cerevisiae* [18, 24] has also shown enhanced ROS production providing further support for the hypothesis that ROS underlies the complex II mutations-associated carcinogenesis. Indeed, some studies have been conducted on human cell lines using pharmacological and genetic interventions to mimic complex II mutations, but the results are controversial. For example, ROS production from human mitochondrial complex II has been shown by Guzy et al. [25] in intact cells of the hepatoma cell line Hep3B by inhibiting the complex II activity by the Q site inhibitor theonyl trifluoroacetone (TTFA) and by RNA interference of Ip subunit. In contrast, RNA interference of the same subunit of complex II in the same cell line by Cervera et al. have failed to detect ROS production [26].

On the other hand, ROS produced from mitochondrial complex II has received considerable attention as a mediator of "mitocans" (a novel class of mitochondrial targeted anticancer drugs) induced cancer cell death [5]. Interestingly, complex II Q site inhibiting mitocan, α-tocopheryl succinate (α-TOS) has been found to induce ROS only in complex II competent

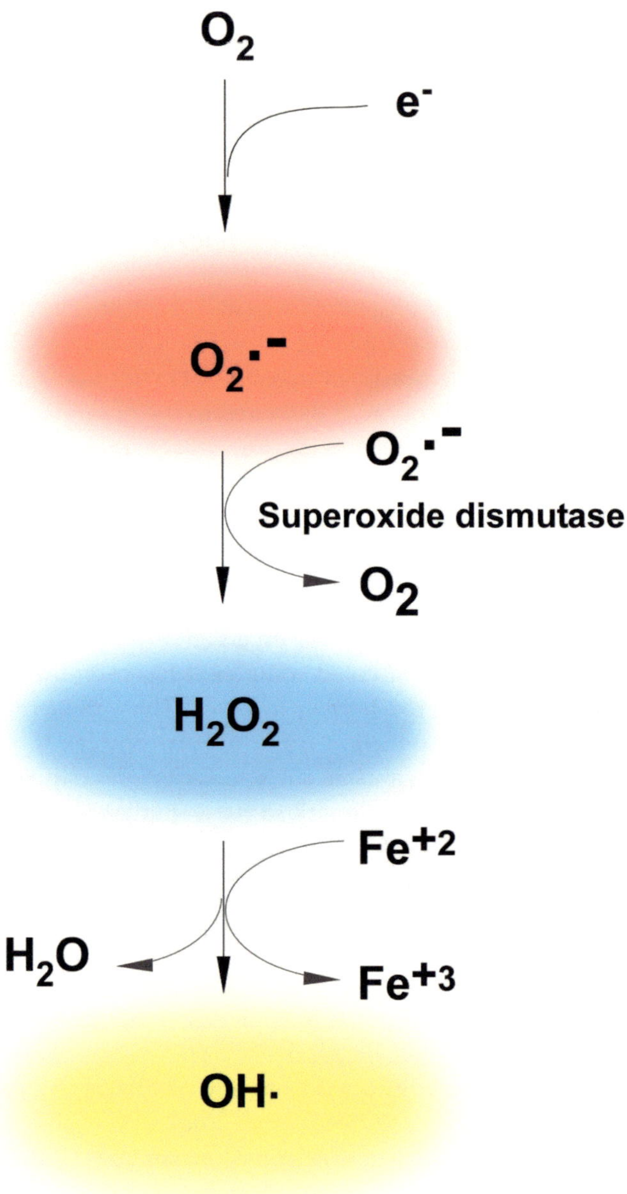

Figure 4. Diagrammatic representation of the production of the reactive oxygen species (ROS). When oxygen is reduced with a single electron, O_2^- is formed. Superoxide is converted to H_2O_2 by the enzyme superoxide dismutase. In the presence of transition metals such as Fe^{2+}, H_2O_2 is converted into hydroxyl radicals ($OH^•$) by the Fenton reaction.

cells but not in complex II mutant cells [27, 28], indicating the importance of a wild-type complex II for its action. More importantly, this complex II inhibitor has caused selective death of cancer cells, but the exact reason for this selectivity is not yet understood [29].

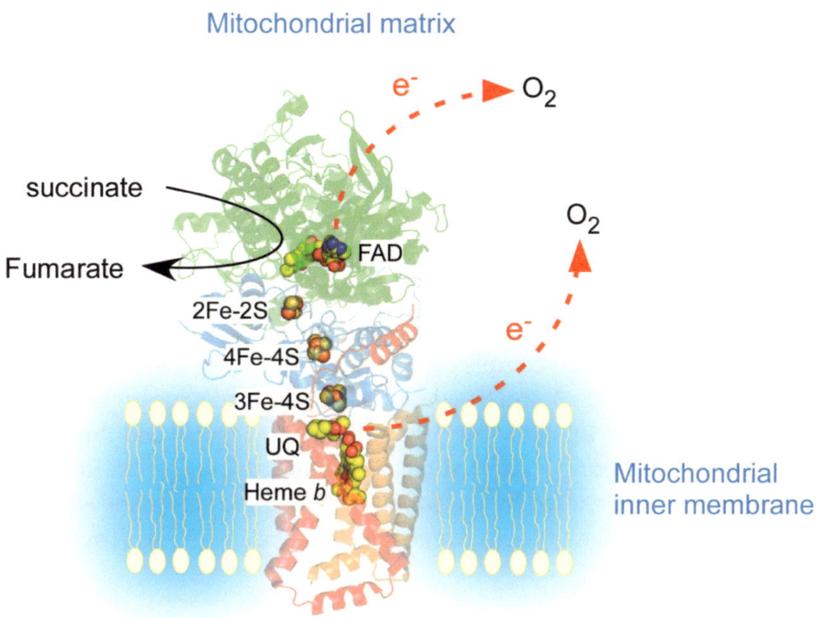

Figure 5. Ribbon model of mitochondrial complex II of *Sus scrofa* (pdb1ZOY) showing the potential ROS production sites. Fp, Ip, Cy*b*L, and Cy*b*S subunits are shown in green, blue, red, and orange, respectively. The redox centers—FAD, iron sulfur clusters, and heme *b*—are labeled in the figure.

In this chapter, we show that the potent and specific complex II Q site inhibitor atpenin A5 [30] can specifically induce ROS production in two human cancer cell lines HT-29, which predominantly express Fp I, and DLD-1, which predominantly express Fp II in the mitochondrial complex II but not in the noncancerous tissue, human dermal fibroblasts that predominantly express Fp I. This difference in ROS production may be attributed to the difference in the post-translational modifications of the wild-type mitochondrial complex II's in normal cells and cancer cells. This finding highlights new avenues in developing complex II-targeted mitocans with considerable promise.

2. Materials and methods

2.1. Culture of cells

Human colon cancer cell lines HT-29, which predominantly express Fp I in its complex II, and DLD-1, which predominantly express Fp II in its complex II, were obtained from ETCC and grown in glucose-free Roswell Park Memorial Institute (RPMI) medium supplemented with 1 g/L of glucose with 10% heated fetal bovine serum, 100 units/mL penicillin, 100 μg/mL streptomycin, and 0.25 μg/mL amphotericin B at 37°C and 5% CO_2 in a humidified incubator. The medium was renewed in 48 h intervals, and the cells were harvested at 70% confluence.

Human dermal fibroblasts, which predominantly express Fp I in its complex II, were obtained from Cell Applications Inc., Japan, and grown in Dulbecco's Modified Eagle Medium Nutrient Mixture F-12 (DMEM-F12).

2.2. Analysis of complex II isoform expression

Analysis of complex II isoform expression was carried out as described previously [8]. Briefly, total RNA was isolated from cultured cells using TRIzol LS reagent (Invitrogen) according to the manufacturer's instructions. After removal of residual DNA by treating with DNAse, cDNA was synthesized from total RNA using ReverTraAce (Toyobo, Japan) and an oligo (dT) primer. DNA sequence of the Fp I subunit of the complex II was amplified using Taq DNA polymerase with the sense primer 5′tacggagcaggca 3′ and the antisense primer 5′aatggtggcgggac 3′ and that of the Fp II subunit was amplified with the sense primer 5′cggacagaggcg3′ and the antisense primer 5′aatggctggcgggat3′. The resulting PCR products were subjected to agarose gel electrophoresis, and the two isoforms were identified by the size of the PCR products in the ethidium bromide-stained agarose gels scanned with the electronic transilluminator FAS III (Toyobo, Japan).

2.3. Isolation of mitochondria

Cells cultured in three 225 cm^2 flasks were harvested by trypsinization. The cells were suspended in mitochondria preparation buffer (250 mM sucrose, 20 mM HEPES, 3 mM EDTA, and 1 mM sodium malonate), pH 7.5, and homogenized with a power-driven glass-teflon Potter-Elvehjem homogenizer (20 passes). The homogenate was centrifuged at 700 × g for 15 min to pellet the cell debris and nuclei. The resulting supernatant was centrifuged at 14,000 × g for 15 min to sediment the mitochondria. The pellet was washed thrice with the mitochondria isolation buffer without sodium malonate, resuspended in the same buffer, and stored on ice until analysis. Integrity of the mitochondria was analyzed by citrate synthase activity in the presence and absence of 0.05% sucrose monolaurate (SML) in the assay mixture.

2.4. H_2O_2 assay in isolated mitochondria

Hydrogen peroxide-mediated oxidation of the fluorescent probe Amplex Red (10-acetyl-3,7-dihydroxyphenoxazine) to resorufin was used to determine the H_2O_2 generation rate of the isolated mitochondria as described previously [31, 32]. Since Amplex Red does not enter the mitochondria, polyethylene glycol-conjugated SOD (PEG-SOD), a membrane permeable form of SOD, was added to the reaction mixture to convert the O_2^- produced in the mitochondrial matrix into H_2O_2, which is subsequently released to the cytosol. The assay was performed in a 96-well plate maintained at 25°C. The resorufin formation rate was measured in SpectraMax Plus spectroflourometer (Molecular Devices, Sunnyvale, CA) at an excitation wavelength of 540 nm and emission wavelength of 590 nm. The H_2O_2 generation rate was calculated using a standard curve (0–1000 nmol/ml). To eliminate the fluorescence increment due to nonspecific oxidation of Amplex Red, a parallel assay was performed in the presence of catalase, an enzyme that scavenges H_2O_2, and the result was obtained by subtracting the amount of H_2O_2 produced in the presence of catalase from that in the absence of catalase.

H_2O_2 generation assays were also performed in the presence of respiratory chain inhibitors-10 mM nitropropionic acid (NPA), which blocks the dicarboxylate-binding site of complex II; 10 μM atpenin A5, which blocks the Q site of complex II; and 10 μM antimycin A, which blocks the Qi site of complex III in order to dissect the specific ROS-producing site of the respiratory chain.

2.5. Superoxide assay in intact cells

MitoSOX Red is a fluorescent probe that is targeted to the mitochondria of intact cells and oxidized by O_2^- produced within mitochondria. This probe was used to detect O_2^- production in the intact cells as previously described with slight modifications [33, 34]. Briefly, DLD-1 and HT-29 colon epithelial cells and the human dermal fibroblasts were cultured on cover slips and loaded with 5 μM MitoSOX Red and 50 nM MitoTracker Green (Molecular Probes, Eugene, OR) in the dark at 37°C in the CO_2 incubator for 15 min. After washing the cells for three times with prewarmed phosphate-buffered saline (PBS), three cover slip cultures each from DLD-1 and HT-29 cells were treated with the vehicle (0.2% DMSO), PEG-SOD or 10 mM NPA and incubated for 30 min. Thereafter, 10 μM atpenin A5 was added to all the cover slip cultures and imaged at 488 nm/455 nm excitation and emission wavelengths for MitoTracker Green and 633/650 nm for MitoSOX Red immediately (0 min images) and after 30 min (30 min images), using a confocal laser scanning microscope (LSM 510, Carl Zeiss, Germany). The two cover slip cultures of dermal fibroblasts were treated with 0.2% DMSO for 30 min, and subsequently one was treated with 10 μM atpenin A5 and the other one was treated with 1 μM antimycin A. Image acquisition of dermal fibroblasts was done similar to those of DLD-1 and HT-29 cells.

2.6. Statistical analysis

Results of the H_2O_2 assay are expressed as means ± SEM of three independent experiments. The data were analyzed using Shapiro-Wilks test followed by one way ANOVA. Subsequently, Levene's test and Tuckey's post hoc tests were performed. The level of significance was $P < 0.05$. Graph Pad Prism software (version 7, USA) was used for the analysis.

3. Results

3.1. Complex II isoforms in cell lines

cDNA from the two cancer cell lines (HT-29 and DLD-1) and the normal cell line (dermal fibroblasts) were amplified using Fp I- and Fp II-specific primers to analyze the degree of expression of the two Fp types in complex II isoforms. As shown in **Figure 6**, the results revealed that HT-29 and DLD-1 cells predominantly express Fp I and Fp II, respectively, in their complex II, whereas dermal fibroblasts predominantly express Fp I.

3.2. H_2O_2 production from the complex II in isolated mitochondria

As shown by the first bar of **Figure 7a–c**, mitochondria isolated from all three cell lines generated H_2O_2 when incubated with succinate in the absence of any respiratory chain inhibitors. This result

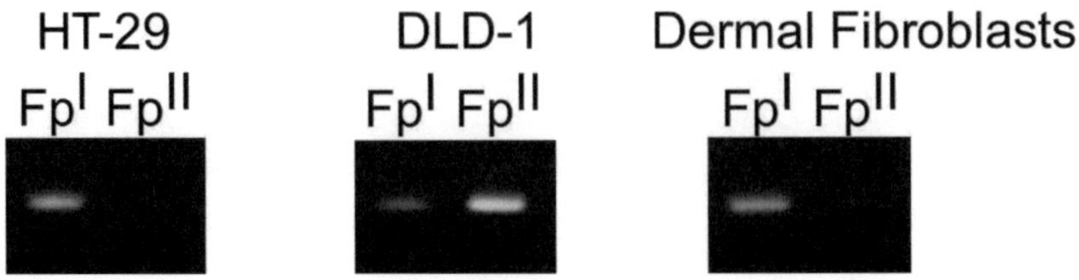

Figure 6. Mitochondrial complex II isoforms expression pattern in HT-29, DLD-1, and dermal fibroblasts. Ethidium bromide-stained agarose gels show the RT-PCR products obtained with Fp-specific primers using the RNA isolated from HT-29, DLD-1, and dermal fibroblasts. Isoform I is comprised of Fp I and isoform II is comprised of Fp II.

shows that mitochondrial complex II in all three cell lines under investigation can rapidly oxidize succinate and feed electrons to their respiratory chains and a portion of those electrons are leaked to O_2 to generate ROS.

The second bar in **Figure 7a–c** shows that addition of atpenin A5, an inhibitor of the Q-binding site of complex II, increases the H_2O_2 production in mitochondria isolated from HT-29 and DLD-1 cells but not in the mitochondria isolated from dermal fibroblasts. It shows that when electron flow through the Q-binding site is blocked, increase in the proton motive force in the respiratory chain proximal to the complex II Q site leads to leakage of electrons from the respiratory chain to oxygen in mitochondria isolated from cancer cells but not in mitochondria isolated from normal cells. This observation implies that a site proximal to the Q-binding site of complex II is responsible for leakage of electrons in cancer cell respiratory chains, which is different from that in normal cells. As shown by the third bar of the **Figure 7a–c**, addition of NPA, an inhibitor of the dicarboxylate-binding site of the mitochondrial complex II, along with atpenin A5 almost completely abolished the succinate-dependent H_2O_2 production in all three cell types. According to this observation, the increment in H_2O_2 production from the mitochondria isolated from cancer cells in the presence of atpenin A5 is attributed to a leakage of electrons from a site upstream of the Q site and downstream of the dicarboxylate-binding site. However, one can argue that the difference observed in H_2O_2 production between mitochondria of cancer cells and normal cells in the presence of atpenin A5 is due to the difference in the antioxidant defense systems between the two cell types. Therefore, we observed the H_2O_2 production in isolated mitochondria in the presence of antimycin A, an inhibitor of the Qi site of complex III that is reported to induce ROS generation from the respiratory chain complex III [32]. As shown by the fourth bar of **Figure 7a–c**, addition of antimycin A to the reaction mixture could increase the H_2O_2 production from mitochondria isolated from cancer cells as well as from the normal cells, indicating that the difference in the antioxidant levels is not the case.

3.3. Superoxide production from the complex II in live cells

When HT-29 and DLD-1 cells grown in RPMI medium containing glucose were treated with atpenin A5, their confocal images showed a clear red fluorescence in the cytoplasm while the untreated cells were devoid of such red fluorescence. To verify the localization of this fluorescence to mitochondria, the cells were simultaneously loaded with MitoTracker Green, a

http://dx.doi.org/10.5772/intechopen.71638

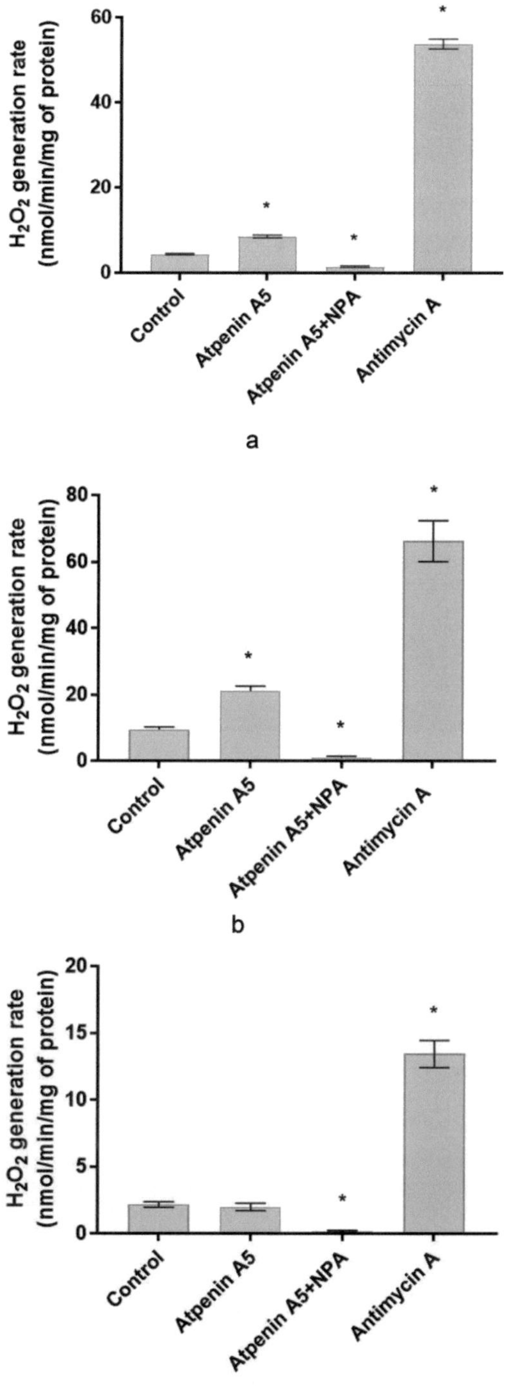

Figure 7. H_2O_2 production from the mitochondria isolated from HT-29 cells (a), DLD-1 cells (b), and dermal fibroblasts (c) oxidizing 0.75 mM succinate. Results are expressed as mean ± SEM of three independent experiments. *Significantly different from control cells ($P < 0.05$).

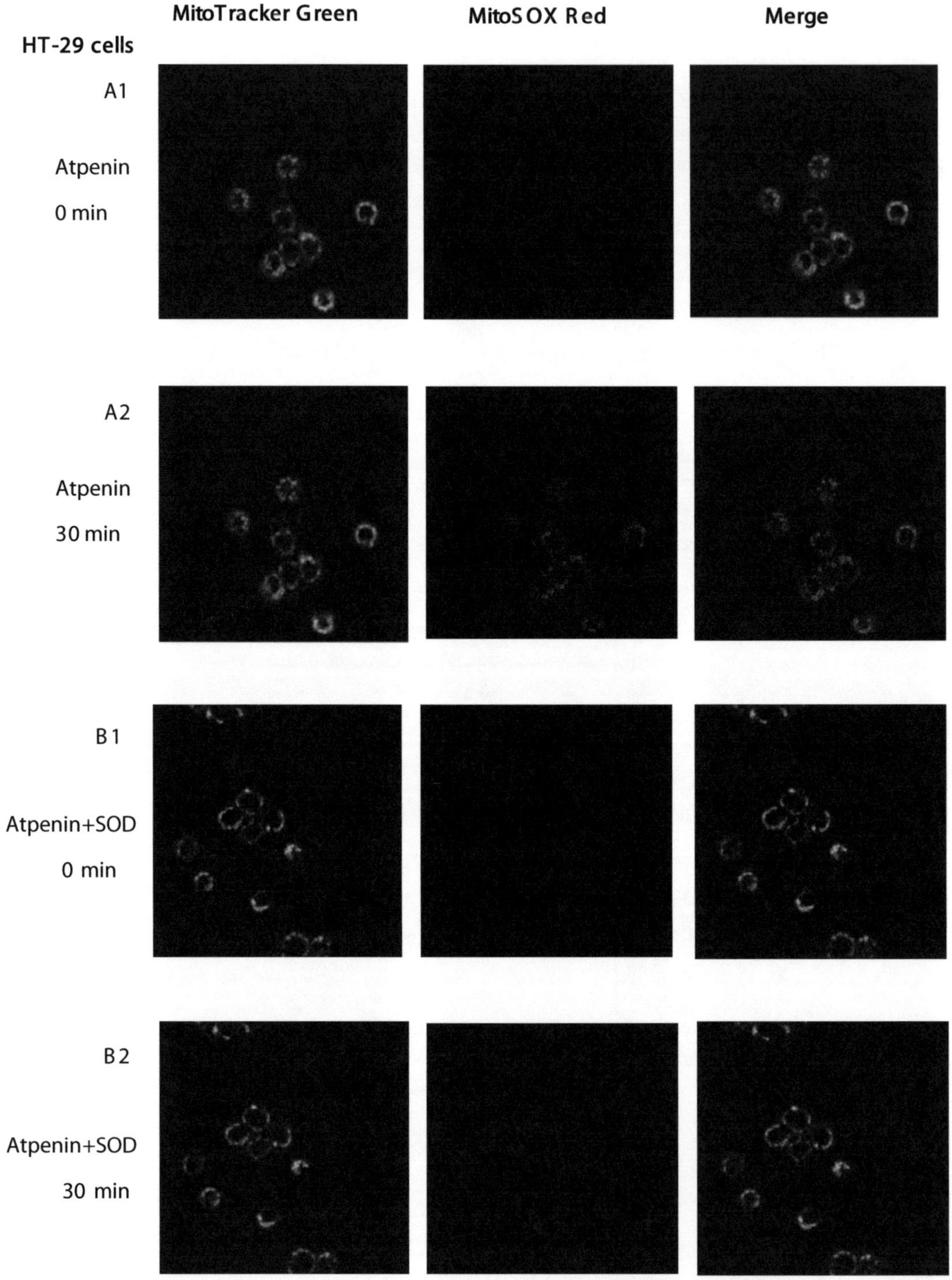
MitoTracker Green
MitoSOX Red
Merge
HT-29 cells
A1
Atpenin
0 min
A2
Atpenin
30 min
B1
Atpenin+SOD
0 min
B2
Atpenin+SOD
30 min

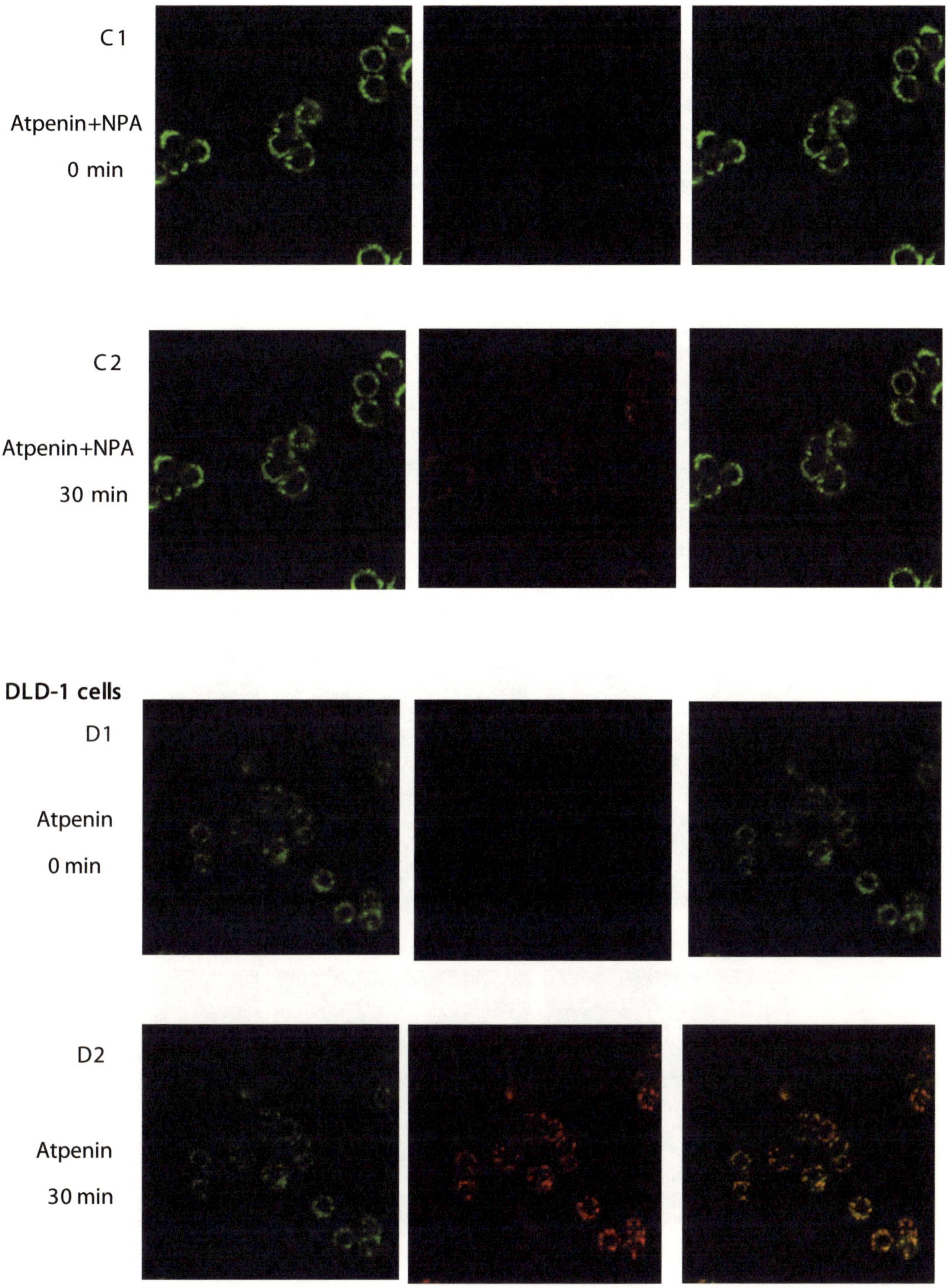
C1
Atpenin+NPA
0 min
C2
Atpenin+NPA
30 min
DLD-1 cells
D1
Atpenin
0 min
D2
Atpenin
30 min

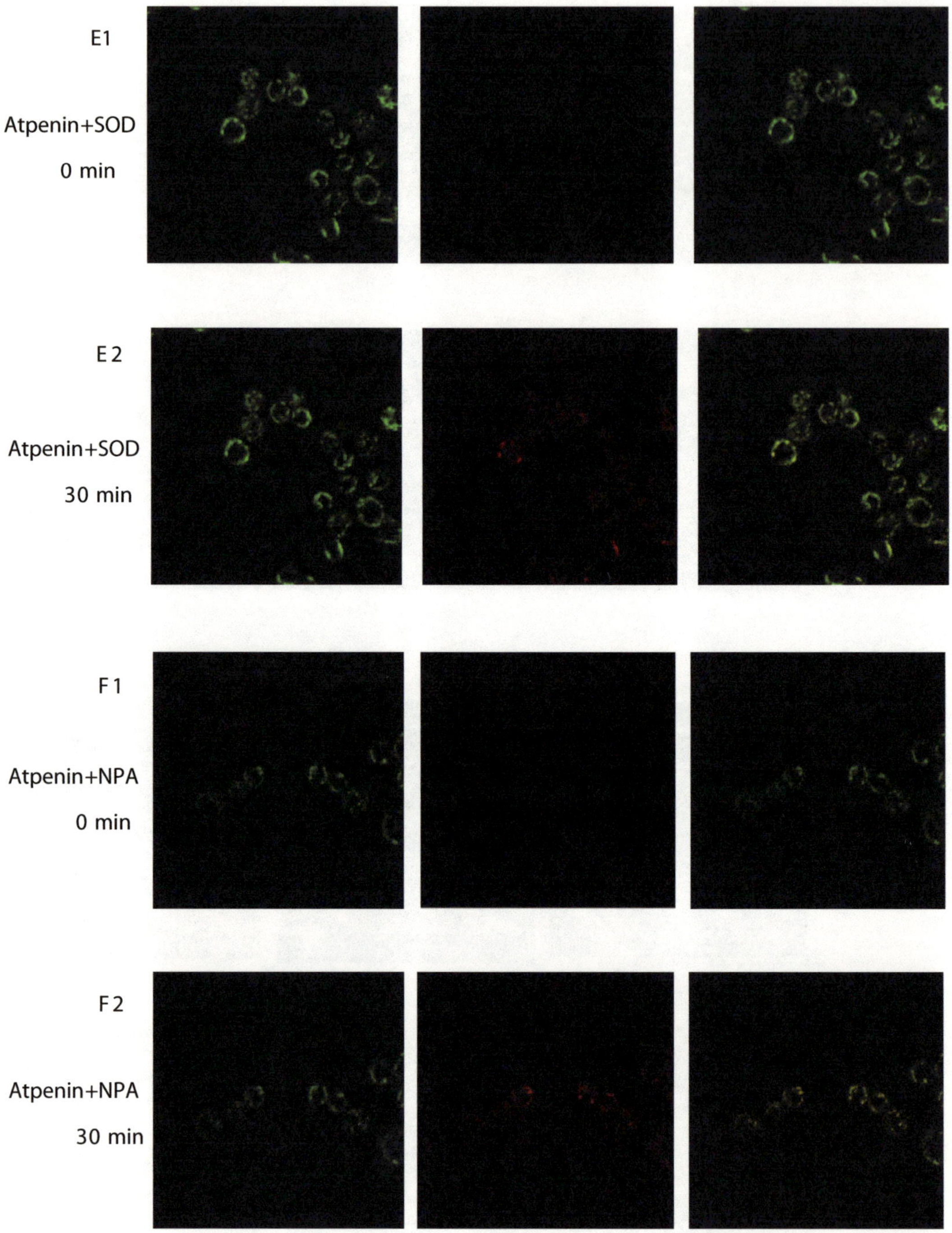
E1
Atpenin+SOD
0 min
E2
Atpenin+SOD
30 min
F1
Atpenin+NPA
0 min
F2
Atpenin+NPA
30 min

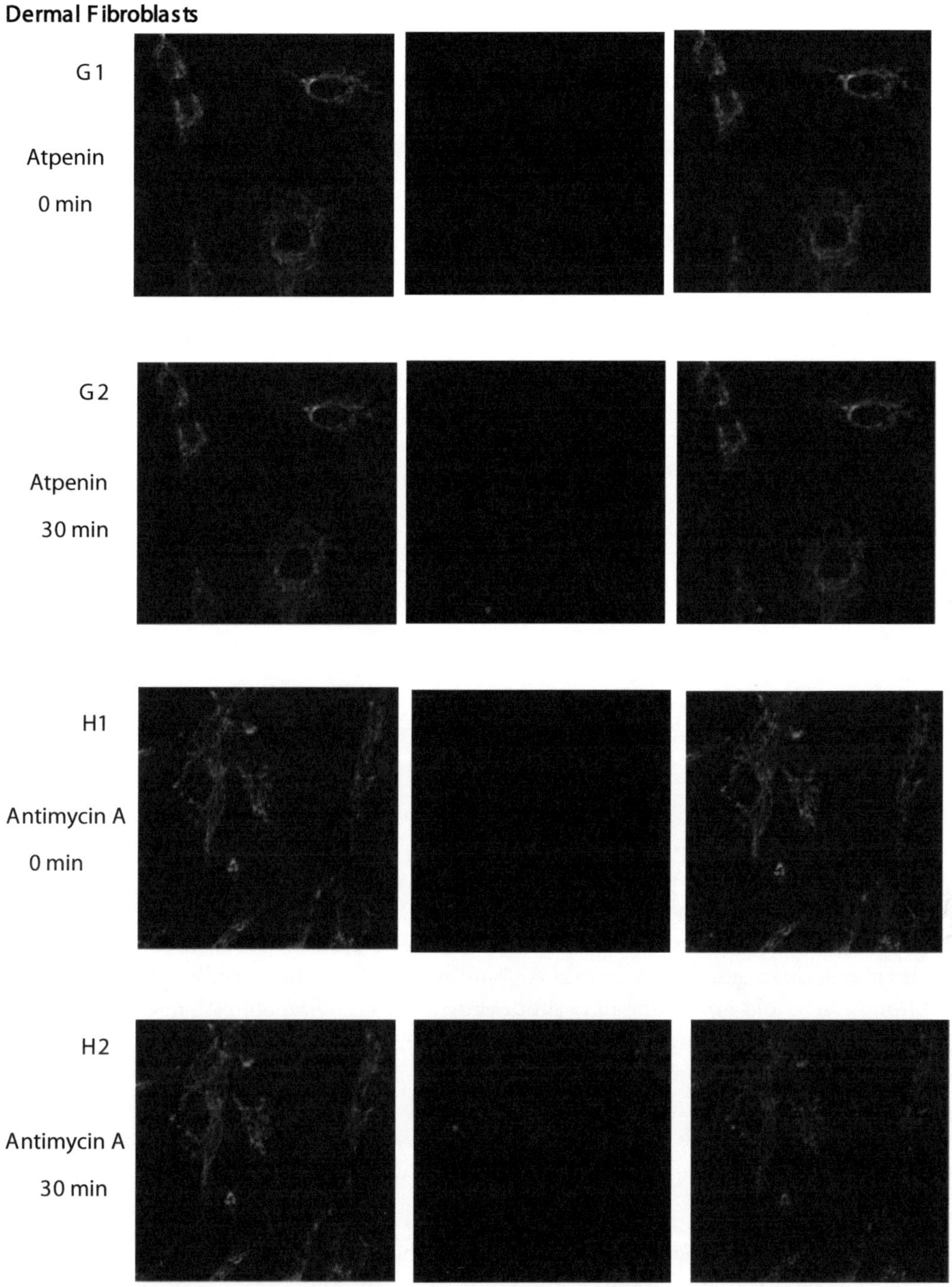

Figure 8. Confocal laser scanning microscopic images showing the O_2^- production from the mitochondrial complex II in live cells. Panels A, D, and G show the time lapse images of the cells preincubated with DMSO and treated with atpenin A5. Panels B and E show the cells preincubated with SOD-PEG and treated with atpenin A5. Panels C and F show the cells preincubated with NPA and treated with atpenin A5. Cells treated with antimycin A are shown in panel H. The cells in the first column have a green florescence. The cells in the second column have a red florescence. Out of the cells in the third column, A2, D2 and H2 panels have a dark orange florescence and B2, C2 and E2 panels have a light orange florescence and other panels have a green florescence.

fluorescent probe that is specifically targeted to mitochondria. The resulting confocal images revealed that the green fluorescence of MitoTracker Green colocalize with the red fluorescence of MitoSOX Red indicating that MitoSOX Red is oxidized within mitochondria (**Figure 8**). To determine whether MitoSOX oxidation is a superoxide-dependent process, the cells were preincubated with PEG-SOD, which can scavenge O_2^- generated within cells. In the presence of PEG-SOD, MitoSOX Red fluorescence was negligible (**Figure 8**, panels B and E). This result indicates that the majority of the atpenin A5-induced MitoSOX fluorescence is superoxide dependent. Next, we attempted to determine whether the atpenin A5-induced O_2^- production is a succinate-dependent process by preincubating the cells with NPA before adding atpenin A5. As shown in **Figure 8** panels C and F, the MitoSOX Red fluorescence intensity in the NPA-treated cells was markedly reduced indicating that the atpenin A5-induced MitoSOX Red oxidation is a succinate-dependent event. Collectively, these data indicate that atpenin A5 induces succinate-dependent O_2^- production from the mitochondrial complex II within intact DLD-1 and HT-29 cells. In agreement with the results from the isolated mitochondria, addition of atpenin A5 to the MitoSOX Red-loaded dermal fibroblasts did not display any red fluorescence (**Figure 8** panel G) indicating that atpenin A5 does not induce O_2^- production in mitochondria of dermal fibroblasts. But dermal fibroblasts showed an increment in red fluorescence with antimycin A (**Figure 8** panel H). This observation shows that the mitochondria of the dermal fibroblasts can produce O_2^- when the Q site of complex III is inhibited by antimycin A.

4. Discussion

ROS are produced from the mitochondrial complex II of the cancer cells (DLD-1 and HT-29) but not from the normal cells (dermal fibroblasts) when the entry of electrons to its quinone-binding site is blocked with 10 μM atpenin A5. However, previous studies in our laboratory have revealed that quinone reduction in the mitochondrial complex II can be completely inhibited at the tested concentration of atpenin A5 [8, 10]. Therefore, the difference in ROS production between cancer cells and normal cells may be attributed to a difference in the complex IIs that is upstream of the atpenin A5-binding site. Since the dicarboxylate-binding site inhibitor, NPA, could inhibit the ROS production induced by atpenin A5 in cancer cells, it is concluded that the ROS-producing site must be within the complex II, upstream of the atpenin A5 inhibition site(Q site) and downstream of NPA-binding site (dicarboxylate-binding site). According to previous evidence, the most likely ROS-producing sites of mitochondrial complex II are FAD [35–37] site and the Q site [37–39]. Observations of this study show that the ROS-generating site of complex II in atpenin A5-treated cancer cells is FAD but not Q site.

In order to explain this observation, we analyzed the published data on the crystal structures of flavoproteins, which are available in both the substrate bound and unbound forms [40–42]. They have shown that the capping domain in Fp subunit rotates during the enzyme catalysis. When the active site is not occupied by the substrate, the capping domain is rotated away from the active site creating a solvent channel linking the active site and the surrounding aqueous environment. In the substrate bound state, the capping domain is rotated inward concealing the active site, preventing the access of solvent to the active site [37]. Thus, closed conformation acquired during enzyme catalysis appears to be vital for preventing the electron leak into oxygen. It appears that differences in the three-dimensional structure of the capping domain of the enzyme contribute to the difference in ROS production in cancer cells and normal cells. In fact, previous studies in our laboratory have shown that DLD-1 and HT-29 cells display FRD activity associated with the phosphorylation status of the Fp subunit of complex II and the degree of phosphorylation has been increased under hypoxic and hypoglycemic conditions [11]. If phosphorylation of amino acid residues in the Fp subunit can affect the correct movement of the capping domain during succinate oxidation, it will be possible for the electrons to leak to oxygen from the FAD site.

Our observation of a 1.5-fold higher ROS production from isolated mitochondria of DLD-1 cells than that of HT-29 cells may also have resulted due to the difference in the phosphorylation status of the two isoforms because the amino acids, which differ in the two isoforms, are found in the C-terminal domain of the Fp subunit, which plays an important role in opening and closing of the active site of the complex II enzymes [9] Substitution of tyrosine 629 in Fp I with phenylalanine in Fp II may affect the phosphorylation state of the C-terminal domain since tyrosine is a possible phosphorylation site while phenylalanine is not. This difference may affect the closing of the active site in Fp II during enzyme catalysis and allow more electrons to leak to oxygen from FAD. However, it is essential to resolve the crystal structure of the two isoforms of the human mitochondrial complex II with both the open and closed states of the capping domain and to establish the relationship between the phosphorylation status of the Fp subunit and the ROS production.

In summary, complex II Q site inhibitor atpenin A5 differentially affects the ROS production in normal cells and cancer cells. This difference may be utilized for selective destruction of cancer cells using complex II-inhibiting mitocans. We hypothesize that the difference in ROS production observed in this study is attributed to the difference in posttranslational modifications of mitochondrial complex II between normal cells and cancer cells, which may be more pronounced under hypoxic and hypoglycemic tumor microenvironments.

Acknowledgements

Ministry of Education, Culture and Sports in Japan is gratefully acknowledged for their financial support.

Author details

Madhavi P. Paranagama[1]* and Kiyoshi Kita[2]

*Address all correspondence to: madhaviparanagama@gmail.com

1 Department of Basic Sciences, Faculty of Dental Sciences, University of Peradeniya, Peradeniya, Sri Lanka

2 School of Tropical Medicine and Global Health, Nagasaki University, Nagasaki, Japan

References

[1] Alston CL, Rocha MC, Lax NZ, Turnbull DM, Taylor RW. The genetics and pathology of mitochondrial disease. The Journal of Pathology. 2017;**241**(2):236-250

[2] Hoekstra AS, Bayley JP. The role of complex II in disease. Biochimica et Biophysica Acta. 2013;**1827**(5):543-551

[3] Kita K, Shiomi K, Omura S. Advances in drug discovery and biochemical studies. Trends in Parasitology. 2007;**23**(5):223-229

[4] Sakai C, Tomitsuka E, Esumi H, Harada S, Kita K. Mitochondrial fumarate reductase as a target of chemotherapy: From parasites to cancer cells. Biochimica et Biophysica Acta. 2012;**1820**(5):643-651

[5] Kluckova K, Bezawork-Geleta A, Rohlena J, Dong L, Neuzil J. Mitochondrial complex II, a novel target for anti-cancer agents. Biochimica et Biophysica Acta. 2013;**1827**(5):552-564

[6] Ackrell BA. Progress in understanding structure-function relationships in respiratory chain complex II. FEBS Letters. 2000;**466**(1):1-5

[7] Iverson TM. Catalytic mechanisms of complex II enzymes: A structural perspective. Biochimica et Biophysica Acta. 2013;**1827**(5):648-657

[8] Tomitsuka E, Goto Y, Taniwaki M, Kita K. Direct evidence for expression of type II flavoprotein subunit in human complex II (succinate-ubiquinone reductase). Biochemical and Biophysical Research Communications. 2003;**311**(3):774-779

[9] Tomitsuka E, Hirawake H, Goto Y, Taniwaki M, Harada S, Kita K. Direct evidence for two distinct forms of the flavoprotein subunit of human mitochondrial complex II (succinate-ubiquinone reductase). Journal of Biochemistry. 2003;**134**(2):191-195

[10] Sakai C, Tomitsuka E, Miyagishi M, Harada S, Kita K. Type II Fp of human mitochondrial respiratory complex II and its role in adaptation to hypoxia and nutrition-deprived conditions. Mitochondrion. 2013;**13**(6):602-609

[11] Tomitsuka E, Kita K, Esumi H. Regulation of succinate-ubiquinone reductase and fumarate reductase activities in human complex II by phosphorylation of its flavoprotein subunit. Proceedings of the Japan Academy. Series B, Physical and Biological Sciences. 2009;**85**(7):258-265

[12] Cecchini G. Function and structure of complex II of the respiratory chain. Annual Review of Biochemistry. 2003;**72**:77-109

[13] Kita K, Takamiya S. Electron-transfer complexes in Ascaris mitochondria. Advances in Parasitology. 2002;**51**:95-131

[14] Hirayama A, Kami K, Sugimoto M, Sugawara M, Toki N, Onozuka H, et al. Quantitative metabolome profiling of colon and stomach cancer microenvironment by capillary electrophoresis time-of-flight mass spectrometry. Cancer Research. 2009;**69**(11):4918-4925

[15] Murphy MP. How mitochondria produce reactive oxygen species. The Biochemical Journal. 2009;**417**(1):1-13

[16] Jezek P, Hlavata L. Mitochondria in homeostasis of reactive oxygen species in cell, tissues, and organism. The International Journal of Biochemistry & Cell Biology. 2005;**37**(12):2478-2503

[17] Messner KR, Imlay JA. Mechanism of superoxide and hydrogen peroxide formation by fumarate reductase, succinate dehydrogenase, and aspartate oxidase. The Journal of Biological Chemistry. 2002;**277**(45):42563-42571

[18] Guo J, Lemire BD. The ubiquinone-binding site of the *Saccharomyces cerevisiae* succinate-ubiquinone oxidoreductase is a source of superoxide. The Journal of Biological Chemistry. 2003;**278**(48):47629-47635

[19] Ishii N, Fujii M, Hartman PS, Tsuda M, Yasuda K, Senoo-Matsuda N, et al. A mutation in succinate dehydrogenase cytochrome b causes oxidative stress and ageing in nematodes. Nature. 1998;**394**(6694):694-697

[20] Senoo-Matsuda N, Yasuda K, Tsuda M, Ohkubo T, Yoshimura S, Nakazawa H, et al. A defect in the cytochrome b large subunit in complex II causes both superoxide anion overproduction and abnormal energy metabolism in *Caenorhabditis elegans*. The Journal of Biological Chemistry. 2001;**276**(45):41553-41558

[21] Ishii T, Yasuda K, Akatsuka A, Hino O, Hartman PS, Ishii NA. Mutation in the SDHC gene of complex II increases oxidative stress, resulting in apoptosis and tumorigenesis. Cancer Research. 2005;**65**(1):203-209

[22] Huang J, Lemire BD. Mutations in the *C. elegans* succinate dehydrogenase iron-sulfur subunit promote superoxide generation and premature aging. Journal of Molecular Biology. 2009;**387**(3):559-569

[23] Zhao Z, Rothery RA, Weiner JH. Effects of site-directed mutations in *Escherichia coli* succinate dehydrogenase on the enzyme activity and production of superoxide radicals. Biochemistry and Cell Biology. 2006;**84**(6):1013-1021

[24] Szeto SS, Reinke SN, Sykes BD, Lemire BD. Ubiquinone-binding site mutations in the *Saccharomyces cerevisiae* succinate dehydrogenase generate superoxide and lead to the accumulation of succinate. The Journal of Biological Chemistry. 2007;**282**(37):27518-27526

[25] Guzy RD, Sharma B, Bell E, Chandel NS, Schumacker PT. Loss of the SdhB, but not the SdhA, subunit of complex II triggers reactive oxygen species-dependent hypoxia-inducible factor activation and tumorigenesis. Molecular and Cellular Biology. 2008;**28**(2):718-731

[26] Cervera AM, Apostolova N, Crespo FL, Mata M, McCreath KJ. Cells silenced for SDHB expression display characteristic features of the tumor phenotype. Cancer Research. 2008;**68**(11):4058-4067

[27] Dong LF, Low P, Dyason JC, Wang XF, Prochazka L, Witting PK, et al. Alpha-tocopheryl succinate induces apoptosis by targeting ubiquinone-binding sites in mitochondrial respiratory complex II. Oncogene. 2008;**27**(31):4324-4335

[28] Dong LF, Freeman R, Liu J, Zobalova R, Marin-Hernandez A, Stantic M, et al. Suppression of tumor growth in vivo by the mitocan alpha-tocopheryl succinate requires respiratory complex II. Clinical Cancer Research. 2009;**15**(5):1593-1600

[29] Angulo-Molina A, Reyes-Leyva J, Lopez-Malo A, Hernandez J. The role of alpha tocopheryl succinate (alpha-TOS) as a potential anticancer agent. Nutrition and Cancer. 2014;**66**(2):167-176

[30] Miyadera H, Shiomi K, Ui H, Yamaguchi Y, Masuma R, Tomoda H, et al. Atpenins, potent and specific inhibitors of mitochondrial complex II (succinate-ubiquinone oxidoreductase). Proceedings of the National Academy of Sciences of the United States of America. 2003;**100**(2):473-477

[31] Mohanty JG, Jaffe JS, Schulman ES, Raible DG. A highly sensitive fluorescent microassay of H_2O_2 release from activated human leukocytes using a dihydroxyphenoxazine derivative. Journal of Immunological Methods. 1997;**202**(2):133-141

[32] Chen Q, Vazquez EJ, Moghaddas S, Hoppel CL, Lesnefsky EJ. Production of reactive oxygen species by mitochondria: Central role of complex III. The Journal of Biological Chemistry. 2003;**278**(38):36027-36031

[33] Mukhopadhyay P, Rajesh M, Hasko G, Hawkins BJ, Madesh M, Pacher P. Simultaneous detection of apoptosis and mitochondrial superoxide production in live cells by flow cytometry and confocal microscopy. Nature Protocols. 2007;**2**(9):2295-2301

[34] Robinson KM, Janes MS, Beckman JS. The selective detection of mitochondrial superoxide by live cell imaging. Nature Protocols. 2008;**3**(6):941-947

[35] Ohnishi T, King TE, Salerno JC, Blum H, Bowyer JR, Maida T. Thermodynamic and electron paramagnetic resonance characterization of flavin in succinate dehydrogenase. The Journal of Biological Chemistry. 1981;**256**(11):5577-5582

[36] Maklashina E, Iverson TM, Sher Y, Kotlyar V, Andrell J, Mirza O, et al. Fumarate reductase and succinate oxidase activity of *Escherichia coli* complex II homologs are perturbed differently by mutation of the flavin binding domain. The Journal of Biological Chemistry. 2006;**281**(16):11357-11365

[37] Paranagama MP, Sakamoto K, Amino H, Awano M, Miyoshi H, Kita K. Contribution of the FAD and quinone binding sites to the production of reactive oxygen species from *Ascaris suum* mitochondrial complex II. Mitochondrion. 2010;**10**(2):158-165

[38] Salerno JC, Ohnishi T. Studies on the stabilized ubisemiquinone species in the succinate-cytochrome c reductase segment of the intact mitochondrial membrane system. The Biochemical Journal. 1980;**192**(3):769-781

[39] Tran QM, Rothery RA, Maklashina E, Cecchini G, Weiner JH. The quinone binding site in *Escherichia coli* succinate dehydrogenase is required for electron transfer to the heme b. The Journal of Biological Chemistry. 2006;**281**(43):32310-32317

[40] Yamashita T, Ino T, Miyoshi H, Sakamoto K, Osanai A, Nakamaru-Ogiso E, et al. Rhodoquinone reaction site of mitochondrial complex I, in parasitic helminth, *Ascaris suum*. Biochimica et Biophysica Acta. 2004;**1608**(2-3):97-103

[41] Yankovskaya V, Horsefield R, Tornroth S, Luna-Chavez C, Miyoshi H, Leger C, et al. Architecture of succinate dehydrogenase and reactive oxygen species generation. Science. 2003;**299**(5607):700-704

[42] Yu L, Xu JX, Haley PE, Yu CA. Properties of bovine heart mitochondrial cytochrome b560. The Journal of Biological Chemistry. 1987;**262**(3):1137-1143

Chapter 5

A New Insight into the Development of Novel Anti-Cancer Drugs that Improve the Expression of Mitochondrial Function-Associated Genes

Fumiaki Uchiumi, Jun Arakawa, Yutaka Takihara,
Motohiro Akui, Hiroshi Hamada and
Sei-ichi Tanuma

Additional information is available at the end of the chapter

http://dx.doi.org/10.5772/intechopen.71095

Abstract

Recent analyses of the whole genome sequencing data enable us to predict cancer incidence for healthy people at present. In addition, metabolome analyses rediscovered that "cancer is a metabolic disease". Importantly, it has been suggested that mitochondrial dysfunction might precede the metabolic change. In this chapter, we would discuss if "cancer is a transcriptional disease". Analyzing 5′-upstream non-protein-encoding regions of the human mitochondrial function-associated genes, we speculate that mitochondrial functions could be recovered or improved at a transcriptional level. In the near future, novel chemo-/gene-therapies might be applied to treat cancer patient converting cancerous cells into normal differentiated cells.

Keywords: cancer, CTCF (CCCTC-binding factor), DNA repair, ETS (E26 transformation specific), gene expression, GGAA, HMGB (High mobility group box), ISG (Interferon stimulated gene), metabolism, mitochondria, NAD^+, PARP inhibitors, poly (ADP-ribosyl) ation, PARP (poly(ADP-ribose) polymerase), transcription, transcription factors, Warburg effect

1. Introduction

We have already learned that "cancer is a genetic disease". Recent high-impact research has shown the genomic/genetic differences between cancer and normal cells using methods such as next-generation sequencing [1, 2]. The analysis of the whole genome sequencing data will even enable us to predict the incidence of cancer in healthy individuals [3]. More importantly, recent metabolome analyses have led to the rediscovery that metabolites could be biomarkers for cancer and its development [4]. The "Warburg effect", which was shown by Dr Otto Warburg over 60 years ago, is the most essential discovery in the field of cancer science [5]. The "Warburg effect" refers to abnormal metabolism in cancer, which mainly utilizes glucose to produce ATP by glycolysis. In this regard, "cancer is a metabolic disease". This is not only important as an indicator of tumors, but also as one of the essential characteristics of cancer [6, 7]. A number of lines of evidence, including dysregulated TCA (Krebs/Citrate)-cycle progression and the insufficient oxidative phosphorylation in cancer cells, suggest that mitochondrial dysfunction might precede the metabolic change [8]. Thus, "cancer must be a mitochondrial disease". In this chapter, which focuses on the causative factors that lead to mitochondrial dysfunction, we discuss whether "cancer is a transcriptional disease". Most of the genes (99%) that encode mitochondria or their function-associated proteins are contained in nuclear genomes [9]. The mitochondrial functions might be recovered or improved at a transcriptional level. In this chapter, we propose the establishment of novel chemo-/gene-therapies with no side effects, to force cancerous cells to regenerate into their normal differentiated state.

2. The relevance of duplicated GGAA-motifs in the 5′-upstream regions of human genes to the regulation of biological events

2.1. The transcription factors that recognize and bind to the GGAA-containing motifs

The most widely known transcription factors (TFs) that selectively recognize the GGAA-core-containing sequences are the ETS (E26 transformation specific) family proteins, which consist of at least 27 members [10, 11]. Moreover, a genome-wide ChIP-seq analysis estimated that the promoter regions of human genes are very frequently occupied by ETS family or GGAA-binding proteins [12]. The duplication of the GGAA-motif could be advantageous to organisms, as it would allow the transcription of various genes to be controlled in a manner that is mainly dependent on the expression profile of the GGAA-binding proteins in the cells [13, 14]. Besides ETS family proteins, several TFs could bind to the motif. For example, some of the duplicated GGAA-motifs would be identical to IFN-stimulated response element (ISRE), the consensus sequence of which is 5′-GGAAANNGAAACT-3′ [15], if one of the Ns was G. The double-stranded sequence, 5′-AACTTT-3′, which is a core binding motif of the IRF1 [16], could be generated if CT was inserted between GGAA and TTCC. Moreover, NF-κB p65 (RELA) homodimer binds to two symmetric sequences, 5′-GGAATTTCC-3′ and 5′-GGAATTCCC-3′ [17]. IRF8 (ICSBP) either positively or negatively regulates transcription through binding to ISRE [18, 19].

Importantly, the ETS family proteins and other TFs cooperatively regulate the expression of various genes. For instance, STAT1 plays a role in the regulation of the expression of interferon (IFN)-stimulated genes (ISGs) with ETS family proteins [20, 21]. Sp1 and Ets1 interact with each other to regulate mouse *Npr1* gene expression [22]. The ETS-binding consensus sequence is frequently found with a second ETS-binding sequence and with the Sp1-binding sequence, but not with a TATA element [23], implying the exclusive role of the GGAA- and TATA elements. The human

VEGFR1 promoter region, which contains overlapping GGAA-motifs, is also regulated by CREB and EGR-binding elements [24]. Furthermore, the mouse *Ppp2r1a* gene promoter, which carries duplicated TTCC motifs, is regulated by Creb, Ets1, Ap2 alpha, and Sp1proteins [25]. Thus, multiple elements adjacent to duplicated GGAA-motifs may recruit various TFs to form a pre-initiation complex on the transcription start site (TSS) of TATA-less promoters. The transcription initiation system might be advantageous for a rapid response to stresses in a TATA-independent manner.

2.2. The duplicated GGAA-motifs that are contained in the 5′-upstream regions of immune response factor-encoding human genes

Duplicated GGAA-motifs are found in the 5′-upstream of the ISGs [20, 26, 27]. The GGAA-motifs are also harbored in the IFN-stimulated response element (ISRE)-like sequences [28, 29]. Thus, the duplicated GGAA-motifs near TSSs may play roles in controlling the expression of ISGs. The ISG-encoded proteins include TFs, immune modulators, apoptosis mediators, and anti-viral factors [30]. Previously, the duplicated GGAA-motifs in the regulatory regions of ISGs have been analyzed [31]. We surveyed the 5′-upstream regions in a number of ISGs to find GGAA-motifs within 500-bp upstream from the TSSs [32], and reported that IFNβ-inducible human *OAS1* promoter activity is regulated by binding of ELF-1 (which belongs to the ETS family proteins) to a duplicated GGAA-motif, and by its interaction with Sp1 and Rb proteins [33].

Collectively, the majority of the promoter regions from ISGs contain duplicated GGAA-motifs but rarely with TATA element. This suggests that the mechanism by which transcription is initiated differs from that of the house-keeping genes or genes that are essentially required, such as those that encode cell structure components. IFNs, the expression of which should be suppressed under normal conditions, only play important roles when it is necessary to fight against viral infection and oncogenesis. The duplicated GGAA-motifs might have contributed, through evolution, to the development of an immune response at the transcriptional level. In addition, GGAA-binding factors, which are associated with other TFs around TSSs, facilitate the expression of each ISG as appropriate, depending on the different signals that are induced by IFN.

2.3. The duplicated GGAA-motifs in the 5′-upstream regions of the human DNA repair factor-encoding genes

The duplicated GGAA (TTCC) motif is present adjacent to the TSS of the human *TP53* gene [34], the expression of which is regulated by IFN-α and β [35]. IRF1 was reported to be a negative regulator of the human *TERT* promoter in response to IFN-γ [36]. In addition, IRF-5 has been shown to upregulate the expression of DNA repair/apoptosis-associated genes [37]. Moreover, DNA damage initiates an immune response that regulates DNA repair-associated genes [38]. These observations suggest that the immune responses and DNA damage responses might be co-dependent, and that the duplicated GGAA-motifs have important roles in controlling the expression of genes that encode DNA repair-associated factors in response to IFN-induced signals.

It should be noted that the duplicated GGAA-motif is present in the promoter regions of the human *Poly(ADP-ribose) polymerase 1*(*PARP1*) [39, 40] and *XRCC1* [41] genes. The duplicated GGAA-motifs are present near the TSS of the *ADPRHL2* (*ARH3*) and the *ZC3HAV1* genes, which encode mitochondria-localizing poly(ADP-ribose) (PAR) degrading enzyme [42] and an anti-viral RNA-binding protein PARP13 [43, 44], respectively. These findings suggest that the expression of genes encoding single-strand DNA break repair factors is commonly regulated by the duplicated GGAA-motifs.

The promoter activities of the human *WRN* and *TERT* genes, both encoding telomere maintenance factors, positively respond to both 2-deoxy-D-glucose (2DG) [45] and *trans*-resveratrol (Rsv) [46], which are caloric restriction (CR) mimetic drugs that have been shown to prolong the life span of several organisms [47]. The natural compound Rsv upregulates the expression of the *HELB* gene [46, 48], which encodes DNA replication and DNA double strand break repair-helicase HELB (HDHB) [49–52]. Moreover, the 5′-regulatory regions of the genes that encode DNA repair factors, such as *XPB, RB1, RTEL1, ATR, TP53,* and *CDKN1A (p21),* contain GGAA duplications near the TSS [53]. Several of the DNA repair factors are localized in the mitochondria and may also regulate the mitochondrial functions [53].

2.4. The surveillance of regulatory regions adjacent to the TSSs of human mitochondrial function-associated genes

The surveillance of a human genomic DNA database suggested putative TPA-responsive elements in the 5′-upstream regions of the *MRPL32, NDUFB3, NDUFS3, SDHB,* and *SDHAF2* genes contain GGAA duplication [54]. The duplicated GGAA-motifs are present in the upstream regions of human genes encoding mitochondrial ribosomal proteins and enzymes or components that function in the TCA cycle and oxidative phosphorylation (OXPHOS) [54].

Mitochondrial dysfunction is thought to cause either cellular senescence or oncogenesis [55–58]. Remarkably, TCA cycle enzymes, fumarate hydratase (FH), and succinate dehydrogenase (SDH) have been suggested as tumor suppressors [59]. Hence, mutations of the TCA cycle factor-encoding genes give rise to abnormal mitochondrial respiration, which is one of the characteristics of tumors and cancer [60, 61]. Mutations of the *IDH1* and *IDH2* genes have been identified in human brain cancer cells [62, 63]. A recent study demonstrated that the mutation of IDH2 could lead to the generation of sarcoma [64]. Duplicated GGAA-motifs are contained in the upstream region of the *NAMPT* (*NmPRT*), encoding a nicotinamide phosphoribosyltransferase that catalyzes the first rate-limiting step of (nicotinamide adenine dinucleotides) NAD^+ synthesis from nicotinamide [65–67]. Depending on the NAD^+ level, NAMPT could modulate the TCA cycle, poly(ADP-ribosyl)ation, and sirtuin-mediated de-acetylation [66, 67]. The duplicated GGAA-motifs are present near the TSSs of the human TCA cycle enzyme-encoding *ACLY, ACO2, CS, FH, IDH1, IDH3A, IDH3B, SDHAF2, SDHB, SDHD,* and *SUCLG1* genes [68].

A duplicated GGAA-motif is present in the bidirectional promoter of the *PDHX* [54], which encodes one of the components of the PDH enzyme to metabolize pyruvate to acetyl-CoA. Aberrant pyruvate metabolism is thought to play a prominent role in cancer [69]. The genomic deletion of *ME2,* which encodes malic enzyme 2 (an NAD^+-dependent malate decarboxylase that converts malate into pyruvate), is found in pancreatic ductal adenocarcinoma [70]. The GGAA-duplication is not only found near the TSSs of the human *ME2* gene, but also the *MDH2* gene (which encodes NAD⁺-dependent malate dehydrogenase), suggesting that duplicated GGAA-dependent transcription could affect the metabolism of malate in the mitochondria.

3. The possible roles of metabolic states that can alter transcription profiles

Recently, a study using a CAP-SELEX analysis showed that different transcription factors, such as FOXO1 and ETS family proteins, are mediated by a DNA that contains a GGAA-core motif [71]. As described above, a number of promoters or regulatory regions of human genes that encode immune response-/DNA repair-/mitochondrial function-associated proteins contain overlapping or duplicated GGAA-containing motifs. Thus, the alteration of the profile of the GGAA-motif-binding proteins or their associated protein factors may allow for the control of appropriate cellular responses against viral infection, DNA damage, and oxidative/nutrient/metabolic stress. Importantly, the DNA damage responses affect the transcriptional state [72] through oxidative stress, which is mainly produced by the mitochondria [73, 74]. NF-κB- and p53-dependent transcription, which regulates the expression of the ISGs and DNA repair factor-encoding genes, is also affected by oxidative stress [75]. Thus, metabolites that are mainly produced by respiration or mitochondrial functions may influence the transcription control system [76, 77].

3.1. The transcription profile may be controlled by the NAD^+/NADH balance

We have reported that the promoter regions of the human *TP53*, *HELB*, and telomere maintenance factor-encoding genes respond positively to Rsv [46, 48, 78]. Rsv not only activates SIRT1, which is an NAD^+-dependent deacetylase [79], but also inhibits phosphodiesterase [80]. Importantly, low-dose Rsv activates mitochondrial complex I [81] to upregulate the NAD^+/NADH ratio, to induce the expression of duplicated GGAA-motif-driven genes. The transcription of the bidirectional promoter-driven *BRCA1/NBR2* genes, which contain a duplication of the GGAA-motif, may be regulated by the NAD^+/NADH ratio [82]. Notably, the C terminal-binding protein (CtBP) [83, 84] has a central role in this regulation as a metabolic sensor. Moreover, PARP1 poly(ADP-ribosyl)ates transcription elongation factor NELF to release the paused RNA pol II-dependent transcription [85], suggesting that PARP1 itself contributes to NAD^+-sensitive transcription. Recently, it was reported that nuclear PAR can be utilized by NUDIX5 to supply ATP molecules, which are required for chromatin remodeling [86]. Thus, the accumulation of NAD^+ molecules or NAD^+/NADH ratio-sensitive proteins, including GGAA-motif binding TFs, might affect the transcription of ISGs/DNA repair/mitochondrial function-associated genes in response to metabolic stress.

It should be noted that PARP activity is upregulated in tumors and cancer cells [44]. Because the duplicated GGAA-motifs are present in the 5′-upstream regions of the human *PARP* and *PARG* genes [40], subtle changes in the quality/quantity profile of the GGAA-binding TFs may modulate the PAR synthesis/degradation ratio at the transcription level. The accumulation of NAD^+ molecules in cells might be transiently caused by mitochondrial dysfunction, which is usually accompanied by insufficient OXPHOS or aberrant respiration [87, 88]. However, when DNA damage eventually activates PARP, NAD^+ molecules will be consumed to synthesize PAR polymer in the nuclei or mitochondria. Thus, the decrease in the NAD^+/NADH ratio would not only reduce the activities but also the expression of enzymes that function in the NAD^+-dependent TCA cycle progression. At this point, cells will have to produce ATP in a mitochondria-independent manner. This metabolic change would be observed as the "Warburg effect" in cancer cells [5, 6].

3.2. The regulation of TFs and nucleotide binding proteins by poly(ADP-ribosyl)ation

PARP inhibitors, such as talazoparib, niraparib, rucaparib, olaparib, and veliparib, are clinically used for the treatment of cancer, especially when *BRCA1* and *BRCA2* gene mutations are present [89]. They all interact with the NAD^+-binding site of the catalytic domain of PARP1 and PARP2. A recent study indicated that the NAD^+-binding pocket of the PARP1 regulates interaction with DBC1, which is deleted in breast cancer 1, which is a known SIRT1 inhibitor protein [90]. A decrease in the NAD^+ will upregulate the interaction between DBC1 and PARP1, leading to the suppression of its activity. This might partly explain why DNA repair declines with aging [91]. The poly(ADP-ribosyl)ation of proteins not only initiates the response to DNA damage, but also regulates the transcription of specific genes [92]. The poly(ADP-ribosyl)ation of C/EBPβ by PARP-1 modulates its transcriptional activity to enhance the expression of the genes encoding factors that regulate adipogenesis [93]. A recent study showed that the poly(ADP-ribosyl)ation of an RNA-binding protein HuR by PARP1 stabilizes *Cxcl2* gene transcripts [94]. Moreover, the poly(ADP-ribosyl)ation of FoxO3 suppresses its transcriptional activity and leads to cardiac hypertrophy [95]. Taken together, poly(ADP-ribosyl)ation, which consumes NAD^+ as a substrate for PAR synthesis, may regulate transcription to respond to DNA damage-induced signals. Thus, it should be noted that PARP inhibitors not only limit the DNA damage response to lead to the death of cancerous cells, but also reduce the consumption of NAD^+ molecules to modulate the transcription of specific genes.

4. Epigenetic alterations in chromosomal DNAs and proteins

Epigenetic alterations are frequently found in cancer, implying that "cancer is an epigenetic disease" [96]. It has been hypothesized that epigenetic and/or transcriptional changes play a role in determining the chromatin state in tumor cells [97]. Epigenetic regulation is mainly driven by modifications of chromosomal DNAs and histone proteins [98]. The biological relevance between cellular metabolites and the gene expression has been proposed as the RNA/enzyme/metabolite (REM) networking system [99]. The metabolites, NAD^+, S-adenosylmethionine (AdoMet), and acetyl-CoA, are the substrates for poly (ADP-ribosyl) ation, methylation, and acetylation, respectively [76], suggesting that these metabolic state-dependent molecules play important roles in the epigenetic regulation.

4.1. The possible functions of poly(ADP-ribosyl)ation on epigenetic regulation

NAD^+ not only plays important roles in DNA repair, mitochondrial functions, and cellular senescence [72, 100], but also affects the modification of chromatin proteins [77] and modulates the gene expression regulatory system [101]. More importantly, NAD^+ is a substrate for the PARP enzyme to synthesize PAR macromolecules, which modify both PARP itself and chromosomal proteins and DNA repair factors [67]. Histones and HMGB (High mobility group box) proteins can be poly(ADP-ribosyl)ated [102–105], suggesting that modifications by such macromolecules on chromosomes affect the epigenetic regulation of the gene expression system. Moreover, poly(ADP-ribosyl)ation on the chromosomal insulator protein CTCF (CCCTC-binding factor) may be involved in epigenetic regulation [106, 107]. Recently, it was shown that CTCF binds directly to PAR to be recruited at DNA lesion sites, indicating that the CTCF also plays a role in the DNA damage response [108]. It has been suggested that poly(ADP-ribosyl)ation affects the methylation patterns in chromosomal DNAs [109, 110]. A recent study showed that the transcriptional regulation of the *EZH2* gene, which encodes the catalytic subunit of the polycomb repressive complex 2 (PRC2), by PARP1 [111], affects the methylation of chromatin proteins [112]. Because the incidence of cancer increases with aging [113], a decline in the cellular level of NAD^+, which might accompany the decrease in PARP activity [114]. SIRT1, which depends on the NAD^+ molecule to de-acetylate histone proteins, plays important roles in the aging process [115]. Taken together, these observations imply that NAD^+ and its polymerized form, PAR, are involved in epigenetic regulation, and that it may be altered in line with the aging process.

4.2. The DNA methylation of chromosomal DNAs

The methylation of promoter regions of specific genes in human chromosomes can be used as biomarkers in various cancers [116]. The DNA methylation reaction is catalyzed by methyltransferases (DNMTs), which utilize AdoMet as a methyl group donor [117]. A recent study showed that intragenic DNA methylation, which is carried out by Dnmt3b in mouse embryonic stem cells, protects the gene body from the entry of spurious RNA pol II and the initiation of cryptic transcription [118]. The extended data showed that the ETS factor binding regions are sensitive to the knock out of the *Dnmt3b* gene, suggesting that the occupation of the GGAA (TTCC)-motifs by GGAA-motif binding proteins could be epigenetically controlled by methylation. Furthermore, the regulation of demethylation by ten-eleven translocation (TET)-family enzymes [119], the activity of which is reduced by hypoxia, should not be ignored. Hypoxia-induced hyper methylation has been demonstrated to occur on the promoter regions of the DNA repair factor-encoding genes, including *BRCA1*, *FANCD2*, *FANCF*, *POLL*, and *UNG* [120]. Of note, the duplicated GGAA-motifs are contained in these gene promoters [53]. A methylation sensitive SELEX analysis showed that ETS-binding was inhibited by mCpG, though NFAT, which also recognizes the GGAA-core motif sequence and preferentially binds to methylated DNA [121]. The observation suggests that GGAA-motif recognizing TFs could be classified into two groups according to their preference to DNA methylation.

The SET protein is an epigenetic regulatory factor that promotes loss of methylation through direct interaction with hypo-acetylated histones [122]. A genome-wide analysis showed that DNA hypermethylation is apparently induced in old male adults, relative to young male adults, suggesting a relationship between DNA methylation and aging [123–125]. Moreover, the methylation and demethylation of the lysine residues of histones might affect the regulation of transcription [126]. In summary, AdoMet, a methyl group donor, plays an important role in epigenetic control.

4.3. The acetylation of histones could regulate the generation or progression of cancers

Acetyl-CoA is required for acetylation on the lysine residue of histones [127]. This process is catalyzed by acetyltransferases (HATs), including KAT2A (GCN5), KAT2B (CAF), KAT5 (ESA1), KAT7 (HBO1), and KAT8 (MOF) [128], which can be classified into two major groups: the GCNT and MYST families [129]. At least 11 enzymes are known to be histone deacetylases (HDACs) [130]. Because the increased or aberrant expression of HDACs has been reported in various cancers, inhibitors or modulators of HDACs are expected to be effective as anticancer drugs [131]. On the other hand, the lysine acetylation is negatively regulated by sirtuin proteins, including SIRT1 [116], which de-acetylate proteins, utilizing NAD^+ as an acceptor of the acetyl group [127]. It is hypothesized that a reduction in nutrient levels could induce the accumulation of NAD^+ to activate sirtuins. Histone de-acetylation is consistent with the finding that CR mimetics prolong the life span [131–133]. In cancer cells, if mitochondrial dysfunction occurs with a reduction in the NAD^+ level or the hindrance of the progression of the TCA cycle, acetyl-CoA might only be converted to citrate to be used as an acetyl group donor for histones in the nuclei. If so, an increase in histone acetylation would occur naturally in the course of oncogenesis. The activation of HDACs in cancer cells might be the response to the aberrant hyper-acetylation of histone proteins that could lead to the abnormal transcription of various genes, including the mitochondrial function-associated genes.

To summarize, key metabolites, NAD^+ and acetyl-CoA could regulate DNA methylation and histone acetylation directly or indirectly, and play essential roles in epigenetic control.

5. Mitonuclear communication regulates apoptosis, DNA repair, and aging

The mechanisms by which nuclear DNA damage signaling causes the mitochondrial dysfunctions that accelerate aging and aging-related diseases including cancer have been investigated in a review [134]. This process can be referred to as "mitonuclear communication" [135], suggesting that DNA repair systems are integrated into the mitochondrial functions. Given that α proteobacteria are the putative ancestors of the mitochondria [136], they need to take care of the nuclear DNAs that contain almost all (99%) of their essential protein-encoding genes [9]. Thus, the mitochondria might have developed a nuclear genome monitoring system, especially when DNA damage is induced. Several TCA cycles or metabolic enzymes functions as tumor suppressors [59, 64, 137], suggesting that mitochondrial dysfunction may lead to cancerous states.

5.1. The mitochondria play the role of judge in the decision to induce cell death

The execution of apoptosis is mediated by the mitochondria in response to various stresses, including DNA damage and immunological stress signals [138–140]. Thus, the mitochondria are known to serve as master regulators of danger signaling to determine cell death or survival [141]. Several mechanisms, including the regulation of the regulators of apoptosis [142, 143] and miRNAs [144], are involved in the induction of apoptosis. The surveillance of the human genomic DNA database indicated the presence of the duplicated GGAA-motifs in the 5′-regulatory regions of the human *PDCD1, DFFA, BCL2, FAS, FASL, ATG12/AP3S1, APOPT1/BAG5,* and *HTRA2/AUP1* genes [13, 53, 54]. These observations suggest that the expression of the apoptosis regulating factor-encoding genes is modulated by the GGAA-duplicated sequences. In this context, apoptosis or programmed cell death, which is controlled by the mitochondria, partly depends on the GGAA-motif binding TFs.

5.2. The localization of p53 and other DNA repair factors in the mitochondria and the regulation of their gene expression

Recent studies have shown that the p53 protein not only acts as a "guardian of the genome", but also serves as a regulator of metabolism [145, 146]. Moreover, p53 has been reported to accumulate in the mitochondria in response to stress [147]. Besides p53, a number of widely known DNA repair factors, including ATM, BRCA1, PARP, PARG, and RB, localize in the mitochondria or regulate their functions [148–152]. The surveillance of the 5′-upstream regions of these DNA repair factor-encoding genes revealed that they commonly possess duplicated GGAA-motifs [53, 78].

GGAA-motif duplications are found in the bidirectional *APEX1/OSGEP* promoter region. The *APEX1* encodes apurinic/apyrimidinic endonuclease 1 (APE1) that regulates both the base excision repair (BER) and the mitochondrial DNA repair systems [75, 153]. The GGAA-duplication is contained in the regulatory region of the head–head configured *ACO2/PHF5A* genes [54]. The *ACO2* gene encodes aconitase, which plays an important role in the TCA cycle to produce citrate and isocitrate, and which also serves as a mitochondrial redox-sensor [154]. Importantly, aconitase and mitochondrial BER enzyme OGG1 (8-oxoguanine DNA glycosylase) cooperatively preserve mitochondrial DNA integrity [155]. We also confirmed that the duplicated GGAA-motifs were present in the 5′-upstream regions of the genes associated with Fanconi's anemia (FA) [53], which encode the DNA repair factors that are shown to regulate nucleotide excision repair and genome stability [156]. Interestingly, it was shown that mitochondrial dysfunction forces FA cells to produce energy by glycolysis [157], suggesting that FA proteins might be involved in the metabolic switch system in cancer cells. Additionally, Cockayne syndrome proteins CSA and CSB, which play roles in nucleotide excision repair (NER), accumulate in the mitochondria under oxidative stress [158]. In KRAS/LKB1-mutant lung cancer cells, carbamoyl phosphate synthetase-1 (CPS1), which is localized in mitochondria and which eliminates NH_4 to initiate the urea cycle, also plays a role in controlling the pyrimidine/purine balance to regulate the integrity of nuclear DNAs [159]. In this circumstance, the silencing of the *CPS1* gene expression leads to an incomplete S-phase or apoptotic cell death due to increased DNA damage. As expected, the duplicated GGAA is present in the *CPS1/LANCL1* bidirectional promoter region. However, no such element is found near the TSSs of either the *CAD* or *ASS1* genes, which encode cytoplasmic enzymes carbamoyl phosphate syntetase-2 and argininosuccinate synthase, respectively. These observations suggest that expression of the mitochondria-localizing, DNA repair-associated protein-encoding genes could be cooperatively regulated by duplicated GGAA-motif binding TFs, supporting the hypothesis that mitochondrial dysfunction causes oncogenesis [8].

5.3. The communication between telomeres and mitochondria may depend on the NAD+/ NADH ratio

The telomeres and mitochondria are thought to communicate with each other [160]. Several nuclear DNA repair factors play roles in the maintenance of mtDNAs, and damaged mtDNAs in turn exert signals to regulate nuclear transcription [74]. The system by which DNA repair/ energy production is monitored might be mediated by the balance of the NAD+/NADH ratio, which is regulated by a number of enzymes in the nuclei, mitochondria, and cytosol [161]. In breast cancer cells, the crosstalk between BRCA1 and PARP1 maintains the stability of the DNA repair ability, which would be partly sensitive to the NAD+ concentration [162].

The mitochondria might have conveniently deposited their function-associated genes into the nuclei, but need to take care, especially when DNA damage occurs. However, high-dose or repeated DNA damage may eventually activate the PARP enzyme, which consumes NAD+ as a substrate for the synthesis of PAR, to initiate the DNA repair system [66]. The decrease in the NAD+ level will subsequently cause incomplete TCA cycle progression and the dysregulation of respiration/OXPHOS, accompanied by the reduced expression of the mitochondrial function-associated genes. At this stage, the "Warburg effect" can be observed (**Figure 1**).

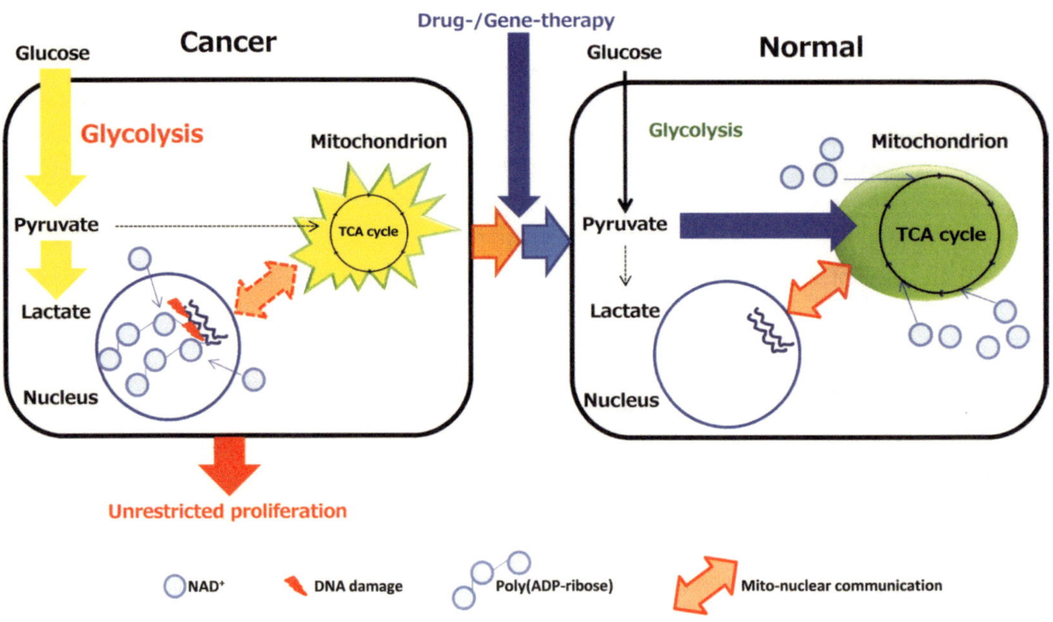

Figure 1. Toward the establishment of a novel cancer therapy. Cellular NAD+ molecules will decrease in accordance with aging or increased levels of various types of stress, especially DNA damage, which activates the PARP enzyme, which synthesizes PAR to consume NAD+ as a substrate. Subsequently, alterations in the transcriptional profile might occur, leading to a reduction or the mismanagement of the mitochondrial functions. In these circumstances, energy producing mitochondrial respiratory systems will decline or be dysregulated, while glycolysis will be enhanced providing ATP molecules that allow cells to proliferate in an unrestricted manner. Novel cancer therapies should be based on the concept that they will never kill cancer cells; rather, they should force the cells to regain their normal respiratory systems, including the TCA cycle and OXPHOS. The recovery of these mitochondria might also lead to the restoration of the mitonuclear communication system. In order to establish a gene therapy, it is necessary to reveal the molecular mechanisms that control the transcription of the mitochondrial function-associated genes.

6. The involvement of nicotinamide adenine dinucleotide (NAD^+) in oncogenesis and the aging process

The biological relevance of the NAD^+ molecule, especially in relation to its pivotal roles in metabolism and the protection of chromosomal DNAs, has been discussed in detail [66, 67]. A recent study showed that nuclear PAR can be utilized by NUDIX5 to supply ATP molecules, which are required for chromatin remodeling [86]. Moreover, NAD^+ and its precursor nicotinamide have been reported to ameliorate metabolism or the mitochondrial functions [163–165]. The repletion of NAD^+ improves the mitochondrial functions to prolong the life span of adult mouse stem cells [166]. Conversely, decreased concentrations of NAD^+ could cause aging or aging-related diseases [75]. These observations suggest that the NAD^+ level may be correlated with mitohormesis [167], and that nutrient sensing molecules may control aging [57].

6.1. NAD^+ restricts the generation and development of cancer by supporting the mitochondrial functions

Several drugs that induce an increase in the intracellular NAD^+ level are expected to contribute to the establishment of novel therapeutics for treating age-related diseases, including cancer [168]. Mitochondrial dysfunction has been suggested to be associated with the development of tumors or cancerous cells [169, 170]. In breast cancer cells, the knockdown of the subunit NDUFV1 leads to an aberration in complex I, which was shown to enhance aggressiveness or metastasis [171]. An increase in the cellular level of NAD^+ may be associated with the improvement of the mitochondrial integrity to suppress oncogenesis. PGC-1α, which upregulates mitochondrial biogenesis, drives NAD^+ biosynthesis and thereby induces stress resistance [172]. A recent study showed that PGC-1α suppresses the metastasis of melanoma, acting on the transcription program, namely the PGC-1α-ID2-TCF-integrin axis [173].

A loss of CSB, which can localize in the mitochondria [158], activates PARP1 to synthesize PAR [174], suggesting that the dysregulation of the mitochondrial functions to regulate DNA repair system may reduce the NAD^+/NADH molecular ratio.

6.2. NAD^+-dependent transcription of DNA repair factor-encoding genes

It is worth noting again that the NAD^+ molecule is the substrate for the PARP enzyme, which is required for the DNA damage response and the DNA repair system [66, 67]. The inhibition of the PARP1 enzyme ameliorates the mitochondrial metabolism through the activation of SIRT1 [175]. Conversely, the over-activation of the PARP1 enzyme can lead to mitochondrial dysfunction [176]. The *PARP1* gene expression was found to be negatively regulated when poly(ADP-ribose) glycohydrolase (PARG) siRNAs were introduced into HeLa S3 cells [40], suggesting that the degradation of the PAR macromolecule is required for the transcription of the *PARP1* gene. Because the 5′-upstream regions of both the human *PARP1* and *PARG* genes commonly contain the duplicated GGAA-motifs [53, 54], these two genes may be regulated by an NAD^+-sensitive mechanism. The results support the concept that PARP1 is involved in the NAD^+-sensitive transcription system [85]. In summary, the NAD^+/NADH ratio not only contributes to the DNA repair, but also to the fine-tuning of the transcription of genes that encode the NAD^+ metabolism-associated DNA repair factors.

As described previously, the promoter regions of a number of genes that encode TCA cycle enzymes and DNA repair factors contain duplicated GGAA (TTCC) motifs [53, 54]. Thus, the fine-tuning of the transcription of mitochondrial function-associated factor- and DNA repair factor-encoding genes would be required for cells to conduct mitochondria in response to DNA damage-inducing stress.

7. The development of novel cancer therapeutics to improve mitochondrial functions

In cancer cells, the mitochondrial functions are downregulated but glycolysis is upregulated [7, 8]. Thus, inhibitors of glycolysis/PDHK1/PARP, which target the metabolic switch in cancer cells, could be effective anti-cancer drugs [59]. In general, glycolysis- or glycolytic pathway-targeting drugs are expected to kill cancer cells specifically. For example, 2-deoxy-D-glucose, cisplatin and 5-FU—which have an inhibitory effect on glycolysis—are used to treat cancer in the clinical setting [177]. However, glycolysis is one of the most essential biological reactions. Thus, glycolysis inhibitors may be harmful or toxic to normal cells. Given that mitochondrial dysfunction is another essential cause of oncogenesis, the improvement of the mitochondria might provide clues that can be used to design innovative next-generation cancer therapies.

7.1. Chemicals that will initiate the recovery of mitochondria

Our previous *in vitro* studies showed that Rsv moderately upregulates the expression of various duplicated GGAA-motif-driven genes, including *TP53* and *HELB* [46, 48, 78]. Given that the increase in the NAD^+/NADH ratio can improve the mitochondrial functions, the introduction of the redox reaction-associated genes may be applied in cancer treatment. PARP inhibitors, which are especially effective for treating cancer with BRCA1 and BRCA2 mutations by disrupting specific types of DNA repair systems, are clinically approved drugs [89]. Another compound is TEMPOL, an antioxidant that has a suppressive effect on tumor cell proliferation [178], which increases the cellular NAD^+ level, supporting the DNA repair system [179, 180]. A number of compounds that target mitochondria have been tested in clinical trials [181]. Tocotrienols and their analogues target mitochondria and the immune system, causing the death of cancer cells [182]. Metformin and rapamycin are also expected to be novel anti-cancer/aging drugs that effectively suppress mTOR signaling [183]. Activators of mTOR, AMPK, and PGC-1α have been shown to have a synergistic effect with PD-1 blockade therapy [184], suggesting that mitochondrial activation can augment the immune response.

7.2. Possible gene-therapies that improve the mitochondrial functions

PGC-1α, which is encoded by the *PPARGC1A* gene, has been shown to be involved in the *de novo* synthesis of the NAD^+ [172]. Recently, it was reported that lactamase β (LACTB) is a multifunctional protein, which suppresses tumors through its effects on the mitochondrial lipid metabolism [185]. LACTB is included in mitochondrial complex I and treatment of fibroblast cells with its siRNA reduces complex I activity [186]. It therefore works as an upregulator of NAD^+. As expected, multiple duplications of the GGAA-motif are present in the bidirectional promoter region between the *LACTB* (*MRPL56*) gene and the bidirectional partner *LOC107987798*. We confirmed that the duplicated GGAA-motif is present near the TSS of the human *PDSS2* gene, which encodes prenyl-diphosphatase synthase subunit 2, which is a modulator of the complex I–III and II–III [133]. The PDSS2 is required for the integrity of Coenzyme Q (CoQ) or ubiquinone, which can improve the mitochondrial functions [187]. Thus, PDSS2 would be one of the targets for novel anticancer agents [188, 189]. The introduction of the *LbNOX* gene, which encodes bacterial NADH oxidase, into HeLa cells via a lentiviral vector ameliorates the proliferative and metabolic defects caused by the impairment of the electron transport chain (ETC) [190].These lines of evidence suggest that NAD^+ metabolism regulator encoding genes, including *PARP*, *PARG*, and *NAMPT*, as well as the *PPARGC1A*, *LACTB*, *PDSS2*, and *LbNOX* genes, could be applied or targeted in anti-cancer gene therapy.

Alternatively, TF-encoding genes can be applied to anti-cancer therapies that aid in the recovery of mitochondria. First, the transcription modulator CtBP might be artificially controlled to suppress oncogenesis or cancer progression [83, 84]. Second, because duplicated GGAA-motifs are present in the 5′-upstream regions of a number of DNA repair factor- and mitochondrial factor-encoding genes, GGAA-motif binding factors could upregulate the mitochondrial functions at the transcriptional level. Recently, it was reported that mouse Gabp, which is an ETS family protein, is required for mitochondrial biogenesis through the regulation of the *Tfb1m* gene [191], suggesting that a *GABP* expression vector might be designed and constructed for cancer treatment. The 5′-upstream regions of a number of human genes contain the GGAA-duplication, and it is a GC-box that is very frequently found near the GGAA-core motif [12]. Recently, it was reported that mutations on the ETS family protein-encoding *ERF* and *ERG* genes play roles in prostate oncogenesis [192], implying that imbalances in GGAA-binding TFs could lead to aberrant gene expression. In order to determine which TF-encoding genes should be chosen, the mechanisms through which each of these genes is differently regulated during tumorigenesis should be elucidated.

8. Conclusions and future prospects

In this article, we focused on the transcription mechanism that regulates the mitochondrial functions and the DNA repair systems, both of which decline with aging. Although the molecular mechanisms underlying the regulation of the expression of these genes are not yet fully understood, several lines of evidence suggest that it is dependent on the NAD^+/NADH balance.

The anti-cancer drugs that are currently in use, including metabolism inhibitors, telomerase inhibitors, and apoptosis inducers, were developed with the common intention of killing cancer cells. Although immune receptor target drugs have been applied in the clinical setting, they are similar in that they force cancer cells to die. The anti-cancer drugs that are currently in use damage both malignant cancer cells and normal healthy cells. Importantly, the undesired effects of these anti-cancer drugs are problematic with regard to the quality of life (QOL) of cancer patients, especially those who are too old to endure severe adverse effects that occur during the course of chemotherapy. In order to avoid lethal side effects, individual whole genome sequencing to identify drug sensitivities, the development of a side-effect monitoring system, and the improvement of treatment policies could be adapted. These are the burdens that are necessitated by the intrinsic concept underlying the development and creation of most anti-cancer drugs.

In the near future, novel anti-cancer drugs or therapies must be developed and established. These drugs should not kill cancer cells; rather they should give them a chance to regain the right mitochondrial functions and DNA repair systems, and immunological responses. Natural or chemical compounds can ameliorate the NAD^+/NADH level to improve the mitochondrial functions, DNA repair systems, and even immune responses. Alternatively, specific TF expression vector(s) could be introduced into cancer cells to lead them to recover to a healthy state. A number of promoter regions of the mitochondrial function-, DNA repair-, and anti-viral/tumor factor-encoding genes have duplicated GGAA-motifs with GC-boxes. Needless to say, it is necessary to determine the TFs that should and should not be applied prior to their clinical use. Based on this novel concept, the design of anticancer/tumor drugs or gene transfer vector(s) will contribute to the prevention of aging and its associated diseases, including cancer.

Acknowledgements

The authors are grateful to Asuka Shinozaki, Akiko Kawahara, Erisa Murayama, and Mayu Yamamura for their discussion and outstanding technical assistance.

Abbreviations

CR	caloric restriction
FA	Fanconi's anemia
HDAC	histone deacetylase
IFN	interferon
ISG	interferon-stimulated gene
OXPHOS	oxidative phosphorylation
PAR	poly(ADP-ribose)
PARG	poly(ADP-ribose) glycohydrolase
PARP	poly(ADP-ribose) polymerase
TF	transcription factor
TSS	transcription start site

Author details

Fumiaki Uchiumi[1]*, Jun Arakawa[1], Yutaka Takihara[1], Motohiro Akui[1], Hiroshi Hamada[1] and Sei-ichi Tanuma[2]

*Address all correspondence to: uchiumi@rs.noda.tus.ac.jp

1 Department of Gene Regulation, Faculty of Pharmaceutical Sciences, Tokyo University of Science, Noda, Chiba-ken, Japan

2 Department of Biochemistry, Faculty of Pharmaceutical Sciences, Tokyo University of Science, Noda, Chiba-ken, Japan

References

[1] Kandoth C, McLellan MD, Vandin F, Ye K, Niu B, Lu C, et al. Mutational landscape and significance across 12 major cancer types. Nature. 2013;**502**(7471):333-339

[2] Rahman N. Realizing the promise of cancer predisposition genes. Nature. 2014;**505**(7483):302-308

[3] Aronson S, Rehm H. Building the foundation for genomics in precision medicine. Nature. 2015;**526**(7573):336-342

[4] Wishart DS, Mandal R, Stanislaus A, Ramirez-Gaona M. Cancer metabolomics and the human metabolome database. Metabolomics. 2016;**6**(1):E10

[5] Warburg O. On the origin of cancer cells. Science. 1956;**123**(3191):309-314

[6] Vander Heiden MG, Cantley LC, Thompson CB. Understanding the Warburg effect: The metabolic requirements of cell proliferation. Science. 2009;**324**(5930):1029-1033

[7] Seyfried TN, Flores RE, Poff AM, D'Agostino DP. Cancer as a metabolic disease: Implications for novel therapeutics. Carcinogenesis. 2014;**35**(3):515-527

[8] Seyfried TN. Cancer as a mitochondrial metabolic disease. Frontiers in Cell and Developmental Biology. 2015;**3**:43

[9] Vafai SB, Mootha VK. Mitochondrial disorders as windows into an ancient organelle. Nature. 2012;**491**(7424):374-383

[10] Oikawa T, Yamada T. Molecular biology of the Ets family of transcription factors. Gene. 2003;**303**:11-34

[11] Hsu T, Trojanowska M, Watson DK. Ets proteins in biological control and cancer. Journal of Cellular Biochemistry. 2004;**91**(5):896-903

[12] Hollenhorst PC, Shah AA, Hopkins C, Graves BJ. Genome-wide analyses reveal properties of redundant and specific promoter occupancy within the *ETS* gene family. Genes & Development. 2007;**21**(15):1882-1894

[13] Uchiumi F, Miyazaki S, Tanuma S. The possible functions of duplicated *ets* (GGAA) motifs located near transcription start sites of various human genes. Cellular and Molecular Life Sciences. 2011;**68**(12):2039-2051

[14] Uchiumi F, Miyazaki S, Tanuma S. Biological functions of the duplicated GGAA-motifs in various human promoter regions. Yakugaku Zasshi. 2011;**1311**(12):1787-1800

[15] Kerr IM, Stark GR. The control of interferon-inducible gene expression. FEBS Letters. 1991;**285**(2):194-198

[16] Sheikh SZ, Kobayashi T, Matsuoka K, Onyiah JC, Plevy SE. Characterization of an interferon-stimulated response element (ISRE) in the *Il23a* promoter. The Journal of Biological Chemistry. 2011;**286**(2):1174-1180

[17] Chen YQ, Sengchanthalangsy LL, Hackett A, Ghosh G. NF-kappaB p65 (RelA) homodimer uses distinct mechanisms to recognize DNA targets. Structure. 2000;**8**(4):419-428

[18] Nelson N, Marks MS, Driggers PH, Ozato K. Interferon consensus sequence-binding protein, a member of the interferon regulatory factor family, suppresses interferon-induced gene transcription. Molecular and Cellular Biology. 1993;**13**(1):588-599

[19] Wang IM, Contursi C, Masumi A, Ma X, Trinchieri G, Ozato K. An IFN-γ-inducible transcription factor, IFN consensus sequence binding protein (ICSBP), stimulates IL12 p40 expression in macrophages. Journal of Immunology. 2000;**165**(1):271-279

[20] Nguyen VT, Benveniste EN. Involvement of STAT-1 and Ets family members in interferon-γ induction of CD40 transcription in microglia/macrophages. The Journal of Biological Chemistry. 2000;**275**(31):23674-23684

[21] Aittomäki S, Yang J, Scott EW, Simon MC, Silvennoinen O. Molecular basis of Stat1 and PU.1 cooperation in cytokine-induced Fcg receptor 1 promoter activation. International Immunology. 2004;**16**(2):265-274

[22] Kumar P, Garg R, Bolden G, Pandey KN. Interactive roles of Ets-1, Sp1, and acetylated histones in the retinoic acid-dependent activation of guanylyl cyclase/atrial natriuretic peptide receptor-A gene transcription. The Journal of Biological Chemistry. 2010;**285**(48):37521-37530

[23] FitzGerald PC, Shlyakhtenko A, Mir AA, Vinson C. Clustering of DNA sequences in human promoters. Genome Research. 2004;**14**(8):1562-1574

[24] Jin E, Liu J, Suehiro J, Yuan L, Okada Y, Nikolova-Krstevski V, et al. Differential roles for ETS, CREB, and EGR binding sites in mediating VEGF receptor 1 expression in vivo. Blood. 2009;**114**(27):5557-5566

[25] Chen HG, Han WJ, Deng M, Qin J, Yuan D, Liu JP, et al. Transcriptional regulation of PP2A-A alpha is mediated by multiple factors including AP-2alpha, CREB, ETS-1, and SP-1. PLoS One. 2009;**4**(9):e7019

[26] Perry DJ, Austin KJ, Hansen TR. Cloning of interferon-stimulated gene 17: The promoter and nuclear proteins that regulate transcription. Molecular Endocrinology. 1999;**13**(7):1197-1206

[27] Rouyez MC, Lestingi M, Charon M, Fichelson S, Buzyn A, Dusanter-Fourt I. IFN regulatory factor-2 cooperates with STAT1 to regulate transporter associated with antigen processing-1 promoter activity. Journal of Immunology. 2005;**174**(7):3948-3958

[28] Masumi A, Hamaguchi I, Kuramitsu M, Mizukami T, Takizawa K, Momose H, et al. Interferon regulatory factor-2 induces megakaryopoiesis in mouse bone marrow hematopoietic cells. FEBS Letters. 2009;**583**(21):3493-3500

[29] Cho HY, Lee SW, Seo SK, Choi IW, Choi I, Lee SW. Interferon-sensitive response element (ISRE) is mainly responsible for IFN-α-induced upregulation of programmed death-1 (PD-1) in macrophages. Biochimica et Biophysica Acta. 2008;**1779**(12):811-819

[30] De Veer MJ, Holko M, Frevel M, Walker E, Der S, Paranjape JM, et al. Functional classification of interferon-stimulated genes identified using microarrays. Journal of Leukocyte Biology. 2001;**69**(6):912-920

[31] Schoggins JW, Wilson SJ, Panis M, Murphy MY, Jones CT, Bieniasz P, et al. A diverse range of gene products are effectors of the type I interferon antiviral response. Nature. 2011;**472**(7344):481-485

[32] Uchiumi F, Larsen S, Masumi A, Tanuma S. The putative implications of duplicated GGAA-motifs located in the human interferon regulated genes (ISGs). In: Genomics I-Humans, Animals and Plants. Hong Kong: iConcept Press Ltd; 2013. p. 87-105

[33] Larsen S, Kawamoto S, Tanuma S, Uchiumi F. The hematopoietic regulator, ELF-1, enhances the transcriptional response to Interferon-β of the OAS1 anti-viral gene. Scientific Reports. 2015;**5**:17497

[34] Sementchenko VI, Watson DK. Ets target genes: Past, present and future. Oncogene. 2000;**19**(55):6533-6548

[35] Takaoka A, Hayakawa S, Yanai H, Stoiber D, Negishi H, Kikuchi H, et al. Integration of interferon-α/β signaling to p53 responses in tumor suppression and antiviral defense. Nature. 2003;**424**(6948):516-523

[36] Lee SH, Kim JW, Lee HW, Cho YS, Oh SH, Kim YJ, et al. Interferon regulatory factor-1 (IRF-1) is a mediator for interferon-gamma induced attenuation of telomerase activity and human telomerase reverse transcriptase (hTERT) expression. Oncogene. 2003;**22**(3):381-391

[37] Barnes BJ, Kellum MJ, Pinder KE, Frisancho JA, Pitha PM. Interferon regulatory factor 5, a novel mediator of cell cycle arrest and cell death. Cancer Research. 2003;**63**(19):6424-6431

[38] Xiong GM, Gasser S. Integration of the DNA damage response with innate immune pathways. In: Vengrova S, editor. DNA Repair and Human Health. InTech OPEN: Rijeka, Croatia; 2011. p. 715-742

[39] Yokoyama Y, Kawamoto T, Mitsuuchi Y, Kurosaki T, Toda K, Ushiro H, et al. Human poly(ADP-ribose) polymerase gene. Cloning of the promoter region. European Journal of Biochemistry. 1990;**194**(2):521-526

[40] Uchiumi F, Watanabe T, Ohta R, Abe H, Tanuma S. *PARP1* gene expression is downregulated by knockdown of PARG gene. Oncology Reports. 2013;**29**(5):1683-1688

[41] Wei L, Nakajima S, Hsieh CL, Kanno S, Masutani M, Levine AS, et al. Damage response of XRCC1 at sites of DNA single strand breaks is regulated by phosphorylation and ubiquitylation after degradation of poly(ADPribose). Journal of Cell Science. 2013;**126**(Pt 19):4414-4423

[42] Niere M, Mashimo M, Agledal L, Dölle C, Kasamatsu A, Kato J, et al. ADP-ribosylhydrolase 3 (ARH3), not poly(ADP-ribose) glycohydrolase (PARG) isoforms, is responsible for degradation of mitochondrial matrix associated poly(ADP-ribose). The Journal of Biological Chemistry. 2012;**287**(20):16088-16102

[43] Leung A, Todorova T, Ando Y, Chang P. Poly(ADP-ribose) regulate post-transcriptional gene regulation in the cytoplasm. RNA Biology. 2012;**9**(5):542-548

[44] Gibson BA, Kraus WL. New insights into the molecular and cellular functions of poly(ADP-ribose) and PARPs. Nature Reviews. Molecular Cell Biology. 2012;**13**(7):411-424

[45] Zhou B, Ikejima T, Watanabe T, Iwakoshi K, Idei Y, Tanuma S, et al. The effect of 2-deoxy-D-glucose on Werner syndrome RecQ helicase gene. FEBS Letters. 2009;**583**(8):1331-1336

[46] Uchiumi F, Watanabe T, Hasegawa S, Hoshi T, Higami Y, Tanuma S. The effect of Resveratrol on the Werner Syndrome RecQ helicase gene and telomerase activity. Current Aging Science. 2011;**4**(1):1-7

[47] Ingram DK, Zhu M, Mamczarz J, Zou S, Lane MA, Roth GS, et al. Calorie restriction mimetics: An emerging research field. Aging Cell. 2006;**5**(2):97-108

[48] Uchiumi F, Arakawa J, Iwakoshi K, Ishibashi S, Tanuma S. Characterization of the 5′-flanking region of the human DNA helicase B (*HELB*) gene and its response to trans-resveratrol. Scientific Reports. 2016;**6**:24510

[49] Taneja P, Gu J, Peng R, Carrick R, Uchiumi F, Ott RD, et al. A dominant-negative mutant of human DNA helicase B blocks the onset of chromosomal DNA replication. The Journal of Biological Chemistry. 2002;**277**(43):40853-40861

[50] Gu J, Xia X, Yan P, Liu H, Podust VN, Reynolds AB, et al. Cell cycle-dependent regulation of a human DNA helicase that localizes in DNA damage foci. Molecular Biology of the Cell. 2004;**15**(7):3320-3332

[51] Guler GD, Liu H, Vaithiyalingam S, Arnett DR, Kremmer E, Chazin WJ, et al. Human DNA helicase B (HDHB) binds to replication protein A and facilitates cellular recovery from replication stress. The Journal of Biological Chemistry. 2012;**287**(9):6469-6481

[52] Tkáč J, Xu G, Adhikary H, Young JT, Gallo D, Escribano-Díaz C, et al. HELB is a feedback inhibitor of DNA end resection. Molecular Cell. 2016;**61**(3):405-418

[53] Uchiumi F, Larsen S, Tanuma S. Transcriptional regulation of the human genes that encode DNA repair- and mitochondrial function-associated proteins. In: Chen C, editor. Advances in DNA Repair. Rijeka, Croatia: InTech OPEN; 2015. p. 129-167

[54] Uchiumi F, Fujikawa M, Miyazaki S, Tanuma S. Implication of bidirectional promoters containing duplicated GGAA motifs of mitochondrial function-associated genes. AIMS Molecular Science. 2013;**1**(1):1-26

[55] Seyfried TN, Shelton LM. Cancer as a metabolic disease. Nutrition and Metabolism. 2010;**7**:7

[56] Schultze A, Harris AL. How cancer metabolism is tuned for proliferation and vulnerable to disruption. Nature. 2012;**491**(7424):364-373

[57] López-Otín C, Serrano M, Partridge L, Blasco MA, Kroemer G. The hallmarks of aging. Cell. 2013;**153**(6):1194-1217

[58] Gomes AP, Price NL, Ling AJY, Mosiehi JJ, Montgomery MK, Rajman L, et al. Declining NAD^+ induces a pseudohypoxic state disrupting nuclear-mitochondrial communication during aging. Cell. 2013;**155**(7):1624-1638

[59] Pollard PJ, Brière JJ, Alam NA, Barwell J, Barclay E, Wortham NC, et al. Accumulation of Krebs cycle intermediates and over-expression of HIFalpha in tumors which result from germline FH and SDH mutations. Human Molecular Genetics. 2005;**14**(15):2231-2239

[60] Hoekstra AS, de Graaff MA, Briaire-de Bruijn IH, Ras C, Seifar RM, van Minderhout I, et al. Inactivation of SDH and FH cause loss of 5hmC and increased H3K9me3 in paraganglioma/pheochromocytoma and smooth muscle tumors. Oncotarget. 2015;**6**(36):38777-38788

[61] Desideri E, Vegliante R, Ciriolo MR. Mitochondrial dysfunctions in cancer: Genetic defects and oncogenic signaling impinging on TCA cycle activity. Cancer Letters. 2015;**356**(2 Pt A): 217-223

[62] Dang L, White DW, Gross S, Bennett BD, Bittinger MA, Driggers EM, et al. Cancer-associated IDH1 mutations produce 2-hydroxyglutarate. Nature. 2009;**462**(7274):739-744

[63] Yan H, Parsons DW, Jin G, McLendon R, Rasheed BA, Yuan W, et al. IDH1 and IDH2 mutations in gliomas. The New England Journal of Medicine. 2009;**360**(8):765-773

[64] Lu C, Ward PS, Kapoor GS, Rohle D, Turcan S, Abdel-Wahab O, et al. IDH mutation impairs histonedemethylation and results in a block to cell differentiation. Nature. 2012;**483**(7390):474-478

[65] Tan B, Young DA, Lu Z-H, Meier TI, Shepard RL, Roth K, et al. Pharmacological inhibition of nicotinamide phosphoribosyltransferase (NAMPT), an enzyme essential for NAD^+ biosynthesis, in human cancer cells. The Journal of Biological Chemistry. 2012;**288**(5):3500-3511

[66] Maruta H, Okita N, Takasawa R, Uchiumi F, Hatano T, Tanuma S. The Involvement of ATP produced via (ADP-Ribose)(n) in the maintenance of DNA replication apparatus during DNA Repair. Biological & Pharmaceutical Bulletin. 2007;**30**(3):447-450

[67] Tanuma S, Sato A, Oyama T, Yoshimori Y, Abe H, Uchiumi F. New insights into the roles of NAD^+-poly(ADP-ribose) metabolism and poly(ADP-ribose) glycohydrolase. Current Protein & Peptide Science. 2016;**17**(7):668-682

[68] Uchiumi F, Larsen S, Tanuma S. Possible roles of a duplicated GGAA motif as a driver cis-element for cancer-associated genes. In: Understand Cancer – Research and Treatment. Hong Kong, iConcept Press Ltd; 2016. p. 1-25

[69] Gray LR, Tompkins SC, Taylor EB. Regulation of pyruvate metabolism and human disease. Cellular and Molecular Life Sciences. 2014;**71**(14):2577-2604

[70] Dey P, Baddour J, Muller F, Wu CC, Wang H, Liao WT, et al. Genomic deletion of malic enzyme 2 confers collateral lethality in pancreatic cancer. Nature. 2017;**542**(7639):119-123

[71] Jolma A, Yin Y, Nitta KR, Dave K, Popov A, Taipale M, et al. DNA-dependent formation of transcription factor pairs alters their binding specificity. Nature. 2016;**527**(7578):384-388

[72] Wolters S, Schumacher B. Genome maintenance and transcription integrity in aging and disease. Frontiers in Genetics. 2013;**4**:19

[73] Pohjoismäki JLO, Boettger T, Liu Z, Goffart S, Szibor M, Braun T. Oxidative stress during mitochondrial biogenesis compromises mtDNA integrity in growing hearts and induces a global DNA repair response. Nucleic Acids Research. 2012;**40**(14):6595-6607

[74] Kazak L, Reyes A, Holt IJ. Minimizing the damage: Repair pathways keep mitochondrial DNA intact. Nature Reviews. Molecular Cell Biology. 2012;**13**(11):659-671

[75] Rehmani I, Liu F, Liu A. Chemistry, mechanisms, and disease pathogenesis. In: Villamena FA, editor. Molecular Basis of Oxidative Stress. Hoboken, NJ: John Wiley & Sons; 2013. p. 179-201

[76] Gut P, Verdin E. The nexus of chromatin regulation and intermediary metabolism. Nature. 2013;**502**(7472):489-498

[77] Liu J, Kim J, Oberdoerffer P. Metabolic modulation of chromatin: Implications for DNA repair and genomic integrity. Frontiers in Genetics. 2013;**4**:182

[78] Uchiumi F, Shoji K, Sasaki Y, Sasaki M, Sasaki Y, Oyama T, et al. Characterization of the 5′-flanking region of the human *TP53* gene and its response to the natural compound, Resveratrol. Journal of Biochemistry. 2016;**159**(4):437-447

[79] Wood JG, Rogina B, Lavu S, Howitz K, Helfand SL, Tatar M, et al. Sirtuin activators mimic caloric restriction and delay aging in metazoans. Nature. 2004;**430**(7000):686-689

[80] Park SJ, Ahmad F, Philp A, Baar K, Williams T, Luo H, et al. Resveratrol ameliorates aging-related metabolic phenotypes by inhibiting cAMP phosphodiesterases. Cell. 2012; **148**(3):421-433

[81] Gueguen N, Desquiret-Dumas V, Leman G, Chupin S, Baron S, Nivet-Antoine V, et al. Resveratroldirectly binds to mitochondrial complex I and increases oxidative stress in brain mitochondria of aged mice. PLoS One. 2015;**10**(12):e0144290

[82] Di LJ, Fernandez AG, de Siervi A, Longo DL, Gardner K. Transcriptional regulation of BRCA1 expression by a metabolic switch. Nature Structural & Molecular Biology. 2010;**17**(12):1406-1413

[83] Chinnadurai G. CtBP, an unconventional transcription corepressor in development and oncogenesis. Molecular Cell. 2002;**9**(2):213-224

[84] Chinnadurai G. The transcription corepressor CtBP: A foe of multiple tumor suppressors. Cancer Research. 2009;**69**(3):731-734

[85] Gibson BA, Zhang Y, Jiang H, Hussey KM, Shrimp JH, Lin H, et al. Chemical genetic discovery of PARP targets reveals a role for PARP-1 in transcription elongation. Science. 2016;**353**(6294):45-50

[86] Wright RH, Lioutas A, Le Dily F, Soronellas D, Pohl A, Bonet J, et al. ADP-ribose-derived nuclear ATP synthesis by NUDIX5 is required for chromatin remodeling. Science. 2016;**352**(6290):1221-1225

[87] Porporato PE, Payen VL, Baselet B, Sonveaux P. Metabolic changes associated with tumor metastasis, part 2: Mitochondria, lipid and amino acid metabolism. Cellular and Molecular Life Sciences. 2016;**73**(7):1349-1363

[88] Gentric G, Mieulet V, Mechta-Grigoriou F. Heterogeneity in cancer metabolism: New concepts in an old field. Antioxidants & Redox Signaling. 2017;**26**(9):462-485

[89] Lord CJ, Ashworth A. PARP inhibitors: Synthetic lethality in the clinic. Science. 2017; **355**(6330):1152-1158

[90] Li J, Bonkowski MS, Moniot S, Zhang D, Hubbard BP, Ling AJY, et al. A conserved NAD^+ binding pocket that regulates protein-protein interactions during aging. Science. 2017;**355**(6331):1312-1317

[91] Gorbunova V, Seluanov A, Mao Z, Hine C. Changes in DNA repair during aging. Nucleic Acids Research. 2007;**35**(22):7466-7474

[92] Kraus WL, Lis JT. PARP goes transcription. Cell. 2003;**113**(6):677-683

[93] Luo X, Ryu KW, Kim DS, Nandu T, Medina CJ, Gupte R, et al. PARP-1 controls the adipogenic transcriptional program by PARylating C/EBPβ and modulating its transcriptional activity. Molecular Cell. 2017;**65**(2):260-271

[94] Ke Y, Han Y, Guo X, Wen J, Wang K, Jiang X, et al. PARP1 promotes gene expression at the post-transcriptional level by modulating the RNA-binding protein HuR. Nature Communications. 2017;**8**:14632

[95] Lu J, Zhang R, Hong H, Yang Z, Sun D, Sun S, et al. The poly(ADP-ribosyl)ation of FoxO3 mediated by PARP1 participates in isoproterenol-induced cardiac hypertrophy. Biochimica et Biophysica Acta. 2016;**1863**(12):3027-3039

[96] McDevitt MA. Clinical applications of epigenetics. In: Fraga M, Fernández AF, editors. Epigenomics in health and disease. San Diego, CA: Academic Press; 2016. p. 271-295

[97] Suvà ML, Riggi N, Bernstein BE. Epigenetic reprogramming in cancer. Science. 2013;**339**(6127):1567-1570

[98] Blakey CA, Litt MD. Epigenetic gene expression-an introduction. In: Huang S, Litt MD, Ann Blakey C, editors. Epigenetic Gene Expression and Regulation. San Diego, CA: Academic Press; 2016. p. 1-19

[99] Hentze MW, Preiss T. The REM phase of gene regulation. Trends in Biochemical Sciences. 2010;**35**(8):423-426

[100] Verdin E. NAD^+ in aging, metabolism, and neurodegeneration. Science. 2015;**350**(6265): 1208-1213

[101] Pearce EL, Poffenberger MC, Chang CH, Jones RG. Fueling immunity: Insights into metabolism and lymphocyte function. Science. 2013;**342**(6155):1242454

[102] Tanuma S, Johnson GS. ADP-ribosylation of nonhistone high mobility group proteins in intact cells. The Journal of Biological Chemistry. 1983;**258**(7):4067-4070

[103] Tanuma S, Johnson LD, Johnson GS. ADP-ribosylation of chromosomal proteins and mouse mammary tumor virus gene expression. The Journal of Biological Chemistry. 1983;**258**(24):15371-15375

[104] Ogata N, Ueda K, Hayaishi O. ADP-ribosylation of histone H2B. Identification of glutamic acid residue 2 as the modification site. The Journal of Biological Chemistry. 1980; **255**(16):7610-7615

[105] Ogata N, Ueda K, Kagamiyama H, Hayaishi O. ADP-ribosylation of histone H1. Identification of glutamic acid residue 2, 14, and the COOH-terminal lysine residue as modification sites. The Journal of Biological Chemistry. 1980;**255**(16):7616-7620

[106] Yu W, Ginjala V, Pant V, Chernukhin I, Whitehead J, Docquier F, et al. Poly(ADP-ribosyl)ation regulates CTCF-dependent chromatin insulation. Nature Genetics. 2004;**36**(10):1105-1110

[107] Klenova E, Ohlsson R. Poly(ADP-ribosyl)ation and epigenetics. Is CTCF PARt of the plot? Cell Cycle. 2005;**4**(1):96-101

[108] Han D, Chen Q, Shi J, Zhang F, Yu X. CTCF participates in DNA damage response via poly(ADP-ribosyl)ation. Scientific Reports. 2017;**7**:43530

[109] Reale A, Matteis GD, Galleazzi G, Zampieri M, Caiafa P. Modulation of DNMT1 activity by ADP-ribose polymers. Oncogene. 2005;**24**(1):13-19

[110] Caiafa P, Guastafierro T, Zampieri M. Epigenetics: Poly(ADP-ribosyl)ation of PARP-1 regulates genomic methylation patterns. The FASEB Journal. 2009;**23**(3):672-678

[111] Martin KA, Cesaroni M, Denny MF, Lupey LN, Tempera I. Global transcriptome analysis reveals that poly(ADP-ribose) polymerase 1 regulates gene expression through EZH2. Molecular and Cellular Biology. 2015;**35**(23):3934-3944

[112] Cao R, Wang L, Wang H, Xia L, Erdjument-Bromage H, Tempst P, et al. Role of histone H3 lysine 27 methylation in polycomb-group silencing. Science. 2002;**298**(5595):1039-1043

[113] Vijg J. From genome to phenome. In: Vijg J, editor. Aging of the Genome. The Dual Role of DNA in Life and Death. New York, NY: Oxford University Press; 2007. p. 233-288

[114] Grube K, Bürkle A. Poly(ADP-ribose) polymerase activity in mononuclear leukocytes of 13 mammalian species correlates with species-specific life span. Proceedings of the National Academy of Sciences of the United States of America. 1992;**89**(24):11759-11763

[115] Houtkooper RH, Pirinen E, Auwerx J. Sirtuins as regulators of metabolism and health-span. Nature Reviews. Molecular Cell Biology. 2012;**13**(4):225-238

[116] Neidhart M. DNA methylation and epigenetic biomarkers in cancer. In: Neidhart M, editor. DNA Methylation and Complex Human Disease. San Diego, CA: Academic Press; 2016. p. 9-27

[117] Neidhart M. DNA methylation in metabolic diseases. In: Neidhart M, editor. DNA Methylation and Complex Human Disease. San Diego, CA: Academic Press; 2016. p. 201-214

[118] Neri F, Rapelli S, Krepelova A, Incarnato D, Parlato C, Basile G, et al. Intragenic DNA methylation prevents spurious transcription initiation. Nature. 2017;**543**(7643):72-77

[119] Hu X, Chen Y, Zhao ZJ. Structure, regulation, and function of TET family proteins. In: Huang S, Litt MD, Ann Blakey C, editors. Epigenetic Gene Expression and Regulation. San Diego, CA: Academic Press; 2016. p. 379-395

[120] Thienpont B, Steinbacher J, Zhao H, D'Anna F, Kuchnio A, Ploumakis A, et al. Tumor hypoxia causes DNA hyper-methylation by reducing TET activity. Nature. 2016; **537**(7618):763-768

[121] Yin Y, Morgunova E, Jolma A, Kaasinen E, Sahu B, Khund-Sayeed S, et al. Impact of cyto-sine methylation on DNA binding specificities of human transcription factors. Science. 2017;**356**(6337):aaj2239

[122] Almeida LO, Neto MPC, Sousa LO, Tannous MA, Curti C, Leopoldino AM. SET onco-protein accumulation regulates transcription through DNA methylation and histone hypoacetylation. Oncotarget. 2017;**8**(16):26802-26818

[123] Zykovich A, Hubbard A, Flynn JM, Tarnopolsky M, Fraga MF, Kerksick C, et al. Genome-wide DNA methylation changes with age in disease-free human skeletal mus-cle. Aging Cell. 2014;**13**(2):360-366

[124] Florath I, Butterbach K, Müller H, Bewerunge-Hudler M, Brenner H. Cross-sectional and longitudinal changes in DNA methylation with age: An epigenome-wide analy-sis revealing over 60 novel age-associated CpG sites. Human Molecular Genetics. 2014;**23**(5):1186-1201

[125] Tang M, Luo H, Lu J. Genetically altered cancer epigenome. In: Huang S, Litt MD, Ann Blakey C, editors. Epigenetic Gene Expression and Regulation. San Diego, CA: Academic Press; 2016. p. 265-289

[126] Youn HD. Methylation and demethylation of DNA and histones in chromatin: The most complicated epigenetic marker. Experimental & Molecular Medicine. 2017;**49**(4):e321

[127] Choudhary C, Weinert BT, Nishida Y, Verdin E, Mann M. The growing landscape of lysine acetylation links metabolism and cell signalling. Nature Reviews. Molecular Cell Biology. 2014;**15**(8):536-550

[128] Verdin E, Ott M. 50 years of protein acetylation: From gene regulation to epigenetics, metabolism and beyond. Nature Reviews. Molecular Cell Biology. 2015;**16**(4):258-264

[129] Blakey CA, Litt MD. Histone modifications-models and mechanisms. In: Huang S, Litt MD, Ann Blakey C, editors. Epigenetic Gene Expression and Regulation. San Diego, CA: Academic Press; 2016. p. 21-42

[130] Yan B, Li X, Johnson A, Yang Y, Jian W, Qui Y. Epigenetic drugs for cancer therapy. In: Huang S, Litt MD, Blakey CA, editors. Epigenetic Gene Expression and Regulation. San Diego, CA: Academic Press; 2016. p. 397-423

[131] Chung JH, Manganiello V, Dyck JR. Resveratrol as a calorie restriction mimetic: Therapeutic implications. Trends in Cell Biology. 2012;**22**(10):546-554

[132] Roth GS, Ingram DK. Manipulation of health span and function by dietary caloric restriction mimetics. Annals of the New York Academy of Sciences. 2016;**1363**:5-10

[133] Uchiumi F, Arakawa J, Takihara Y, Akui M, Ishibashi S, Tanuma S. The effect of *trans*-resveratrol on the expression of the human DNA-repair associated genes. International Journal of Molecular Medicine. 2016;**3**(5):783-792

[134] Fang EF, Scheibye-Knudsen M, Chua KF, Mattson MP, Croteau DL, et al. Nuclear DNA damage signaling to mitochondria in aging. Nature Reviews. Molecular Cell Biology. 2016;**17**(5):308-321

[135] Quiros PM, Mottis A, Auwerx J. Mitonuclear communication in homeostasis and stress. Nature Reviews. Molecular Cell Biology. 2016;**17**(4):213-226

[136] Ku C, Nelson-Sathi S, Roettger M, Sousa FL, Lockhart PJ, Bryant D, et al. Endosymbiotic origin and differential loss of eukaryotic genes. Nature. 2015;**524**(7566):427-432

[137] Vogelstein B, Papadopoulos N, Velculescu VE, Zhou S, Diaz LA Jr, Kinzler KW. Cancer genome landscapes. Science. 2013;**339**(6127):1546-1558

[138] Tait SW, Green DR. Mitochondria and cell death: Outer membrane permeabilization and beyond. Nature Reviews. Molecular Cell Biology. 2010;**11**(9):621-632

[139] Estaquier J, Vallette F, Vayssiere JL, Mignotte B. The mitochondrial pathways of apoptosis. In: Scatena R, Bottoni P, Giardina B, editors. Advances in Mitochondrial Medicine. Dordrecht, Germany: Springer Science+Business Media BV; 2012. p. 157-183

[140] Kroemer G. Mitochondrial implication in apoptosis. Towards an endosymbiont hypothesis of apoptosis evolution. Cell Death and Differentiation. 1997;**4**(6):443-456

[141] Galluzzi L, Kepp O, Kroemer G. Mitochondria: Master regulators of danger signaling. Nature Reviews. Molecular Cell Biology. 2012;**13**(12):780-788

[142] Shankar S, Chen Q, Sarva K, Siddiqui I, Srivastava RK. Sensitization of TRAIL-resistant LNCaP cells by resveratrol (3, 4′, 5 tri-hydroxystilbene): Molecular mechanisms and therapieutic potential. Journal of Molecular Signaling. 2007;**2**:7

[143] Shankar S, Siddiqui I, Srivastava RK. Molecular mechanisms of resveratrol (3,4,5-tri-hydroxy-trans-stilbene) and its interaction with TNF-related apoptosis inducing ligand (TRAIL) in androgen-insensitive prostate cancer cells. Molecular and Cellular Biochemistry. 2007;**304**(1-2):273-285

[144] Venkatadri R, Muni T, Iyer AK, Yakisich JS, Azad N. Role of apoptosis-related miRNAs in resveratrol-induced breast cancer cell death. Cell Death Disease. 2016;**7**:e2104

[145] Vousden KH, Lane DP. p53 in health and disease. Nature Reviews. Molecular Cell Biology. 2007;**8**(4):275-283

[146] Vousden KH, Ryan KM. p53 and metabolism. Nature Reviews. Cancer. 2009;**9**(10):691-700

[147] Green DR, Kroemer G. Cytoplasmic functions of the tumor suppressor p53. Nature. 2009;**458**(7242):1127-1130

[148] King MC. "The race" to clone BRCA1. Science. 2014;**343**(6178):1462-1465

[149] Sharma NK, Lebedeva M, Thomas T, Kovalenko OA, Stumpf JD, Shadel G, et al. Intrinsic mitochondrial DNA repair defects in Ataxia Telangiectasia. DNA Repair (Amst). 2014;**13**:22-31

[150] Whatcott CJ, Meyer-Ficca ML, Meyer RG, Jacobson MK. A specific isoform of poly(ADP-ribose) glycohydrolase is targeted to the mitochondrial matrix by a N-terminal mitochondrial targeting sequence. Experimental Cell Research. 2009;**315**(20):3477-3485

[151] Rossi MN, Carbone M, Mostocotto C, Mancone C, Tripodi M, Maione R, et al. Mitochondrial localization of PARP-1 requires interaction with mitofilin and is involved in the maintenance of mitochondrial DNA integrity. The Journal of Biological Chemistry. 2009;**284**(46):31616-31624

[152] Moiseeva O, Bourdeau V, Roux A, Deschênes-Simard X, Ferbeyre G. Mitochondrial dysfunction contributes to oncogene-induced senescence. Molecular and Cellular Biology. 2009;**29**(16):4495-4507

[153] Mohan V, Madhusuden S. DNA base excision repair: Evolving biomarkers for personalized therapies in cancer. In: Chen C, editor. New Research Directions in DNA Repair. Rijeka, Croatia: InTechOPEN; 2013. p. 529-557

[154] Liu G, Kamp DW. Mitochondrial DNA damage: Role of Ogg1 and aconitase. In: Kruman I, editor. DNA Repair. Rijeka, Croatia: InTechOPEN; 2011. p. 85-102

[155] Kim SJ, Cheresh P, Williams D, Cheng Y, Ridge K, Schumacker PT, et al. Mitochondria-targeted Ogg1 and aconitase-2 prevent oxidant-induced mitochondrial DNA damage in Alveolar Epithelial cells. The Journal of Biological Chemistry. 2014;**289**(9):6165-6176

[156] Ceccaldi R, Sarangi P, D'Andrea AD. The Fanconi anaemia pathway: New players and new functions. Nature Reviews. Molecular Cell Biology. 2016;**17**(6):337-349

[157] Cappelli E, Cuccarolo P, Stroppiana G, Miano M, Bottega R, Cossu V, et al. Defects in mitochondrial energetic function compels Fanconi Anaemia cells to glycolytic metabolism. Biochimica et Biophysica Acta. 2017;**1863**(6):1214-1221

[158] Kamenisch Y, Fousteri M, Knoch J, von Thaler AK, Fehrenbacher B, Kato H, et al. Proteins of nucleotide and base excision repair pathways interact in mitochondria to protect from loss of subcutaneous fat, a hallmark of aging. The Journal of Experimental Medicine. 2010;**207**(2):379-390

[159] Kim J, Hu Z, Cai L, Li K, Choi E, Faubert B, et al. CPS1 maintains pyrimidine pools and DNA synthesis in KRAS/LKB1-mutant lung cancer cells. Nature. 2017;**546**(7656):168-172

[160] Sahin E, DePinho R. A axis of aging: Telomerase, p53 and mitochondria. Nature Reviews. Molecular Cell Biology. 2012;**13**(6):397-404

[161] Cantó C, Menzies KJ, Auwerx J. NAD^+ metabolism and the control of energy homeostasis: A balancing act between mitochondria and the nucleus. Cell Metabolism. 2015; **22**(1):31-53

[162] Li D, Bi FF, Chen NN, Cao JM, Sun WP, Zhou YM, et al. A novel crosstalk between BRCA1 and poly(ADP-ribose) polymerase 1 in breast cancer. Cell Cycle. 2014;**13**(21):3442-3449

[163] Cantó C, Houtkooper RH, Pirinen E, Youn DY, Oosterveer MH, Cen Y, et al. The NAD^+ precursor nicotinamide riboside enhances oxidative metabolism and protects against high-fat diet-induced obesity. Cell Metabolism. 2012;**15**(6):838-847

[164] Han X, Tai H, Wang X, Wang Z, Zhou J, Wei X, et al. AMPK activation protects cells from oxidative stress-induced senescence via autophagic flux restoration and intracellular NAD elevation. Aging Cell. 2016;**15**(3):416-427

[165] Yang Y, Sauve AA. NAD^+ metabolism: Bioenergetics, signaling and manipulation for therapy. Biochimica et Biophysica Acta. 2016;**1864**(12):1787-1800

[166] Zhang H, Ryu D, Wu Y, Gariani K, Wang X, Luan P, et al. NAD^+ repletion improves mitochondrial and stem cell function and enhances life span in mice. Science. 2016;**352** (6292):1436-1443

[167] Yun J, Finkel T. Mitohormesis. Cell Metabolism. 2014;**19**(5):757-766

[168] Mouchiroud L, Houtkooper RH, Auwerx J. NAD^+ metabolism, a therapeutic target for age-related metabolic disease. Critical Reviews in Biochemistry and Molecular Biology. 2013;**48**(4):397-408

[169] Seyfried TN, Flores RE, Poff AM, D'Agostino DP. Cancer as a metabolic disease: Implications for novel therapeutics. Carcinogenesis. 2013;**35**(3):515-527

[170] Vyas S, Zaganjor E, Haigis MC. Mitochondria and cancer. Cell. 2016;**166**(3):555-566

[171] Santidrian AF, Matsuno-Yagi A, Ritland M, Seo BB, LeBoeuf SE, Gay LJ, et al. Mitochondrial complex I activity and NAD^+/NADH balance regulate breast cancer progression. The Journal of Clinical Investigation. 2013;**123**(3):1068-1081

[172] Tran MT, Zsengeller ZK, Berg AH, Khankin EV, Bhasin MK, Kim W, et al. PGC1α drives NAD biosynthesis linking oxidative metabolism to renal protection. Nature. 2016; **531**(7595):528-532

[173] Luo C, Lim JH, Lee Y, Granter SR, Thomas A, Vazquez F, et al. PGC1α-mediated transcriptional axis suppresses melanoma metastasis. Nature. 2016;**537**(7620):422-426

[174] Guarente L. Linking DNA damage, NAD^+/SIRT1, and aging. Cell Metabolism. 2014;**20**(4):706-707

[175] Bai P, Cantó C, Oudart H, Brunyanszki A, Cen Y, Thomas C, et al. PARP-1 inhibition increases mitochondrial metabolism through SIRT1 activation. Cell Metabolism. 2011;**13**(4):461-468

[176] Baxter P, Chen Y, Xu Y, Swanson RA. Mitochondrial dysfunction induced by nuclear poly(ADP-ribose) polymerase-1: A treatable cause of cell death in stroke. Translational Stroke Research. 2014;**5**(1):136-144

[177] Zhao Y, Butler EB, Tan M. Targeting cellular metabolism to improve cancer therapeutics. Cell Death & Disease. 2013;**4**:e532

[178] Georgakilas AG, Redon CE, Ferguson NF, Kryston TB, Parekh P, Dickey JS, et al. Systemic DNA damage accumulation under in vivo tumor growth can be inhibited by the antioxidant Tempol. Cancer Letters. 2014;**353**(2):248-257

[179] Khabour OF, Alzoubi KH, Mfady DS, Alasseiri M, Hasheesh TF. Tempol protects human lymphocytes from genotoxicity induced by cisplatin. International Journal of Clinical and Experimental Medicine. 2014;**7**(4):982-988

[180] Yamato M, Kawano K, Yamanaka Y, Saiga M, Yamada K. TEMPOL increases NAD^+ and improves redox imbalance in obese mice. Redox Biology. 2016;**8**:316-322

[181] Chen G, Pelicano H, Ogasawara MA, Wang F, Huang P. Targeting mitochondria of cancer cells: Mechanisms and compounds. In: Neuzil J, Pervaiz S, Fulda S, editors. Mitochondria: The Anti-cancer Target for the Third Millenium. Dordrecht, Germany: Springer Science+Business Media BV; 2014. p. 183-210

[182] Dong LF, Neuzil J. Vitamin E analogues as prototypic mitochondria-targeting anti-cancer agents. In: J. Neuzil, S. Pervaiz, S. Fulda, editors. Mitochondria: The Anti-cancer Target for the Third Millennium. Dordrecht, Germany: Springer Science+Business Media BV; 2014. p. 151-181

[183] Halicka HD, Zhao H, Li J, Lee YS, Hsieh TC, Wu JM, et al. Potential anti-aging agents suppress the level of constitutive mTOR- and DNA damage-signaling. Aging. 2012;**4**(12):952-965

[184] Chamoto K, Chowdhury PS, Kumar A, Sonomura K, Matsuda F, Fagarasan S, et al. Mitochondrial activation chemicals synergize with surface receptor PD-1 blockade for T cell-dependent antitumor activity. Proceedings of the National Academy of Sciences of the United States of America. 2017;**114**(5):E761-E770

[185] Keckesova Z, Donaher JL, De Cock J, Freinkman E, Lingrell S, Bachovchin DA, et al. LACTB is a tumor suppressor that modulates lipid metabolism and cell state. Nature. 2017;**543**(7647):681-686

[186] Pagliarini DJ, Calvo SE, Chang B, Sheth SA, Vafai SB, Ong SE, et al. A mitochondrial protein compendium elucidates complex I disease biology. Cell. 2008;**134**(1):112-123

[187] Wang Y, Oxer D, Hekimi S. Mitochondrial function and lifespan of mice with controlled ubiquinone biosynthesis. Nature Communications. 2015;**6**:6393

[188] Chen P, Yu J, Knecht J, Chen Q. Decrease of PDSS2 expression, a novel tumor suppressor, in non-small cell lung cancer. Cancer Epidemiology. 2013;**37**(2):166-171

[189] Kanda M, Sugimoto H, Nomoto S, Oya H, Shimizu D, Takami H, et al. Clinical utility of PDSS2 expression to stratify patients at risk for recurrence of hepatocellular carcinoma. International Journal of Oncology. 2014;**45**(5):2005-2012

[190] Titov DV, Cracan V, Goodman RP, Peng J, Grabarek Z, Mootha VK. Complementation of mitochondrial electron transport chain by manipulation of the NAD^+/NADH ratio. Science. 2016;**352**(6282):231-235

[191] Yang ZF, Drumea K, Mott S, Wang J, Rosmarin AG. GABP transcription factor (nuclear respiratory factor 2) is required for mitochondrial biogenesis. Molecular and Cellular Biology. 2014;**34**(17):3194-3201

[192] Bose R, Karthaus WR, Armenia J, Abida W, Iaquinta PJ, Zhang Z, et al. ERF mutations reveal a balance of ETS factors controlling prostate oncogenesis. Nature. 2017;**546**(7660): 671-675

Section 3

Mitochondrial Dysfunction and Neuronal Disorders

Chapter 6

Mitochondria at the Base of Neuronal Innate Immunity in Alzheimer's and Parkinson's Diseases

A. Raquel Esteves, Diana F. Silva, Daniel Santos, Emanuel Candeias, Filipa Filipe and Sandra M. Cardoso

Additional information is available at the end of the chapter

http://dx.doi.org/10.5772/intechopen.72612

Abstract

Mitochondria are exceptionally primed to play a key role in neuronal cell survival since they are involved in energy production and function as the metabolic center of cells. Several findings provide evidence for the role of mitochondria in neurodegeneration associated with Alzheimer's and Parkinson's diseases (AD and PD). Recent data highlight the role of mitochondrial proteins and mitochondrial reactive oxygen species in the intracellular signaling that regulates innate immunity and inflammation. In this chapter, we will discuss the relevance of the interplay between mitochondria and innate immunity, focusing on mitochondrial damage-associated molecular patterns (DAMPs) and how they can activate innate immunity and elicit AD and PD neurodegenerative process.

Keywords: mitochondria, neuronal innate immunity, Alzheimer's disease, Parkinson's disease, damage-associated molecular patterns

1. Introductory remarks

Mitochondria, derived from an ancestral bacterial endosymbiosis, are important cellular organelles in all cell types, but particularly important in the nervous system, since they are the major source of energy for the brain. Mitochondria are essential for neuronal function and neuronal processes, such as calcium (Ca^{2+}) homeostasis, maintenance of plasma membrane potential, apoptosis, axonal and dendritic transport, release and re-uptake of neurotransmitters at synapses, among others [1, 2]. The brain is particularly vulnerable to oxidative stress due to its high lipid content, its high oxygen demand and its low levels of antioxidant defenses. Therefore, any abnormalities in mitochondria function may impact the aging process and also potentiate the onset of age-dependent neurodegenerative disorders [3, 4].

In Alzheimer's disease (AD) and Parkinson's disease (PD), it has been described that mitochondrial metabolism and dynamics are affected not only in susceptible brain areas but also in peripheral cell models, namely platelets, fibroblasts and lymphocytes. Additionally, it was shown in AD and PD cellular and animal models that mitochondrial network is highly fragmented. Mitochondrial fission is required to selectively target dysfunctional mitochondria for degradation by the lysosome in a process called mitophagy [5, 6]. Nevertheless, it was recently proven that mitochondrial fission leads to the exposure of the inner membrane phospholipid, cardiolipin, which serves an important defensive function for the elimination of damaged mitochondria [7]. Since cardiolipin is found only in mitochondrial and bacterial membranes, it is considered a mitochondrial-derived damage-associated molecular pattern (DAMP) that is detected by a Nod-like receptor (NLR), the nucleotide-binding domain and leucine-rich repeat pyrin domain containing 3 (NLRP3) inflammasome Nlrp3 [8]. NLR and toll-like receptors (TLR) are pattern-recognition receptors that recognize pathogen-associated molecular patterns (PAMPs), such as lipopolysaccharide and short-chain fatty acids, and DAMPs that are responsible for the initiation of innate immune responses. NLR and TLR activation trigger the production of proinflammatory cytokines and antimicrobial peptides (AMPs) [9]. So, it is perceived that also neuronal cells are able to mount an innate immune response. Neurons express critical Toll/interleukin-1 receptor (TIR) domain-containing adaptors that transduce signals of TLR, regulating the expression of various cytokines. Indeed, TLR 3 and 7, localized in the neuronal endosomal compartment, play a role in neurite outgrowth. It is assumed that the cytokines produced by neurons may be just enough to recruit and activate local microglia and may not cause global brain inflammation [10].

Overall, mitochondria play a central role in metabolism, thus allowing the maintenance of cellular homeostasis. In this chapter, we will discuss how mitochondria can regulate neuronal innate immunity and how this impact age-related neurodegenerative disorders, such as AD and PD.

2. Alzheimer's disease hallmarks

AD is one of the most frequent age-related neurodegenerative disorder, characterized by neuronal loss and gradual cognitive demise. It is the major cause of dementia in the elderly [11], predominantly affects more women than men [12], and is expected that the number of people with AD will triple by the year 2050 [13]. Patients with AD show an impaired ability to perform everyday tasks and often experience psychiatric, emotional and personality disturbances [14]. Two well-known abnormal protein aggregates in the brain of the patients, cerebral cortex and hippocampus, characterize AD pathologically: the neuritic plaques that are extracellular and composed of insoluble amyloid β peptides (Aβ) and neurofibrillary tangles that are intracellular aggregates, mostly consisted of phosphorylated tau, a microtubule-associated protein [15]. It is assumed that oligomers can induce toxicity for neurons causing synaptic dysfunction, neuroinflammation and oxidative stress [16, 17].

Several authors have mentioned that mitochondrial dysfunction and oxidative damage occur in the AD brain before the onset of Aβ pathology. Mitochondrial dysfunction was reported in brain neurons, platelets and fibroblasts from AD patients and in transgenic AD mice models. These mitochondrial abnormalities have been reported in neurons and astrocytes, suggesting that both types of cell might be affected in brains of AD patients [18]. For example, it has been described in post-mortem AD brains, a deficit of cytochrome c oxidase (COX) in hippocampus, frontal, temporal, occipital and parietal lobes [3]. Additionally, it is recognized that mitochondrial DNA (mtDNA) is also involved in the mitochondrial dysfunction having a determinant role in AD pathogenesis. When patient's mtDNA is transferred into mtDNA-deficient cell lines, the originated 'cybrids' reproduce the respiratory enzyme deficiency that occurs in the brain and other tissues in AD, suggesting this defect is carried in part by mtDNA abnormalities [19].

Neuroinflammation has been implicated in AD etiology, but its contribution to disease progression is still not yet understood [20]. Astrocytes and microglial cells are the main type of cells involved in inflammatory responses in the central nervous system (CNS) after infection or injury occurs. Indeed, in this process, cellular and molecular immune components, such as cytokines, are important players, which may lead to the activation of glial cells (microglia and astrocytes) [21]. Several studies have described that Aβ, pathogenic infection or cellular debris triggers an initial inflammatory stimulus, which activates the microglia, allowing the maintenance of neuronal plasticity and synaptic connectivity [22]. Data suggest that microglia internalize and degrade Aβ deposits, helping its clearance from the brain. However, during disease process, microglia acquire a 'toxic' phenotype due to chronic activation and continue the production of proinflammatory mediators [23]. In animal models and human brain tissue, both neuritic plaques and neurofibrillary tangles colocalize with activated glial cells. Different studies have reported pathological astrogliosis, in both AD patients and transgenic animal models brains, characterized by an increased glial fibrillary acidic protein (GFAP) and distinct cellular hypertrophy, which is correlated somehow with the severity of cognitive impairment in AD patients [24].

2.1. The role of mitochondrial dysfunction in Alzheimer's disease etiology

Despite its elusive origin, mitochondrial dysfunction is long recognized as a striking feature of sporadic AD, mediating cell pathways that sustain the disorder progression. Brain bioenergetic function is compromised in AD. Images from fluorodeoxyglucose positron emission tomography (FDG-PET) scan show that glucose utilization is significantly lower in AD subjects as compared to age-matched controls in the cortex and the posterior cingulate brain regions [25]. This bioenergetic compromise correlates with decreased COX activities measured in post-mortem brain tissue from AD patients [26]. Mitochondrial deficits in AD have been described not only in the brain but also in peripheral tissues. COX activity was found decreased in platelets and lymphocytes from AD subjects [27–30]. This COX deficiency correlates with decreased oxygen consumption first described in AD subject's brain, where PET scans showed decreased cerebral metabolic rate of oxygen (CMRO2) [31]. Mitochondrial respiration is also compromised in peripheral blood mononuclear cells [32], and in cytoplasmic hybrid (cybrid) cell lines [33], generated by the fusion of mitochondrial DNA (mtDNA) depleted cells with platelets from AD subjects [34]. These cell lines elucidated on the relevance of mtDNA in AD pathology, since the main features of the disease are recapitulated [33, 35, 36]. The same observation was made in a number of transgenic mice models that carry mutations linked to AD familial forms [37–39].

Along with impaired mitochondrial function, it has been widely demonstrated that mitochondria from AD tissues and models have decreased mitochondrial membrane potential ($\Delta\Psi$mit) [40]. Cumulative evidence consistently showed a positive correlation between $\Delta\Psi$mit and reactive oxygen species (ROS) production [41]. In the case of neurodegenerative disorders, such as AD, associated with dysfunctions of the respiratory chain components, lower $\Delta\Psi$mit and decreased activity of the respiratory chain are observed with a simultaneous increase in ROS production [42]. The primary ROS in mitochondria is the superoxide radical anion $O_2^{-\cdot}$, mainly produced at complexes I and III [43], which is rapidly converted to H_2O_2 by mitochondrial dismutases, superoxide dismutase (SOD). Regardless the contradictory data on the contribution of COX deficiency to ROS production [44, 45], oxidative damage is an utterly feature of AD, from human samples to cellular and animal models [36, 46–48]. Evidence show that mitochondrial dysfunction and ROS production are accentuated by Aβ, a 4 kDa protein, derived from a larger protein, amyloid β-protein precursor (βAPP), that is overproduced during AD progression. Aβ interacts with mitochondrial proteins, namely ABAD, causing increased ROS production, mitochondrial dysfunction and neuronal death [49, 50]. These changes in mitochondrial metabolism seem to be related with morphological alteration of mitochondria of AD tissues and models. Electron microscopy images from AD brain tissue show mitochondria with reduced dimensions and disrupted *cristae* [51]. Similarly, mitochondria from AD subjects transferred to mtDNA depleted cell into cybrids at an ultrastructural level are small and have a swollen-like structure [52], with a fragmented mitochondrial network that correlates with increased mitochondrial content of dynamin-related protein 1 (DRP1) [53] a key protein for mitochondrial division [54]. Concerning mitochondrial content/mass in AD neurons, the matter is not as straight forward [55]. Vulnerable neurons have a decrease in functional mitochondria, but mtDNA is increased [51]. In accordance it was observed, in AD cybrids, an increase in mtDNA content [33]. This increment was first explained as a compensatory response to counteract the loss of mtDNA transcription efficiency [51], but data gathered on the subject point to decreased mitochondria degradation through autophagy (mitophagy), with imprisoned mitochondria within autophagic vacuoles that are accessible for mtDNA detection [53]. A number of studies have shown autophagy dysfunction as a driving force of AD progression, with important impact on Aβ deposition and plaque formation [56–60]. In human brain samples, it could be observed a massive accumulation of autophagic vacuoles and lysosome-related vesicles, which led to the conclusion of simultaneous induction and impairment of autophagy [56, 61]. Purified autophagic vesicles contain βAPP and the proteases responsible for its cleavage [56]. Aβ peptides are produced by sequential proteolytic processing of βAPP by β-secretase (BACE) and γ-secretase complex (presenilin and nicastrin) [62, 63]. These accumulated vacuoles cause swellings along dystrophic neurites and potentiate Aβ production and aggregation [64], which gradually form the extracellular amyloid plaques, one of the most prominent brain pathological hallmarks of AD. It is reasonable to argue that stimulating autophagy would clear the cell waste materials. Although some contradictory data were published, in opposition of ameliorating Aβ pathology, stimulating autophagy, either chemically or starvation-induced, fails to degrade accumulating Aβ and worsens cell function in *in vivo* models [65]. The driver of such failure is the microtubule network, along which autophagic vesicles are transported towards lysosomes, for degradation of cell waste. Mitochondrial metabolism failure compromises microtubule proper dynamics. Destabilized microtubule cytoskeleton negatively impacts autophagic vesicles retrograde transport towards lysosomes and promotes microtubule-associated protein Tau to detach and undergo phosphorylation [5]. Tau is the main component of paired helical filaments (PHF) that form neurofibrillary tangles found in AD brains [66] and is a microtubule-associated protein (MAP) that promotes microtubule assembly and stabilization [67–69]. Ultrastructural analysis performed in AD neurons found that the number and total length of microtubules are decreased in AD subjects [70]. In AD cybrids, microtubule network is disrupted with increased free tubulin content, and this correlates with increased Tau phosphorylation, comparing with control cybrids [53]. Targeting microtubule stability is able to protect cells from Tau and Aβ-induced toxicity and restores autophagy function in a variety of AD models [71, 72].

2.2. Immune response in Alzheimer's disease

The role of neuroinflammation in AD dates back to 1907, to the original report of Alois Alzheimer, with microglia surrounding Aβ plaques, thus showing a close relation between the pathway and the disease [73]. Twenty-five years after the postulation of Selkoe and Hardy, the amyloid cascade hypothesis is still the main hypothesis for AD pathogenesis. It is a fact that all AD patients undergo progressive Aβ deposition, and moreover, the sequence of major pathogenic events leading to AD proposed by the amyloid cascade hypothesis is perfectly aligned with the dominantly inherited forms of AD. However, different mechanisms have to be considered to explain the development of AD in sporadic cases, which constitute the vast majority of the cases [74]. Even though Aβ peptide and tau protein oligomers are considered the major contributors to disease progression and the deposition of Aβ occurs decades before any other alterations, there are some missing links between the accumulation and oligomerization of Aβ and tau pathology, synaptic dysfunction and cognitive decline [15, 75]. In this follow-up, neuroinflammation is consistently reported to be deregulated in AD and to facilitate disease progression [76, 77]. Indeed, various forms of Aβ oligomers and aggregates are detected by numerous receptors (TLRs), receptor for advanced glycated end-products (RAGE), CD14, CD36, CD47, α6β1 integrin, class A scavenger receptor and NOD-like receptor family pyrin domains (NLRP) that activate innate immunity response (mainly via MAPK/Erk and NF-κB-mediated signaling) [22, 78–80]. In neurodegenerative diseases, such as AD, the inflammatory response starts by innate immune system activating monocytes (in periphery) and microglial cells, astrocytes and perivascular cells (in the CNS) [81].

Microglia, the resident macrophages of the CNS, play an active role surveying the brain for pathogens and maintaining neuronal plasticity and synaptic connectivity [82]. In AD, stimulation of microglia involves the microglial polarization to a M1 phenotype that triggers the production of proinflammatory cytokines (TNF-α, IL-1, IL-6, IL-12 and IL-18) [83, 84] and chemokines (CCL2, CCR3, CCR5) [85, 86] and is accompanied by impaired phagocytic capacity [87]. Interestingly, deregulation of Aβ clearance from the CNS is a key pathogenic mechanism in pathology progression, whereas microglial phagocytosis activation plays a crucial role (in combination with the endolysosomal pathway, being Aβ enzymatically digested by neprilysin, insulin-degrading enzyme and matrix metalloprotease proteases) and is controlled by two microglial cell surface receptors: TREM2 (positive regulator) and CD33 (negative regulator) [88, 89]. Moreover, caspases are known mediators of apoptosis, but they also regulate inflammation. Upon binding of Aβ to NLRP, there is an inflammasome-dependent activation of caspase-1 that mediates the production of mature IL-1β by cleavage of an inactive pro-IL-1β peptide [90, 91]. Therefore, elevated concentrations of active caspase 1 detected in the brains of patients with AD [92] are in accordance with the increased NLRP3 activation observed in monocytes from AD patients [93]. In addition, mitochondrial DAMPs were shown to increase AD-associated biomarkers, such as App mRNA, APP protein and $A\beta_{1-42}$ levels, in SH-SY5Y and mice brains [94, 95]. Together, these studies suggest that mitochondria and mitochondrial DAMPs have the potential to promote inflammation in the brain, with important consequences relevant for neurodegenerative disorders such as AD.

Pathological responses of astrocytes include reactive astrogliosis directed at recovery of injured neural tissue and neuroprotection [96]. In AD, astrocytes, like microglia, are a major source of cytokines (TNF-α and IL-1β are readily released upon astrocytic Aβ detection) [97, 98] and chemokines. Indeed CCL4 has been detected in reactive astrocytes near Aβ plaques [99] and has a high capacity to degrade $Aβ_{1-42}$ in a more efficient way than their microglial counterparts [100]. In addition, post-mortem brains from AD patients are characterized by hypertrophic reactive astrocytes, elevated GFAP and S100B expression surrounding senile plaques [101]. Interestingly, studies have shown that reactive astrogliosis occurs early in the course of pathogenesis and correlates with the severity of cognitive impairment in AD patients [102]. Furthermore, resident microglia and astrocytes in AD have been shown to stimulate inducible nitric oxide synthase (iNOS) and NADPH oxidase [103]. These upregulations lead to the production of high concentrations of ROS (such as nitric oxide, superoxide, hydrogen peroxide, peroxynitrite), which not only further promote microglia activation but also lead to post-translational modifications (nitration, S-nitrosylation, and dityrosine formation), including Aβ nitration leading to a higher propensity to aggregate and seriously suppress hippocampal LTP [103–105]. Likewise, the complement system is another major constituent of the innate immune system that shows enhanced levels in disease settings. In the brain, activated microglia and astrocytes are responsible for the production of proteins of the complement system, which in turn are associated with Aβ deposits [106]. Additionally, complement receptor 1 (CR1) modulates the impact of the APOE ε4 allele on brain fibrillar amyloid burden [107]. Furthermore, there are other players with neuroinflammatory actions in AD, such as perivascular macrophages promoting Aβ clearance [108], endothelial cells contributing to the transport of Aβ species between the brain and the periphery [109, 110], oligodendrocytes [111] and neurons [112] that contribute to neuroinflammation by expressing complement components.

In the end, the recruited microglia and astrocytes fail to resolve the Aβ insult effectively, resulting in an excessive proinflammatory cytokine and chemokine production, as well as enhancing DAMPs secretion, ultimately leading to deleterious microglial and astrocytic reactivity [113]. This chronic neuroinflammatory environment thus starts a vicious cycle altering APP processing towards a further increase in Aβ production, culminating in neuronal loss and perpetuating inflammation, which with the advance of the disease compromises blood-brain barrier (BBB) permeability, allowing the invasion of peripheral inflammatory cells that exacerbate the deleterious neuroinflammation and facilitate neurodegeneration [114]. Therefore, neuroinflammation in AD was firstly attributed exclusively to these innate immune sensors of Aβ, contributing to the exacerbation of the disease and viewed only as a response, but in reality the pathway is much more complex.

A decade ago, a significant change in this thought was brought by Wyss-Coray who reviewed the hypothesis that inflammation may serve as a cause and driving force for AD [115]. As seen by the significant immune response later on in the disease and as a response to the Aβ accumulation, it is accurate to state that inflammatory pathways are a driving force in AD. However, for a causative role, inflammation should have an early impact or precede the pathogenesis of the disease [81]. In support of inflammation as a primary contributor for the disease, recent genome-wide association studies (GWASs) of sporadic AD cases (or LOAD—late-onset AD) have found associations between AD and genes that are involved in cholesterol metabolism and in innate immunity [116]. Surprisingly, even Selkoe and Hardy drew attention to the importance of the innate immune system in AD on their update on the status of the amyloid hypothesis [74]. Accordingly, three risk genes have been highlighted: TREM2, CD33 and CR1, and all are involved in some way in microglial response, being upregulated during Aβ plaque development [117–119]. Another important aspect is the timeline involvement of the immune system response in AD's development. Analyses from both patients with early AD and mild cognitive impairment (MCI), which precedes AD stage, have identified a correlation between clinical symptoms and the presence of inflammatory markers in the cerebrospinal fluid (CSF), suggesting a much early involvement of the immune system in the disease [120, 121]. Noteworthy, a study in wild-type mice found that chronic inflammatory conditions triggered the development of AD-like neuropathology during aging, demonstrating a case where immune response not only precedes fibrillary Aβ plaque deposition and neurofibrillary tangle formations but also is responsible for their induction [122]. Thus, the possibility to manipulate inflammatory pathways, thereby changing the course of the disease, is yet another indication of the role of inflammation as a driving force of AD pathology. The questions we should make previously of that said manipulation are: Which cells and immune molecules should be modulated? And when should modulation occur? As the activation of microglia and the neuroinflammatory environment are constantly changing depending on the stage of the disease, the time window for modulation and for therapeutically potential is very important [81]. Inefficiency in clinical trials with nonsteroidal anti-inflammatory drugs (NSAIDs) in AD could be largely due to wrong timing of intervention [123], since epidemiological and preclinical studies show a reduction up to 80% in the risk of AD onset and decrease in microglial activation and amyloid burden with NSAID use [124, 125].

As aforementioned, there is an uncontrolled production of cytokines and chemokines that may be used as effective tools for inflammatory biomarkers in AD. Early assessment of neuroinflammation in the AD patients may be an important preventive strategy to act before the detrimental aspects of neuroinflammation, thus averting or delaying any cognitive decline [126]. Several studies have investigated the levels of proinflammatory and anti-inflammatory markers in the CSF, plasma and serum of AD patients. IL-1β, TNF-α and IL-6 have been observed to be altered in the three types of samples in AD, although the results vary according to the time point of sampling [126]. Once again, the stage of the disease is a crucial factor for any therapeutic intervention. Moreover, an increase in TGF-β [127] and S100B [128] levels in the CSF from AD compared to controls has also been reported. Regarding blood-based biomarkers of inflammation, α-1-antichymotrypsin (ACT) [129] and C-reactive protein (CRP) [130] have been shown to be increased in AD. Noteworthy, α-2-macroglobulin (α-2 M) [131] and clusterin (or apolipoprotein J) [132] have been implicated in the pathology of AD, with significant increases in patients, showing promising results as potential plasma biomarkers of AD. Interestingly, many of these inflammatory mediators are also altered in MCI subjects. The levels of IL-8, monocyte chemoattractant protein-1 and interferon-γ-inducible protein 10 are found to be increased in CSF, while IL-1β and TNF-α are increased and apolipoprotein A-1 and complement C1 inhibitor are decreased in blood [126]. Besides the detection of neuroinflammatory markers, inflammation may be also monitored through imaging methods. In patients with AD or MCI subjects, increased microglia activation has been detected by PET scans [133].

The induction of neuroinflammatory effects is not restricted to factors of the CNS and can result from systemic influences [125]. On the one hand, traumatic brain injury is an example of a CNS-intrinsic neuroinflammatory condition that facilitates the development of AD pathology [134]; on the other hand,systemic inflammation may be induced from several chronic diseases [135], such as obesity and T2D, all characterized by CNS inflammation and microglia activation [136, 137]. Therefore, in AD, neuroinflammation can cause and drive pathogenesis [22].

3. Parkinson's disease hallmarks

PD is the most common movement neurodegenerative disorder characterized by numerous motor symptoms, including tremor, bradykinesia, rigidity and postural instability [138]. PD is twice as common in men than in women, and about 2% of the population above the age of 60 is affected by the disease [139]. PD is characterized by the severe loss of dopaminergic neurons in the substantia nigra pars compacta (SNpc) and by the presence of intracytoplasmatic proteinaceous inclusions called Lewy bodies, which are primarily composed of fibrillary α-synuclein (SNCA), and ubiquitinated proteins within some remaining nigral neurons [140, 141].

Several evidences from autopsy studies showed that multiple processes are involved in cell death, including oxidative stress, mitochondrial dysfunction, neuroinflammation, excitotoxicity and accumulation of misfolded proteins due to proteasomal and autophagic impairment [142].

Data show that mitochondrial deficits occur in PD patient's brain neurons, platelets and lymphocytes [139],which play a critical role in the loss of dopaminergic neurons [143]. Furthermore, data suggest that mitochondrial dysfunction can be potentiated by defects in mitochondrial biogenesis caused by the deregulation of transcription factors, such as peroxisome proliferator-activated receptor gamma coactivator1-alpha (PGC-1α) [144], which levels are decreased in post-mortem brains of PD and in white blood cells [139]. Recent studies in post-mortem PD brain tissue showed that nigrostriatal axon terminals are dysfunctional, which can alter normal axonal transport. Also, the generation of ROS induces the damage of complexes I and III and protein oxidation in mitochondria and in cytoplasmic proteins, leading to mitochondrial dysfunction [145].

Several studies obtained in post-mortem PD brain tissue, human clinical imaging and fluid biomarker have demonstrated that neuroinflammation is a salient feature and probably an essential contributor to PD pathogenesis [145]. Inflammation associated with oxidative stress and cytokine-dependent toxicity has been described and can lead to both innate and adaptive immune responses. Immune responses can act a secondary response to cellular damage and/ or neuronal loss in the affected regions of the nervous system. These mechanisms imply not only a complex crosstalk between the CNS and the peripheral immune system but also interactions between the brain resident immune cells (microglial cells) and other brain cells (neurons, astrocytes, endothelial cells) [146]. Indeed, it has been described that PD brains show microglial activation and lymphocyte infiltration in the areas of degeneration and an increased expression of inflammatory cytokines with alterations in the composition of peripheral immune cells, suggesting the key role of neuroinflammation in PD.

3.1. The role of mitochondrial dysfunction in Parkinson's disease etiology

Mitochondrial dysfunction relevance in PD was first documented when 1-methyl-4-phenyl-1,2,3,6-tetrahydropyridine (MPTP) was associated with parkinsonian syndrome in humans [147].

MPTP is able to cross the blood-brain barrier, is metabolized to 1-methyl-4-phenylpyridinium (MPP^+) and is uptaken by dopaminergic neurons, inhibiting mitochondrial respiration at complex I [148]. Complex I activity was shown to be decreased in PD brain samples [149], in peripheral tissues namely platelets and lymphocytes [150] and in PD cybrids [151]. The inhibition of complex I, with MPTP and rotenone, is widely used as *in vitro* and *in vivo* models of PD since these recapitulate the main features of the disease [152–154]. Mitochondrial dysfunction in PD tissues and models is also characterized by a decrease in $\Delta\Psi$mit [52, 155, 156]. Accordingly, at a functional level, brain bioenergetics is compromised in PD where PET scans showed glucose utilization are decreased in PD individuals in the occipital cortex compared to control individuals [157].

Oxidative damage driven by mitochondria malfunctioning is a prominent aspect in PD [158]. Mitochondrial complex I is one of the most important sites of ROS production in the cell, primarily O_2^- [159]. The consequences of oxidative damage are such in PD that oxidative stress was proposed as the cause for dopaminergic neurons death in the SNpc [160, 161]. The same authors found in post-mortem samples from PD subjects increased lipid peroxidation whereas glutathione pathway, an antioxidant defense, is impaired [160]. Mitochondria are the main producers and are also the primary targets of ROS. PD brain biopsies revealed complex I itself is oxidatively damaged, which prevents its proper assembly and function [149]. Although it is incontestable that oxidative stress contributes to PD pathology, it is now generally accepted that ROS are a by-product of mitochondrial dysfunction that contributes to worsen cell demise [162].

Familial forms of PD bearing mutations in mitochondrial proteins reinforced the involvement of mitochondrial dysfunction in PD etiology and shed light into the mechanisms leading to neuronal death, unifying both familial and sporadic cases. Rare mutations causing juvenile PD are related to mitochondrial degradation by mitophagy created an opportunity for clarification of the disease mechanisms. The first identified mutation in *PARK2* (Parkin), an E3 ubiquitin ligase, cause early onset PD [163]. The second mutation was identified in *PARK6,* PTEN-induced kinase 1 (PINK1) and a mitochondrial kinase [164]. PINK1 and Parkin act together in a tightly regulated process to target dysfunctional mitochondria for degradation, named mitophagy. This process is crucial for the maintenance of a healthy pool of mitochondria, potentially protecting cells in early stages of mitochondrial dysfunction [165]. In healthy mitochondria, PINK1 levels are maintained low as this protein is degraded within mitochondrial matrix after its import from cytosol [166]. When mitochondria lose their membrane potential, PINK1 is stabilized at their surface recruiting Parkin that, in turn, ubiquitinates and targets mitochondria to undergo mitophagy [167–169]. PD caused by PINK1 and Parkin mutations is not clinically differentiated from idiopathic PD [170]. Morphologically, PINK1 mutations have drastic repercussions in mitochondria from *Drosophila melanogaster* to mouse models, with larger, swollen and disrupted cristae [171, 172]. In cybrids from sporadic PD subjects, mitochondria also present abnormal structure with enlarged and scarce cristae [52, 173]. Mitochondrial network images show that in PD models it presents a fragmented structure. From PD cybrids [174] to dopaminergic neurons treated with MPTP [175], a number of models show early mitochondrial fragmentation that precedes cell death. Although DRP1 has been implicated in the fragmentation of mitochondria in PD [174], studies point to SNCA directly interacting with mitochondria inducing fragmentation, in a process that does not require DRP1 [176]. Recently, it was found a common mechanism for mitophagy failure, besides Pink1-Parkin axis, that is shared by familial and sporadic PD, with potential of an early biomarker [177]. In fibroblasts isolated from patients that carry PD mutations and idiopathic PD subjects, it was found an impairment in RHOT1 degradation that in turn delays mitochondria immobilization and consequent degradation [178]. RHOT1 is a mitochondrial kinesin adaptor protein that, upon mitochondrial damage, interacts with PINK1 and Parkin to target mitochondria for proteasomal degradation [179]. Consequently, abnormal levels of autophagy markers were found in brain tissue preparations from PD patients, both sporadic and early onset [180, 181]. This impairment in autophagy has been related to the decreased transport along microtubules and fusion of autophagic vesicles with the lysosomes rather than a defect in cell waste recognition by autophagy machinery [173]. Mitochondrial dysfunction is intimately connected to microtubule instability and, thus, autophagy impairment in PD models. In PD cybrids, intracellular transport of autophagosomes and mitochondria is compromised [173]. Accordingly, MPP^+-treated cells have disrupted microtubule network and a decrease in mitochondrial trafficking [182]. Also, there are some data pointing that Parkin can bind to microtubules contributing to their stabilization, whereas ablation of Parkin causes reduced microtubule mass [183, 184]. Accumulation of non-degraded mitochondria and other autophagic substrates, such as SNCA aggregates, increments cell demise and contributes to Lewy body-like structure formation. Oxidative stress provoked by mitochondrial malfunctioning is able to induce proteasomal subunit disassembly, leading to the accumulation of degrading substrates, such as ubiquitin [185], contributing to Lewy body formation and cell death. In fact, ubiquitin accumulation, impaired ubiquitin proteasome system (UPS) function and mitochondrial dysfunction have been proposed to be intimately associated [186].

3.2. Immune response in Parkinson's disease

Despite PD is characterized by a slow and progressive degeneration of dopaminergic neurons in the SNpc, the cause of this neuronal loss is still poorly understood. Nevertheless, neuroinflammatory mechanisms, such as microglial activation, astrogliosis and lymphocytic infiltration have been postulated to contribute to the cascade of events leading to neuronal degeneration [187].

A growing body of evidence suggests a role of autoimmune and neuroinflammatory mechanisms in the etiopathogenesis of PD [188]. Peripheral immune responses can trigger inflammation and exacerbate neurodegeneration in several neurodegenerative disorders including PD. Indeed, peripheral inflammation in early stages of disease appears to accompany the development of preclinical non-motor symptoms, including olfactory and gastrointestinal dysfunction, providing a possible association between autoimmunity and PD [189]. Strikingly, chronic constipation, which occurs many years before the first motor symptoms of PD, is casually linked to peripheral inflammation [190].

Inflammation is a defense mechanism aimed at counteracting with diverse insults. In neurodegenerative disorders, such as PD, inflammation could results from the activation of innate immunity by PAMPs; DAMPs or protein aggregates. Other than the activation of inflammatory responses, there is also the ability of the immune system to detect harmful agents. Mounting evidence indicates that dopaminergic cell death is influenced by the innate immune system and neuroinflammatory processes in PD. Soreq and coworkers described an altered expression of neuroimmune signaling-related transcripts in early stages of PD [191].

Remarkably, epidemiological studies showed that non-steroidal anti-inflammatory drugs, such as ibuprofen lowers the risk of PD further supporting the contribution of inflammation to disease process [192–194]. Interestingly, the SNpc (main area affected in PD) exhibit high sensitivity to proinflammatory compounds, whereas the hippocampus appears to be more resistant, which can be explained due to the differences in the number of microglial cells between both areas [195]. In fact, numerous evidences that came from experimental PD models suggest that dopaminergic neurons are extremely vulnerable to inflammatory challenge [196, 197]. Moreover, stereotaxic injection of lipopolysaccharide (LPS, a Gram-negative bacteriotoxin that activates microglial cells) into the SNpc induced degeneration of dopaminergic neurons while sparing GABAergic and serotonergic neurons, suggesting selective dopaminergic neurons vulnerability to PAMPs [198].

There are several factors that may be underlying this selectivity. Dying neurons release substances that are recognized by glial cells, activating them, such as dopamine, neuromelanin and SNCA [199]. Dopamine seems to play a role in the inflammatory response induced by LPS, since depletion of this neurotransmitter prevents gliosis and reduces peripheral macrophages infiltration and dopaminergic neuronal death induced by 6-hydroxydopamine (6-OHDA) [200]. Recently, Dominguez-Meijide and colleagues observed that the decrease in dopamine levels observed in early stages of PD promotes neuroinflammation and disease progression via glial renin-angiotensin system exacerbation [201]. Neuromelanin is able to activate microglia cells leading to neuroinflammatory processes and degeneration of dopaminergic neurons [202, 203]. Extracellular and misfolded SNCA prompts microglia activation and production of proinflammatory molecules [204–206].

Further support for a role of innate immunity activation in PD pathogenesis come from genetic studies showing that polymorphisms in some proinflammatory cytokines may influence the risk of developing PD. Indeed, there is an association between genetic variations in the human leukocyte antigen (HLA) region and sporadic PD [207, 208]. HLA isalso called human MHC molecules, which presentation activates CD+4 T cells and CD+8 cytotoxic lymphocytes. Remarkably, in a GWA study, several susceptibility loci have been identified as strong risk factors that are related to both innate and adaptive immune functions [209]. Moreover, PD-linked genes such as LRRK2 and SNCA are also known to stimulate inflammatory responses and immunological regulation [210]. In fact, Harms and colleagues reported that accumulation of pathological SNCA in PD brain leads to T cell infiltration, microglial activation and increased production of inflammatory cytokines and chemokines [211]. Furthermore, transgenic mice with overexpression of wild-type or mutated SNCA showed an early microglial activation [212, 213]. Beraud and colleagues demonstrated that misfolded SNCA directly activates microglia, inducing production and release of TNFα and increasing expression of Nfr2-dependent antioxidant enzymes [214]. Aggregated and nitrated SNCA also stimulates microglia activation triggering innate and adaptive immune responses [215]. Intranigral injection of SNCA resulted in the upregulation of mRNA expression of proinflammatory cytokines and the expression of endothelial markers of inflammation and microglial activation [216, 217]. Multiple immune cells show high levels of LRRK2 expression [218, 219]. R1441G LRRK2 mutation was shown to increase proinflammatory cytokine release from activated microglial cells [220, 221]. Moreover, LPS-mediated neuroinflammation is attenuated in murine *lrrk2*-knockdown brain microglia [222].

The first evidence for a neuroinflammatory processes in PD came in 1988 when McGeer and co-workers observed the presence of activated microglial cells and inflammatory macrophages, as well as, proinflammatory cytokines in post-mortem brain samples of the SNpc of PD patients [223]. Similarly, Langston and coworkers reported an accumulation of activated microglia around dopaminergic neurons in post-mortem human brains with MPTP-induced parkinsonism [224]. Later, several authors corroborated this result and further observed the presence of other markers such as HLA-DP, HLA-DQ, HLADR (CR3/43), CD68 (EBM11, a low-density lipoprotein binding glycoprotein, equivalent to macrosialin in mice) and ferritin in the SNpc and putamen [225–227]. In addition, intercellularadhesion molecule-1-positive glia levels are also increased in the SNpc of PD brains, indicating activation of cells of the innate immune system, in particular, in areas with neuronal loss and extracellular melanin accumulation [228]. Furthermore, Damien and colleagues used glutathione peroxidase as an astrocytic marker and observed that the density of astrocytes in the SNpc is low when compared to the ventral tegmental area. This indicates that vulnerable neurons in patients with PD have less surrounding astroglial cells and as a result reduced detoxification of oxygen-free radicals by glutathione peroxidase [229]. McGeer and colleagues described for the first time the presence of cytotoxic T lymphocytes (CD8+) in the substantia nigra from one patient with PD [223]. Moreover, several reports found alterations in the population of blood T lymphocytes in PD patients [230–232]. In addition, cytotoxic infiltration of CD8+ and CD4+ T cells into the brain parenchyma of both post-mortem human PD specimens and in the MPTP mouse model of PD was described during the course of neuronal degeneration [233, 234]. Interestingly, these markers were not detected in the red nucleus suggesting that this infiltration is selective for the injured brain areas. Furthermore, these cells were in close contact with blood vessels and near to melanized dopaminergic neurons. These data indicate that cells migrate from the bloodstream and suggest an interaction between the lymphocytes and the dopaminergic neurons during the neurodegenerative process. Hence, alterations in the BBB might occur in the brains of PD patients. Not only during aging but also in PD, a BBB disruption can occur, leading to an invasion of immune cells, peripheral mediators, toxins and elements of adaptive immunity to the brain parenchyma potentiating the degenerative process [235]. Additionally, PD patients have increased permeability of the intestinal epithelial barrier and a chronic gut inflammation characterized by increased expression levels of proinflammatory cytokines and inflammatory markers [236, 237]. Moreover, several studies reported increase in TNFα, β2-microglobulin, epidermal growth factor (EGF), transforming growth factor α (TGFα), TGFβ1 and interleukins 1β, 6 and 2 levels in the striatum of PD patients and increasein TNFα, interleukin 1β and interferon γ levels in the SN of PD patients [238–243]. Interestingly, dopaminergic neurons express the receptors for these cytokines, suggesting that they are sensitive to these cytokines [244, 245]. Proinflammatory cytokines, such as TNFα, interleukin 1β, and interferon γ, can induce the expression of the inducible form of nitric oxide synthase (iNOS) or cyclo-oxygenase 2 (COX2), which are known to produce toxic reactive species. To corroborate the previous studies, a CD23-mediated increase in iNOS in the SN of PD patients was found. Furthermore, enzymes that are involved in neuroinflammatory processes mediated by oxidative stress, such as NADPH oxidase, COX2 and myeloperoxidase, are also increased in PD patients [239, 246, 247]. This may indicate that the inflammation-derived oxidative stress could contribute to dopaminergic neuronal degeneration.

The results obtained in post-mortem studies were further corroborated by studies carried out in biological fluids (serum or CSF) of patients suffering from PD. Serum samples from PD patients indicated that the expression of certain cytokines such as IL-1β, IL-2, IL-4, IL-6, IL-8, IL-10, IL-12,

TNFα, TNFR1 and RANTES is increased [248–254]. Interestingly, RANTES levels were correlated with the severity and duration of the disease [255]. Additionally, studies analyzing CSF from PD patients reported proinflammatory changes such as the presence of TNFα [238] and interleukin 1β [225, 256, 257] and osteopontin (a member of the integrins family) [258]. Moreover, PET scan analysis also reported the presence of PK-11195 in PD samples, which is indicative of microglia activation [259, 260]. PET analysis using radioligand ^{11}C-PK-11195 corroborated these results in the SNpc of sporadic PD patients within a year from clinical onset [261]. More recently, microglial activation in PD has been observed with PET by using [18F]-FEPPA [262]. Moreover, it was found a significantly increase numbers of T-helper 17 cells and myeloid-derived suppressor cells in peripheral circulation in PD patients compared with controls [263]. This suggests that a microglial-mediated inflammatory process occurs early in PD process.

It has also been demonstrated that mitochondrial toxins, such as 6-OHDA, MPTP and rotenone, trigger an immune reaction in the striatum and SNpc suggesting that a primary damage to the mitochondrial respiratory chain represents, per se, a trigger for microglial activation and neuroinflammatory processes [264–267]. This reaction includes activation of microglia and infiltration of CD4+ and CD8+ T cells. Rotenone administration was shown to cause microglial activation not only in rodent models [268] but also in human microglial cell lines [269]. Similarly, a significant increase in the number of activated microglial cells was detected in the brain of 6-OHDA rats, at both nigral and striatal areas [233, 270]. Moreover, in the same model CD+3, CD+4 and CD+8 T cells were abundant and migrated from blood vessels into the SNpc [271]. Additionally, in the brains of both monkeys and mice after systemic injection of MPTP, an activated microglia and infiltration of T-lymphocytes has been observed [197]. Microglial activation was also observed in mice that overexpress SNCA [213], in the SNpc and striatum of rats exposed to 6-OHDA [272, 273] and to MPTP [274].

Interestingly, intranigral or systemic injection of LPS in animals can selectively kill dopaminergic neurons [200, 275–279]. Furthermore, injection of LPS into pregnant female rats led to offspring with less and abnormal dopaminergic neurons and increased levels of TNFα in the striatum when compared to the controls [280]. Remarkably, the offspring in adulthood were also more susceptible to the effects of parkinsonian toxins than were the controls [281, 282]. Furthermore, the injection of other proinflammatory compounds such as thrombin within the SNpc also induced the death of dopaminergic neurons [283, 284]. These studies suggest that microglia-mediated inflammation underlies the neuronal cell death in the SNpc.

As previously mentioned, microglial cells when activated produce and release toxic oxygen-derived and nitrogen-derived products, which rely on the regulated induction of several enzymatic systems such as NADPH oxidase and iNOS.Indeed, the expression of these biocatalytic systems within the SNpc is significantly increased in PD patient's post-mortem samples as well as in PD animal models [239, 247]. Oxygen and nitrogen-derived products such as NO, O_2^- and $ONOO^-$ can directly cross membranes and enter dopaminergic neurons, which can cause oxidative damage in tyrosine hydroxylase decreasing its enzymatic activity and in SNCA promoting its aggregation [285, 286]. Additionally, activated microglia can release inflammatory cytokines and chemokines, such as TNFα, interleukin 1β and interferon,whichcan induce neurotoxicity via a direct mechanism through receptor binding on dopaminergic neurons or an indirect mechanism through glial-cell activation and expression of inflammatory factors. In fact, chronic adenoviral expression of TNFα in the SNpc of rats can cause time-dependent dopaminergic cell death [287].

4. The interplay between mitochondria and innate immunity

In response to microbial infection, the mammalian innate immune system recognizes invading microorganisms and orchestrates a proinflammatory immune response to eliminate the undesired pathogens and infected cells. The sensing of the infection by the innate immune system is mediated by a variety of pattern recognition receptors (PRRs), which recognize molecular patterns conserved among microbial species known as PAMPs. For detailed information regarding the different families of receptors, respective PAMPs recognition, and the intracellular signaling cascades triggered, see reference [288]. Interestingly, even in the absence of microbial infection, PRRs sense and orchestrate inflammatory responses through recognition of intracellular molecules known as DAMPs. DAMPs are endogenous molecules sequestered within cellular compartments of healthy cells, which, upon injury or stress, are released to trigger sterile proinflammatory immune responses.

Recent insights revealed that mitochondria are an important source of DAMPs. Interestingly, upon injury, both mtDNA and N-formylated peptides can act as DAMPs. This is due to the fact that mitochondria and bacteria display some similarities in that both possess circular DNA, N-formylated proteins and are double-membrane structures—evidence used in support of the endosymbiotic theory. mtDNA is similar to bacterial DNA in that it contains CpG motifs, which activate the TLR9 [289, 290]. Moreover, mitochondrial protein synthesis is initiated with the residue N-formyl methionine, similar to bacterial protein synthesis [291]. The resulting bacterial N-formylated peptides are known to act as PAMPs by binding and activating G protein-coupled formyl peptide receptors (FPRs) [292], while the mitochondrial N-formylated peptides act as DAMPs through activation of the formyl peptide receptor 1 [290]. Therefore, upon injury, release of these mitochondrial DAMPs activates the innate immune system, much like bacterial PAMPs, to promote sterile inflammatory responses [290].

Several studies have now described a crucial role for mitochondria in the regulation and activation of the inflammasome, specifically the NLRP3 inflammasome [293]. The inflammasomes are intracellular molecular platforms activated upon cellular infection or sterile stressors, which activate the proinflammatory cytokines, interleukin-1β (IL-1β) and IL-18, to trigger pyroptotic cell death (reviewed in [294, 295]). A variety of insults, resulting from cellular infection or stress, can promote mitochondrial dysfunction and activate the NLRP3 inflammasome [293]; however, the molecular mechanisms underlying the contribution of mitochondria to the activation of the NLRP3 inflammasome have only recently been described. While initial studies showed that mitochondrial dysfunction and mtROS production are required for NLRP3 inflammasome activation [296, 297], further evidence has shown that mtDNA translocation to the cytosol plays an active role in this process [297, 298], where it can directly bind to and activate the NRLP3 inflammasome [298]. In addition, the mitochondrial lipid cardiolipin—a phospholipid located exclusively in mitochondrial inner and bacterial membranes, regarded as evidence for symbiogenesis [299, 300]—is also required for NLRP3 inflammasome activation, by directly binding to NLRP3, downstream of mitochondrial dysfunction [301]. Altogether, mitochondria and mitochondrial DAMPs (such as mtDNA and cardiolipin) play a critical role in NLRP3 inflammasome activation and regulation. Moreover, by sensing mitochondrial DAMPs, the NLRP3 inflammasome plays a critical role in integrating mitochondrial dysfunction in a proinflammatory signaling response, thus explaining the association of mitochondrial damage with inflammatory diseases.

Despite the great number of studies describing mitochondria as a source of DAMPs during inflammation in the periphery, the potential for mitochondrial DAMPs to trigger, or exacerbate, inflammation in the brain is now being explored. In recent studies, this potential was tested by treating different brain cell types with mitochondrial components and measuring markers of inflammation afterwards. Neuronal and microglial cell lines exposed to mitochondrial lysates displayed increased markers of inflammation, with mtDNA being identified as the candidate DAMP responsible for the inflammatory changes [95]. While SH-SY5Y neuronal cells treated with mitochondrial lysates showed increased TNFα mRNA, decreased IκBα protein and increased NF-κB protein, microglial cells treated with mitochondrial lysates showed increased TNFα mRNA, increased IL-8 mRNA and redistribution of NF-κB to the nucleus [95]. In a different study, extracellular recombinant Tfam treatment of different models of human microglia, in combination with IFN-Υ, was shown to induce secretions that were toxic to SH-SY5Y neuronal cells [302]. Recombinant Tfam treatment induced the expression of proinflammatory cytokines, such as IL-1β, IL-6 and IL-18, supporting the hypothesis that Tfam may also act as a proinflammatory intercellular signaling molecule recognized by brain microglia [302]. Moreover, mice injected with isolated mitochondria into the brain also revealed increased markers of inflammation such as increased Tnfα, increased NF-κB phosphorylation, increased GFAP protein and decreased Trem2 mRNA [94]. Despite these novel findings describing a role for extracellular mitochondrial DAMPs as proinflammatory signaling molecules in the brain, little is known about the mechanisms by which mitochondria act as a transcellular signaling platforms in the CNS. Recent research revealed that neurons and astrocytes can exchange mitochondria as a potential mode of cell-to-cell signaling [303, 304]. Whilean initial study showed that retinal ganglion cell axons can transfer mitochondria to adjacent astrocytes for degradation [303], mitochondria can also be transferred from astrocytes to adjacent neurons during ischemia to amplify cell survival signals [304], thus representing a neuroprotective strategy or a more efficient way to dispose/recycle mitochondria. However, during neurodegeneration, increased disposal of damaged mitochondria by compromised neurons (e.g. due to compromised mitochondrial quality control mechanisms) or its inefficient uptake by the recipient astrocytes (e.g. due to the presence of extracellular protein aggregates) might result in extracellular accumulation of mitochondrial DAMPs and, as a result, exacerbating neuroinflammation. Further research is necessary to test this hypothesis and identify the PRRs in the brain that are responsible for recognizing extracellular mitochondrial DAMPs; nevertheless, these studies suggest that mitochondria play an active role in neuroglial crosstalk during cellular homeostasis and stress.

5. Concluding comments

Although the innate immune system has specialized in the recognition of molecular patterns foreign to the host cells, cellular injury or stress may result in the release of endogenous molecular patterns, which trigger sterile inflammatory responses. Given its bacterial origin, mitochondria display some similarities with bacteria and represent an important source of DAMPs (including lipids, nucleic acids and proteins) with immunostimulatory potential. While under healthy conditions these DAMPs are sequestered within mitochondria, pathological insults resulting in mitochondrial and cellular damage promote the release of these danger signals to cause inflammation mediated by the innate immune system. Recent studies have shown that mitochondrial DAMPs have the potential to mediate inflammatory signaling in the brain; therefore, its contribution to the neuroinflammatory process in neurodegenerative disorders characterized by impaired mitochondrial function represents an emerging and promising field of research (**Figure 1**).

Further understanding of neuronal innate immunity-induced chronic mild neuroinflammation and its impact on age-related neurodegenerative disorders should focus on new studies addressing not only mitochondrial dysfunction and protein oligomerization but also mild inflammation, nutritional states, among others. The development of new biomarkers focusing on the inflammatory process and the identification of protective inflammatory processes should be pursuit. Additionally, exploiting the effect of mutations, epigenetic and the microbiome on immune-related modifications affecting the AD and PD phenotypes will be of paramount relevance to understand etiology of both diseases.

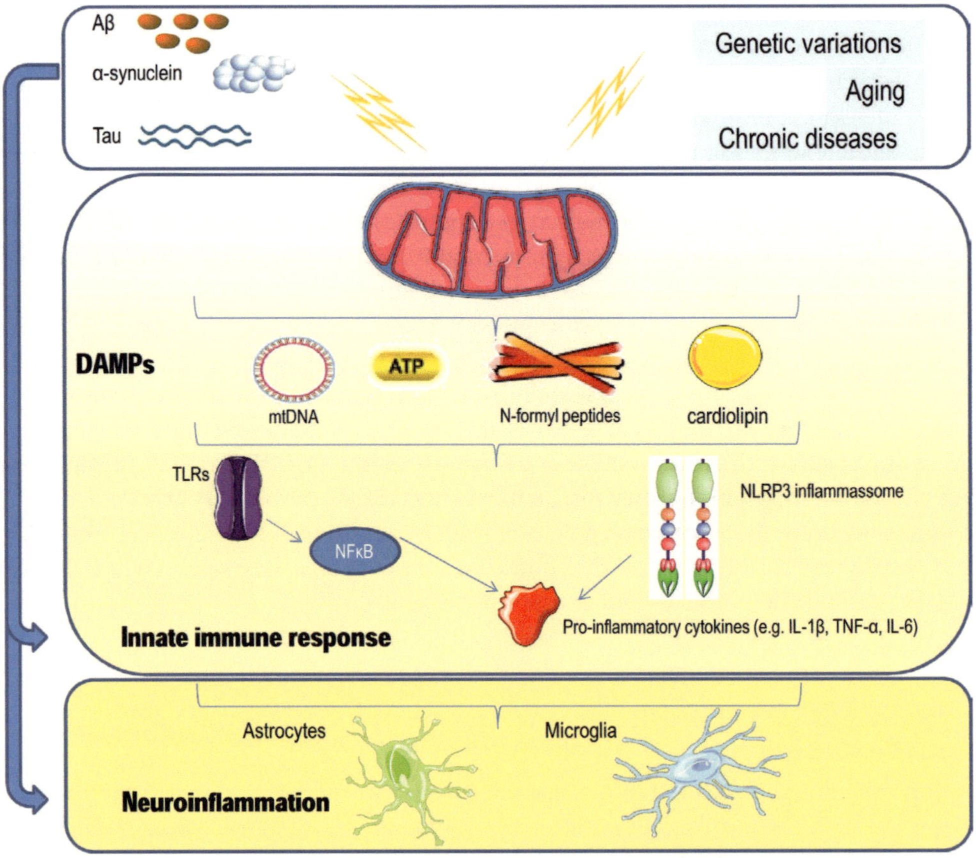

Figure 1. Mitochondria are primary targets of cellular peptides, such as Aβ, tau and SNCA, overproduced during AD and PD pathogenesis. Damaged mitochondria are a source of DAMPs that activate the NLRP3 inflammasome and TLRs leading to the intraneuronal production of cytokines. These proinflammatory cytokines are released and activate innate immune response through microglia and astrocytes. This chronic inflammation impacts neurons exacerbating peptides formation and mitochondrial damage.

Acknowledgements

Work in our laboratories is supported by Fundação para a Ciência e a Tecnologia (FCT) and by EU-FEDER funding through the Operational Competitiveness Programme—COMPETE grant UID/NEU/04539/2013 and by Prémio Santa Casa Neurociências Mantero Belard MB-40-2016.

Author details

A. Raquel Esteves[1,2], Diana F. Silva[1,2], Daniel Santos[1,2], Emanuel Candeias[1,2], Filipa Filipe[1,2] and Sandra M. Cardoso[1,2,3]*

*Address all correspondence to: cardoso.sandra.m@gmail.com

1 CNC–Center for Neuroscience and Cell Biology, University of Coimbra, Coimbra, Portugal

2 CNC-IBILI, University of Coimbra, Coimbra, Portugal

3 Institute of Cellular and Molecular Biology, Faculty of Medicine, University of Coimbra, Coimbra, Portugal

References

[1] Knott AB, Perkins G, Schwarzenbacher R, Bossy-Wetzel E. Mitochondrial fragmentation in neurodegeneration. Nature Reviews Neuroscience. 2008;**9**:505-518. DOI: 10.1038/nrn2417

[2] Lobet E, Letesson JJ, Arnould T. Mitochondria: A target for bacteria. Biochemical Pharmacology. 2015;**94**:173-185. DOI: 10.1016/j.bcp.2015.02.007

[3] Hawking ZL. Alzheimer's disease: The role of mitochondrial dysfunction and potential new therapies. Bioscience Horizons: The International Journal of Student Research. 2016;**9**:1-11

[4] Lionaki E, Markaki M, Palikaras K, Tavernarakis N. Mitochondria, autophagy and age-associated neurodegenerative diseases: New insights into a complex interplay. Biochimica et Biophysica Acta. 2015;**1847**:1412-1423. DOI: 10.1016/j.bbabio.2015.04.010

[5] Silva DF, Esteves AR, Oliveira CR, Cardoso SM. Mitochondria: The common upstream driver of amyloid-beta and tau pathology in Alzheimer's disease. Current Alzheimer Research. 2011;**8**:563-572

[6] Arduino DM, Esteves AR, Oliveira CR, Cardoso SM. Mitochondrial metabolism modulation: A new therapeutic approach for Parkinson's disease. CNS & Neurological Disorders Drug Targets. 2010;**9**:105-119

[7] Chu CT, Ji J, Dagda RK, Jiang JF, Tyurina YY, Kapralov AA, Tyurin VA, Yanamala N, Shrivastava IH, Mohammadyani D, Wang KZQ, Zhu J, Klein-Seetharaman J, Balasubramanian K, Amoscato AA, Borisenko G, Huang Z, Gusdon AM, Cheikhi A, Steer EK, Wang R, Baty C, Watkins S, Bahar I, Bayir H, Kagan VE. Cardiolipin

externalization to the outer mitochondrial membrane acts as an elimination signal for mitophagy in neuronal cells. Nature Cell Biology. 2013;**15**:1197-1205. DOI: 10.1038/ncb2837

[8] He Y, Hara H, Nunez G. Mechanism and regulation of NLRP3 inflammasome activation. Trends in Biochemical Sciences. 2016;**41**:1012-1021. DOI: 10.1016/j.tibs.2016.09.002

[9] Lampron A, Elali A, Rivest S. Innate immunity in the CNS: Redefining the relationship between the CNS and its environment. Neuron. 2013;**78**:214-232. DOI: 10.1016/j.neuron.2013.04.005

[10] Liu HY, Chen CY, Hsueh YP. Innate immune responses regulate morphogenesis and degeneration: Roles of toll-like receptors and Sarm1 in neurons. Neuroscience Bulletin. 2014;**30**:645-654. DOI: 10.1007/s12264-014-1445-5

[11] Vinters HV. Emerging concepts in Alzheimer's disease. Annual Review of Pathology: Mechanisms of Disease. 2015;**10**:291-319. DOI: 10.1146/annurev-pathol-020712-163927

[12] Candeias E, Duarte AI, Sebastião I, Fernandes MA, Plácido AI, Carvalho C, Correia S, Santos RX, Seiça R, Santos MS, Oliveira CR, Moreira PI. Middle-aged diabetic females and males present distinct susceptibility to Alzheimer disease-like pathology. Molecular Neurobiology. 2016;**54**(8):6471-6489. DOI: 10.1007/s12035-016-0155-1

[13] Huang Y, Mucke L. Alzheimer mechanisms and therapeutic strategies. Cell. 2012;**148**:1204-1222. DOI: 10.1016/j.cell.2012.02.040

[14] Tarawneh R, Holtzman DM, Tarawneh R, Holtzman DM. The clinical problem of symptomatic Alzheimer disease and mild cognitive impairment. Cold Spring Harbor Perspectives in Medicine. 2012;**2**:a006148-a006148. DOI: 10.1101/cshperspect.a006148

[15] Jack CR, Holtzman DM. Biomarker modeling of alzheimer's disease. Neuron. 2013;**80**:1347-1358. DOI: 10.1016/j.neuron.2013.12.003

[16] Irvine GB, El-Agnaf OM, Shankar GM, Walsh DM. Protein aggregation in the brain: The molecular basis for Alzheimer's and Parkinson's diseases. Molecular Medicine. 2008;**14**(7-8):451-64. DOI: 10.2119/2007-00100

[17] Gowrishankar S, Yuan P, Wu Y, Schrag M, Paradise S, Grutzendler J, De Camilli P, Ferguson SM. Massive accumulation of luminal protease-deficient axonal lysosomes at Alzheimer's disease amyloid plaques. Proceedings of the National Academy of Sciences of the United States of America. 2015;**112**:E3699-E3708. DOI: 10.1073/pnas.1510329112

[18] Reddy PH, Beal MF. Amyloid beta, mitochondrial dysfunction and synaptic damage: Implications for cognitive decline in aging and Alzheimer's disease. Trends in Molecular Medicine. 2008;**14**:45-53. DOI: 10.1016/j.molmed.2007.12.002

[19] Lin MT, Beal MF. Mitochondrial dysfunction and oxidative stress in neurodegenerative diseases. Nature. 2006;**443**:787-795. DOI: 10.1038/nature05292

[20] Walters A, Phillips E, Zheng R. Evidence for neuroinflammation in Alzheimer's disease. Progress in Neurology and Psychiatry. 2016;**20**:25-31. DOI: 10.1002/pnp.444

[21] Morales I, Guzmán-Martínez L, Cerda-Troncoso C, Farías GA, Maccioni RB. Neuroinflammation in the pathogenesis of Alzheimer's disease. A rational framework for the search of novel therapeutic approaches. Frontiers in Cellular Neuroscience. 2014;**8**:1-9. DOI: 10.3389/fncel.2014.00112

[22] Minter MR, Taylor JM, Crack PJ. The contribution of neuroinflammation to amyloid toxicity in Alzheimer's disease. Journal of Neurochemistry. 2016;**136**:457-474. DOI: 10.1111/jnc.13411

[23] Hamelin L, Lagarde J, Dorothée G, Leroy C, Labit M, Comley RA, De Souza LC, Corne H, Dauphinot L, Bertoux M, Dubois B, Gervais P, Colliot O, Potier MC, Bottlaender M, Sarazin M. Early and protective microglial activation in Alzheimer's disease: A prospective study using 18F-DPA-714 PET imaging. Brain. 2016;**139**:1252-1264. DOI: 10.1093/brain/aww017

[24] Bronzuoli MR, Steardo L, Scuderi C. Targeting neuroinflammation in Alzheimer's disease. Journal of Inflammation Research. 2016:199-208. DOI: 10.2147/JIR.S86958

[25] Swerdlow RH, Koppel S, Weidling I, Hayley C, Ji Y, Wilkins HM. Mitochondria, Cybrids, aging, and Alzheimer's disease. Progress in Molecular Biology and Translational Science. 2017;**146**:259-302. DOI: 10.1016/bs.pmbts.2016.12.017

[26] Mutisya EM, Bowling AC, Beal MF. Cortical cytochrome oxidase activity is reduced in Alzheimer's disease. Journal of Neurochemistry. 1994;**63**:2179-2184

[27] Bosetti F, Brizzi F, Barogi S, Mancuso M, Siciliano G, Tendi EA, Murri L, Rapoport SI, Solaini G. Cytochrome c oxidase and mitochondrial F1F0-ATPase (ATP synthase) activities in platelets and brain from patients with Alzheimer's disease. Neurobiology of Aging. 2002;**23**:371-376

[28] Cardoso SM, Proenca MT, Santos S, Santana I, Oliveira CR. Cytochrome c oxidase is decreased in Alzheimer's disease platelets. Neurobiology of Aging. 2004;**25**:105-110

[29] Parker WD Jr, Mahr NJ, Filley CM, Parks JK, Hughes D, Young DA, Cullum CM. Reduced platelet cytochrome c oxidase activity in Alzheimer's disease. Neurology. 1994;**44**:1086-1090

[30] Molina JA, deBustos F, Jimenez-Jimenez FJ, Benito-Leon J, Gasalla T, Orti-Pareja M, Vela L, Bermejo F, Martin MA, Campos Y, Arenas J. Respiratory chain enzyme activities in isolated mitochondria of lymphocytes from patients with Alzheimer's disease. Neurology. 1997;**48**:636-638

[31] Fukuyama H, Ogawa M, Yamauchi H, Yamaguchi S, Kimura J, Yonekura Y, Konishi J. Altered cerebral energy metabolism in Alzheimer's disease: A PET study. Journal of Nuclear Medicine. 1994;**35**:1-6

[32] Maynard S, Hejl AM, Dinh TS, Keijzers G, Hansen AM, Desler C, Moreno-Villanueva M, Burkle A, Rasmussen LJ, Waldemar G, Bohr VA. Defective mitochondrial respiration, altered dNTP pools and reduced AP endonuclease 1 activity in peripheral blood mononuclear cells of Alzheimer's disease patients. Aging (Albany NY). 2015;**7**:793-815. DOI: 10.18632/aging.100810

[33] Silva DF, Selfridge JE, Lu JEL, Roy N, Hutfles L, burns JM, Michaelis EK, Yan S, Cardoso SM, Swerdlow RH. Bioenergetic flux, mitochondrial mass and mitochondrial

morphology dynamics in AD and MCI cybrid cell lines. Human Molecular Genetics. 2013;**22**:3931-3946. DOI: 10.1093/hmg/ddt247

[34] King MP, Attardi G. Human cells lacking mtDNA: Repopulation with exogenous mitochondria by complementation. Science. 1989;**246**:500-503

[35] Ghosh SS, Swerdlow RH, Miller SW, Sheeman B, Parker WD Jr, Davis RE. Use of cytoplasmic hybrid cell lines for elucidating the role of mitochondrial dysfunction in Alzheimer's disease and Parkinson's disease. Annals of the New York Academy of Sciences. 1999;**893**:176-191

[36] Silva DF, Santana I, Esteves AR, Baldeiras I, Arduino DM, Oliveira CR, Cardoso SM. Prodromal metabolic phenotype in MCI cybrids: Implications for Alzheimer's disease. Current Alzheimer Research. 2013;**10**:180-190

[37] Caspersen C, Wang N, Yao J, Sosunov A, Chen X, Lustbader JW, Xu HW, Stern D, McKhann G, Yan SD. Mitochondrial Abeta: A potential focal point for neuronal metabolic dysfunction in Alzheimer's disease. The FASEB Journal. 2005;**19**:2040-2041. DOI: 10.1096/fj.05-3735fje

[38] Schuh RA, Jackson KC, Schlappal AE, Spangenburg EE, Ward CW, Park JH, Dugger N, Shi GL, Fishman PS. Mitochondrial oxygen consumption deficits in skeletal muscle isolated from an Alzheimer's disease-relevant murine model. BMC Neuroscience. 2014;**15**:24. DOI: 10.1186/1471-2202-15-24

[39] Chowdhury SR, Djordjevic J, Albensi BC, Fernyhough P. Simultaneous evaluation of substrate-dependent oxygen consumption rates and mitochondrial membrane potential by TMRM and safranin in cortical mitochondria. Bioscience Reports. 2015;**36**:e00286. DOI: 10.1042/BSR20150244

[40] Onyango IG, Dennis J, Khan SM. Mitochondrial dysfunction in Alzheimer's disease and the rationale for bioenergetics based therapies. Aging & Disease. 2016;**7**:201-214. DOI: 10.14336/AD.2015.1007

[41] Suski JM, Lebiedzinska M, Bonora M, Pinton P, Duszynski J, Wieckowski MR. Relation between mitochondrial membrane potential and ROS formation. Methods in Molecular Biology. 2012;**810**:183-205. DOI: 10.1007/978-1-61779-382-0_12

[42] Lebiedzinska M, Karkucinska-Wieckowska A, Giorgi C, Karczmarewicz E, Pronicka E, Pinton P, Duszynski J, Pronicki M, Wieckowski MR. Oxidative stress-dependent p66Shc phosphorylation in skin fibroblasts of children with mitochondrial disorders. Biochimica et Biophysica Acta. 2010;**1797**:952-960. DOI: 10.1016/j.bbabio.2010.03.005

[43] McLennan HR, Degli Esposti M. The contribution of mitochondrial respiratory complexes to the production of reactive oxygen species. Journal of Bioenergetics and Biomembranes. 2000;**32**:153-162

[44] Pickrell AM, Fukui H, Moraes CT. The role of cytochrome c oxidase deficiency in ROS and amyloid plaque formation. Journal of Bioenergetics and Biomembranes. 2009;**41**:453-456. DOI: 10.1007/s10863-009-9245-3

[45] Paradies G, Petrosillo G, Pistolese M, Ruggiero FM. The effect of reactive oxygen species generated from the mitochondrial electron transport chain on the cytochrome c oxidase

activity and on the cardiolipin content in bovine heart submitochondrial particles. FEBS Letters. 2000;**466**:323-326

[46] Lyras L, Cairns NJ, Jenner A, Jenner P, Halliwell B. An assessment of oxidative damage to proteins, lipids, and DNA in brain from patients with Alzheimer's disease. Journal of Neurochemistry. 1997;**68**:2061-2069

[47] Han BH, Zhou ML, Johnson AW, Singh I, Liao F, Vellimana AK, Nelson JW, Milner E, Cirrito JR, Basak J, Yoo M, Dietrich HH, Holtzman DM, Zipfel GJ. Contribution of reactive oxygen species to cerebral amyloid angiopathy, vasomotor dysfunction, and microhemorrhage in aged Tg2576 mice. Proceedings of the National Academy of Sciences of the United States of America. 2015;**112**:E881-E890. DOI: 10.1073/pnas.1414930112

[48] Leutner S, Schindowski K, Frolich L, Maurer K, Kratzsch T, Eckert A, Muller WE. Enhanced ROS-generation in lymphocytes from Alzheimer's patients. Pharmacopsychiatry. 2005;**38**:312-315. DOI: 10.1055/s-2005-916186

[49] Lustbader JW, Cirilli M, Lin C, Xu HW, Takuma K, Wang N, Caspersen C, Chen X, Pollak S, Chaney M, Trinchese F, Liu S, Gunn-Moore F, Lue LF, Walker DG, Kuppusamy P, Zewier ZL, Arancio O, Stern D, Yan SS, Wu H. ABAD directly links Abeta to mitochondrial toxicity in Alzheimer's disease. Science. 2004;**304**:448-452. DOI: 10.1126/science.1091230

[50] Manczak M, Anekonda TS, Henson E, Park BS, Quinn J, Reddy PH. Mitochondria are a direct site of a beta accumulation in Alzheimer's disease neurons: Implications for free radical generation and oxidative damage in disease progression. Human Molecular Genetics. 2006;**15**:1437-1449. DOI: 10.1093/hmg/ddl066

[51] Hirai K, Aliev G, Nunomura A, Fujioka H, Russell RL, Atwood CS, Johnson AB, Kress Y, Vinters HV, Tabaton M, Shimohama S, Cash AD, Siedlak SL, Harris PL, Jones PK, Petersen RB, Perry G, Smith MA. Mitochondrial abnormalities in Alzheimer's disease. The Journal of Neuroscience. 2001;**21**:3017-3023

[52] Trimmer PA, Swerdlow RH, Parks JK, Keeney P, Bennett Jr JP, Miller SW, Davis RE, Parker WD Jr. Abnormal mitochondrial morphology in sporadic Parkinson's and Alzheimer's disease cybrid cell lines. Experimental Neurology. 2000;**162**:37-50. DOI: 10.1006/exnr.2000.7333

[53] Silva DF, Esteves AR, Oliveira CR, Cardoso SM. Mitochondrial metabolism power SIRT2-dependent deficient traffic causing Alzheimer's-disease related pathology. Molecular Neurobiology. 2016. DOI: 10.1007/s12035-016-9951-x

[54] Smirnova E, Griparic L, Shurland DL, van der Bliek AM. Dynamin-related protein Drp1 is required for mitochondrial division in mammalian cells. Molecular Biology of the Cell. 2001;**12**:2245-2256

[55] SilvaDF, SelfridgeJE, Lu JEL, Cardoso SM, Swerdlow RH. Mitochondrial abnormalities in Alzheimer's disease: Possible targets for therapeutic intervention. Advances in Pharmacology.2012;**64**:83-126. DOI: 10.1016/B978-0-12-394816-8.00003-9

[56] Yu WH, Cuervo AM, Kumar A, Peterhoff CM, Schmidt SD, Lee JH, Mohan PS, Mercken M, Farmery MR, Tjernberg LO, Jiang Y, Duff K, Uchiyama Y, Naslund J, Mathews PM,

Cataldo AM, Nixon RA. Macroautophagy--a novel Beta-amyloid peptide-generating pathway activated in Alzheimer's disease. The Journal of Cell Biology. 2005;**171**:87-98. DOI: 10.1083/jcb.200505082

[57] Cardoso SM, Pereira CF, Moreira PI, Arduino DM, Esteves AR, Oliveira CR. Mitochondrial control of autophagic lysosomal pathway in Alzheimer's disease. Experimental Neurology. 2010;**223**:294-298. DOI: 10.1016/j.expneurol.2009.06.008

[58] Cai Z, Zhou Y, Liu Z, Ke Z, Zhao B. Autophagy dysfunction upregulates beta-amyloid peptides via enhancing the activity of gamma-secretase complex. Neuropsychiatric Disease and Treatment. 2015;**11**:2091-2099. DOI: 10.2147/NDT.S84755

[59] Nilsson P, Saido TC. Dual roles for autophagy: Degradation and secretion of Alzheimer's disease Abeta peptide. BioEssays. 2014;**36**:570-578. DOI: 10.1002/bies.201400002

[60] Nilsson P, Loganathan K, Sekiguchi M, Matsuba Y, Hui K, Tsubuki S, Tanaka M, Iwata N, Saito T, Saido TC. Abeta secretion and plaque formation depend on autophagy. Cell Reports. 2013;**5**:61-69. DOI: 10.1016/j.celrep.2013.08.042

[61] Nixon RA, Wegiel J, Kumar A, WH Y, Peterhoff C, Cataldo A, Cuervo AM. Extensive involvement of autophagy in Alzheimer disease: An immuno-electron microscopy study. Journal of Neuropathology and Experimental Neurology. 2005;**64**:113-122

[62] Marks N, Berg MJ. BACE and gamma-secretase characterization and their sorting as therapeutic targets to reduce amyloidogenesis. Neurochemical Research. 2010;**35**:181-210. DOI: 10.1007/s11064-009-0054-1

[63] Yu WH, Kumar A, Peterhoff C, Shapiro Kulnane L, Uchiyama Y, Lamb BT, Cuervo AM, Nixon RA. Autophagic vacuoles are enriched in amyloid precursor protein-secretase activities: Implications for beta-amyloid peptide over-production and localization in Alzheimer's disease. The International Journal of Biochemistry & Cell Biology. 2004;**36**:2531-2540. DOI: 10.1016/j.biocel.2004.05.010

[64] Nixon RA. Autophagy, amyloidogenesis and Alzheimer disease. Journal of Cell Science. 2007;**120**:4081-4091. DOI: 10.1242/jcs.019265

[65] Chen X, Kondo K, Motoki K, Homma H, Okazawa H. Fasting activates macroautophagy in neurons of Alzheimer's disease mouse model but is insufficient to degrade amyloid-beta. Scientific Reports. 2015;**5**:12115. DOI: 10.1038/srep12115

[66] Kosik KS, Joachim CL, Selkoe DJ. Microtubule-associated protein tau (tau) is a major antigenic component of paired helical filaments in Alzheimer disease. Proceedings of the National Academy of Sciences of the United States of America. 1986;**83**:4044-4048

[67] Ma RH, Zhang Y, Hong XY, Zhang JF, Wang JZ, Liu GP. Role of microtubule-associated protein tau phosphorylation in Alzheimer's disease. Journal of Huazhong University of Science and Technology. Medical Sciences. 2017;**37**:307-312. DOI: 10.1007/s11596-017-1732-x

[68] Takemura R, Okabe S, Umeyama T, Kanai Y, Cowan NJ, Hirokawa N. Increased microtubule stability and alpha tubulin acetylation in cells transfected with microtubule-associated proteins MAP1B, MAP2 or tau. Journal of Cell Science. 1992;**103**(Pt 4):953-964

[69] Michaelis ML, Dobrowsky RT, Li G. Tau neurofibrillary pathology and microtubule stability. Journal of Molecular Neuroscience. 2002;**19**:289-293. DOI: 10.1385/JMN:19:3:289

[70] Cash AD, Aliev G, Siedlak SL, Nunomura A, Fujioka H, Zhu X, Raina AK, Vinters HV, Tabaton M, Johnson AB, Paula-Barbosa M, Avila J, Jones PK, Castellani RJ, Smith MA, Perry G. Microtubule reduction in Alzheimer's disease and aging is independent of tau filament formation. The American Journal of Pathology. 2003;**162**:1623-1627

[71] Silva DF, Esteves AR, Arduino DM, Oliveira CR, Cardoso SM. Amyloid-beta-induced mitochondrial dysfunction impairs the autophagic lysosomal pathway in a tubulin dependent pathway. Journal of Alzheimer's Disease. 2011;**26**:565-581. DOI: 10.3233/JAD-2011-110423

[72] Matsuoka Y, Jouroukhin Y, Gray AJ, Ma L, Hirata-Fukae C, Li HF, Feng L, Lecanu L, Walker BR, Planel E, Arancio O, Gozes I, Aisen PS. A neuronal microtubule-interacting agent, NAPVSIPQ, reduces tau pathology and enhances cognitive function in a mouse model of Alzheimer's disease. The Journal of Pharmacology and Experimental Therapeutics. 2008;**325**:146-153. DOI: 10.1124/jpet.107.130526

[73] Alzheimer A, Stelzmann RA, Schnitzlein HN, Murtagh FR. An English translation of Alzheimer's 1907 paper, "Uber eine eigenartige Erkankung der Hirnrinde". Clinical Anatomy. 1995;**8**:429-431. DOI: 10.1002/ca.980080612

[74] Selkoe DJ, Hardy J. The amyloid hypothesis of Alzheimer's disease at 25 years. EMBO Molecular Medicine. 2016;**8**:595-608. DOI: 10.15252/emmm.201606210

[75] Morris GP, Clark IA, Vissel B. Inconsistencies and controversies surrounding the amyloid hypothesis of Alzheimer's disease. Acta Neuropathologica Communications. 2014;**2**:135. DOI: 10.1186/s40478-014-0135-5

[76] Jack CR Jr, Knopman DS, Jagust WJ, Petersen RC, Weiner MW, Aisen PS, Shaw LM, Vemuri P, Wiste HJ, Weigand SD, Lesnick TG, Pankratz VS, Donohue MC, Trojanowski JQ. Tracking pathophysiological processes in Alzheimer's disease: An updated hypothetical model of dynamic biomarkers. Lancet Neurology. 2013;**12**:207-216. DOI: 10.1016/S1474-4422(12)70291-0

[77] McGeer PL, McGeer EG. The amyloid cascade-inflammatory hypothesis of Alzheimer disease: Implications for therapy. Acta Neuropathologica. 2013;**126**:479-497. DOI: 10.1007/s00401-013-1177-7

[78] Stewart CR, Stuart LM, Wilkinson K, vanGils JM, Deng J, Halle A, Rayner KJ, Boyer L, Zhong R, Frazier WA, Lacy-Hulbert A, ElKhoury J, Golenbock DT, Moore KJ. CD36 ligands promote sterile inflammation through assembly of a toll-like receptor 4 and 6 heterodimer. Nature Immunology. 2010;**11**:155-161. DOI: 10.1038/ni.1836

[79] Koenigsknecht J, Landreth G. Microglial phagocytosis of fibrillar beta-amyloid through a beta1 integrin-dependent mechanism. The Journal of Neuroscience. 2004;**24**:9838-9846. DOI: 10.1523/JNEUROSCI.2557-04.2004

[80] Bamberger ME, Harris ME, McDonald DR, Husemann J, Landreth GEA. Cell surface receptor complex for fibrillar beta-amyloid mediates microglial activation. The Journal of Neuroscience. 2003;**23**:2665-2674

[81] Heppner FL, Ransohoff RM, Becher B. Immune attack: The role of inflammation in Alzheimer disease. Nature Reviews. Neuroscience. 2015;**16**:358-372. DOI: 10.1038/nrn3880

[82] Prokop S, Miller KR, Heppner FL. Microglia actions in Alzheimer's disease. Acta Neuropathologica. 2013;**126**:461-477

[83] Francois A, Rioux Bilan A, Quellard N, Fernandez B, Janet T, Chassaing D, Paccalin M, Terro F, Page G. Longitudinal follow-up of autophagy and inflammation in brain of APPswePS1dE9 transgenic mice. Journal of Neuroinflammation. 2014;**11**:139. DOI: 10.1186/s12974-014-0139-x

[84] Patel NS, Paris D, Mathura V, Quadros AN, Crawford FC, Mullan MJ. Inflammatory cytokine levels correlate with amyloid load in transgenic mouse models of Alzheimer's disease. Journal of Neuroinflammation. 2005;**2**:9. DOI: 10.1186/1742-2094-2-9

[85] Xia MQ, Qin SX, LJ W, Mackay CR, Hyman BT. Immunohistochemical study of the beta-chemokine receptors CCR3 and CCR5 and their ligands in normal and Alzheimer's disease brains. The American Journal of Pathology. 1998;**153**:31-37

[86] Ishizuka K, Kimura T, Igata-yi R, Katsuragi S, Takamatsu J, Miyakawa T. Identification of monocyte chemoattractant protein-1 in senile plaques and reactive microglia of Alzheimer's disease. Psychiatry and Clinical Neurosciences. 1997;**51**:135-138

[87] Mawuenyega KG, Sigurdson W, Ovod V, Munsell L, Kasten T, Morris JC, Yarasheski KE, Bateman RJ. Decreased clearance of CNS beta-amyloid in Alzheimer's disease. Science. 2010;**330**:1774. DOI: 10.1126/science.1197623

[88] Griciuc A, Serrano-Pozo A, Parrado AR, Lesinski AN, Asselin CN, Mullin K, Hooli B, Choi SH, Hyman BT, Tanzi RE. Alzheimer's disease risk gene CD33 inhibits microglial uptake of amyloid beta. Neuron. 2013;**78**:631-643. DOI: 10.1016/j.neuron.2013.04.014

[89] Lee CY, Landreth GE. The role of microglia in amyloid clearance from the AD brain. Journal of Neural Transmission (Vienna). 2010;**117**:949-960. DOI: 10.1007/s00702-010-0433-4

[90] Monteleone M, Stow JL, Schroder K. Mechanisms of unconventional secretion of IL-1 family cytokines. Cytokine. 2015;**74**:213-218. DOI: 10.1016/j.cyto.2015.03.022

[91] Winkler S, Rosen-Wolff A. Caspase-1: An integral regulator of innate immunity. Seminars in Immunopathology. 2015;**37**:419-427. DOI: 10.1007/s00281-015-0494-4

[92] Heneka MT, Kummer MP, Stutz A, Delekate A, Schwartz S, Vieira-Saecker A, Griep A, Axt D, Remus A, Tzeng TC, Gelpi E, Halle A, Korte M, Latz E, Golenbock DT. NLRP3 is activated in Alzheimer's disease and contributes to pathology in APP/PS1 mice. Nature. 2013;**493**:674-678. DOI: 10.1038/nature11729

[93] Saresella M, La Rosa F, Piancone F, Zoppis M, Marventano I, Calabrese E, Rainone V, Nemni R, Mancuso R, Clerici M. The NLRP3 and NLRP1 inflammasomes are activated in Alzheimer's disease. Molecular Neurodegeneration. 2016;**11**:23. DOI: 10.1186/s13024-016-0088-1

[94] Wilkins HM, Koppel SJ, Weidling IW, Roy N, Ryan LN, Stanford JA, Swerdlow RH. Extracellular mitochondria and mitochondrial components act as damage-associated molecular pattern molecules in the mouse brain. Journal of Neuroimmune Pharmacology. 2016;**11**:622-628. DOI: 10.1007/s11481-016-9704-7

[95] Wilkins HM, Carl SM, Weber SG, Ramanujan SA, Festoff BW, Linseman DA, Swerdlow RH. Mitochondrial lysates induce inflammation and Alzheimer's disease-relevant changes in microglial and neuronal cells. Journal of Alzheimer's Disease. 2015;**45**:305-318. DOI: 10.3233/JAD-142334

[96] Sofroniew MV, Vinters HV. Astrocytes: Biology and pathology. Acta Neuropathologica. 2010;**119**:7-35. DOI: 10.1007/s00401-009-0619-8

[97] Hennessy E, Griffin EW, Cunningham C. Astrocytes are primed by chronic Neurodegeneration to produce exaggerated chemokine and cell infiltration responses to acute stimulation with the cytokines IL-1beta and TNF-alpha. The Journal of Neuroscience. 2015;**35**:8411-8422. DOI: 10.1523/JNEUROSCI.2745-14.2015

[98] Carrero I, Gonzalo MR, Martin B, Sanz-Anquela JM, Arevalo-Serrano J, Gonzalo-Ruiz A. Oligomers of beta-amyloid protein (Abeta1-42) induce the activation of cyclooxygenase-2 in astrocytes via an interaction with interleukin-1beta, tumour necrosis factor-alpha, and a nuclear factor kappa-B mechanism in the rat brain. Experimental Neurology. 2012;**236**:215-227. DOI: 10.1016/j.expneurol.2012.05.004

[99] Smits HA, Rijsmus A, vanLoon JH, Wat JW, Verhoef J, Boven LA, Nottet HS. Amyloid-beta-induced chemokine production in primary human macrophages and astrocytes. Journal of Neuroimmunology. 2002;**127**:160-168

[100] Nielsen HM, Mulder SD, Belien JA, Musters RJ, Eikelenboom P, Veerhuis R. Astrocytic a beta 1-42 uptake is determined by a beta-aggregation state and the presence of amyloid-associated proteins. Glia. 2010;**58**:1235-1246. DOI: 10.1002/glia.21004

[101] Edwards MM, Robinson SR. TNF alpha affects the expression of GFAP and S100B: Implications for Alzheimer's disease. Journal of Neural Transmission (Vienna). 2006;**113**:1709-1715. DOI: 10.1007/s00702-006-0479-5

[102] Simpson JE, Ince PG. Lace G, Forster G, Shaw PJ, Matthews F, Savva G, Brayne C, Wharton SB, function MRCC, and ageing neuropathology study G. Astrocyte phenotype in relation to Alzheimer-type pathology in the ageing brain. Neurobiology of Aging. 2010;**31**:578-590. DOI: 10.1016/j.neurobiolaging.2008.05.015

[103] Heneka MT, Carson MJ, El Khoury J, Landreth GE, Brosseron F, Feinstein DL, Jacobs AH, Wyss-Coray T, Vitorica J, Ransohoff RM, Herrup K, Frautschy SA, Finsen B, Brown GC, Verkhratsky A, Yamanaka K, Koistinaho J, Latz E, Halle A, Petzold GC, Town T, Morgan D, Shinohara ML, Perry VH, Holmes C, Bazan NG, Brooks DJ, Hunot S, Joseph B, Deigendesch N, Garaschuk O, Boddeke E, Dinarello CA, Breitner JC, Cole GM, Golenbock DT, Kummer MP. Neuroinflammation in Alzheimer's disease. Lancet Neurology. 2015;**14**:388-405. DOI: 10.1016/S1474-4422(15)70016-5

[104] Thiabaud G, Pizzocaro S, Garcia-Serres R, Latour JM, Monzani E, Casella L. Heme binding induces dimerization and nitration of truncated beta-amyloid peptide Abeta16 under oxidative stress. Angewandte Chemie (International Ed. in English). 2013;**52**:8041-8044. DOI: 10.1002/anie.201302989

[105] Butterfield DA, Reed TT, Perluigi M, De Marco C, Coccia R, Keller JN, Markesbery WR, Sultana R. Elevated levels of 3-nitrotyrosine in brain from subjects with amnestic mild cognitive impairment: Implications for the role of nitration in the progression of Alzheimer's disease. Brain Research. 2007;**1148**:243-248. DOI: 10.1016/j.brainres.2007.02.084

[106] Wyss-Coray T, Rogers J. Inflammation in Alzheimer disease-a brief review of the basic science and clinical literature. Cold Spring Harbor Perspectives in Medicine. 2012;**2**:a006346. DOI: 10.1101/cshperspect.a006346

[107] Thambisetty M, An Y, Nalls M, Sojkova J, Swaminathan S, Zhou Y, Singleton AB, Wong DF, Ferrucci L, Saykin AJ, Resnick SM. Baltimore longitudinal study of A, and the Alzheimer's disease neuroimaging I. Effect of complement CR1 on brain amyloid burden during aging and its modification by APOE genotype. Biological Psychiatry. 2013;**73**:422-428. DOI: 10.1016/j.biopsych.2012.08.015

[108] Hawkes CA, McLaurin J. Selective targeting of perivascular macrophages for clearance of beta-amyloid in cerebral amyloid angiopathy. Proceedings of the National Academy of Sciences of the United States of America. 2009;**106**:1261-1266. DOI: 10.1073/pnas.0805453106

[109] Sagare AP, Bell RD, Zlokovic BV. Neurovascular dysfunction and faulty amyloid beta-peptide clearance in Alzheimer disease. Cold Spring Harbor Perspectives in Medicine. 2012;**2**:a011452. DOI: 10.1101/cshperspect.a011452

[110] Vukic V, Callaghan D, Walker D, Lue LF, Liu QY, Couraud PO, Romero IA, Weksler B, Stanimirovic DB, Zhang W. Expression of inflammatory genes induced by beta-amyloid peptides in human brain endothelial cells and in Alzheimer's brain is mediated by the JNK-AP1 signaling pathway. Neurobiology of Disease. 2009;**34**:95-106. DOI: 10.1016/j.nbd.2008.12.007

[111] Yamada T, Akiyama H, McGeer PL. Complement-activated oligodendroglia: A new pathogenic entity identified by immunostaining with antibodies to human complement proteins C3d and C4d. Neuroscience Letters. 1990;**112**:161-166

[112] Walker DG, Dalsing-Hernandez JE, Campbell NA, Lue LF. Decreased expression of CD200 and CD200 receptor in Alzheimer's disease: A potential mechanism leading to chronic inflammation. Experimental Neurology. 2009;**215**:5-19. DOI: 10.1016/j.expneurol.2008.09.003

[113] Latta CH, Brothers HM, Wilcock DM. Neuroinflammation in Alzheimer's disease; a source of heterogeneity and target for personalized therapy. Neuroscience. 2015;**302**:103-111. DOI: 10.1016/j.neuroscience.2014.09.061

[114] Cai Z, Hussain MD, Yan LJ. Microglia, neuroinflammation, and beta-amyloid protein in Alzheimer's disease. The International Journal of Neuroscience. 2014;**124**:307-321. DOI: 10.3109/00207454.2013.833510

[115] Wyss-Coray T. Inflammation in Alzheimer disease: Driving force, bystander or beneficial response? Nature Medicine. 2006;**12**:1005-1015. DOI: 10.1038/nm1484

[116] Jones L, Holmans PA, Hamshere ML, Harold D, Moskvina V, Ivanov D, Pocklington A, Abraham R, Hollingworth P, Sims R, Gerrish A, Pahwa JS, Jones N, Stretton A, Morgan AR, Lovestone S, Powell J, Proitsi P, Lupton MK, Brayne C, Rubinsztein DC, Gill M, Lawlor B, Lynch A, Morgan K, Brown KS, Passmore PA, Craig D, McGuinness B, Todd S, Holmes C, Mann D, Smith AD, Love S, Kehoe PG, Mead S, Fox N, Rossor M, Collinge J, Maier W, Jessen F, Schurmann B, Heun R, Kolsch H, van den Bussche H, Heuser I, Peters O, Kornhuber J, Wiltfang J, Dichgans M, Frolich L, Hampel H, Hull M, Rujescu D, Goate AM, Kauwe JS, Cruchaga C, Nowotny P, Morris JC, Mayo K, Livingston G, Bass NJ, Gurling H, McQuillin A, Gwilliam R, Deloukas P, Al-Chalabi A, Shaw CE, Singleton AB, Guerreiro R, Muhleisen TW, Nothen MM, Moebus S, Jockel KH, Klopp N, Wichmann HE, Ruther E, Carrasquillo MM, Pankratz VS, Younkin SG, Hardy J, O'Donovan MC, Owen MJ, Williams J. Genetic evidence implicates the immune system and cholesterol metabolism in the aetiology of Alzheimer's disease. PLoS One. 2010;**5**:e13950. DOI: 10.1371/journal.pone.0013950

[117] Bradshaw EM, Chibnik LB, Keenan BT, Ottoboni L, Raj T, Tang A, Rosenkrantz LL, Imboywa S, Lee M, Von Korff A, Alzheimer Disease Neuroimaging Initiative, Morris MC, Evans DA, Johnson K, Sperling RA, Schneider JA, Bennett DA, De Jager PL. CD33 Alzheimer's disease locus: Altered monocyte function and amyloid biology. Nature Neuroscience. 2013;**16**:848-850. DOI:10.1038/nn.3435

[118] Guerreiro R, Wojtas A, Bras J, Carrasquillo M, Rogaeva E, Majounie E, Cruchaga C, Sassi C, Kauwe JS, Younkin S, Hazrati L, Collinge J, Pocock J, Lashley T, Williams J, Lambert JC, Amouyel P, Goate A, Rademakers R, Morgan K, Powell J, St George-Hyslop P, Singleton A, Hardy J, Alzheimer Genetic Analysis Group. TREM2 variants in Alzheimer's disease. The New England Journal of Medicine. 2013;**368**:117-127. DOI: 10.1056/NEJMoa1211851

[119] Lambert JC, Heath S, Even G, Campion D, Sleegers K, Hiltunen M, Combarros O, Zelenika D, Bullido MJ, Tavernier B, Letenneur L, Bettens K, Berr C, Pasquier F, Fievet N, Barberger-Gateau P, Engelborghs S, De Deyn P, Mateo I, Franck A, Helisalmi S, Porcellini E, Hanon O, European Alzheimer's Disease Initiative I, de Pancorbo MM, Lendon C, Dufouil C, Jaillard C, Leveillard T, Alvarez V, Bosco P, Mancuso M, Panza F, Nacmias B, Bossu P, Piccardi P, Annoni G, Seripa D, Galimberti D, Hannequin D, Licastro F, Soininen H, Ritchie K, Blanche H, Dartigues JF, Tzourio C, Gut I, Van Broeckhoven C, Alperovitch A, Lathrop M, Amouyel P. Genome-wide association study identifies variants at CLU and CR1 associated with Alzheimer's disease. Nature Genetics. 2009;**41**:1094-1099. DOI: 10.1038/ng.439

[120] Brosseron F, Krauthausen M, Kummer M, Heneka MT. Body fluid cytokine levels in mild cognitive impairment and Alzheimer's disease: A comparative overview. Molecular Neurobiology. 2014;**50**:534-544. DOI: 10.1007/s12035-014-8657-1

[121] Tarkowski E, Andreasen N, Tarkowski A, Blennow K. Intrathecal inflammation precedes development of Alzheimer's disease. Journal of Neurology, Neurosurgery, and Psychiatry. 2003;**74**:1200-1205

[122] Krstic D, Madhusudan A, Doehner J, Vogel P, Notter T, Imhof C, Manalastas A, Hilfiker M, Pfister S, Schwerdel C, Riether C, Meyer U, Knuesel I. Systemic immune challenges trigger and drive Alzheimer-like neuropathology in mice. Journal of Neuroinflammation. 2012;**9**:151. DOI: 10.1186/1742-2094-9-151

[123] Group ADC, Bentham P, Gray R, Sellwood E, Hills R, Crome P, Raftery J. Aspirin in Alzheimer's disease (AD2000): A randomised open-label trial. Lancet Neurology. 2008;**7**:41-49. DOI: 10.1016/S1474-4422(07)70293-4

[124] Szekely CA, Breitner JC, Fitzpatrick AL, Rea TD, Psaty BM, Kuller LH, Zandi PP. NSAID use and dementia risk in the cardiovascular health study: Role of APOE and NSAID type. Neurology. 2008;**70**:17-24. DOI: 10.1212/01.wnl.0000284596.95156.48

[125] VanItallie TB. Alzheimer's disease: Innate immunity gone awry? Metabolism. 2017;**69S**: S41-S49. DOI: 10.1016/j.metabol.2017.01.014

[126] Bhamra MS, Ashton NJ. Finding a pathological diagnosis for Alzheimer's disease: Are inflammatory molecules the answer? Electrophoresis. 2012;**33**:3598-3607. DOI: 10.1002/elps.201200161

[127] Swardfager W, Lanctot K, Rothenburg L, Wong A, Cappell J, Herrmann N. A meta-analysis of cytokines in Alzheimer's disease. Biological Psychiatry. 2010;**68**:930-941. DOI: 10.1016/j.biopsych.2010.06.012

[128] Petzold A, Jenkins R, Watt HC, Green AJ, Thompson EJ, Keir G, Fox NC, Rossor MN. Cerebrospinal fluid S100B correlates with brain atrophy in Alzheimer's disease. Neuroscience Letters. 2003;**336**:167-170

[129] Licastro F, Pedrini S, Caputo L, Annoni G, Davis LJ, Ferri C, Casadei V, Grimaldi LM. Increased plasma levels of interleukin-1, interleukin-6 and alpha-1-antichymotrypsin in patients with Alzheimer's disease: Peripheral inflammation or signals from the brain? Journal of Neuroimmunology. 2000;**103**:97-102

[130] Helmy AA, Naseer MM, Shafie SE, Nada MA. Role of interleukin 6 and alpha-globulins in differentiating Alzheimer and vascular dementias. Neurodegenerative Diseases. 2012;**9**:81-86. DOI: 10.1159/000329568

[131] Thambisetty M, Hye A, Foy C, Daly E, Glover A, Cooper A, Simmons A, Murphy D, Lovestone S. Proteome-based identification of plasma proteins associated with hippocampal metabolism in early Alzheimer's disease. Journal of Neurology. 2008;**255**:1712-1720. DOI: 10.1007/s00415-008-0006-8

[132] Schrijvers EM, Koudstaal PJ, Hofman A, Breteler MM. Plasma clusterin and the risk of Alzheimer disease. Journal of the American Medical Association. 2011;**305**:1322-1326. DOI: 10.1001/jama.2011.381

[133] Yasuno F, Kosaka J, Ota M, Higuchi M, Ito H, Fujimura Y, Nozaki S, Takahashi S, Mizukami K, Asada T, Suhara T. Increased binding of peripheral benzodiazepine receptor in mild cognitive impairment-dementia converters measured by positron emission tomography with [(1)(1)C]DAA1106. Psychiatry Research. 2012;**203**:67-74. DOI: 10.1016/j.pscychresns.2011.08.013

[134] Djordjevic J, Sabbir MG, Albensi BC. Traumatic brain injury as a risk factor for Alzheimer's disease: Is inflammatory Signaling a key player? Current Alzheimer Research. 2016;**13**:730-738

[135] Holmes C, Cunningham C, Zotova E, Woolford J, Dean C, Kerr S, Culliford D, Perry VH. Systemic inflammation and disease progression in Alzheimer disease. Neurology. 2009; **73**:768-774. DOI: 10.1212/WNL.0b013e3181b6bb95

[136] Verdile G, Keane KN, Cruzat VF, Medic S, Sabale M, Rowles J, Wijesekara N, Martins RN, Fraser PE, Newsholme P. Inflammation and oxidative stress: The molecular connectivity between insulin resistance, obesity, and Alzheimer's disease. Mediators of Inflammation. 2015;**2015**:105828. DOI: 10.1155/2015/105828

[137] De Felice FG, Ferreira ST. Inflammation, defective insulin signaling, and mitochondrial dysfunction as common molecular denominators connecting type 2 diabetes to Alzheimer disease. Diabetes. 2014;**63**:2262-2272. DOI: 10.2337/db13-1954

[138] Lotharius J, Brundin P. Pathogenesis of parkinson's disease: Dopamine, vesicles and α-synuclein. Nature Reviews Neuroscience. 2002;**3**:932-942. DOI: 10.1038/nrn983

[139] Bose A, Beal MF. Mitochondrial dysfunction in Parkinson's disease. Journal of Neurochemistry. 2016;**139**:216-231. DOI: 10.1111/jnc.13731

[140] Esteves AR, Arduíno DM, Swerdlow RH, Oliveira CR, Cardoso SM. Oxidative stress involvement in α–Synuclein Oligomerization in Parkinson's disease Cybrids. Antioxidants & Redox Signaling. 2009;**11**:439-448. DOI: 10.1089/ars.2008.2247

[141] McNaught KS, Jenner P. Proteasomal function is impaired in substantia nigra in Parkinson's disease. Neuroscience Letters. 2001;**297**:191-194

[142] Olanow CW. The pathogenesis of cell death in Parkinson's disease – 2007. Movement Disorders. 2007;**22**:S335-S342. DOI: 10.1002/mds.21675

[143] Ryan BJ, Hoek S, Fon EA, Wade-martins R. Mitochondrial dysfunction and mitophagy in Parkinson ' s : From familial to sporadic disease. Trends in Biochemical Sciences. 2015;**40**: 200-210. DOI: 10.1016/j.tibs.2015.02.003

[144] Hu Q, Wang G. Mitochondrial dysfunction in Parkinson's disease. Translational Neurodegeneration. 2016;**5**:14-14. DOI: 10.1186/s40035-016-0060-6

[145] Poewe W, Seppi K, Tanner CM, Halliday GM, Brundin P, Volkmann J, Schrag A-E, Lang AE. Parkinson disease. Nature Reviews Disease Primers. 2017;**3**:17013-17013. DOI: 10.1038/nrdp.2017.13

[146] Hirsch EVS, Hunot S. Neuroinflammation in Parkinson's disease. Journal of Neuroimmune Pharmacology. 2012:S210-S212. DOI: 10.1007/s11481-009-9176-0

[147] Exner N, Lutz AK, Haass C, Winklhofer KF. Mitochondrial dysfunction in Parkinson's disease: Molecular mechanisms and pathophysiological consequences. The EMBO Journal. 2012;**31**:3038-3062. DOI: 10.1038/emboj.2012.170

[148] Langston JW, Langston EB, Irwin I. MPTP-induced parkinsonism in human and non-human primates--clinical and experimental aspects. Acta Neurologica Scandinavica. Supplementum. 1984;**100**:49-54

[149] Keeney PM, Xie J, Capaldi RA, Bennett JP Jr. Parkinson's disease brain mitochondrial complex I has oxidatively damaged subunits and is functionally impaired and misassembled. The Journal of Neuroscience. 2006;**26**:5256-5264. DOI: 10.1523/JNEUROSCI.0984-06.2006

[150] Yoshino H, Nakagawa-Hattori Y, Kondo T, Mizuno Y. Mitochondrial complex I and II activities of lymphocytes and platelets in Parkinson's disease. Journal of Neural Transmission. Parkinson's Disease and Dementia Section. 1992;**4**:27-34

[151] Esteves AR, Lu J, Rodova M, Onyango I, Lezi E, Dubinsky R, Lyons KE, Pahwa R, Burns JM, Cardoso SM, Swerdlow RH. Mitochondrial respiration and respiration-associated proteins in cell lines created through Parkinson's subject mitochondrial transfer. Journal of Neurochemistry. 2010;**113**:674-682. DOI: 10.1111/j.1471-4159.2010.06631.x

[152] Bove J, Prou D, Perier C, Przedborski S. Toxin-induced models of Parkinson's disease. NeuroRx. 2005;**2**:484-494. DOI: 10.1602/neurorx.2.3.484

[153] Xiong N, Long X, Xiong J, Jia M, Chen C, Huang J, Ghoorah D, Kong X, Lin Z, Wang T. Mitochondrial complex I inhibitor rotenone-induced toxicity and its potential mechanisms in Parkinson's disease models. Critical Reviews in Toxicology. 2012;**42**:613-632. DOI: 10.3109/10408444.2012.680431

[154] Meredith GE, Rademacher DJ. MPTP mouse models of Parkinson's disease: An update. Journal of Parkinson's Disease. 2011;**1**:19-33. DOI: 10.3233/JPD-2011-11023

[155] Esteves AR, Domingues AF, Ferreira IL, Januario C, Swerdlow RH, Oliveira CR, Cardoso SM. Mitochondrial function in Parkinson's disease cybrids containing an nt2 neuron-like nuclear background. Mitochondrion. 2008;**8**:219-228. DOI: 10.1016/j.mito.2008.03.004

[156] Mann VM, Cooper JM, Krige D, Daniel SE, Schapira AH, Marsden CD. Brain, skeletal muscle and platelet homogenate mitochondrial function in Parkinson's disease. Brain. 1992;**115**(Pt 2):333-342

[157] Bohnen NI, Minoshima S, Giordani B, Frey KA, Kuhl DE. Motor correlates of occipital glucose hypometabolism in Parkinson's disease without dementia. Neurology. 1999;**52**:541-546

[158] Schapira AH. Mitochondria in the aetiology and pathogenesis of Parkinson's disease. Lancet Neurology. 2008;**7**:97-109. DOI: 10.1016/S1474-4422(07)70327-7

[159] Lenaz G. The mitochondrial production of reactive oxygen species: Mechanisms and implications in human pathology. IUBMB Life. 2001;**52**:159-164. DOI: 10.1080/15216540152845957

[160] Jenner P, Dexter DT, Sian J, Schapira AH, Marsden CD. Oxidative stress as a cause of nigral cell death in Parkinson's disease and incidental Lewy body disease. The Royal Kings and Queens Parkinson's Disease Research Group. Annals of Neurology. 1992;**32**(Suppl): S82-S87

[161] Fahn S, Cohen G. The oxidant stress hypothesis in Parkinson's disease: Evidence supporting it. Annals of Neurology. 1992;**32**:804-812. DOI: 10.1002/ana.410320616

[162] Blesa J, Trigo-Damas I, Quiroga-Varela A, Jackson-Lewis VR. Oxidative stress and Parkinson's disease. Frontiers in Neuroanatomy. 2015;**9**:91. DOI: 10.3389/fnana.2015.00091

[163] Kitada T, Asakawa S, Hattori N, Matsumine H, Yamamura Y, Minoshima S, Yokochi M, Mizuno Y, Shimizu N. Mutations in the parkin gene cause autosomal recessive juvenile parkinsonism. Nature. 1998;**392**:605-608. DOI: 10.1038/33416

[164] Valente EM, Abou-Sleiman PM, Caputo V, Muqit MM, Harvey K, Gispert S, Ali Z, Del Turco D, Bentivoglio AR, Healy DG, Albanese A, Nussbaum R, Gonzalez-Maldonado R, Deller T, Salvi S, Cortelli P, Gilks WP, Latchman DS, Harvey RJ, Dallapiccola B, Auburger G, Wood NW. Hereditary early-onset Parkinson's disease caused by mutations in PINK1. Science. 2004;**304**:1158-1160. DOI: 10.1126/science.1096284

[165] Wu W, Xu H, Wang Z, Mao Y, Yuan L, Luo W, Cui Z, Cui T, Wang XL, Shen YH. PINK1-parkin-mediated Mitophagy protects mitochondrial integrity and prevents metabolic stress-induced endothelial injury. PLoS One. 2015;**10**:e0132499. DOI: 10.1371/journal.pone.0132499

[166] Thomas RE, Andrews LA, Burman JL, Lin WY, Pallanck LJ. PINK1-parkin pathway activity is regulated by degradation of PINK1 in the mitochondrial matrix. PLoS Genetics. 2014;**10**:e1004279. DOI: 10.1371/journal.pgen.1004279

[167] Narendra DP, Jin SM, Tanaka A, Suen DF, Gautier CA, Shen J, Cookson MR, Youle RJ. PINK1 is selectively stabilized on impaired mitochondria to activate parkin. PLoS Biology. 2010;**8**:e1000298. DOI: 10.1371/journal.pbio.1000298

[168] Bingol B, Sheng M. Mechanisms of mitophagy: PINK1, parkin, USP30 and beyond. Free Radical Biology & Medicine. 2016;**100**:210-222. DOI: 10.1016/j.freeradbiomed.2016.04.015

[169] Nguyen TN, Padman BS, Lazarou M. Deciphering the molecular signals of PINK1/parkin Mitophagy. Trends in Cell Biology. 2016;**26**:733-744. DOI: 10.1016/j.tcb.2016.05.008

[170] Narendra D, Walker JE, Youle R. Mitochondrial quality control mediated by PINK1 and parkin: Links to parkinsonism. Cold Spring Harbor Perspectives in Biology. 2012;**4**: a011338. DOI: 10.1101/cshperspect.a011338

[171] Kitada T, Pisani A, Porter DR, Yamaguchi H, Tscherter A, Martella G, Bonsi P, Zhang C, Pothos EN, Shen J. Impaired dopamine release and synaptic plasticity in the striatum of

PINK1-deficient mice. Proceedings of the National Academy of Sciences of the United States of America. 2007;**104**:11441-11446. DOI: 10.1073/pnas.0702717104

[172] Park J, Lee SB, Lee S, Kim Y, Song S, Kim S, Bae E, Kim J, Shong M, Kim JM, Chung J. Mitochondrial dysfunction in drosophila PINK1 mutants is complemented by parkin. Nature. 2006;**441**:1157-1161. DOI: 10.1038/nature04788

[173] Arduino DM, Esteves AR, Cortes L, Silva DF, Patel B, Grazina M, Swerdlow RH, Oliveira CR, Cardoso SM. Mitochondrial metabolism in Parkinson's disease impairs quality control autophagy by hampering microtubule-dependent traffic. Human Molecular Genetics. 2012;**21**:4680-4702. DOI: 10.1093/hmg/dds309

[174] Santos D, Esteves AR, Silva DF, Januario C, Cardoso SM. The impact of mitochondrial fusion and fission modulation in sporadic Parkinson's disease. Molecular Neurobiology. 2015;**52**:573-586. DOI: 10.1007/s12035-014-8893-4

[175] Wiemerslage L, Ismael S, Lee D. Early alterations of mitochondrial morphology in dopaminergic neurons from Parkinson's disease-like pathology and time-dependent neuroprotection with D2 receptor activation. Mitochondrion. 2016;**30**:138-147. DOI: 10.1016/j.mito.2016.07.004

[176] Nakamura K, Nemani VM, Azarbal F, Skibinski G, Levy JM, Egami K, Munishkina L, Zhang J, Gardner B, Wakabayashi J, Sesaki H, Cheng Y, Finkbeiner S, Nussbaum RL, Masliah E, Edwards RH. Direct membrane association drives mitochondrial fission by the Parkinson disease-associated protein alpha-synuclein. The Journal of Biological Chemistry. 2011;**286**:20710-20726. DOI: 10.1074/jbc.M110.213538

[177] Lahiri V, Klionsky DJ. Functional impairment in RHOT1/Miro1 degradation and mitophagy is a shared feature in familial and sporadic Parkinson disease. Autophagy. 2017;**13**(8):1259-1261. DOI: 10.1080/15548627.2017.1327512

[178] Hsieh CH, Shaltouki A, Gonzalez AE, Bettencourt da Cruz A, Burbulla LF, St Lawrence E, Schule B, Krainc D, palmer TD, Wang X. Functional impairment in miro degradation and mitophagy is a shared feature in familial and sporadic Parkinson's disease. Cell Stem Cell. 2016;**19**:709-724. DOI: 10.1016/j.stem.2016.08.002

[179] Wang X, Winter D, Ashrafi G, Schlehe J, Wong YL, Selkoe D, Rice S, Steen J, LaVoie MJ, Schwarz TL. PINK1 and parkin target Miro for phosphorylation and degradation to arrest mitochondrial motility. Cell. 2011;**147**:893-906. DOI: 10.1016/j.cell.2011.10.018

[180] Huang Y, Chegini F, Chua G, Murphy K, Gai W, Halliday GM. Macroautophagy in sporadic and the genetic form of Parkinson's disease with the A53T alpha-synuclein mutation. Transl Neurodegener. 2012;**1**:2. DOI: 10.1186/2047-9158-1-2

[181] Nixon RA. The role of autophagy in neurodegenerative disease. Nature Medicine. 2013;**19**:983-997. DOI: 10.1038/nm.3232

[182] Cartelli D, Ronchi C, Maggioni MG, Rodighiero S, Giavini E, Cappelletti G. Microtubule dysfunction precedes transport impairment and mitochondria damage in MPP+ –induced neurodegeneration. Journal of Neurochemistry. 2010;**115**:247-258. DOI: 10.1111/j.1471-4159.2010.06924.x

[183] Cappelletti G, Casagrande F, Calogero A, De Gregorio C, Pezzoli G, Cartelli D. Linking microtubules to Parkinson's disease: The case of parkin. Biochemical Society Transactions. 2015;**43**:292-296. DOI: 10.1042/BST20150007

[184] Scarffe LA, Stevens DA, Dawson VL, Dawson TM. Parkin and PINK1: Much more than mitophagy. Trends in Neurosciences. 2014;**37**:315-324. DOI: 10.1016/j.tins.2014.03.004

[185] Livnat-Levanon N, Kevei E, Kleifeld O, Krutauz D, Segref A, Rinaldi T, Erpapazoglou Z, Cohen M, Reis N, Hoppe T, Glickman MH. Reversible 26S proteasome disassembly upon mitochondrial stress. Cell Reports. 2014;**7**:1371-1380. DOI: 10.1016/j.celrep.2014.04.030

[186] Ross JM, Olson L, Coppotelli G. Mitochondrial and ubiquitin proteasome system dysfunction in ageing and disease: Two sides of the same coin? International Journal of Molecular Sciences. 2015;**16**:19458-19476. DOI: 10.3390/ijms160819458

[187] McKenzie JA, Spielman LJ, Pointer CB, Lowry JR, Bajwa E, Lee CW, Klegeris A. Neuroinflammation as a common mechanism associated with the modifiable risk factors for Alzheimer's and Parkinson's diseases. Current Aging Science. 2017;**10**(3):158-176. DOI: 10.2174/1874609810666170315113244

[188] Subramaniam SR, Federoff HJ. Targeting microglial activation states as a therapeutic avenue in Parkinson's disease. Frontiers in Aging Neuroscience. 2017;**9**:176. DOI: 10.3389/fnagi.2017.00176

[189] Hawkes CH, DelTredici K, Braak H. A timeline for Parkinson's disease. Parkinsonism & Related Disorders. 2010;**16**:79-84. DOI: 10.1016/j.parkreldis.2009.08.007

[190] Savica R, Carlin JM, Grossardt BR, Bower JH, Ahlskog JE, Maraganore DM, Bharucha AE, Rocca WA. Medical records documentation of constipation preceding Parkinson disease: A case-control study. Neurology. 2009;**73**:1752-1758. DOI: 10.1212/WNL.0b013e3181c34af5

[191] Soreq L, Israel Z, Bergman H, Soreq H. Advanced microarray analysis highlights modified neuro-immune signaling in nucleated blood cells from Parkinson's disease patients. Journal of Neuroimmunology. 2008;**201-202**:227-236. DOI: 10.1016/j.jneuroim.2008.06.019

[192] Rees K, Stowe R, Patel S, Ives N, Breen K, Clarke CE, Ben-Shlomo Y. Non-steroidal anti-inflammatory drugs as disease-modifying agents for Parkinson's disease: Evidence from observational studies. Cochrane Database of Systematic Reviews. 2011;**9**:CD008454. DOI: 10.1002/14651858.CD008454.pub2

[193] Chen H, Zhang SM, Hernan MA, Schwarzschild MA, Willett WC, Colditz GA, Speizer FE, Ascherio A. Nonsteroidal anti-inflammatory drugs and the risk of Parkinson disease. Archives of Neurology. 2003;**60**:1059-1064. DOI: 10.1001/archneur.60.8.1059

[194] Samii A, Etminan M, Wiens MO, Jafari S. NSAID use and the risk of Parkinson's disease: Systematic review and meta-analysis of observational studies. Drugs & Aging. 2009;**26**:769-779. DOI: 10.2165/11316780-000000000-00000

[195] Espinosa-Oliva AM, de Pablos RM, Villaran RF, Arguelles S, Venero JL, Machado A, Cano J. Stress is critical for LPS-induced activation of microglia and damage in the rat hippocampus. Neurobiology of Aging. 2011;**32**:85-102. DOI: 10.1016/j.neurobiolaging.2009.01.012

[196] Pott Godoy MC, Ferrari CC, Pitossi FJ. Nigral neurodegeneration triggered by striatal AdIL-1 administration can be exacerbated by systemic IL-1 expression. Journal of Neuroimmunology. 2010;**222**:29-39. DOI: 10.1016/j.jneuroim.2010.02.018

[197] McGeer PL, McGeer EG. Glial reactions in Parkinson's disease. Movement Disorders. 2008;**23**:474-483. DOI: 10.1002/mds.21751

[198] Liu M, Bing G. Lipopolysaccharide animal models for Parkinson's disease. Journal of Parkinson's Disease. 2011;**2011**:327089. DOI: 10.4061/2011/327089

[199] Herrera AJ, Espinosa-Oliva AM, Carrillo-Jimenez A, Oliva-Martin MJ, Garcia-Revilla J, Garcia-Quintanilla A, dePablos RM, Venero JL. Relevance of chronic stress and the two faces of microglia in Parkinson's disease. Frontiers in Cellular Neuroscience. 2015;**9**:312. DOI: 10.3389/fncel.2015.00312

[200] dePablos RM, Herrera AJ, Espinosa-Oliva AM, Sarmiento M, Munoz MF, Machado A, Venero JL. Chronic stress enhances microglia activation and exacerbates death of nigral dopaminergic neurons under conditions of inflammation. Journal of Neuroinflammation. 2014;**11**:34. DOI: 10.1186/1742-2094-11-34

[201] Dominguez-Meijide A, Rodriguez-Perez AI, Diaz-Ruiz C, Guerra MJ, Labandeira-Garcia JL. Dopamine modulates astroglial and microglial activity via glial renin-angiotensin system in cultures. Brain, Behavior, and Immunity. 2017;**62**:277-290. DOI: 10.1016/j.bbi.2017.02.013

[202] Karlsson O, Lindquist NG. Melanin affinity and its possible role in neurodegeneration. Journal of Neural Transmission (Vienna). 2013;**120**:1623-1630. DOI: 10.1007/s00702-013-1062-5

[203] Viceconte N, Burguillos MA, Herrera AJ, De Pablos RM, Joseph B, Venero JL. Neuromelanin activates proinflammatory microglia through a caspase-8-dependent mechanism. Journal of Neuroinflammation. 2015;**12**:5. DOI: 10.1186/s12974-014-0228-x

[204] Lema Tome CM, Tyson T, Rey NL, Grathwohl S, Britschgi M, Brundin P. Inflammation and alpha-synuclein's prion-like behavior in Parkinson's disease--is there a link? Molecular Neurobiology. 2013;**47**:561-574. DOI: 10.1007/s12035-012-8267-8

[205] Klegeris A, Pelech S, Giasson BI, Maguire J, Zhang H, McGeer EG, McGeer PL. Alpha-synuclein activates stress signaling protein kinases in THP-1 cells and microglia. Neurobiology of Aging. 2008;**29**:739-752. DOI: 10.1016/j.neurobiolaging.2006.11.013

[206] Zhang W, Wang T, Pei Z, Miller DS, Wu X, Block ML, Wilson B, Zhang W, Zhou Y, Hong JS, Zhang J. Aggregated alpha-synuclein activates microglia: A process leading to disease progression in Parkinson's disease. The FASEB Journal. 2005;**19**:533-542. DOI: 10.1096/fj.04-2751com

[207] Hamza TH, Zabetian CP, Tenesa A, Laederach A, Montimurro J, Yearout D, Kay DM, Doheny KF, Paschall J, Pugh E, Kusel VI, Collura R, Roberts J, Griffith A, Samii A, Scott WK, Nutt J, Factor SA, Payami H. Common genetic variation in the HLA region is associated with late-onset sporadic Parkinson's disease. Nature Genetics. 2010;**42**:781-785. DOI: 10.1038/ng.642

[208] International Parkinson Disease Genomics Consortium, Nalls MA, Plagnol V, Hernandez DG, Sharma M, Sheerin UM, Saad M, Simon-Sanchez J, Schulte C, Lesage S, Sveinbjornsdottir S, Stefansson K, Martinez M, Hardy J, Heutink P, Brice A, Gasser T, Singleton AB, Wood NW. Imputation of sequence variants for identification of genetic risks for Parkinson's disease: A meta-analysis of genome-wide association studies. Lancet. 2011;**377**:641-649. DOI: 10.1016/S0140-6736(10)62345-8

[209] Pihlstrom L, Axelsson G, Bjornara KA, Dizdar N, Fardell C, Forsgren L, Holmberg B, Larsen JP, Linder J, Nissbrandt H, Tysnes OB, Ohman E, Dietrichs E, Toft M. Supportive evidence for 11 loci from genome-wide association studies in Parkinson's disease. Neurobiology of Aging. 1708;**2013**(34):e1707-e1713. DOI: 10.1016/j.neurobiolaging.2012.10.019

[210] Russo I, Bubacco L, Greggio E. LRRK2 and neuroinflammation: Partners in crime in Parkinson's disease? Journal of Neuroinflammation. 2014;**11**:52. DOI: 10.1186/1742-2094-11-52

[211] Harms AS, Cao S, Rowse AL, Thome AD, Li X, Mangieri LR, Cron RQ, Shacka JJ, Raman C, Standaert DG. MHCII is required for alpha-synuclein-induced activation of microglia, CD4 T cell proliferation, and dopaminergic neurodegeneration. The Journal of Neuroscience. 2013;**33**:9592-9600. DOI: 10.1523/JNEUROSCI.5610-12.2013

[212] Su X, Maguire-Zeiss KA, Giuliano R, Prifti L, Venkatesh K, Federoff HJ. Synuclein activates microglia in a model of Parkinson's disease. Neurobiology of Aging. 2008;**29**:1690-1701. DOI: 10.1016/j.neurobiolaging.2007.04.006

[213] Su X, Federoff HJ, Maguire-Zeiss KA. Mutant alpha-synuclein overexpression mediates early proinflammatory activity. Neurotoxicity Research. 2009;**16**:238-254. DOI: 10.1007/s12640-009-9053-x

[214] Beraud D, Hathaway HA, Trecki J, Chasovskikh S, Johnson DA, Johnson JA, Federoff HJ, Shimoji M, Mhyre TR, Maguire-Zeiss KA. Microglial activation and antioxidant responses induced by the Parkinson's disease protein alpha-synuclein. Journal of Neuroimmune Pharmacology. 2013;**8**:94-117. DOI: 10.1007/s11481-012-9401-0

[215] Reynolds AD, Glanzer JG, Kadiu I, Ricardo-Dukelow M, Chaudhuri A, Ciborowski P, Cerny R, Gelman B, Thomas MP, Mosley RL, Gendelman HE. Nitrated alpha-synuclein-activated microglial profiling for Parkinson's disease. Journal of Neurochemistry. 2008;**104**:1504-1525. DOI: 10.1111/j.1471-4159.2007.05087.x

[216] Couch Y, Alvarez-Erviti L, Sibson NR, Wood MJ, Anthony DC. The acute inflammatory response to intranigral alpha-synuclein differs significantly from intranigral lipopolysaccharide and is exacerbated by peripheral inflammation. Journal of Neuroinflammation. 2011;**8**:166. DOI: 10.1186/1742-2094-8-166

[217] Rahmani F, Kamalian A, Aarabi MH. New evidence comes to light: How is alpha-synuclein aggregation related to mitochondrial protein import in Parkinson's disease? Movement Disorders. 2017;**32**:107. DOI: 10.1002/mds.26889

[218] Maekawa T, Kubo M, Yokoyama I, Ohta E, Obata F. Age-dependent and cell-population-restricted LRRK2 expression in normal mouse spleen. Biochemical and Biophysical Research Communications. 2010;**392**:431-435. DOI: 10.1016/j.bbrc.2010.01.041

[219] Miklossy J, Arai T, Guo JP, Klegeris A, Yu S, McGeer EG, McGeer PL. LRRK2 expression in normal and pathologic human brain and in human cell lines. Journal of Neuropathology and Experimental Neurology. 2006;**65**:953-963. DOI: 10.1097/01.jnen.0000235121.98052.54

[220] Gillardon F, Schmid R, Draheim H. Parkinson's disease-linked leucine-rich repeat kinase 2(R1441G) mutation increases proinflammatory cytokine release from activated primary microglial cells and resultant neurotoxicity. Neuroscience. 2012;**208**:41-48. DOI: 10.1016/j.neuroscience.2012.02.001

[221] Lopez de Maturana R, Aguila JC, Sousa A, Vazquez N, Del Rio P, Aiastui A, Gorostidi A, Lopez de Munain A, Sanchez-Pernaute R. Leucine-rich repeat kinase 2 modulates cyclooxygenase 2 and the inflammatory response in idiopathic and genetic Parkinson's disease. Neurobiology of Aging. 2014;**35**:1116-1124. DOI: 10.1016/j.neurobiolaging.2013.11.018

[222] Kim B, Yang MS, Choi D, Kim JH, Kim HS, Seol W, Choi S, Jou I, Kim EY, Joe EH. Impaired inflammatory responses in murine Lrrk2-knockdown brain microglia. PLoS One. 2012;**7**:e34693. DOI: 10.1371/journal.pone.0034693

[223] McGeer PL, Itagaki S, Akiyama H, McGeer EG. Rate of cell death in parkinsonism indicates active neuropathological process. Annals of Neurology. 1988;**24**:574-576. DOI: 10.1002/ana.410240415

[224] Langston JW, Forno LS, Tetrud J, Reeves AG, Kaplan JA, Karluk D. Evidence of active nerve cell degeneration in the substantia nigra of humans years after 1-methyl-4-phenyl-1,2,3,6-tetrahydropyridine exposure. Annals of Neurology. 1999;**46**:598-605

[225] Banati RB, Daniel SE, Blunt SB. Glial pathology but absence of apoptotic nigral neurons in long-standing Parkinson's disease. Movement Disorders. 1998;**13**:221-227. DOI: 10.1002/mds.870130205

[226] Mirza B, Hadberg H, Thomsen P, Moos T. The absence of reactive astrocytosis is indicative of a unique inflammatory process in Parkinson's disease. Neuroscience. 2000;**95**:425-432

[227] Imamura K, Hishikawa N, Sawada M, Nagatsu T, Yoshida M, Hashizume Y. Distribution of major histocompatibility complex class II-positive microglia and cytokine profile of Parkinson's disease brains. Acta Neuropathologica. 2003;**106**:518-526. DOI: 10.1007/s00401-003-0766-2

[228] Miklossy J, Doudet DD, Schwab C, Yu S, McGeer EG, McGeer PL. Role of ICAM-1 in persisting inflammation in Parkinson disease and MPTP monkeys. Experimental Neurology. 2006;**197**:275-283. DOI: 10.1016/j.expneurol.2005.10.034

[229] Damier P, Hirsch EC, Zhang P, Agid Y, Javoy-Agid F. Glutathione peroxidase, glial cells and Parkinson's disease. Neuroscience. 1993;**52**:1-6

[230] Fiszer U, Mix E, Fredrikson S, Kostulas V, Link H. Parkinson's disease and immunological abnormalities: Increase of HLA-DR expression on monocytes in cerebrospinal fluid and of CD45RO+ T cells in peripheral blood. Acta Neurologica Scandinavica. 1994;**90**:160-166

[231] Bas J, Calopa M, Mestre M, Mollevi DG, Cutillas B, Ambrosio S, Buendia E. Lymphocyte populations in Parkinson's disease and in rat models of parkinsonism. Journal of Neuroimmunology. 2001;**113**:146-152

[232] Baba Y, Kuroiwa A, Uitti RJ, Wszolek ZK, Yamada T. Alterations of T-lymphocyte populations in Parkinson disease. Parkinsonism & Related Disorders. 2005;**11**:493-498. DOI: 10.1016/j.parkreldis.2005.07.005

[233] Brochard V, Combadiere B, Prigent A, Laouar Y, Perrin A, Beray-Berthat V, Bonduelle O, Alvarez-Fischer D, Callebert J, Launay JM, Duyckaerts C, Flavell RA, Hirsch EC, Hunot S. Infiltration of CD4+ lymphocytes into the brain contributes to neurodegeneration in a mouse model of Parkinson disease. The Journal of Clinical Investigation. 2009;**119**:182-192. DOI: 10.1172/JCI36470

[234] Stone DK, Reynolds AD, Mosley RL, Gendelman HE. Innate and adaptive immunity for the pathobiology of Parkinson's disease. Antioxidants & Redox Signaling. 2009;**11**:2151-2166. DOI: 10.1089/ARS.2009.2460

[235] Cabezas R, Avila M, Gonzalez J, El-Bacha RS, Baez E, Garcia-Segura LM, Jurado Coronel JC, Capani F, Cardona-Gomez GP, Barreto GE. Astrocytic modulation of blood brain barrier: Perspectives on Parkinson's disease. Frontiers in Cellular Neuroscience. 2014;**8**:211. DOI: 10.3389/fncel.2014.00211

[236] Forsyth CB, Shannon KM, Kordower JH, Voigt RM, Shaikh M, Jaglin JA, Estes JD, Dodiya HB, Keshavarzian A. Increased intestinal permeability correlates with sigmoid mucosa alpha-synuclein staining and endotoxin exposure markers in early Parkinson's disease. PLoS One. 2011;**6**:e28032. DOI: 10.1371/journal.pone.0028032

[237] Devos D, Lebouvier T, Lardeux B, Biraud M, Rouaud T, Pouclet H, Coron E, Bruley des Varannes S, Naveilhan P, Nguyen JM, Neunlist M, Derkinderen P. Colonic inflammation in Parkinson's disease. Neurobiology of Disease. 2013;**50**:42-48. DOI: 10.1016/j.nbd.2012.09.007

[238] Mogi M, Harada M, Riederer P, Narabayashi H, Fujita K, Nagatsu T. Tumor necrosis factor-alpha (TNF-alpha) increases both in the brain and in the cerebrospinal fluid from parkinsonian patients. Neuroscience Letters. 1994;**165**:208-210

[239] Hunot S, Dugas N, Faucheux B, Hartmann A, Tardieu M, Debre P, Agid Y, Dugas B, Hirsch EC. FcepsilonRII/CD23 is expressed in Parkinson's disease and induces, in vitro, production of nitric oxide and tumor necrosis factor-alpha in glial cells. The Journal of Neuroscience. 1999;**19**:3440-3447

[240] Mogi M, Harada M, Kondo T, Riederer P, Inagaki H, Minami M, Nagatsu T. Interleukin-1 beta, interleukin-6, epidermal growth factor and transforming growth factor-alpha are elevated in the brain from parkinsonian patients. Neuroscience Letters. 1994;**180**:147-150

[241] Mogi M, Harada M, Kondo T, Narabayashi H, Riederer P, Nagatsu T. Transforming growth factor-beta 1 levels are elevated in the striatum and in ventricular cerebrospinal fluid in Parkinson's disease. Neuroscience Letters. 1995;**193**:129-132

[242] Mogi M, Harada M, Narabayashi H, Inagaki H, Minami M, Nagatsu T. Interleukin (IL)-1 beta, IL-2, IL-4, IL-6 and transforming growth factor-alpha levels are elevated in ventricular cerebrospinal fluid in juvenile parkinsonism and Parkinson's disease. Neuroscience Letters. 1996;**211**:13-16

[243] Mogi M, Kondo T, Mizuno Y, Nagatsu T. p53 protein, interferon-gamma, and NF-kappaB levels are elevated in the parkinsonian brain. Neuroscience Letters. 2007;**414**:94-97. DOI: 10.1016/j.neulet.2006.12.003

[244] Boka G, Anglade P, Wallach D, Javoy-Agid F, Agid Y, Hirsch EC. Immunocytochemical analysis of tumor necrosis factor and its receptors in Parkinson's disease. Neuroscience Letters. 1994;**172**:151-154

[245] Mogi M, Togari A, Kondo T, Mizuno Y, Komure O, Kuno S, Ichinose H, Nagatsu T. Caspase activities and tumor necrosis factor receptor R1 (p55) level are elevated in the substantia nigra from parkinsonian brain. Journal of Neural Transmission (Vienna). 2000;**107**:335-341. DOI: 10.1007/s007020050028

[246] Knott C, Stern G, Wilkin GP. Inflammatory regulators in Parkinson's disease: iNOS, lipocortin-1, and cyclooxygenases-1 and -2. Molecular and Cellular Neurosciences. 2000;**16**:724-739. DOI: 10.1006/mcne.2000.0914

[247] Choi DK, Pennathur S, Perier C, Tieu K, Teismann P, Wu DC, Jackson-Lewis V, Vila M, Vonsattel JP, Heinecke JW, Przedborski S. Ablation of the inflammatory enzyme myeloperoxidase mitigates features of Parkinson's disease in mice. The Journal of Neuroscience. 2005;**25**:6594-6600. DOI: 10.1523/JNEUROSCI.0970-05.2005

[248] Stypula G, Kunert-Radek J, Stepien H, Zylinska K, Pawlikowski M. Evaluation of interleukins, ACTH, cortisol and prolactin concentrations in the blood of patients with parkinson's disease. Neuroimmunomodulation. 1996;**3**:131-134

[249] Dobbs RJ, Charlett A, Purkiss AG, Dobbs SM, Weller C, Peterson DW. Association of circulating TNF-alpha and IL-6 with ageing and parkinsonism. Acta Neurologica Scandinavica. 1999;**100**:34-41

[250] Rentzos M, Nikolaou C, Andreadou E, Paraskevas GP, Rombos A, Zoga M, Tsoutsou A, Boufidou F, Kapaki E, Vassilopoulos D. Circulating interleukin-15 and RANTES chemokine in Parkinson's disease. Acta Neurologica Scandinavica. 2007;**116**:374-379. DOI: 10.1111/j.1600-0404.2007.00894.x

[251] Rentzos M, Nikolaou C, Andreadou E, Paraskevas GP, Rombos A, Zoga M, Tsoutsou A, Boufidou F, Kapaki E, Vassilopoulos D. Circulating interleukin-10 and interleukin-12 in Parkinson's disease. Acta Neurologica Scandinavica. 2009;**119**:332-337. DOI: 10.1111/j.1600-0404.2008.01103.x

[252] Dufek M, Hamanova M, Lokaj J, Goldemund D, Rektorova I, Michalkova Z, Sheardova K, Rektor I. Serum inflammatory biomarkers in Parkinson's disease. Parkinsonism & Related Disorders. 2009;**15**:318-320. DOI: 10.1016/j.parkreldis.2008.05.014

[253] Scalzo P, Kummer A, Cardoso F, Teixeira AL. Increased serum levels of soluble tumor necrosis factor-alpha receptor-1 in patients with Parkinson's disease. Journal of Neuroimmunology. 2009;**216**:122-125. DOI: 10.1016/j.jneuroim.2009.08.001

[254] Reale M, Iarlori C, Thomas A, Gambi D, Perfetti B, Di Nicola M, Onofrj M. Peripheral cytokines profile in Parkinson's disease. Brain, Behavior, and Immunity. 2009;**23**:55-63. DOI: 10.1016/j.bbi.2008.07.003

[255] Tang P, Chong L, Li X, Liu Y, Liu P, Hou C, Li R. Correlation between serum RANTES levels and the severity of Parkinson's disease. Oxidative Medicine and Cellular Longevity. 2014;**2014**:208408. DOI: 10.1155/2014/208408

[256] Blum-Degen D, Muller T, Kuhn W, Gerlach M, Przuntek H, Riederer P. Interleukin-1 beta and interleukin-6 are elevated in the cerebrospinal fluid of Alzheimer's and de novo Parkinson's disease patients. Neuroscience Letters. 1995;**202**:17-20

[257] Gonzalez-Scarano F, Baltuch G. Microglia as mediators of inflammatory and degenerative diseases. Annual Review of Neuroscience. 1999;**22**:219-240. DOI: 10.1146/annurev.neuro.22.1.219

[258] Maetzler W, Berg D, Schalamberidze N, Melms A, Schott K, Mueller JC, Liaw L, Gasser T, Nitsch C. Osteopontin is elevated in Parkinson's disease and its absence leads to reduced neurodegeneration in the MPTP model. Neurobiology of Disease. 2007;**25**:473-482. DOI: 10.1016/j.nbd.2006.10.020

[259] Gerhard A, Pavese N, Hotton G, Turkheimer F, Es M, Hammers A, Eggert K, Oertel W, Banati RB, Brooks DJ. In vivo imaging of microglial activation with [11C](R)-PK11195 PET in idiopathic Parkinson's disease. Neurobiology of Disease. 2006;**21**:404-412. DOI: 10.1016/j.nbd.2005.08.002

[260] Ouchi Y, Yoshikawa E, Sekine Y, Futatsubashi M, Kanno T, Ogusu T, Torizuka T. Microglial activation and dopamine terminal loss in early Parkinson's disease. Annals of Neurology. 2005;**57**:168-175. DOI: 10.1002/ana.20338

[261] Iannaccone S, Cerami C, Alessio M, Garibotto V, Panzacchi A, Olivieri S, Gelsomino G, Moresco RM, Perani D. In vivo microglia activation in very early dementia with Lewy bodies, comparison with Parkinson's disease. Parkinsonism & Related Disorders. 2013;**19**:47-52. DOI: 10.1016/j.parkreldis.2012.07.002

[262] Ghadery C, Koshimori Y, Coakeley S, Harris M, Rusjan P, Kim J, Houle S, Strafella AP. Microglial activation in Parkinson's disease using [18F]-FEPPA. Journal of Neuroinflammation. 2017;**14**:8. DOI: 10.1186/s12974-016-0778-1

[263] Yang L, Guo C, Zhu J, Feng Y, Chen W, Feng Z, Wang D, Sun S, Lin W, Wang Y. Increased levels of pro-inflammatory and anti-inflammatory cellular responses in

Parkinson's disease patients: Search for a disease indicator. Medical Science Monitor. 2017;**23**:2972-2978

[264] He Y, Appel S, Le W. Minocycline inhibits microglial activation and protects nigral cells after 6-hydroxydopamine injection into mouse striatum. Brain Research. 2001;**909**: 187-193

[265] McGeer PL, Schwab C, Parent A, Doudet D. Presence of reactive microglia in monkey substantia nigra years after 1-methyl-4-phenyl-1,2,3,6-tetrahydropyridine administration. Annals of Neurology. 2003;**54**:599-604. DOI: 10.1002/ana.10728

[266] Depino AM, Earl C, Kaczmarczyk E, Ferrari C, Besedovsky H, delRey A, Pitossi FJ, Oertel WH. Microglial activation with atypical proinflammatory cytokine expression in a rat model of Parkinson's disease. The European Journal of Neuroscience. 2003;**18**:2731-2742

[267] Barcia C, Sanchez Bahillo A, Fernandez-Villalba E, Bautista V, Poza YPM, Fernandez-Barreiro A, Hirsch EC, Herrero MT. Evidence of active microglia in substantia nigra pars compacta of parkinsonian monkeys 1 year after MPTP exposure. Glia. 2004;**46**:402-409. DOI: 10.1002/glia.20015

[268] Sherer TB, Betarbet R, Kim JH, Greenamyre JT. Selective microglial activation in the rat rotenone model of Parkinson's disease. Neuroscience Letters. 2003;**341**:87-90

[269] Shaikh SB, Nicholson LF. Effects of chronic low dose rotenone treatment on human microglial cells. Molecular Neurodegeneration. 2009;**4**:55. DOI: 10.1186/1750-1326-4-55

[270] Armentero MT, Levandis G, Nappi G, Bazzini E, Blandini F. Peripheral inflammation and neuroprotection: Systemic pretreatment with complete Freund's adjuvant reduces 6-hydroxydopamine toxicity in a rodent model of Parkinson's disease. Neurobiology of Disease. 2006;**24**:492-505. DOI: 10.1016/j.nbd.2006.08.016

[271] Wheeler CJ, Seksenyan A, Koronyo Y, Rentsendorj A, Sarayba D, Wu H, Gragg A, Siegel E, Thomas D, Espinosa A, Thompson K, Black K, Koronyo-Hamaoui M, Pechnick R, Irvin DK. T-lymphocyte deficiency exacerbates behavioral deficits in the 6-OHDA unilateral lesion rat model for Parkinson's disease. Journal of Neurology & Neurophysiology. 2014;**5**(3):209. DOI: 10.4172/2155-9562.1000209

[272] Rodrigues RW, Gomide VC, Chadi G. Astroglial and microglial reaction after a partial nigrostriatal degeneration induced by the striatal injection of different doses of 6-hydroxydopamine. The International Journal of Neuroscience. 2001;**109**:91-126

[273] Rodrigues RW, Gomide VC, Chadi G. Astroglial and microglial activation in the wistar rat ventral tegmental area after a single striatal injection of 6-hydroxydopamine. The International Journal of Neuroscience. 2004;**114**:197-216. DOI: 10.1080/00207450490249338

[274] Breidert T, Callebert J, Heneka MT, Landreth G, Launay JM, Hirsch EC. Protective action of the peroxisome proliferator-activated receptor-gamma agonist pioglitazone in a mouse model of Parkinson's disease. Journal of Neurochemistry. 2002;**82**:615-624

[275] Herrera AJ, Castano A, Venero JL, Cano J, Machado A. The single intranigral injection of LPS as a new model for studying the selective effects of inflammatory reactions on dopaminergic system. Neurobiology of Disease. 2000;**7**:429-447. DOI: 10.1006/nbdi.2000.0289

[276] Qin L, Wu X, Block ML, Liu Y, Breese GR, Hong JS, Knapp DJ, Crews FT. Systemic LPS causes chronic neuroinflammation and progressive neurodegeneration. Glia. 2007;**55**:453-462. DOI: 10.1002/glia.20467

[277] Castano A, Herrera AJ, Cano J, Machado A. Lipopolysaccharide intranigral injection induces inflammatory reaction and damage in nigrostriatal dopaminergic system. Journal of Neurochemistry. 1998;**70**:1584-1592

[278] Kim WG, Mohney RP, Wilson B, Jeohn GH, Liu B, Hong JS. Regional difference in susceptibility to lipopolysaccharide-induced neurotoxicity in the rat brain: Role of microglia. The Journal of Neuroscience. 2000;**20**:6309-6316

[279] Xie X, Luo X, Liu N, Li X, Lou F, Zheng Y, Ren Y. Monocytes, microglia, and CD200-CD200R1 signaling are essential in the transmission of inflammation from the periphery to the central nervous system. Journal of Neurochemistry. 2017;**141**:222-235. DOI: 10.1111/jnc.13972

[280] Carvey PM, Chang Q, Lipton JW, Ling Z. Prenatal exposure to the bacteriotoxin lipopolysaccharide leads to long-term losses of dopamine neurons in offspring: A potential, new model of Parkinson's disease. Frontiers in Bioscience. 2003;**8**:s826-s837

[281] Ling Z, Gayle DA, Ma SY, Lipton JW, Tong CW, Hong JS, Carvey PM. Utero bacterial endotoxin exposure causes loss of tyrosine hydroxylase neurons in the postnatal rat midbrain. Movement Disorders. 2002;**17**:116-124

[282] Ling Z, Chang QA, Tong CW, Leurgans SE, Lipton JW, Carvey PM. Rotenone potentiates dopamine neuron loss in animals exposed to lipopolysaccharide prenatally. Experimental Neurology. 2004;**190**:373-383. DOI: 10.1016/j.expneurol.2004.08.006

[283] Arguelles S, Herrera AJ, Carreno-Muller E, dePablos RM, Villaran RF, Espinosa-Oliva AM, Machado A, Cano J. Degeneration of dopaminergic neurons induced by thrombin injection in the substantia nigra of the rat is enhanced by dexamethasone: Role of monoamine oxidase enzyme. Neurotoxicology. 2010;**31**:55-66. DOI: 10.1016/j.neuro.2009.12.001

[284] Carreno-Muller E, Herrera AJ, de Pablos RM, Tomas-Camardiel M, Venero JL, Cano J, Machado A. Thrombin induces in vivo degeneration of nigral dopaminergic neurones along with the activation of microglia. Journal of Neurochemistry. 2003;**84**:1201-1214

[285] Ara J, Przedborski S, Naini AB, Jackson-Lewis V, Trifiletti RR, Horwitz J, Ischiropoulos H. Inactivation of tyrosine hydroxylase by nitration following exposure to peroxynitrite and 1-methyl-4-phenyl-1,2,3,6-tetrahydropyridine (MPTP). Proceedings of the National Academy of Sciences of the United States of America. 1998;**95**:7659-7663

[286] Przedborski S, Chen Q, Vila M, Giasson BI, Djaldatti R, Vukosavic S, Souza JM, Jackson-Lewis V, Lee VM, Ischiropoulos H. Oxidative post-translational modifications of alpha-synuclein in the 1-methyl-4-phenyl-1,2,3,6-tetrahydropyridine (MPTP) mouse model of Parkinson's disease. Journal of Neurochemistry. 2001;**76**:637-640

[287] De Lella Ezcurra AL, Chertoff M, Ferrari C, Graciarena M, Pitossi F. Chronic expression of low levels of tumor necrosis factor-alpha in the substantia nigra elicits progressive neurodegeneration, delayed motor symptoms and microglia/macrophage activation. Neurobiology of Disease. 2010;**37**:630-640. DOI: 10.1016/j.nbd.2009.11.018

[288] Takeuchi O, Akira S. Pattern recognition receptors and inflammation. Cell. 2010;**140**:805-820. DOI: 10.1016/j.cell.2010.01.022

[289] West AP, Koblansky AA, Ghosh S. Recognition and signaling by toll-like receptors. Annual Review of Cell and Developmental Biology. 2006;**22**:409-437. DOI: 10.1146/annurev.cellbio.21.122303.115827

[290] Zhang Q, Raoof M, Chen Y, Sumi Y, Sursal T, Junger W, Brohi K, Itagaki K, Hauser CJ. Circulating mitochondrial DAMPs cause inflammatory responses to injury. Nature. 2010;**464**:104-107. DOI: 10.1038/nature08780

[291] Taanman JW. The mitochondrial genome: Structure, transcription, translation and replication. Biochimica et Biophysica Acta. 1999;**1410**:103-123

[292] Rabiet MJ, Huet E, Boulay F. The N-formyl peptide receptors and the anaphylatoxin C5a receptors: An overview. Biochimie. 2007;**89**:1089-1106. DOI: 10.1016/j.biochi.2007.02.015

[293] Gurung P, Lukens JR, Kanneganti TD. Mitochondria: Diversity in the regulation of the NLRP3 inflammasome. Trends in Molecular Medicine. 2015;**21**:193-201. DOI: 10.1016/j.molmed.2014.11.008

[294] Latz E, Xiao TS, Stutz A. Activation and regulation of the inflammasomes. Nature Reviews. Immunology. 2013;**13**:397-411. DOI: 10.1038/nri3452

[295] Schroder K, Tschopp J. The inflammasomes. Cell. 2010;**140**:821-832. DOI: 10.1016/j.cell.2010.01.040

[296] Zhou R, Yazdi AS, Menu P, Tschopp J. A role for mitochondria in NLRP3 inflammasome activation. Nature. 2011;**469**:221-225. DOI: 10.1038/nature09663

[297] Nakahira K, Haspel JA, Rathinam VA, Lee SJ, Dolinay T, Lam HC, Englert JA, Rabinovitch M, Cernadas M, Kim HP, Fitzgerald KA, Ryter SW, Choi AM. Autophagy proteins regulate innate immune responses by inhibiting the release of mitochondrial DNA mediated by the NALP3 inflammasome. Nature Immunology. 2011;**12**:222-230. DOI: 10.1038/ni.1980

[298] Shimada K, Crother TR, Karlin J, Dagvadorj J, Chiba N, Chen S, Ramanujan VK, Wolf AJ, Vergnes L, Ojcius DM, Rentsendorj A, Vargas M, Guerrero C, Wang Y, Fitzgerald KA, Underhill DM, Town T, Arditi M. Oxidized mitochondrial DNA activates the NLRP3 inflammasome during apoptosis. Immunity. 2012;**36**:401-414. DOI: 10.1016/j.immuni.2012.01.009

[299] deAndrade RI, Einicker-Lamas M, Roney Bernardo R, Previatto LM, Mohana-Borges R, Morgado-Diaz JA, Benchimol M. Cardiolipin in hydrogenosomes: Evidence of symbiotic origin. Eukaryotic Cell. 2006;**5**:784-787. DOI: 10.1128/EC.5.4.784-787.2006

[300] Kutschera U, Niklas KJ. Endosymbiosis, cell evolution, and speciation. Theory in Biosciences. 2005;**124**:1-24. DOI: 10.1016/j.thbio.2005.04.001

[301] Iyer SS, He Q, Janczy JR, Elliott EI, Zhong Z, Olivier AK, Sadler JJ, Knepper-Adrian V, Han R, Qiao L, Eisenbarth SC, Nauseef WM, Cassel SL, Sutterwala FS. Mitochondrial cardiolipin is required for Nlrp3 inflammasome activation. Immunity. 2013;**39**:311-323. DOI: 10.1016/j.immuni.2013.08.001

[302] Little JP, Simtchouk S, Schindler SM, Villanueva EB, Gill NE, Walker DG, Wolthers KR, Klegeris A. Mitochondrial transcription factor a (Tfam) is a pro-inflammatory extracellular signaling molecule recognized by brain microglia. Molecular and Cellular Neurosciences. 2014;**60**:88-96. DOI: 10.1016/j.mcn.2014.04.003

[303] Davis CH, Kim KY, Bushong EA, Mills EA, Boassa D, Shih T, Kinebuchi M, Phan S, Zhou Y, Bihlmeyer NA, Nguyen JV, Jin Y, Ellisman MH, Marsh-Armstrong N. Transcellular degradation of axonal mitochondria. Proceedings of the National Academy of Sciences of the United States of America. 2014;**111**:9633-9638. DOI: 10.1073/pnas.1404651111

[304] Hayakawa K, Esposito E, Wang X, Terasaki Y, Liu Y, Xing C, Ji X, Lo EH. Transfer of mitochondria from astrocytes to neurons after stroke. Nature. 2016;**535**:551-555. DOI: 10.1038/nature18928

Section 4

Mitochondrial Components and Their Roles in Diseases

Chapter 7

Protein Kinases and Regulation of Mitochondrial Function in Ischemia/Reperfusion Injury

Grażyna Nowak

Additional information is available at the end of the chapter

http://dx.doi.org/10.5772/intechopen.71094

Abstract

Ischemic heart disease and stroke are the leading causes of death worldwide. Nonetheless, our understanding of the molecular mechanisms regulating cardiac and cerebral ischemic injury is very modest and our ability to develop therapies arresting and/or reversing detrimental events that spread from the ischemic core to the surrounding tissue is limited. Ischemia occurs when oxygen is unavailable to tissues due to occlusion of an artery (myocardial infarction, stroke, and pulmonary embolism), hemorrhage, organ transplantation, or hypotension in septic shock. The mitochondrion is a key target of ischemia. Alterations in mitochondrial morphology, dynamics, and functions result in energy deficits and contribute to the pathogenesis of ischemic injury. Phosphorylations of mitochondrial proteins and protein kinases that mediate them are important regulators of mitochondrial functions and tissue ATP levels. Thus, mitochondrial protein kinases could serve as targets for therapeutic interventions to mitigate the effects of ischemic injury. This will review the mitochondrial proteins regulated by phosphorylation, protein kinases mediating these reactions, and their implications in mitochondrial functions in ischemia/reperfusion (I/R)-induced injury.

Keywords: protein kinases, phosphorylation, mitochondria, mitochondrial dysfunction, ischemia, reperfusion, injury, ATP, oxidative phosphorylation, electron transport chain

1. Introduction

Ischemia (insufficient oxygen and nutrient supply to an organ) can affect all major organs and is often encountered in many clinical and nonclinical settings including myocardial infarction, stroke, pulmonary embolism, major surgery, tissue trauma and hemorrhage, transplantation and organ storage, or hypotension in septic shock. Functional deficits caused by ischemia in major organs result in significant morbidity, disability, and mortality. Mitochondria are double-membrane-bound, dynamic organelles present in most eukaryotic cell types. They require large amounts of oxygen to generate ~90–95% of the total energy in oxidative phosphorylation occurring in a majority of cells [1]. Therefore, mitochondria are the key subcellular targets of ischemia, which undergo pathological changes that trigger cellular and tissue damage when oxygen is unavailable. Mitochondria perform several major cellular functions including energy and intermediary metabolisms, several biosyntheses, regulation of calcium storage, and redox homeostasis [1]. They are also involved in signaling, cell cycle, growth, differentiation, and cell death by apoptosis [2].

2. Major mitochondrial targets of ischemia/reperfusion (I/R)

Proteins of the mitochondrial electron transport chain and oxidative phosphorylation are among the primary targets of ischemia and oxidative stress during reperfusion [3]. Decreases in activities of adenine nucleotide translocase (ANT) and ATP synthase are among the earliest events after the onset of cardiac ischemia [4–7]. Inhibition of NADH:ubiquinone dehydrogenase (complex I) and reduced cytochrome c content occur early during ischemia [5, 8], whereas the damage to ubiquinol:cytochrome c oxidoreductase (complex III) and cytochrome oxidase (complex IV) occurs in prolonged ischemia [5, 8]. Reduced activity of complex I is primarily caused by decreases in NADH dehydrogenase activity [5, 9] due to, in part, oxidative damage to the flavin mononucleotide (FMN) prosthetic groups, which results in electron leakage, superoxide production, and the generation of reactive oxygen species (ROS) in ischemic tissues [5, 10]. Ischemia decreases the activity of complex III by inactivating the iron-sulfur center, which contributes to electron leakage and superoxide production, and exacerbates oxidative stress originating from complex I [11]. The voltage-dependent anion channel (VDAC) and proteins of the mitochondrial permeability transition (MPT) pore are also targeted by I/R, which disrupts the transport of ions and solutes and the membrane potential for ATP synthesis [12, 13].

Mitochondria are dynamic organelles that regularly undergo fission (fragmentation) and fusion (formation of a network of mitochondria) [14]. Fission is mediated by the dynamin-related protein 1 (Drp1) and mitochondrial fission protein 1 (Fis1) [14]. Fusion is regulated by the mitofusins (Mfn1 and Mfn2) and the optic atrophy protein 1 (Opa1) [14]. Drp1 and Opa1 are rapidly activated and translocated to mitochondria after ischemia in major organs. This promotes fission, the permeabilization of the mitochondrial outer membrane, and the release of proteins that initiate the intrinsic cascade of apoptosis [15, 16]. Inhibition of Drp1 inhibits fission and reduces cardiomyocyte death, the size of myocardial infarct, and acute kidney injury after ischemia [17]. Mitochondria also regulate the intrinsic cascade of apoptosis, which is activated after the release of mitochondrial proteins. Therefore, preservation of mitochondrial integrity and function is crucial for organ protection against I/R injury.

http://dx.doi.org/10.5772/intechopen.71094

3. Phosphorylation of mitochondrial proteins as a regulatory mechanism of energy metabolism during ischemia/reperfusion

Numerous mitochondrial proteins (354 reported to date) are phosphoproteins that collectively contain 899 identified and 479 potential novel phosphorylation sites [18, 19]. Consequently, phosphorylation of mitochondrial proteins has emerged as an important mechanism involved in progressive damage of mitochondria in response to metabolic stresses including I/R and the status of these phosphorylations is key to understanding the regulation of mitochondrial functions in disease states [18, 19]. A number of protein kinases localize to mitochondria in response to I/R [19, 20]. Protein phosphorylations by these kinases produce differential outcomes in different tissues depending on the phosphorylation site and the kinase involved. The key proteins of oxidative phosphorylation, TCA cycle, transport, and the cascade of intrinsic apoptosis are regulated by phosphorylation [19–23].

3.1. Phosphorylation of proteins involved in oxidative phosphorylation

The largest group of phosphorylation sites was found among proteins involved in oxidative phosphorylation: respiratory complexes, ATP synthase, ANT, and VDAC [18, 19].

4. NADH-ubiquinone oxidoreductase (complex I)

Dysfunction of complex I is the most common disorder of oxidative phosphorylation in humans. It is often due to defects of the subunit assembly to form the mature complex I. Complex I is a major mitochondrial target of I/R. Its activity decreases as early as 10 minutes into cardiac ischemia [24]. Our studies demonstrated that the activity of complex I in renal cortical mitochondria is decreased after renal ischemia [25]. Changes in the activity of complex I during I/R are also regulated by phosphorylation [4, 26]. Phosphorylations occur on several subunits of complex I. The NDUFA10 subunit is phosphorylated on S59 and S95 [27]. The NDUFS4 and NDUFA10 subunits are phosphorylated by mitochondrial protein kinase A (PKA), which stimulates the activity of complex I [27–29]. Phosphorylations of subunit ESSS on S20 and subunit MWFE (NDUFA1) on S55 regulate complex I assembly. Blocking these phosphorylations inhibits assembly of subunits to form a mature complex I and reduces its activity [26, 30]. Tyrosine phosphorylation of the NDUFB10 subunit by Src kinases also increases the activity of complex I, possibly by increasing its affinity toward NADH or increasing assembly of subunits into the fully active complex I [31, 32]. The reduced assembly of subunits leads to decreased levels of complex I [32]. This adaptation shifts fuel utilization from fuels that generate primarily NADH (carbohydrates) to fuels generating more $FADH_2$ (fatty acids) oxidized by complex II. This shift may occur during nutritional restriction or after ischemic injury [32]. Further, complex I is primarily assembled into mitochondrial super-complexes, which increases O_2 consumption and reduces ROS production [33]. Cardiac I/R induces disintegration of mitochondrial super-complexes, which reduces activity of the electron transport chain [34]. Thus, phosphorylation controls the formation, stability, and function of complex I and its assembly into super-complexes.

5. Succinate-ubiquinone oxidoreductase (complex II)

Complex II is an essential regulator of metabolic reprogramming and respiratory adaptation. Mitochondrial Src-type tyrosine kinase Fgr phosphorylates complex II on Y535, Y596, and Y604 when activated by ROS generated by I/R [32]. Phosphorylation of Y604 on the flavoprotein subunit of succinate dehydrogenase (FpSDH) increases activity of complex II and serves as a metabolic adaptation to increased ROS production [32, 34]. Fgr-mediated phosphorylation also reduces the protein levels of complex I, which alters the mitochondrial preference for fuel oxidation from NADH to $FADH_2$, which increases the metabolic capacity of mitochondria to utilize alternative fuels when complex I is impaired [32]. Blocking phosphorylation of FpSDH on Y604 abolishes the capacity of mitochondria to adapt their metabolism after hypoxia/reoxygenation [32]. Mitochondrial phosphatases dephosphorylate Y604 and reverse this metabolic adaptation [32, 34]. In contrast, phosphorylation of FpSDH in cancer cells undergoing hypoxia decreases and dephosphorylation of FpSDH increases SDH activity [35]. Our data show that the activity of complex II in injured renal proximal tubular cells (RPTC) and in the ischemic kidney cortex is unchanged, whereas the activity of complex I is decreased [25, 36]. Supplementing the RPTC with succinate (complex II substrate) ameliorates mitochondrial dysfunction, ATP deficits, oxidative stress, and cell death after injury associated with the generation of ROS and oxidative stress [36].

6. Ubiquinol-cytochrome c oxidoreductase (complex III)

Phosphorylation has been implicated in the regulation of the Rieske iron-sulfur protein of complex III, which is a major target of ischemia and the decreases in its activity lead to increased superoxide production [37]. Several phosphorylation sites have been identified on the subunits of complex III. The tyrosines on the core subunit 1 of complex III are phosphorylated by the Src kinase family, but the functional consequence of this phosphorylation is not yet known [38]. The role of phosphorylation of Rieske iron-sulfur protein is not clear and it was suggested that it regulates the MPTP opening [37].

7. Cytochrome oxidase (complex IV)

To date, 14 phosphorylation sites have been mapped on complex IV [39]. Tyrosine phosphorylation of the specific subunits of complex IV can lead to both inhibition and activation of complex IV activity [39, 40]. Bender and Kadenbach have shown phosphorylation of complex IV subunits I, II/III, and Vb *in vitro* [41]. cAMP-dependent phosphorylation of Y304 on the catalytic subunit I inhibits, whereas tyrosine phosphorylation of subunit II by c-Src kinase activates complex IV [41, 42]. The latter event is required for the normal function of cells, which are dependent on the efficient production of ATP to maintain their functions [42]. Interestingly, phosphorylation of the same subunit by the receptor tyrosine kinase ERBb2 decreases the activity of complex IV and mitochondrial respiration [43, 44]. Complex IV activity is inhibited in a time-dependent manner after myocardial ischemia, which stimulates multiple phosphorylations of complex IV: (1) subunit I on S115 and S116, (2) subunit IVi1 on T52, and (3) subunit Vb on S40 in the heart [38, 45]. These inhibitory phosphorylations are mediated by PKA and inhibition of PKA reduces I/R injury to the myocardial tissue [45]. Phosphorylation of subunit IV-1 on S58 by PKA increases the activity of complex IV by preventing allosteric inhibition of complex IV by ATP [46]. It was proposed that phosphorylation of S58 switches mitochondrial metabolism from energy utilization to energy storage in pathological conditions including I/R-induced injury [46].

8. Cytochrome c

Phosphorylations of serine, threonine, and 2 tyrosine residues have been mapped on cytochrome c [39, 47]. Phosphorylation of T28 results in a partial inhibition of the electron transport chain and respiration [48]. It was suggested that the other phosphorylations regulate the mobility of cytochrome c between complexes, its binding to cardiolipin, and the interaction with Apaf-1 during apoptosis [47].

9. ATP synthase (F_oF_1-ATPase)

Multiple and differential phosphorylations of ATP synthase have been reported in different organisms and tissues. Tyrosine phosphorylations of the ε-subunit (in the F_o domain) and the α- and δ-subunits of the F_1 domain are mediated by Src kinase [49, 50]. The α and e subunits of F_oF_1-ATPase in mammalian brain are phosphorylated on S76 and Y32 [51]. The catalytic β-subunit is extensively phosphorylated on S106, T107, T262/S263, T312, and T368 in mammalian cardiomyocytes, whereas in yeast, the β-subunit is phosphorylated on T58, S213, T262, and T318 [51]. These phosphorylations affect assembly of the F_1 domain and reduce ATP synthase activity [51]. They occur in cardiac preconditioning, which offers protection against ischemia [51]. Phosphorylation of T213 on the β-subunit of skeletal muscle F_oF_1-ATPase downregulates its levels *in vivo* [6, 51]. We have shown serine phosphorylations on the α and/or β- and γ-subunits of ATP synthase in RPTC [52]. These phosphorylations are PKC-α-dependent and preserve the levels of the γ-subunit and F_oF_1-ATPase activity in injured renal cells [52]. Phosphoproteomics demonstrated phosphorylation of S146 on the γ-subunit [52]. Phosphorylation of the γ-subunit is associated with the formation of ATP synthase dimers [52].

10. Adenine nucleotide translocase (ANT)

ANT, an antiporter embedded in the inner mitochondrial membrane that facilitates the exchange of ADP and ATP, is one of the most abundant mitochondrial proteins and a primary target of ischemia [5, 53]. The four human isoforms, ANT1, 2, 3, and 4, are phosphorylated on tyrosines [49]. Phosphorylation of ANT on Y194 and Y190 alters the activity of ADP/ATP translocase and the transport of both nucleotides in the brain [49]. Phosphorylation of ANT1 at Y194 in cardiac tissue is diminished by I/R but maintained by pre- and post-conditioning, which suggests that this phosphorylation plays a protective role against ischemia in the heart and could improve tolerance against injury [54]. Although this phosphorylation improves respiration and mitochondrial function, it is not known whether phosphorylation of Y194 is sufficient for protection of cardiomyocytes from I/R-induced injury [54]. A binding of phosphorylated (inactive) glycogen synthase kinase-3β (GSK-3β) to ANT was also shown, but it is unclear whether GSK-3β directly phosphorylates ANT [55].

11. Voltage-dependent anion channel (VDAC)

VDAC, a channel protein localized to the outer mitochondrial membrane, conducts a variety of small metabolites (NAD^+/NADH, ADP, and ATP) and ions across the outer membrane and is a key regulator of energy metabolism [56]. VDAC forms a complex with ANT, which facilitates influx of ADP into mitochondria and the efflux of ATP to the cytoplasm [56–58]. VDAC1 closure leads to hyperpolarization of mitochondria, disruption of ADP/ATP exchange, decrease in ATP synthesis, and metabolic dysfunction, and rupture of mitochondria [56–58]. The four known VDAC isoforms present in the outer mitochondrial membrane are phosphorylated on multiple serines and threonines [21, 22]. A total of 19 distinct phosphorylations were identified in VDAC isoforms [21, 65]. These phosphorylations are mediated by different kinases including PKA, PKC, tyrosine kinase, hexokinase, GSK-3β, Akt, JNK3, and p38 [59]. The phosphorylation of neuronal and hepatic VDAC1 by PKA and ischemia-activated GSK-3β and JNK induces its closure, disrupts formation of the complex with ANT, and decreases ATP synthesis [59]. In contrast, phosphorylation of cardiac VDAC1 by protein kinase C-ε (PKC-ε) promotes formation of the VDAC-ANT complex, prevents the opening of MPTP, and protects mitochondrial integrity after I/R injury [60]. Phosphorylation of VDAC1 by never-in-mitosis A related kinase 1 (Nek1) on S193 closes the channel in RPTC, blocks release of cytochrome c, and prevents cell death by apoptosis [61]

11.1. Phosphorylation of enzymes of the tricarboxylic acid cycle (TCA)

Phosphoproteomic analyses revealed that most enzymes of the TCA cycle are phosphorylated/dephosphorylated [62]. These include aconitase, isocitrate and oxo-ketoglutarate dehydrogenases, succinyl-coenzyme A synthetase, succinate dehydrogenase, fumarate hydratase, and mitochondrial malate dehydrogenase [62, 63]. Although the functional role of these phosphorylations and the protein kinases that mediate them are not yet known, data suggest that phosphorylation regulates the activity of these enzymes.

11.2. Pyruvate dehydrogenase complex (PDC)

PDC is composed of multiple copies of three distinct enzymes: (1) pyruvate dehydrogenase (E1), dihydrolipoyl transacetylase (E2), and dihydrolipoyl dehydrogenase (E3), which form a large complex. PDC is the rate-limiting enzyme in the oxidative metabolism of all carbohydrates and its activity is tightly regulated by multiple mechanisms including phosphorylation. Phosphorylation of the PDC by the pyruvate dehydrogenase kinase (PDK) inactivates the complex [64]. The α-subunit of the E1 is phosphorylated at multiple sites, but the most known are phosphorylations of three distinct serines [64]. Although phosphorylation at any of these serines is sufficient to inhibit the activity of PDC, the S293 residue has the highest affinity for phosphate, and phosphorylation of this serine has the greatest impact on the inhibition of activity of PDC [64, 65]. I/R-induced injury in cardiac tissue is associated with a 4–5-fold decrease in the phosphorylation of S293, which results in the activation of PDC [64]. PDC activation protects against ischemic injury and improves cardiac efficiency and contractile capacity in the postischemic heart [65].

11.3. Proteins involved in mitochondrial dynamics

Mitochondrial morphology is dynamically changed by the balance between fusion and fission (fragmentation). Phosphorylations of GTPases, Drp1, Mfn1/2, and Opa1 regulate mitochondrial fission and fusion [66]. Phosphorylation of fission-inducing Drp1 on S616 and S637 can be mediated by cyclin-dependent kinase (cdk)-1, cdk-5, PKA, PKC-δ, and extracellular signal regulated kinase-2 (ERK-2) [66–71]. Phosphorylation of Drp1 at S616 by cdk-1, PKC-δ, and ERK-2 promotes Drp1 translocation to mitochondria and fission whereas phosphorylation of S637 by PKA inhibits Drp1 and mitochondrial fission [67–71]. We have demonstrated that activation of PKC-ε induces the translocation of Drp1 to mitochondria, mitochondrial fission and apoptosis in non-injured RPTC [72]. Drp1-dependent mitochondrial fission is associated with mitochondrial outer membrane permeabilization and apoptosis, whereas elongation of the mitochondria through fusion promotes ATP synthesis and prevents mitochondrial autophagy. When phosphorylated by ERK, Mfn1 has decreased ability to oligomerize and tether mitochondria, which inhibits their fusion, recruitment of Bak to the mitochondria, and apoptosis [73]. Mfn2 is phosphorylated on T111 and S442 by PTEN-induced putative kinase protein 1 (PINK1), which recruits the protein Parkin to depolarized mitochondria and eliminates them by mitophagy [74]. Disruption in the balance between fission and fusion occurs in pathological conditions including I/R, which increases phosphorylation of Drp1, its translocation to mitochondria, and mitochondrial fission in the heart and brain [75]. Inhibition of Drp1 protects the heart and brain against ischemia and has been proposed as a therapeutic target following cardiac arrest [76].

11.4. Proteins of the intrinsic apoptotic cascade

Mitochondrial proteins involved in the intrinsic apoptosis include Bcl-2 family members, AIF, Smac/DIABLO, cytochrome c, and Omi/Htra2. With an exception of one, all are regulated by phosphorylation [20]. Phosphorylation of Bcl-2 at S70 is required to prevent permeabilization of the mitochondrial outer membrane and for Bcl-2's anti-apoptotic activity [77]. Several protein kinases serve as Bcl-2 kinases to inhibit (JNK, p38, and GSK-3) or activate (Akt, PKA, and PKC-α) Bcl-2 [77]. Cardiac and neuronal tissues are protected against I/R when Bcl-2 is active [78–80]. Ischemia-induced acute kidney injury upregulates Bcl-2 and Bcl-XL in the distal and Bax in the proximal tubules [80]. Pro-apoptotic Bax, Bak, Bad, and Bid are phosphorylated on serines and tyrosines, which controls their insertion into the outer mitochondrial membrane and formation of pores that mediate the release of pro-apoptotic AIF, Smac, and cytochrome c from the mitochondria [81]. Smac is phosphorylated by JNK3, which decreases its pro-apoptotic actions [81]. Phosphorylation of Y97 and Y48 on cytochrome c regulates its capacity to form the apoptosome and activate caspase-9 [81]. Thus, phosphorylation of specific amino acids on a mitochondrial protein determines the fate of mitochondria by protecting their integrity and functions or inducing MPT and apoptosis.

12. Role of protein kinases in regulating mitochondrial functions in ischemia/reperfusion

Ischemia rapidly changes activities of different protein kinases including the calcium/calmodulin-dependent protein kinase II (CaMK-II), PKA, protein kinase B (PKB/Akt), PKC, Raf-1, ERK1/2, c-jun N-terminal kinase (JNK), p38 mitogen-activated protein kinase (p38 MAPK), GSK3-β, PINK1, and tyrosine kinases, which suggests their involvement in I/R injury.

12.1. Protein kinases regulating large dehydrogenase complexes

A specific family of protein kinases is exclusively present in the mitochondrial matrix of eukaryotic cells. These kinases have different sequences from the cytosolic protein kinases and they phosphorylate and inactivate large enzymatic complexes in the mitochondrial matrix, the branched-chain α-ketoacid dehydrogenase complex and pyruvate dehydrogenase complex, PDC. Perturbations in PDC activity result in energy deficits, neuronal dysfunction, and brain injury, such as those observed in stroke. Phosphorylation of the E1 α-subunit of PDC by PDK isozymes inhibits, whereas dephosphorylation increases PDC activity [82]. Cardiac and cerebral ischemia has no effect on the activity of PDC; however, reperfusion results in a fast decline in PDC activity in the brain [83]. Increased expression of PDK2 following traumatic brain injury may maintain E1 in the hyperphosphorylated (inactive) state, which impairs glucose oxidation after stroke and traumatic brain injuries [83]. Further, reperfusion-induced oxidative stress activates PKC-δ, which translocates to mitochondria and activates PDK2 leading to inhibition of E1 activity [84]. The inhibition of PDK during reperfusion restores PDC activity and decreases brain injury, demonstrating that phosphorylation by PDK2 mediates inhibition of PDC activity [85]. Infusion of the specific peptide inhibitor of PKC-δ, Tat-δV1-1, prevents the translocation of PKC-δ to mitochondria and maintains PDC activity [84]. Isozymes of PDK are considered attractive targets for therapies to improve PDC activity to diminish the detrimental effects of I/R in tissues that depend on metabolism of glucose, such as neuronal and cardiac tissues.

12.2. Serine/threonine kinases in regulation of mitochondrial functions in ischemia/reperfusion

12.2.1. Protein kinase A

PKA is activated by a signaling pathway originating from G-protein receptors, which produces cAMP. The association of PKA with mammalian mitochondria was documented four decades ago [86]. Mitochondrial PKA is present in the outer and inner mitochondrial membranes as well as in the mitochondrial matrix [28, 87]. Several mitochondrial substrates of PKA with distinct tissue-specific responses have been identified. During myocardial I/R, PKA is activated by increased levels of ROS and translocates to mitochondria [88]. The increase in activity of mitochondrial PKA is independent of mitochondrial levels of cAMP and is due to increased sequestration of the catalytic α-subunit in the mitochondrial matrix [88]. The presence of the catalytic α-subunit of PKA results in phosphorylation of subunits I (on S115 and S116), IVi1 (on T52), and Vb (on S40) of complex IV, followed by their degradation and the loss of activity [38, 40, 88]. Because the identified phosphorylation sites on complex IV are not within PKA consensus sites, it was proposed that PKA activation plays an indirect role in the loss of complex IV activity during myocardial ischemia [39]. These changes are sufficient to disrupt the function of mitochondrial respirasome and increase production of ROS [88]. PKA-mediated phosphorylation regulates ischemia-induced dysfunction of complex IV [38, 45, 88]. Ca^{2+} influx activated by PKA in cardiomyocytes induces mitochondrial permeability transition, which stimulates caspase-9 and apoptosis [89]. Inhibition of PKA prevents the loss of activity of complex IV during cardiac I/R, promotes postischemic cardiac contractile recovery, and decreases the infarct size in the ischemic heart [38, 45, 90]. Thus, PKA inhibitors could serve as candidates for cardioprotective agents [87, 89]. PKA also phosphorylates NDUFS4 and NDUFA10 subunits of complex I and this phosphorylation stimulates the activity of complex I and complex I-driven respiration [28, 29, 91]. Finally, Hsp20, which localizes to mitochondria and is expressed at high levels in cardiac, skeletal, and vascular smooth muscle, is regulated by the β-adrenergic/PKA signaling pathway [92]. PKA-mediated phosphorylation of Hsp20 on S16 increases in ischaemic myocardium and is cardioprotective [92].

In contrast, the activation of PKA during liver IR is cAMP-dependent and plays a protective role against liver injury [93]. The cAMP that activates mitochondrial PKA does not originate from membrane-bound adenylyl cyclase activated by the Gα protein, but is produced inside mitochondria by the carbon dioxide/bicarbonate-regulated soluble adenylyl cyclase in response to metabolically generated carbon dioxide [93]. Mitochondrial PKA regulates mitochondrial biogenesis, normalizes ROS production, and activates complex IV [46]. Inhibition of PKA exacerbates hepatocellular damage, whereas increasing cAMP levels to activate PKA protects the ischemic liver from injury [93]. PKA activation diminishes neutrophil and macrophage infiltration into ischemic liver tissue, reduces production of tumor necrosis factor α, interleukin (IL)-6, and IL-12 by macrophages, increases IL-10 expression, and prevents hepatocyte death [93]. Thus, PKA activation reduces the inflammatory response associated with reperfusion after liver ischemia. Because ischemia is an inherent component of liver transplantation, activation of PKA was proposed as a rationale for novel therapies to combat I/R injury and protect transplants [94]. However, increased cAMP levels in the liver *in vivo* inhibit complex IV due to phosphorylation of Y304 [41]. Because PKA is not a tyrosine kinase, it was proposed that PKA activates a downstream tyrosine kinase, which phosphorylates and inactivates complex IV [41]. Therefore, attempts aimed at activating PKA to protect the liver against ischemia should be treated with great caution.

PKA dysregulation has been implicated in several neurodegenerative disorders. PKA-dependent pathways in different regions of the brain play a role in pathogenesis and cognitive decline in Alzheimer and Parkinson's diseases [94]. The acute phase of cerebral ischemia is accompanied by decreases in affinity of PKA for cAMP and PKA activity [94]. In contrast, the peri-ischemic and less-injured areas exhibit increased PKA-mediated phosphorylation compared to the ischemic core, which suggests that active PKA is associated with the survival of neuronal tissue [94]. Derangement of cAMP-dependent signal transduction is associated with ischemic neuronal damage and activation of the PKA is important for neuronal survival in acute cerebral ischemia [94]. Phosphorylation of Bad at S155 by mitochondria-anchored PKA leads to cytosolic sequestration of Bad and blocks its mitochondrial translocation, the release of cytochrome c, and neuronal apoptosis [77]. Also, PKA-mediated phosphorylation of Drp1 at S637 blocks its translocation to mitochondria and their fission and promotes mitochondrial fusion. In hippocampal neurons, expression of a constitutively active catalytic subunit of PKA targeted to the mitochondrion promotes the fusion of mitochondria into networks [95]. Finally, PKA suppresses autophagy and mitochondrial degradation in neurons by phosphorylating and inhibiting the microtubule-associated protein 1A/1B-light chain 3 (LC3) and increases neurite outgrowth [94, 96].

12.2.2. Protein kinase B (PKB/Akt)

Akt can localize to the mitochondrial matrix and the inner and outer membranes of cardiac, neuronal, and kidney cells [97, 98]. Protein levels of mitochondrial Akt are regulated by a variety of extracellular signals and stresses, which induce rapid translocation of active (phosphorylated) Akt to the mitochondria [97, 98]. Mitochondrial localization of Akt is associated with cardioprotection against ischemic injury and renoprotective actions against chemical toxicity [97–100]. The cardioprotective effect of mitochondrial Akt is attributed to its action on mitoK(ATP) channels and to decreasing apoptosis [99]. Akt phosphorylates pro-apoptotic Bad on S136 and Bax on S184, and prevents MPT in neuronal cells [101]. Phosphorylated Bad associates with 14-3-3 proteins in the cytosol and cannot form complexes with mitochondrial Bcl-2/Bcl-XL to induce permeabilization of the mitochondrial outer membrane and MPT [101]. Bax phosphorylation by Akt promotes dimerization of Bax with Bcl-XL or Mcl-1 proteins, which sequesters Bax away from mitochondria and prevents their permeabilization and apoptosis [101]. Akt prevents the MPT in cardiomyocytes by phosphorylating hexokinase II, stabilizing it in the outer mitochondrial membrane, and promoting its binding to VDAC [102]. Inhibition of Akt or targeted disruption of the association of hexokinase II with mitochondria abolishes cardioprotection [102].

We have identified mitochondria as a subcellular target of protective actions of Akt against necrosis in injured RPTC [98]. Mitochondrial levels of active Akt decrease in injured RPTC and this is associated with mitochondrial dysfunction [98, 100]. Selective activation of Akt increases the levels of Akt in mitochondria, improves state 3 respiration, activities of complexes I and III and F_0F_1-ATPase (ATP synthase), and the mitochondrial membrane potential ($\Delta\Psi_m$), increases ATP production, and reduces ATP deficits [100]. Selective inhibition of Akt exacerbates mitochondrial dysfunction, energy deficits, and necrosis in injured RPTC [100]. These results are consistent with a report that Akt phosphorylates the β-subunit of ATP synthase and improves its activity and increases ATP production to prevent energy deficits in injured cells [97]. Also, active Akt increases activity of PDC and oxidative metabolism of carbohydrates by inhibiting phosphorylation of PDC by GSK-3β [103]. Thus, signals from cell membrane receptors or those generated by metabolic stress have a rapid effect on Akt activation status in mitochondria. Akt could serve as a therapeutic target promoting mitochondrial functions in ischemic organs. However, the application is complicated by the fact that Akt promotes tumor formation by blocking apoptosis.

12.2.3. *Protein kinase C*

PKC plays a key role in mediating I/R injury in the brain, heart, and kidneys; however, elucidation of this role is complicated due to the presence of 11 distinct PKC isozymes, which have unique tissue and cellular localizations and often play quite opposite roles in ischemic injury even within the same organ. Alterations in PKC activity or subcellular localization during ischemia occur in the brain, heart, liver, and kidney [25, 104–106]. Major isozymes of PKC (α, β, γ, δ, ε) translocate to mitochondria in response to ischemia and/or reperfusion and oxidative stress, and have been implicated in regulating mitochondrial functions in ischemic and postischemic tissues [104]. The classical PKC isozymes (α, β, γ) are dependent on Ca^{2+} and 1,2-diacylglycerol, and ischemia increases the levels of both activators through the stimulation of phospholipase C. PKC-α activation has been implicated in ischemia-induced heart failure and cerebral barrier breakdown after ischemic stroke [107, 108]. PKC-α inhibition or deletion protects the heart from decompensation and cardiomyopathy and attenuates cerebral barrier breakdown after ischemia [107, 108]. In contrast, PKC-α translocation to mitochondria is protective against mitochondrial dysfunction, ATP deficits, and cell death caused by ischemia, hypoxia, and oxidative stress in RPTC [109]. We have shown that ATP synthase (F_0F_1-ATPase) is a target of PKC-α, which associates with the α-, β-, and γ-subunits of the F_1 domain of ATP synthase [52]. Injury or inactive PKC-α disrupt, whereas active PKC-α promotes this association and increases the levels of α-, β-, and γ-subunits in injured RPTC [52]. Active PKC-α promotes phosphorylation of the γ-subunit on S146 and F_0F_1-ATPase activity after injury [52]. PKC-α also reduces apoptosis by phosphorylating mitochondrial Bcl-2 on S70 [77, 110]. Thus, activation of PKC-α exerts differential effects in different types of cells and tissues.

PKC-γ is expressed exclusively in neurons of the brain and spinal cord and is activated rapidly during ischemia and inhibited during reperfusion [111–114]. PKC-γ plays a detrimental role in the early stages of ischemia mediating events leading to cell death. PKC-γ knockouts show smaller infarct areas after cerebral ischemia [112]. Also, PKC-γ may directly (or through the activation of a Src tyrosine kinase) phosphorylate NMDA receptors, stimulate their function, and increase the concentration of intracellular Ca^{2+}, which results in mitochondrial dysfunction, ATP deficits, increased ROS formation, and neuronal death [112]. However, after reperfusion, PKC-γ may mediate protection against cell death [112]. Thus, the same PKC isozyme may play opposing roles at different stages of ischemic injury.

PKC-δ is rapidly activated by signaling initiated by reperfusion. PKC-δ plays a detrimental role in ischemic stroke injury and mediates oxidative stress, cell death, and inflammation associated with reperfusion [111, 112]. Selective inhibition or deletion of PKC-δ reduces infarct size and ischemic brain injury caused by middle cerebral artery occlusion, specifically, reperfusion-induced death of parenchymal cells [115, 116]. PKC-δ inhibition activates PKB/Akt, inhibits translocation of Bad to mitochondria, and decreases apoptosis [112]. PKC-δ

mediates neutrophil infiltration, which is responsible for the detrimental effects of PKC-δ during reperfusion [112]. Similarly, reperfusion after cardiac ischemia activates PKC-δ, which translocates to mitochondria and reduces state 3 respiration, TCA cycle, and ATP production, increases generation of mitochondrial ROS, and induces release of cytochrome c and cell death [84, 113, 115, 116]. Selective inhibition of PKC-δ translocation to mitochondria blocks these changes and protects the heart from ischemic injury [117]. PKC-δ is also activated by oxidative stress in the kidney, exacerbates RPTC and kidney injury by activating Bax, inducing cytochrome c release and apoptosis, and blocking autophagy. PKC-δ inhibition protects kidneys from injury by upregulating autophagy [118].

PKC-ε, another novel isozyme, is activated and translocates to mitochondria during I/R. These events have been implicated in the cardio- and neuro-protection against ischemic injury and in the reduction of myocardial infarct [119, 120]. PKC-ε activation is a pivotal signaling event in the cardioprotective mechanisms of ischemic preconditioning, and it is thought that this protection is mediated through mitochondrial and transport mechanisms [120]. Conversely, inhibition of PKC-ε eliminates the cardioprotection [120]. Several substrates of PKC-ε are present in cardiac mitochondria. Active PKC-ε induces opening of the mitoK(ATP) channels, maintains ATP production, and reduces ROS production [120]. Specifically, PKC-ε regulates interactions between conexin43 and the mitoK(ATP) subunit, which leads to mitoK(ATP) opening when ATP levels decrease, resulting in cardioprotection [121]. Active PKC-ε also increases phosphorylation of subunit IV and the activity of complex IV [122]. Thus, the PKC-ε-mediated resistance to cardiac ischemia may also be due to increased activity of the electron transport chain and a greater $\Delta\Psi_m$ for ATP synthesis. Also, PKC-ε phosphorylates VDAC1 on T51, which modifies its gating and interaction with proteins of the MPT pore to inhibit its opening and maintain $\Delta\Psi_m$ and ATP synthesis [60]. These data support protective and prosurvival actions of mitochondrial PKC-ε in cardiac I/R. In contrast, translocation of the active PKC-ε to mitochondria in RPTC results in mitochondrial dysfunction, decreases in ATP levels, mitochondrial fission, and RPTC death [25, 72]. Active PKC-ε produces the classical hallmarks of mitochondrial dysfunction in RPTC: decreases in state 3 respiration and activity of complex I, increases in $\Delta\Psi_m$, ROS production, and mitochondrial fission [25, 72]. Inhibition of PKC-ε protects against mitochondrial dysfunction induced by hypoxia and oxidative stress [72]. Deletion of PKC-ε *in vivo* ameliorates I/R-induced decreases in respiration and activities of complexes I, III, and IV, and reduces oxidant production and morphological damage in ischemic kidneys [25]. Deletion of PKC-ε reduces the inflammatory response and apoptosis, and promotes renal function and survival after I/R-induced acute kidney injury in mice [25, 123]. Thus, in contrast to the cardio- and neuroprotective effects of PKC-ε, activation of this PKC isozyme in the renal cortex is detrimental to mitochondria, cell viability, and kidney functions [25, 123].

12.2.4. Mitogen-activated protein kinases (MAPK)

ERK1/2 localize to the mitochondria of cardiac, brain, and renal epithelial cells. Brain and cardiac ischemia activates ERK1/2, which form signaling modules with PKC-ε and translocate to mitochondria [124–126]. ERK1/2–PKC-ε modules play a role in the phosphorylation and inactivation of Bad, which blocks the intrinsic pathway of apoptosis [126]. Furthermore, active

ERK1/2 associates with the outer mitochondrial membrane and protects against MPTP opening and mitochondrial depolarization [127]. These events are thought to contribute to the cardioprotective effects of ERK1/2 activation against I/R injury. In contrast, ERK1/2 activation is detrimental to mitochondria and cell viability in RPTC [128]. We have shown that ERK1/2 activation and translocation to mitochondria in response to oxidant injury mediates mitochondrial dysfunction and cell death in RPTC [128]. ERK1/2 activation mediates decreases in state 3 respiration, activities of aconitase of the TCA cycle and complex I of the electron transport chain, and ATP production in injured RPTC [128]. ERK1/2 inhibition restores respiration, complex I activity, $\Delta\Psi_m$ and ATP production, and decreases RPTC death [128]. Recently, it was shown that ERK1/2 downregulates mitochondrial function through the EGFR/ERK1/2/FOXO3a/1/PGC-1α pathway by phosphorylating the upstream regulators of PGC-1α and decreasing mitochondrial biogenesis [129]. Similarly, ERK1/2 activation mediates inflammatory changes, infiltration by neutrophils, apoptosis, and severe injury after ischemia in the lung [130].

JNK and p38 MAPK are activated and localize in cardiac mitochondria after ischemia or oxidant exposure and mediate mitochondria-initiated apoptosis [131]. p38 MAPK inhibition attenuates the loss of $\Delta\Psi_m$, mitochondrial swelling, and ultrastructural changes, reduces cardiomyocyte apoptosis and infarct size, and improves left ventricular function after ischemia [131, 132]. Inhibition of p38 MAPK also decreases phosphorylation of p53 and Bax expression and reduces cytochrome c release from mitochondria and the levels of active caspase 3 [132]. These data suggests that active p38 MAPK mediates apoptosis.

12.2.5. Glycogen synthase kinase

GSK3β activated by cardiac I/R docks to mitochondria, phosphorylates VDAC1, and leads to phosphorylation of ANT and cyclophilin D, and MPTP opening [55, 133]. This suggests that GSK3β plays a role in mitochondria-mediated apoptosis in cardiac tissue. GSK3β also regulates mitochondrial oxidative metabolism by phosphorylating and inhibiting PDC [65]. Activation enhances whereas inhibition of GSK3β activates mTOR pathway, inhibits mTOR-dependent autophagy, and reduces myocardial I/R injury [134]. Inhibition of GSK-3β also attenuates brain infarct volume after cerebral I/R-induced injury [135].

12.2.6. PTEN-induced kinase 1

The mitochondrial serine-threonine protein kinase, PTEN (phosphatase and tensin homolog on chromosome 10)-induced kinase 1 (PINK1) localizes to both mitochondrial membranes and regulates mitochondrial function and dynamics [136]. PINK1 phosphorylates mitofusin MFN2, a mitochondrial receptor for Parkin (a protein related to Parkinson's disease) [136]. PINK1 regulates mitochondrial dynamics in ischemic stroke and prevents damage to neurons by reducing mitochondrial translocation of Drp1 and fission, and preventing the collapse of $\Delta\Psi_m$ and ATP synthesis [137, 138]. Deletion of PINK1 causes defects in the turnover of proteins of the electron transport chain, impairs mitochondrial respiration and activity of complex I in cardiomyocytes, induces MPTP opening, decreases production of ATP, exacerbates oxidative stress, and increases the size of ischemic myocardial infarct, which suggests increased susceptibility to I/R injury in PINK1-deficient hearts [139]. Overexpressing PINK1 reduces these changes [139]. Thus, this study suggests mitochondrial PINK1 as a target for cardioprotection against ischemia in the heart.

12.3. Tyrosine kinases and regulation of mitochondrial functions in ischemia/reperfusion

Tyrosine phosphorylation is a crucial mechanism for regulating mitochondrial functions [19, 42]. Tyrosine kinases of the Src family (Lyn, Lck, c-Src, Fyn, and Fgr) localize to mitochondria by binding to specific anchoring proteins present in mitochondria [19, 42]. The primary known role of tyrosine phosphorylation is the regulation of the respiratory chain by c-Src [19]. Phosphorylations of NDUFB10 subunit of complex I at Y193, succinate dehydrogenase of complex II at Y215, and subunit II of complex IV on unknown tyrosine by Src increase activities of complexes I, II, and IV [19, 31, 42]. Targeting of c-Src to mitochondria enhances $\Delta\Psi_m$ and oxidative phosphorylation in a c-Src-dependent manner [19]. Src and Lck phosphorylate ANT1 at Y194 and reduce ischemic injury in preconditioned cardiac cells [54]. Mitochondrial Fgr kinase phosphorylates complex II, which increases complex II activity and regulates NADH/$FADH_2$ balance in mitochondria [32]. Epidermal growth factor receptor (EGFR) translocates to mitochondria when phosphorylated on Y845 by Src [43]. EFR interacts with and phosphorylates subunit II of complex IV thereby decreasing its activity and cellular ATP levels [19, 140].

In conclusions, translocation of protein kinases to mitochondria regulates mitochondrial functions in various disease states including ischemia and reperfusion in major organs such as the brain, heart, and kidneys. These findings suggest that these protein kinases can serve as potential effective therapeutic targets to maintain mitochondrial integrity and functions and prevent or reduce organ damage in these disease states.

Author details

Grażyna Nowak

Address all correspondence to: gnowak@uams.edu

Department of Pharmaceutical Sciences, College of Pharmacy, University of Arkansas for Medical Sciences, Little Rock, AR, United States

References

[1] Erecinska M, Wilson D. Regulation of cellular energy metabolism. The Journal of Membrane Biology. 1982;**70**:4-14

[2] McBride HM, Neuspiel M, Wasiak S. Mitochondria: More than just a powerhouse. Current Biology. 2006;**16**:R551-R560

[3] Musatov A, Robinson NC. Susceptibility of mitochondrial electron-transport complexes to oxidative damage. Focus on cytochrome oxidase. Free Radical Research. 2012; **46**:1313-1326

[4] Rouslin W. Mitochondrial complexes I, II, III, IV, and V in myocardial ischemia and autolysis. American Journal of Physiology. Heart and Circulatory Physiology. 1983; **244**:H743-H748

[5] Duan J, Karmazyn M. Relationship between oxidative phosphorylation and adenine nucleotide translocase activity of two populations of cardiac mitochondria and mechanical recovery of ischemic hearts following reperfusion. Canadian Journal of Physiology and Pharmacology. 1989;**67**:704-709

[6] Højlund K, Wrzesinski K, Larsen PM, Fey SJ, Roepstorff P, Handberg A, et al. Proteome analysis reveals phosporylation of ATP synthase β-subunit in humans skeletal muscle and proteins with roles in type 2 diabetes. The Journal of Biological Chemistry. 2003;**278**:10346-10442

[7] Kane L, Van Eyk J. Post-translational modifications of ATP synthase in the heart: Biology and function. Journal of Bioenergetics and Biomembranes. 2009;**41**:145-150

[8] Lesnefsky E, Tandler B, Ye J. Myocardial ischemia decreases oxidative phosphorylation through cytochrome oxidase in subsarcolemmal mitochondria. The American Journal of Physiology. 1997;**273**:H1544-H1554

[9] Chen Q, Camara AK, Stowe DF, Hoppel CL, Lesnefsky EJ. Modulation of electron transport protects cardiac mitochondria and myocardial injury during ischemia and reperfusion. American Journal of Physiology. Cell Physiology. 2007;**292**:C137-C147

[10] Turrens JF, Boveris A. Generation of superoxide anion by the NADH dehydrogenase of bovine heart mitochondria. The Biochemical Journal. 1980;**191**:421-427

[11] Lesnefsky EJ, Gudz TI, Migita CT, Ikeda-Saito M, Hassan MO, et al. Ischemic injury to mitochondrial electron transport in the aging heart: Damage to the iron-sulfur protein subunit of electron transport complex III. Archives of Biochemistry and Biophysics. 2001;**385**:117-128

[12] Shoshan-Barmatz V, Israelson A, Brdiczka D, Sheu S. The voltage-dependent anion channel (VDAC): Function in intracellular signalling, cell and cell death. Current Pharmaceutical Design. 2006;**12**:2249-2270

[13] Vianello A, Casolo V, Petrussa E, Peresson C, Patui S, Bertolini A, et al. The mitochondrial permeability transition pore (MPTP)—An example of multiple molecular exaptation? Biochimica et Biophysica Acta—Bioenergetics. 2012;**1817**:2072-2086

[14] Dimmer K, Scorrano L. (De)constructing mitochondria: What for? Physiology. 2006; **21**:233-241

[15] Liu W, Tian F, Kurata T, Morimoto N, Abe K. Dynamic changes of mitochondrial fusion and fission proteins after transient cerebral ischemia in mice. Journal of Neuroscience Research. 2012;**90**:1183-1189

[16] Brooks C, Wei Q, Cho S, Dong Z. Regulation of mitochondrial dynamics in acute kidney injury in cell culture and rodent models. The Journal of Clinical Investigation. 2009; **119**:1275-1285

[17] Ong S, Subrayan S, Lim S, Yellon D, Davidson S, Hausenloy D. Inhibiting mitochondrial fission protects the heart against ischemia/reperfusion injury. Circulation. 2010; **121**:2012-2022

[18] Zhao X, León IR, Bak S, Mogensen M, Wrzesinski K, Højlund K, et al. Phosphoproteome analysis of functional mitochondria isolated from resting human muscle reveals extensive phosphorylation of inner membrane protein complexes and enzymes. Molecular & Cellular Proteomics. 2011;**10**:M110.000299

[19] Lim S, Smith KR, Lim ST, Tian R, Lu J, Tan M. Regulation of mitochondrial functions by protein phosphorylation and dephosphorylation. Cell & Bioscience. 2016;**14**:6-25

[20] Harris RA, Popov KM, Zhao Y, Kedishvili NY, Shimomura Y, Crabb DW. A new family of protein kinases—The mitochondrial protein kinases. Advances in Enzyme Regulation. 1995;**35**:147-162

[21] Bera AK, Ghosh S, Das S. Mitochondrial VDAC can be phosphorylated by cyclic AMP-dependent protein kinase. Biochemical and Biophysical Research Communications. 1995;**209**:213-217

[22] Nishihara M, Miura T, Miki T, Tanno M, Yano T, Naitoh K, et al. Modulation of the mitochondrial permeability transition pore complex in GSK-3β-mediated myocardial protection. Journal of Molecular and Cellular Cardiology. 2007;**43**:564-570

[23] Lee I, Bender E, Kadenbach B. Control of mitochondrial membrane potential and ROS formation by reversible phosphorylation of cytochrome c oxidase. Molecular and Cellular Biochemistry. 2002;**234-235**:63-70

[24] Drose S, Stepanova A, Galkin A. Ischemic A/D transition of mitochondrial complex I and its role in ROS generation. Biochimica et Biophysica Acta. 2016;**1857**:946-957

[25] Nowak G, Takacsova-Bakajsova D, Megyesi J. Deletion of protein kinase C-ε attenuates mitochondrial dysfunction and ameliorates ischemic renal injury. American Journal of Physiology. Renal Physiology. 2017;**312**:F109-F120

[26] Chen R, Fearnley IM, Peak-Chew SY, Walker JE. The phosphorylation of subunits of complex I from bovine heart mitochondria. The Journal of Biological Chemistry. 2004; **279**:26036-26045

[27] Schilling B, Aggeler R, Schulenberg B, Murray J, Row RH, Capaldi RA, et al. Mass spectrometric identification of a novel phosphorylation site in subunit NDUFA10 of bovine mitochondrial complex I. FEBS Letters. 2005;**579**:2485-2490

[28] Technikova-Dobrova Z, Sardanelli AM, Speranza F, Scacco S, Signorile A, Lorusso V, et al. Cyclic adenosine monophosphate-dependent phosphorylation of mammalian mitochondrial proteins: Enzyme and substrate characterization and functional role. Biochemistry. 2001;**40**:13941-13947

[29] Papa S, Sardanelli AM, Cocco T, Speranza F, Scacco SC, Technikova-Dobrova Z. The nuclear-encoded 18 kDa (IP) AQDQ subunit of bovine heart complex I is phosphorylated by the mitochondrial cAMP-dependent protein kinase. FEBS Letters. 1996;**379**:299-301

[30] Yadava N, Potluri P, Scheffler IE. Investigations of the potential effects of phosphorylation of the MWFE and ESSS subunits on complex I activity and assembly. The International Journal of Biochemistry & Cell Biology. 2008;**40**:447-460

[31] Hebert-Chatelain E, Jose C, Gutierrez Cortes N, Dupuy J, Rocher C, Dachary-Prigent J, et al. Preservation of NADH ubiquinone-oxidoreductase activity by Src kinase-mediated phosphorylation of NDUFB10. Biochimica et Biophysica Acta. 2012;**1817**:718-725

[32] Acín-Pérez R, Carrascoso I, Baixauli F, Roche-Molina M, Latorre-Pellicer A, Fernández-Silva P, et al. ROS-triggered phosphorylation of complex II by Fgr kinase regulates cellular adaptation to fuel use. Cell Metabolism. 2014;**19**:1020-1033

[33] Lopez-Fabuel I, Le Douce J, Logan A, James AM, Bonvento G, Murphy MP. et al, Complex I assembly into supercomplexes determines differential mitochondrial ROSproduction in neurons and astrocytes. PNAS. 2016;**113**:13063-13068

[34] Salvi M, Morrice NA, Brunati AM, Toninello A. Identification of the flavoprotein of succinate dehydrogenase and aconitase as in vitro mitochondrial substrates of Fgr tyrosine kinase. FEBS Letters. 2007;**581**:5579-5585

[35] Tomitsuka E, Kita K, Esumi H. Regulation of succinate-ubiquinone reductase and fumarate reductase activities in human complex II by phosphorylation of its flavoprotein subunit. Proceedings of the Japan Academy. Series B, Physical and Biological Sciences. 2009;**85**:258-265

[36] Nowak G, Clifton GL, Bakajsova D. Succinate ameliorates energy deficits and prevents dysfunction of complex I in injured renal proximal tubular cells. The Journal of Pharmacology and Experimental Therapeutics. 2008;**324**:1155-1162

[37] He L, Lemasters JJ. Dephosphorylation of the Rieske iron-sulfur protein after induction of the mitochondrial permeability transition. Biochemical and Biophysical Research Communications. 2005;**334**:829-837

[38] Fang J, Prabu SK, Sepuri NB, Raza H, Anandatheerthavarada HK, Galati D, et al. Site specific phosphorylation of cytochrome c oxidase subunits I, IVi1 and Vb in rabbit hearts subjected to ischemia/reperfusion. FEBS Letters. 2007;**581**:1302-1310

[39] Hüttemann M, Helling S, Sanderson TH, Sinkler C, Samavati L, Mahapatra G, et al. Regulation of mitochondrial respiration and apoptosis through cell signaling: Cytochrome c oxidase and cytochrome c in ischemia/reperfusion injury and inflammation. Biochimica et Biophysica Acta—Bioenergetics. 2012;**1817**:598-609

[40] Lee I, Salomon AR, Ficarro S, Mathes I, Lottspeich F, Grossman LI, et al. cAMP-dependent tyrosine phosphorylation of subunit I inhibits cytochrome c oxidase activity. The Journal of Biological Chemistry. 2005;**280**:6094-6100

[41] Bender E, Kadenbach B. The allosteric ATP-inhibition of cytochrome c oxidase activity is reversibly switched on by cAMP-dependent phosphorylation. FEBS Letters. 2000; **466**:130-134

[42] Miyazaki T, Neff L, Tanaka S, Horne WC, Baron R. Regulation of cytochrome c oxidase activity by c-Src in osteoclasts. The Journal of Cell Biology. 2003;**160**:709-718

[43] Boerner JL, Demory ML, Silva C, Parsons SJ. Phosphorylation of Y845 on the epidermal growth factor receptor mediates binding to the mitochondrial protein cytochrome c oxidase subunit II. Molecular and Cellular Biology. 2004;**24**:7059-7071

[44] Ding Y, Liu Z, Desai S, Zhao Y, Liu H, Pannell L, et al. Receptor tyrosine kinase ErbB2 translocates into mitochondria and regulates cellular metabolism. Nature Communications. 2012;**3**:1271

[45] Prabu SK, Anandatheerthavarada HK, Raza H, Srinivasan S, Spear JF, Avadhani NG. Protein kinase A-mediated phosphorylation modulates cytochrome c oxidase function and augments hypoxia and myocardial ischemia-related injury. The Journal of Biological Chemistry. 2006;**281**:2061-2070

[46] Acin-Perez R, Gatti D, Bai Y, Manfredi G. Protein phosphorylation and prevention of cytochrome oxidase inhibition by ATP: Coupled mechanisms of energy metabolism regulation. Cell Metabolism. 2011;**13**:712-719

[47] Lee I, Salomon A, Yu K, Doan J, Grossman L, Hüttemann M. New prospects for an old enzyme: Mammalian cytochrome c is tyrosine-phosphorylated in vivo. Biochemistry. 2006;**45**:9121-9128

[48] Mahapatra G, Varughese A, Ji Q, Lee I, Liu J, Vaishnav A, et al. Phosphorylation of cytochrome c threonine 28 regulates electron transport chain activity in kidney: Implications for AMP kinase. The Journal of Biological Chemistry. 2017;**292**:64-79

[49] Lewandrowski U, Sickmann A, Cesaro L, Brunati A, Toninello A. Salvi M, Identification of new tyrosine phosphorylated proteins in rat brain mitochondria. FEBS Letter. 2008;**582**:104-1110

[50] Ko YH, Pan W, Inoue C, Pedersen PL. Signal transduction to mitochondrial ATP synthase: Evidence that PDGF-dependent phosphorylation of the δ-subunit occurs in several cell lines, involves tyrosine, and is modulated by lysophosphatidic acid. Mitochondrion. 2002;**1**:339-348

[51] Kane LA, Youngman MJ, Jensen RE, Van Eyk JE. Phosphorylation of the F_1Fo ATP synthase β subunit: Functional and structural consequences assessed in a model system. Circulation Research. 2010;**106**:504-513

[52] Nowak G, Bakajsova D. Protein kinase C-α interaction with F_0F_1-ATPase promotes F_0F_1-ATPase activity and reduces energy deficits in injured renal cells. The Journal of Biological Chemistry. 2015;**290**:7054-7066

[53] Shug A, Subramanian R. Modulation of adenine nucleotide translocase activity during myocardial ischemia. Zeitschrift für Kardiologie. 1987;**76**:26-33

[54] Feng J, Zhu M, Schaub M, Gehrig P, Roschitzki B, Lucchinetti E, et al. Phosphoproteome analysis of isoflurane-protected heart mitochondria: Phosphorylation of adenine nucleotide translocator-1 on Tyr194 regulates mitochondrial function. Cardiovascular Research. 2008;**80**:20-29

[55] Cheng Y, Xia Z, Han Y, Rong J. Plant natural product formononetin protects rat cardiomyocyte H9c2 cells against oxygen glucose deprivation and reoxygenation via inhibiting ROS formation and promoting GSK-3β phosphorylation. Oxidative Medicine and Cellular Longevity. 2016 Article ID 2060874

[56] Rostovtseva TK. VDAC structure, function, and regulation of mitochondrial and cellular metabolism. Biochimica et Biophysica Acta (BBA)—Biomembranes. 2012;**1818**:1437

[57] Shoshan-Barmatz V, Gincel D. The voltage-dependent anion channel: Characterization, modulation, and role in mitochondrial function in cell life and death. Cell Biochemistry and Biophysics. 2003;**39**:279-292

[58] Martel C, Wang Z, Brenner C. VDAC phosphorylation, a lipid sensor influencing the cell fate. Mitochondrion. 2014;**11**(Part A):69-77

[59] Azarashvili T, Odinokova V, Krestinina O, Baburina Y, Grachev D, Teplova V, et al. Role of phosphorylation of porin (VDAC) in regulation of mitochondrial outer membrane under normal conditions and alcohol intoxication. Biochemistry (Moscow) Supplement. 2011;**5**:11

[60] Baines CP, Song CX, Zheng YT, Wang GW, Zhang J, Wang OL, et al. Protein kinase Cε interacts with and inhibits the permeability transition pore in cardiac mitochondria. Circulation Research. 2003;**92**:873-880

[61] Chen Y, Craigen WJ, Riley DJ. Nek1 regulates cell death and mitochondrial membrane permeability through phosphorylation of VDAC1. Cell Cycle. 2009;**8**:257-267

[62] Durek P, Schmidt R, Heazlewood J, Jones A, MacLean D, Nagel A, et al. PhosPhAt: The Arabidopsis Thaliana phosphorylation site database. Nucleic Acids Research. 2010; **38**:D828-D834

[63] Distler AM, Kerner J, Hoppel CL. Post-translational modifications of rat liver mitochondrial outer membrane proteins identified by mass spectrometry. Biochimica et Biophysica Acta. 2007;**1774**:628-636

[64] Yeaman S, Hutcheson E, Roche T, Pettit F, Brown J, Reed L, et al. Sites of phosphorylation on pyruvate dehydrogenase from bovine kidney and heart. Biochemistry. 1978; **17**:2364-2370

[65] Ledee D, Kang M, Kajimoto M, Purvine S, Brewer H, Pasa-Tolic L, Portman MA. Quantitative cardiac phosphoproteomics profiling during ischemic/reperfusion in an immature swine model. American Journal of Physiology. Heart and Circulatory Physiology. 2017. DOI: ajpheart.00842.2016

[66] Taguchi N, Ishihara N, Jofuku A, Oka T, et al. Mitotic phosphorylation of dynamin-related GTPase Drp1 participates in mitochondrial fission. The Journal of Biological Chemistry. 2007;**282**:11521-11529

[67] Strack S, Wilson T, Cribbs J. Cyclin-dependent kinases regulate splice-specific targeting of dynamin-related protein 1 to microtubules. The Journal of Cell Biology. 2013; **201**:1037-1051

[68] Chang C, Blackstone C. Cyclic AMP-dependent protein kinase phosphorylation of Drp1 regulates its GTPase activity and mitochondrial morphology. The Journal of Biological Chemistry. 2007;**282**:21583-21587

[69] Qi X, Disatnik MH, Shen N, Sobel RA, Mochly-Rosen D. Aberrant mitochondrial fission in neurons induced by protein kinase Cδ under oxidative stress conditions in vivo. Molecular Biology of the Cell. 2011;**22**:256-265

[70] Cho B, Cho H, Kim H, Jeong J, Park S, Hwang E, et al. CDK5-dependent inhibitory phosphorylation of Drp1 during neuronal maturation. Experimental & Molecular Medicine. 2014;**46**:e105

[71] Kashatus J, Nascimento A, Myers L, Sher A, Byrne F, Hoehn K, et al. Erk2 phosphorylation of Drp1 promotes mitochondrial fission and MAPK-driven tumor growth. Molecular Cell. 2015;**57**:537-551

[72] Nowak G, Bakajsova D, Samarel AM. Protein kinase C-ε activation induces mitochondrial dysfunction and fragmentation in renal proximal tubules. American Journal of Physiology. Renal Physiology. 2011;**301**:F197-F208

[73] Pyakurel A, Savoia C, Hess D, Scorrano L. Extracellular regulated kinase phosphorylates mitofusin 1 to control mitochondrial morphology and apoptosis. Molecular Cell. 2015;**58**:244-254

[74] Chen Y, Dorn GW II. PINK1-phosphorylated mitofusin 2 is a parkin receptor for culling damaged mitochondria. Science. 2013;**340**:471-475

[75] Zepeda KJ, Parra V, Troncoso R, Pennanen C, Riquelme J, Pedrozo Z, et al. Drp1 loss-of-function reduces cardiomyocyte oxygen dependence protecting the heart from ischemia-reperfusion injury. Journal of Cardiovascular Pharmacology. 2014;**63**:477-487

[76] Sharp WW. Dynamin-related protein 1 as a therapeutic target in cardiac arrest. Journal of Molecular Medicine. 2015;**93**:243-252

[77] Ruvolo PP, Deng X, May WS. Phosphorylation of Bcl2 and regulation of apoptosis. Leukemia. 2001;**15**:515-522

[78] Ouyang Y, Giffard RG. Cellular neuroprotective mechanisms in cerebral ischemia: Bcl-2 family proteins and protection of mitochondrial function. Cell Calcium. 2004;**36**:303-311

[79] Tanaka K, Fukuuchi Y, Nogawa S, Nozaki H, Nagata E, Suzuki S, et al. Alteration of cAMP-mediated signal transduction in cerebral ischemia-binding activity of PKA and phosphorylation of CREB. Rinshō Shinkeigaku. 1999;**39**:1298-1299

[80] Gobé G, Zhang X, Cuttle L, Pat B, Willgoss D, Hancock J, et al. Bcl-2 genes and growth factors in pathology of ischaemic acute renal failure. Immunology & Cell Biology. 1999;**77**:279-286

[81] Niemi N, MacKeigan J. Mitochondrial phosphorylation in apoptosis: Flipping the death switch. Antioxidants & Redox Signaling. 2013;**19**:572-582

[82] Teague WM, Pettit FH, Yeaman SJ, Reed LJ. Function of phosphorylation sites on pyruvate dehydrogenase. Biochemical and Biophysical Research Communications. 1979;**87**:244-252

[83] Thibodeau A, Geng X, Previch LE, Ding Y. Pyruvate dehydrogenase complex in cerebral ischemia-reperfusion injury. Brain Circulation. 2016;**2**:61-66

[84] Churchill EN, Murriel CL, Chen CH, Mochly-Rosen D, Szweda LI. Reperfusion-induced translocation of δPKC to cardiac mitochondria prevents pyruvate dehydrogenase reactivation. Circulation Research. 2005;**97**:78-85

[85] Cardell M, Koide T, Wieloch T. Pyruvate dehydrogenase activity in the rat cerebral cortex following cerebral ischemia. Journal of Cerebral Blood Flow & Metabolism. 1989;**9**:350-357

[86] Verdanis A. Protein kinase activity at the inner membrane of mammalian mitochondria. The Journal of Biological Chemistry. 1977;**252**:807-813

[87] Sardanelli AM, Technikova-Dobrova Z, Speranza F, Mazzocca A, Scacco S, Papa S. Topology of the mitochondrial cAMP-dependent protein kinase and its substrates. FEBS Letters. 1996;**396**:276-278

[88] Srinivasan S, Spear J, Chandran K, Joseph J, Kalyanaraman B, Avadhani N. Oxidative stress induced mitochondrial protein kinase a mediates cytochrome c oxidase dysfunction. PLoS One. 2013;**8**:77129

[89] Communal C, Colucci W. The control of cardiomyocyte apoptosis via the β-adrenergic signaling pathways. Archives des Maladies du Coeur et des Vaisseaux. 2005;**98**:236-241

[90] Makaula S LA. H-89, a non-specific inhibitor of protein kinase a, promotes post-ischemic cardiac contractile recovery and reduces infarct size. Journal of Cardiovascular Pharmacology. 2005;**45**:341-347

[91] Papa S, Scacco S, Sardanelli AM, Vergari R, Papa F, Budde S, et al. Mutation in the NDUFS4 gene of complex I abolishes cAMP-dependent activation of the complex in a child with fatal neurological syndrome. FEBS Letters. 2001;**489**:259-262

[92] Edwards HV, Scott JD, Baillie GS. PKA phosphorylation of the small heat-shock protein Hsp20 enhances its cardioprotective effects. Biochemical Society Transactions. 2012;**40**:210-214

[93] Ji H, Shen X, Zhang Y, Gao F, Huang C, Chang W, et al. Activation of cyclic adenosine monophosphate-dependent protein kinase a signaling prevents liver ischemia/reperfusion injury in mice. Liver Transplantation. 2012;**18**:659-670

[94] Dagda R, Banerjee T. Role of PKA in regulating mitochondrial function and neuronal development: Implications to neurodegenerative diseases. Reviews in the Neurosciences. 2015;**26**:359-370

[95] Merrill R, Dagda R, Dickey A, Cribbs J, Green S, Usachev Y, et al. Mechanism of neuroprotective mitochondrial remodeling by PKA/AKAP1. PLoS Biology. 2011;**9**:e1000612

[96] Cherra S, Kulich S, Uechi G, Balasubramani M, Mountzouris J, Day B, et al. Regulation of the autophagy protein LC3 by phosphorylation. The Journal of Cell Biology. 2010;**190**:533-539

[97] Bijur GN, Jope RS. Rapid accumulation of Akt in mitochondria following phosphatidylinositol 3-kinase activation. Journal of Neurochemistry. 2003;**87**:1427-1435

[98] Shaik ZP, Fifer EK, Nowak G. Protein kinase B/Akt modulates nephrotoxicant-induced necrosis in renal cells. American Journal of Physiology. Renal Physiology. 2007;**292**:F292-F303

[99] Ahmad N, Wang Y, Haider KH, Wang B, Pasha Z, Uzun O, et al. Cardiac protection by mitoKATP channels is dependent on Akt translocation from cytosol to mitochondria during late preconditioning. American Journal of Physiology. Heart and Circulatory Physiology. 2006;**290**:H2402-H2408

[100] Shaik ZP, Fifer EK, Nowak G. Akt activation improves oxidative phosphorylation in renal proximal tubular cells following nephrotoxicant injury. American Journal of Physiology. Renal Physiology. 2008;**294**:F423-F432

[101] Sussman MA. Mitochondrial integrity: Preservation through Akt/Pim-1 kinase signaling in the cardiomyocyte. Expert Review of Cardiovascular Therapy. 2009;**7**:929-938

[102] Majewski N, Nogueira V, Bhaskar P, Coy PE, Skeen JE, Gottlob K, et al. Hexokinase-mitochondria interaction mediated by Akt is required to inhibit apoptosis in the presence or absence of Bax and Bak. Molecular Cell. 2004;**16**:819-830

[103] Hoshi M, Takashima A, Noguchi K, Murayama M, Sato M, Kondo S, Saitoh Y, Ishiguro K, Hoshino T, Imahori K. Regulation of mitochondrial pyruvate dehydrogenase activity by tau protein kinase I/glycogen synthase kinase 3beta in brain. Proceedings of the National Academy of Sciences of the United States of America. 1996;**93**:2719-2723

[104] Yoshida K, Hirata T, Akita Y, Mizukami Y, Yamaguchi K, Sorimac Y, et al. Translocation of protein kinase C-α, δ and ε isoforms in ischemic rat heart. Biochimica et Biophysica Acta. 1996;**1317**:36-44

[105] Piccoletti R, Bendinelli P, Arienti D, Bernelli-Zazzera A. State and activity of protein kinase C in postischemic reperfused liver. Experimental and Molecular Pathology. 1992;**56**:219-228

[106] Padanilam BJ. Induction and subcellular localization of protein kinase C isozymes following renal ischemia. Kidney International. 2001;**59**:1789-1797

[107] Hambleton M, York A, Sargent M, Kaiser R, Lorenz J, Robbins J, et al. Inducible and myocyte-specific inhibition of PKCα enhances cardiac contractility and protects against infarction-induced heart failure. The American Journal of Physiology. 2007;**293**:H3768-H3771

[108] Abdullah Z, Bayraktutan U. Suppression of PKC-α attenuates TNF-α-evoked cerebral barrier breakdown via regulations of MMP-2 and plasminogen–plasmin system. Biochimica et Biophysica Acta (BBA)—Molecular Basis of Disease. 2016;**1862**:1354-1366

[109] Nowak G, Bakajsova D. Protein kinase C-α activation promotes recovery of mitochondrial function and cell survival following oxidant injury in renal cells. American Journal of Physiology. Renal Physiology. 2012;**303**:F515-F526

[110] Ruvolo PP, Deng X, Carr BK, May WS. A functional role for mitochondrial PKCα in Bcl2 phosphorylation and suppression of apoptosis. The Journal of Biological Chemistry. 1998;**273**:25436-25442

[111] Wieloch T, Cardell M, Bingren H, Zivin J, Saitoh T. Changes in the activity of protein kinase C and the differential subcellular redistribution of its isozymes in the rat striatum during and following transient forebrain ischemia. Journal of Neurochemistry. 1991;**56**:1227-1235

[112] Bright R, Mochly-Rosen D. The role of protein kinase C in cerebral ischemic and reperfusion injury. Stroke. 2005;**36**:2781-2790

[113] Koponen S, Goldsteins G, Keinanen R, Koistinaho J. Induction of protein kinase C-δ subspecies in neurons and microglia after transient global brain ischemia. Journal of Cerebral Blood Flow & Metabolism. 2000;**20**:93-102

[114] Bright R, Raval A, Dembner J, Perez-Pinzon M, Steinberg G, Yenari M, et al. Protein kinase C δ mediates cerebral reperfusion injury in vivo. The Journal of Neuroscience. 2004;**24**:6880-6888

[115] Murriel CL, Churchill E, Inagaki K, Szweda LI, Mochly-Rosen D. Protein kinase Cδ activation induces apoptosis in response to cardiac ischemia and reperfusion damage: A mechanism involving bad and the mitochondria. The Journal of Biological Chemistry. 2004;**279**:47985-47991

[116] Churchill E, Mochly-Rosen D. The roles of PKC δ and ε isoenzymes in the regulation of myocardial ischaemia/reperfusion injury. Biochemical Society Transactions. 2007;**35**:1040-1042

[117] Inagaki K, Chen L, Ikeno F, Lee F, Imahashi K, Bouley D, et al. Inhibition of δ-protein kinase C protects against reperfusion injury of the ischemic heart in vivo. Circulation. 2003;**108**:2304-2307

[118] Zhang D, Pan J, Xiang X, Liu Y, Dong G, Livingston MJ, et al. Protein kinase Cδ suppresses autophagy to induce kidney cell apoptosis in cisplatin nephrotoxicity. Journal of the American Society of Nephrology. 2017;**28**:1131-1144

[119] Sun X, Budas GR, Xu L, Barreto GE, Mochly-Rosen D, Giffard RG. Selective activation of protein kinase Cε in mitochondria is neuroprotective in vitro and reduces focal ischemic brain injury in mice. Journal of Neuroscience Research. 2013;**91**:799-807

[120] Jaburek M, Costa ADT, Burton JR, Costa CL, Garlid KD. Mitochondrial PKCε and mitochondrial ATP-sensitive K^+ channel copurify and coreconstitute to form a functioning signaling module in proteoliposomes. Circulation Research. 2006;**99**:878-883

[121] Waza AA, Andrabi K, Hussain MU. Protein kinase C (PKC) mediated interaction between conexin43 (Cx43) and K^+(ATP) channel subunit (Kir6.1) in cardiomyocyte

mitochondria: Implications in cytoprotection against hypoxia induced cell apoptosis. Cellular Signalling. 2014;**26**:1909-1917

[122] Ogbi M, Johnson JA. Protein kinase Cε interacts with cytochrome c oxidase subunit IV and enhances cytochrome c oxidase activity in neonatal cardiac myocyte preconditioning. The Biochemical Journal. 2006;**393**:191-199

[123] Rong S, Hueper K, Kirsch T, Greite R, Klemann C, Mengel M, et al. Renal PKC-ε deficiency attenuates acute kidney injury and ischemic allograft injury via TNF-α-dependent inhibition of apoptosis and inflammation. American Journal of Physiology. Renal Physiology. 2014;**307**:F718-F726

[124] Zablocka B, Dluzniewska J, Zajac H, Domanska-Janik K. Opposite reaction of ERK and JNK in ischemia vulnerable and resistant regions of hippocampus: Involvement of mitochondria. Brain Research. Molecular Brain Research. 2003;**110**:245-252

[125] Zhou J, Du T, Li B, Rong Y, Verkhratsky A, Peng L. Crosstalk between MAPK/ERK and PI3K/AKT signal pathways during brain ischemia/reperfusion. ASN Neuro. 2015;**7**:5

[126] Baines CP, Zhang J, Wang GW, Zheng YT, Xiu JX, Cardwell EM, et al. Mitochondrial PKCε and MAPK form signaling modules in the murine heart: Enhanced mitochondrial PKCε-MAPK interactions and differential MAPK activation in PKCε-induced cardioprotection. Circulation Research. 2002;**90**:390-397

[127] Hernández-Reséndiz S, Zazueta C. PHO-ERK1/2 interaction with mitochondria regulates the permeability transition pore in cardioprotective signaling. Life Sciences. 2014;**108**:13-21

[128] Nowak G, Clifton GL, Godwin ML, Bakajsova D. Activation of ERK1/2 pathway mediates oxidant-induced decreases in mitochondrial function in renal cells. American Journal of Physiology. Renal Physiology. 2006;**291**:F840-F855

[129] Collier JB, Whitaker RM, Eblen ST, Schnellmann RG. Rapid renal regulation of peroxisome proliferator-activated receptor γ coactivator-1α by ERK1/2 in physiological and pathological conditions. The Journal of Biological Chemistry. 2016;**291**:26850-26859

[130] Okada M, Yamane M, Iga N, Nishikawa H, Yamamoto S, Otani S, et al. MAPK/ERK pathway activation leads to severe ischemia-reperfusion-induced lung injury. The Journal of Heart and Lung Transplantation. 2013;**32**:S138

[131] Mackay K, Mochly-Rosen D. An inhibitor of p38 mitogen-activated protein kinase protects neonatal cardiac Myocytes from ischemia. The Journal of Biological Chemistry. 1999;**274**:6272-6279

[132] Kumphune S, Surinkaew S, Chattipakorn SC, Chattipakorn N. Inhibition of p38 MAPK activation protects cardiac mitochondria from ischemia/reperfusion injury. Pharmaceutical Biology. 2015;**53**:1831-1841

[133] Juhaszova M, Zorov DB, Kim SH, Pepe S, Fu Q, Fishbein KW, et al. Glycogen synthase kinase-3beta mediates convergence of protection signaling to inhibit the mitochondrial permeability transition pore. The Journal of Clinical Investigation. 2004;**113**:1535-1549

[134] Zhai P, Sciarretta S, Galeotti J, Volpe M, Sadoshima J. Differential roles of GSK-3β during myocardial ischemia and ischemia/reperfusion. Circulation Research. 2011;**109**:502-511

[135] Xiao H, Deng M, Yang B, Tang J, Hu Z. Role of GSK-3 in ischemia-induced blood–brain barrier disruption in aged female rats. Journal of Neurochemistry. 2017;**42**:194-203

[136] Cookson MR. Parkinsonism due to mutations in PINK1, Parkin, and DJ-1 and oxidative stress and mitochondrial pathways. Cold Spring Harbor Perspectives in Medicine. 2012;**2**:a009415

[137] Park J, Lee S, Lee S, Kim Y, Song S. Mitochondrial dysfunction in Drosophila PINK1 mutants is complemented by parkin. Nature. 2006;**441**:1157-1161

[138] Zhao Y, Chen F, Chen S, Liu X, Cui M, Dong Q. The Parkinson's disease-associated gene PINK1 protects neurons from ischemic damage by decreasing mitochondrial translocation of the fission promoter Drp1. Journal of Neurochemistry. 2013;**127**:711-722

[139] Siddall HK, Yellon DM, Ong SB, Mukherjee UA, Burke N, et al. Loss of PINK1 increases the heart's vulnerability to ischemia-reperfusion injury. PLoS One. 2013;**8**:e62400

[140] Demory ML, Boerner JL, Davidson R, Faust W, Miyake T, Lee I, Huttemann M, Douglas R, Haddad G, Parsons SJ. Epidermal growth factor receptor translocation to the mitochondria: Regulation and effect. Journal of Biochemistry. 2009;**284**:36592-36604

Chapter 8

Mitochondrial Trafficking by Prohibitin-Kinesin-Myosin-Cadherin Complex in the Eye

Srinivas R. Sripathi, Weilue He, Johnpaul Offor,
Diana R. Gutsaeva and Wan Jin Jahng

Additional information is available at the end of the chapter

http://dx.doi.org/10.5772/intechopen.75994

Abstract

Disruption of the mitochondrial-nuclear network leads to accelerated aging and age-related diseases, including age-related macular degeneration. The current study tested the hypothesis that mitochondrial morphology could be demonstrated quantitatively using a mathematic model and mitochondrial trafficking complex under stress conditions. To test our hypothesis, normal and aberrant mitochondria were examined quantitatively based on mitochondrial size, shape, position, composition, and dynamics. Adaptation of the mitochondrial network to changes in the intracellular oxidation and reduction milieu is critical for the survival of retinal pigment epithelial cells. Our mitochondrial interactome mapping demonstrated that a positive correlation may exist between oxidative stress-mediated phosphorylation and age-related disease progression. The current interactome may provide a potential therapeutic approach to treat mitochondria-induced neurodegeneration, including age-related macular degeneration.

Keywords: mitochondrial trafficking, prohibitin-cytoskeleton, retinal pigment epithelial cells, mitochondrial dynamics, age-related macular degeneration, protein interactome

1. Introduction

Mitochondria are the highly dynamic cellular organelles that form a dynamic network to regulate calcium balance, energy metabolism, and apoptotic signaling [1–8]. Mitochondria alter their morphology repeatedly through the collective actions of fission as a separation of a single organelle into multiple autonomous structures, fusion as the combination of multiple structures to form single organelle, as well as movement along cytoskeletal paths [5, 9]. These combined actions occur concurrently in major cell types to regulate the cell fate.

To maintain the balance that regulates overall morphology and cytoskeletal stability many specialized molecules including dynamin family of proteins play critical roles [10, 11]. Growing body of evidence demonstrates that disruptions of mitochondrial network lead to multiple human pathologies, including metabolic, genetic, cardiovascular diseases, as well as neurogenerative diseases and cancers [12–15]. Several studies provided the evidence that mitochondria play a critical role in the progression of age-related diseases, including age-related macular degeneration (AMD) [16–21]. The damage of mitochondrial DNA could be the key factor involved in altered vascular endothelial growth factor (VEGF) secretion, retinal pigment epithelium (RPE) dysfunction, and cell death during the progression of AMD [22, 23].

The current study aimed to examine the correlation between alterations in mitochondrial morphology and mitochondrial dysfunction. For quantitative analysis of mitochondrial morphology, we introduced the mitochondrial index that includes network size, mitochondrial content and surface area. Mitochondrial interconnectivity and elongation were determined systematically using a computational model in three dimensions, showing a mitochondrial-endoplasmic reticulum (ER)-nuclear hole as open space for trafficking at the beginning of apoptosis under oxidative stress.

The assessment of average circularity showed mitochondrial elongation which is sensitive to fragmented vs. normal shaped mitochondria. The average area/perimeter ratio showed normal or stressed mitochondria as a highly interconnected mass of reticular network. Previously, we observed that prohibitin translocalizes between the nucleus and mitochondria under oxidative stress conditions to influence mitochondrial dynamics [24]. We observed anterograde signaling from the nucleus to mitochondria using a prohibitin shuttle under stress in the retina, as well as the retrograde shuttling of prohibitin from mitochondria to the nucleus in the RPE. In addition, cytoskeletal reorganization, tubulin/vimentin depolymerization and increased phosphorylations were observed in stressed mitochondria [25–27].

In this study, mitochondrial dynamics was further analyzed in mitochondrial trafficking complex using prohibitin immunoprecipitation. We found a motor-based protein complex that includes kinesin 19 (93 kDa), myosin 9 (110 kDa), and cadherin isoforms (88 kDa) to regulate the mitochondrial-nuclear communication. Finally, we have established a comprehensive mitochondrial interactome map by combining several independent sets of interaction data. Our interactome map provides an integrated information on the hidden apoptotic pathway, cytoskeletal rearrangement, nitric oxide signaling, ubiquitination, and mitochondrial network in neurodegeneration.

2. Materials and methods

2.1. Cell culture and oxidative stress treatment

Retinal pigment epithelial cells (ARPE-19) were purchased from ATCC (Manassas, VA) and cultured in Dulbecco's modified Eagle's medium (DMEM) supplemented with fetal bovine serum (FBS; 10%) and penicillin/streptomycin (1%) at 37°C in a humidified atmosphere of 5% CO_2 in air as suggested by the manufacturer. Cells were used between passages 8–9.

Retinal progenitor cells (HRP) were kindly donated by Dr. Harold J. Sheeldo (University of North Texas Health Science Center) and were cultured at the same condition as ARPE-19 cells.

Prior to all experiments, confluent ARPE-19 cells were incubated with fresh medium for 12 h and washed with phosphate buffered saline (PBS) three times. ARPE-19 cells were incubated with an oxidant, *tert*-butyl hydroperoxide (*t*-BuOOH, 200 μM, Sigma-Aldrich, St.Louis, MO), in serum-free medium for 0.5, 1, 2, 4, 6, 8, 12, and 24 h and representative images were presented. After the treatment, medium was removed, cells were washed with PBS and harvested for future analysis. Cells were lysed for experiments, including, immunoprecipitation, sodium dodecyl sulfate polyacrylamide gel electrophoresis (SDS–PAGE), Western blot analysis, immunocytochemistry, and mass spectrometry analysis.

To compare with other stress environment, ARPE-19 cells were incubated under intense light (210 μmoles/m^2/s photon flux; 7000 lx) for 1 h in serum-free media and analyzed by SDS-PAGE/Western blotting, or immunocytochemistry.

Lipids were extracted from ARPE-19 cells using cholorform/methanol (2:1, v/v) and organic solvent was evaporated under a gentle nitrogen stream and dissolved in chloroform for analysis by HPLC and mass spectrometry.

All experiments were repeated (N = 3–10 biological samples) with technical duplicate or triplicate. Statistical analysis was performed using StatView software and statistical significance was determined by variance (ANOVA) or unpaired Student's t test when appropriate.

2.2. Donor eye tissue and phosphoprotein enrichment

Human postmortem donor eye tissues were used following the tenets of the Declaration of Helsinki. Human AMD retinas (8 mm macular and peripheral punches), RPE (8 mm central and peripheral punches), and age-matched control eyes (N = 9, biological triplicate x technical triplicate) were provided by the Lions Eye Bank (Moran Eye Center, University of Utah). Phosphoproteome of macular (I), peripheral retina (II), central RPE (III), and peripheral RPE (IV) was compared to age-matched control donor eyes to determine region-specific senescence-associated molecular mechanisms during AMD progression. Phosphoproteins were enriched by charge-based spin column chromatography and resolved by 2D gel electrophoresis as previously reported [28]. In addition, trypsin digested phosphopeptides from whole lysates were enriched using Ga^{3+}/TiO_2 immobilized metal ion chromatography. Eluted phosphopeptides were analyzed using mass spectrometry including MALDI-TOF-TOF and ESI MS/MS.

2.3. Immunocytochemical analysis

To analyze mitochondrial morphology, Cells were incubated with 100 nM MitoTracker Orange (Molecular Probes). Cells were fixed using 10% formaldehyde (25 min) and the membrane was permeabilized using 0.2% Triton X-100 (20 min), followed by blocking (0.05% Tween 20, 10% FBS, 1 h) and incubation overnight at 4°C with anti-prohibitin antibody

(1:500; Genemed Synthesis, San Antonio). Prohibitin was visualized using Alexa Fluor 488-secondary IgG antibody (1:700; 1 h at 25°C; Molecular Probes). The nuclei were visualized by incubation with DAPI (4, 6-diamidino-2-phenylindole) added to VECTASHIELD Mounting Medium (Vector Laboratories, Burlingame, CA). A fluorescence microscopy was used for image analysis (Zeiss AxioVert 200 M Apo Tome, 63×).

2.4. Immunoprecipitation

ARPE-19 cells were rinsed (Modified Dulbecco's PBS) and lysed using immunoprecipitation (IP) lysis buffer (pH 7.4) containing Tris (25 mM), NaCl (150 mM), EDTA (1 mM), NP-40 (1%), glycerol glycerol (5%), and protease inhibitor cocktail by incubating on ice for 5 min with periodic sonication (3 × 5 min), followed by centrifugation (13,000 × *g*, 10 min). Proteins (1 mg/mL, 200–400 μL) were loaded for immunoprecipitation and nonspecific bindings were avoided using control agarose resin cross-linked by 4% bead agarose. Amino-linked protein-A beads were used to immobilize anti-prohibitin antibody with a coupling buffer (1 mM sodium phosphate, 150 mM NaCl, pH 7.2), followed by incubation (room temperature, 2 h) with sodium cyanoborohydride (3 μL, 5 M). Columns were washed using a washing buffer (1 M NaCl), and protein lysate was incubated in the protein A-antibody column with gentle rocking overnight at 4°C. The unbound proteins were spun down as flow-through, and the column was washed three times using the washing buffer (1 M NaCl) to remove nonspecific binding proteins. The prohibitin-interacting proteins were eluted by incubating with elution buffer for 5 min at room temperature. The eluted proteins were equilibrated with Laemmli sample buffer (5X, 5% β-mercaptoethanol). Eluted proteins were separated using SDS–PAGE and visualized using Coomassie blue (Pierce, IL) or silver staining kit (Bio-Rad, Hercules, CA). Prohibitin and p53 were visualized using Western blot analysis. Proteins were identified by mass spectrometry analysis.

2.5. Mass spectrometry analysis

Protein bands were excised into 1 × 1 × 1 mm cubes. The Coomassie-stained or silver-stained gel pieces were incubated using a Coomassie destaining buffer (200 μL of 50% MeCN in 25 mM NH_4HCO_3, pH 8.0, room temperature, 20 min) or silver destaining buffer (50% of 30 mM potassium ferricyanide, 50% of 100 mM sodium thiosulfate, 5–10 min). The gel pieces were dehydrated (200 μL, MeCN) and vacuum-dried (Speed Vac, Savant, Holbrook, NY). Proteins were reduced (10 mM DTT, 100 mM NH_4HCO_3, 30 min, 56°C) and were alkylated (55 mM iodoacetamide, 100 mM NH_4HCO_3, 20 min, room temperature in the dark). Proteins were digested using trypsin (13 ng/μL sequencing-grade from Promega, 37°C, overnight) in NH_4HCO_3 (10 mM) containing MeCN (10%). The peptides were enriched using a buffer (50 μL, 50% MeCN in NH_4HCO_3, 5% formic acid, 20 min, 37°C). Dried peptides were dissolved in the mass spectrometry sample buffer (5–10 μL, 75% MeCN in NH_4HCO_3,1% trifluoroacetic acid). Alpha-cyano-4-hydroxycinnamic acid (5 mg/mL, Sigma-Aldrich, St. Louis, MO) was freshly dissolved in a matrix buffer (50% MeCN, 50% NH_4HCO_3, 1% triflouroacetic acid) and centrifuged (13,000× *g*, 5 min). The peptide-matrix mixtures (0.5 μL) were spotted onto the MALDI target plate (Ground steel, Bruker Daltonics, Germany). Mass spectrometer and all spectra were calibrated using a known peptide, including trypsin (842.5099, 2211.105 Da). The mass spectrum was recorded in 800–3000 Da range using Flex MALDI-TOF mass spectrometer (Bruker Daltonics, Germany, 70–75% laser intensity, 100–300 shots). Mass spectrometry data were analyzed using Flex analysis software (Bruker Dal- tonics, Germany). Peptides were identified using the Mascot software (Matrix Science) and NCBI/SwissProt database (zero mismatch cleavage, carbamidomethyl cysteine, methionine oxidation, 50–300 ppm mass tolerance). Peptide identification was evaluated based on Mascot MOWSE score, number of matched peptides, and protein sequence coverage. MOWSE score is expressed as -10logP as a probability value to compute the composite probability P.

2.6. Quantitative analysis of mitochondrial morphology

The connectivity, the number of mitochondrial branch points, and the interactive 3D visualization of isosurfaces were examined to identify the contact area between mitochondria and other organelles.

Mitochondria were stained using MitoTracker Orange/Red or rhodamine 123. Mitochondrial interconnectivity and elongation were analyzed systematically using computational software, including Mito-Morphology macro, Mitograph 2.0, Imaris 8.2.1., and SOAX 3.6.1.

Mitochondrial size and morphology were analyzed using the software connected to Image J software (Ruben Dagda: http://imagejdocu.tudor.lu/doku.php?id=macro:mitpophagy_ mitochondrial_morphology_content_lc3_colocalization_macro). We chose the region of interest using the polygon selection tool to analyze mitochondrial morphology. Individual red, green, and blue channels were obtained from the RGB images, and then the red and blue channels were closed. The grayscale was extracted from the red channel and the pixels were inverted to photographic channel. The Threshold function determined maximal and minimal pixel values. To understand mitochondrial structure and function, 12 mitochondrial indexes, including (1) mitochondrial area, (2) cellular area, (3) mitochondrial content, (4) perimeter, (5) circularity, (6) average perimeter, (7) average mitochondrial area, (8) average circularity, (9) area/perimeter, (10) area/perimeter normalized to minor axis, (11) minor axis, (12) area/perimeter normalized to circularity, were evaluated in ARPE-19 cells under oxidative stress conditions.

Mitochondrial shape, including fused, fragmented, tubular, swollen, branched, uniform, and perinuclear clustering, was examined quantitatively. Mitochondrial filaments in three dimensions and mitochondrial parameters in ARPE-19 cells were calculated mathematically using Image J and Imaris (v8.2.1) software. The connectivity, the number of mitochondrial branch points, and the interactive 3D visualization of isosurfaces were examined to identify the contact between mitochondria and other organelles.

2.7. Mitochondrial mapping in AMD

Mitochondrial signaling in a network-based interactome map between genome, proteome, and metabolome of AMD was established using proteome data and bioinformatics software. The protein-protein interaction was established using the Münich Information Center for Protein Sequence (MIPS), Biomolecular Interaction Network Database (BIND), the Database of

Interacting Proteins (DIP), the Molecular Interaction Database (MINT), the Protein Interaction Database (IntAct), and STRING.

Interaction mapping of prohibitin was determined using immunoprecipitation, followed by mass spectrometry analysis. Prohibitin binding proteins in the RPE were connected using STRING 10.0 software (http://string-db.org/).

Prohibitin interactions were confirmed using eight sources that include neighborhood, gene fusion, co-occurence, high-throughput interaction experiments, databases, homology, conserved co-expression, and published knowledge, including ExPASy (http://www.expasy.org/proteomics /protein–protein_interaction), MIPS (http://mips.helmholtz-muenchen.de/proj/ppi/), and Pubmed database (http://www.ncbi.nlm.nih.gov/pubmed).

AMD and oxidative biomarkers interactome were established using protein–protein interaction map software and databases, including STRING 10.0 (http://string-db.org/), MIPS and iHOP (http://www.ihop-net.org/UniPub/iHOP/) (**Figure 8**). Proteins found in AMD or oxidative stress conditions were added to establish the AMD interactome. Protein interactions were presented using eight categories, including neighborhood (green), gene fusion (red), co-occurrence (dark blue), co-expression (black), binding experiments (purple), databases (blue), text mining (lime), and homology (cyan). Protein interactions were determined and confirmed by genomic context, high-throughput experiments, co-expression, and previous publications in Pubmed. Protein database analysis showed the region-specific phosphorylation of specific proteins in AMD eyes. The interactome between AMD proteome was compared to the retina/RPE proteome under stress conditions.

The genome regulatory network was connected to the proteome network using Uniprobe and JASPAR. Protein phosphorylations were examined by phosphoprotein/peptide enrichment, followed by mass spectrometry analysis. Phosphorylations were compared to Phospho.ELM, and PhosphoSite. The metabolome mapping was established using KEGG and BIGG databases.

3. Results

To understand how mitochondria regulate their morphology and function, we first analyzed mitochondrial morphology quantitatively in ARPE-19 cells subjected to oxidative stress conditions using a systematic computational model (**Figure 1**). Representative mitochondrial images at selected time points (0.5, 1, 8, 24 h) are shown for clear comparison **Figure 1**). We examined mitochondrial area, circularity, perimeter, content as well as cellular area to identify changes between healthy and injured mitochondria. Previously, our *in vitro* data using RPE cells demonstrated the positive correlation between apoptotic signaling and mitochondria-nucleus prohibitin shuttling. Our previous studies suggest that cellular distribution and the total volume of mitochondria could be affected by microtubules, intermediate filaments and cardiolipin [24–27, 29, 30].

http://dx.doi.org/10.5772/intechopen.75994

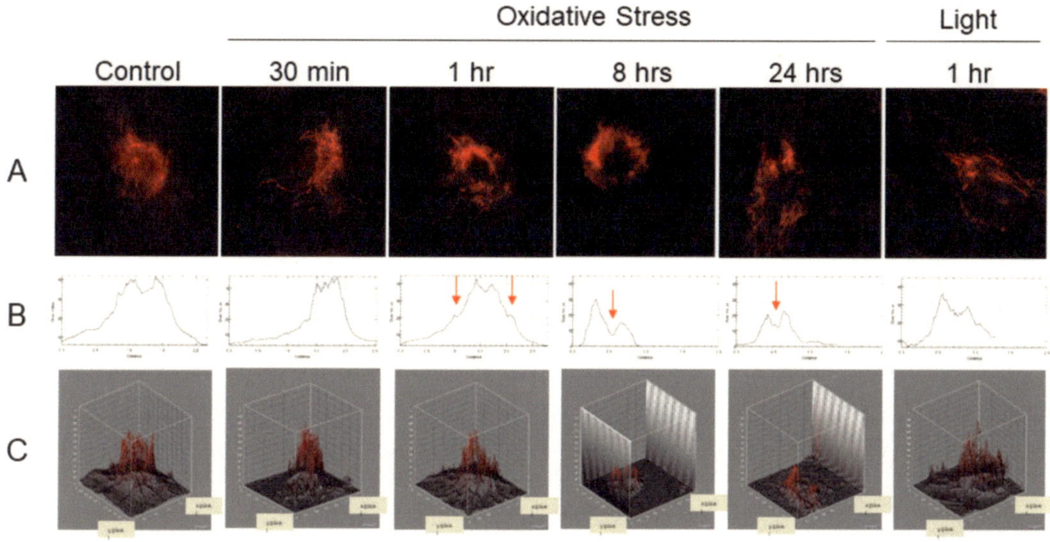

Figure 1. Quantitative analysis of mitochondrial morphology: representative images of MitoTracker Orange-labeled mitochondria from ARPE-19 cells exposed to *t*-BuOOH for 0.5–24 h or light for 1 h are shown here. A. ARPE-19 cells under oxidative stress were analyzed by immunocytochemistry using MitoTracker. B. Mitochondrial content was represented by 2D graph (radius/intensity) showing decreased size and fragmentation pattern under stress conditions. C. Mitochondria in ARPE-19 cells were presented in 3D structure using Image J software.

Our results showed that the connectivity, the number of mitochondrial branch points, and the interactive isosurfaces were altered at the contact sites between mitochondria and other organelles. Under extended oxidative stress (1, 8, 24 h) and intense light (7000 lx, 1 h), we observed a decrease in mitochondrial size, presence of fragmented filaments (red arrows), and holes on the organelle contact sites. Under intense light condition, mitochondria in ARPE-19 cells were decreased and fragmented as shown in oxidative stress (1–8 h).

Next, mitochondrial perimeter vs. circularity was examined to determine the correlation between mitochondrial morphology and oxidative stress (**Figure 2**). We hypothesized that some mitochondrial indexes that include circularity and perimeter ratio may represent mitochondrial dynamics. We calculated mitochondrial area, perimeter, minor axis, and circularity to conclude that specific mitochondrial ratio correlated positively with stress kinetics.

The average mitochondrial area/perimeter ratio normalized to the minor axis suggests that specific conditions may induce mitochondrial swelling (**Figure 3**). Time-dependent decrease of minor axis and mitochondrial area/perimeter normalized to the circularity was noticed under stress condition. Our previous proteomic study demonstrated that tubulin/vimentin depolymerization and phosphorylations increased in stressed mitochondria [25].

To understand mitochondrial dynamics in detail, mitochondrial trafficking complex was examined. Subcellular fractionation, immunoprecipitation using primary prohibitin antibody, native gel, and mass spectrometry analysis suggest that motor protein complex may determine mitochondrial dynamics and retrograde signaling under stress conditions. Molecular motor

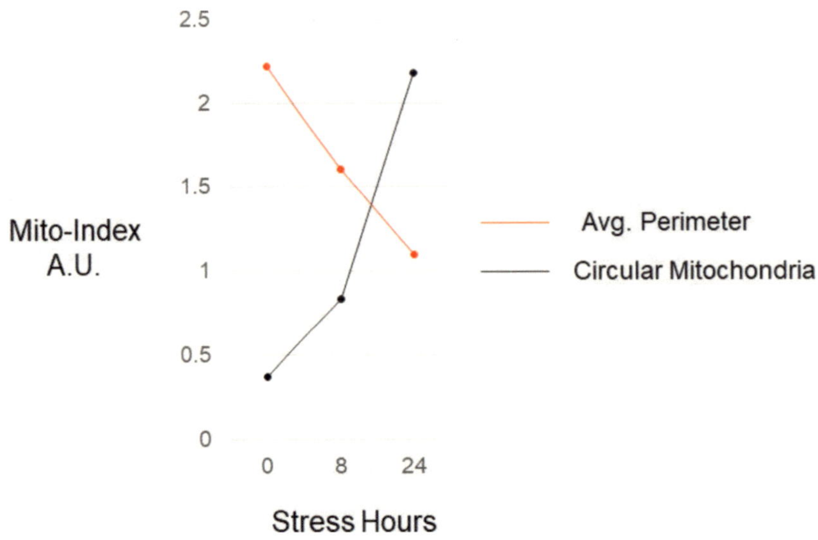

Figure 2. Quantitative analysis of mitochondrial morphology: perimeter vs. circularity. X axis represents time of ARPE-19 cells under oxidative stress and Y axis represents mitochondrial index on perimeter vs. circularity ratio in arbitrary units. Selected time points are 0, 8, 24 h were shown for clarity [24]. Our calculation demonstrated that mitochondria under oxidative stress change their morphology to circular shape for fusion, followed by fragmentation toward greater degree of roundness and circularity. Total area of mitochondria decreased to 40–50% and both perimeter/circular mitochondria were downregulated to 60–70%. Area/perimeter normalized to circularity ratio of mitochondria was decreased to 63% (1 h oxidative stress), showing a positive correlation between mitochondrial morphology changes and apoptotic RPE.

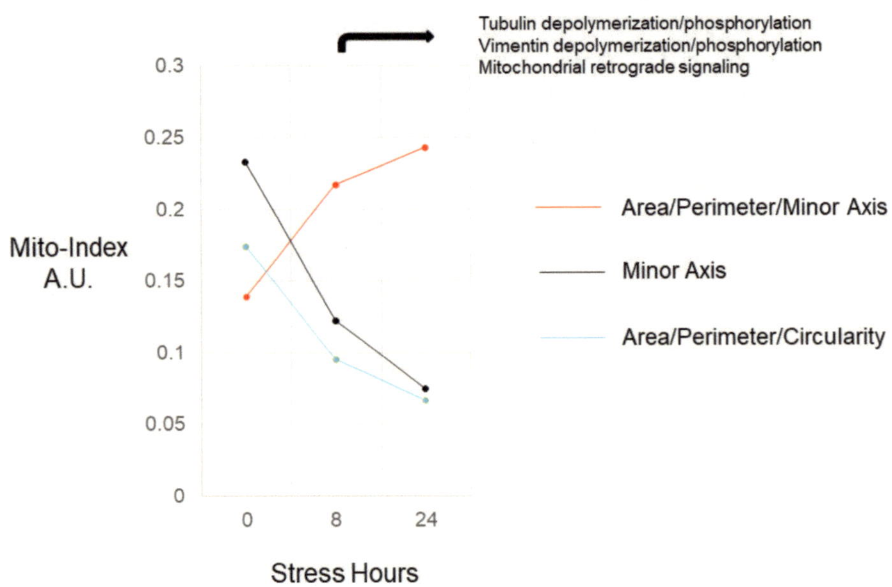

Figure 3. Mitochondrial index: mitochondrial area/perimeter/minor axis vs. minor axis vs. area/perimeter/circularity. X axis represents stressed time (hrs) of ARPE-19 under oxidants and Y axis represents mitochondrial index showing mitochondrial area/perimeter/minor axis (red), compared to mitochondrial minor axis (black), and mitochondrial area/perimeter/mitochondrial circularity (blue) in arbitrary units.

http://dx.doi.org/10.5772/intechopen.75994

complex contains plus-end-directed kinesin 19, myosin 9, protocadherin gA7, and prohibitin (**Figure 4**). The molecular motor/adaptor/receptor complex mediates mitochondrial dynamics. Motor proteins, including kinesin and myosin, facilitate mitochondrial trafficking along the cytoskeleton, mainly microtubules, actin polymers and intermediate filaments (**Figure 5**). Domain analysis of mitochondrial trafficking complex showed that plus-end-directed kinesin 19 (ATP and Mg^{2+} binding domains), myosin 9 (myosin head motor domain, SH3 domain, ATP binding domain), protocadherin gA7 (cadherin repeat and Ca^{2+} binding domain), and prohibitin (PX domain, lipid binding pocket) exist in the trafficking complex.

In order to correlate our *in vitro* findings with human pathology, we analyzed mitochondrial trafficking complex in human postmortem AMD eyes using a proteomic approach (**Figure 6**). RPE and retina tissues (central vs. peripheral) from AMD eyes and age-matching control eyes were analyzed by phosphoproteomics and mass spectrometry analysis. We observed different expression levels of prohibitin, inositol receptor, calponin, ankyrin, guanylate cyclase, and NADP ubiquinone oxidoreductase in the RPE and pyruvate kinase, PP2A, creatine kinase, PAK S/T kinase, vimentin, FES tyrosine kinase and dynamin like protein in the retina from AMD samples compared to control. Our results suggest that mitochondrial trafficking could be a significant determinant of RPE apoptosis by decreased prohibitin. Further, Ca^{2+}, Fe^{2+}, inositide, phosphorylation, and energy imbalance may lead to the accelerated pathogenesis toward AMD.

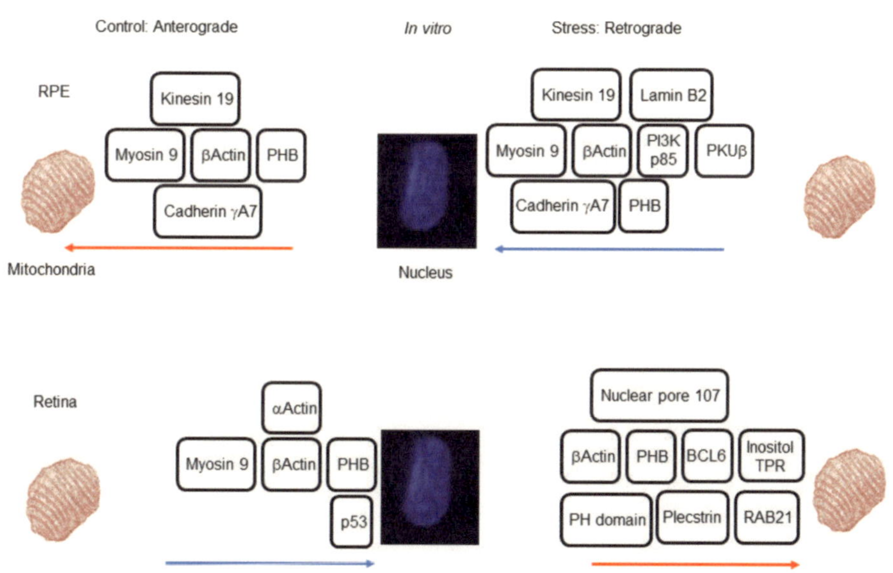

Figure 4. Mitochondrial Trafficking Complex *in vitro*: Retrograde vs. Anterograde Signal. Protein complex in ARPE-19 (RPE) and HRP (retina) cells were analyzed using immunoprecipitation and mass spectrometry. Under normal condition, trafficking complex including prohibitin translocalizes into mitochondria (anterograde) whereas trafficking complex moves into the nucleus (retrograde) under oxidative stress in RPE cells. The molecular motor/adaptor/receptor complex mediates mitochondrial anterograde vs. retrograde signaling. However, in the retina, retrograde signal (mitochondria to the nucleus) is dominant under normal condition, probably due to increased p53 signaling (prohibitin found in the nucleus).

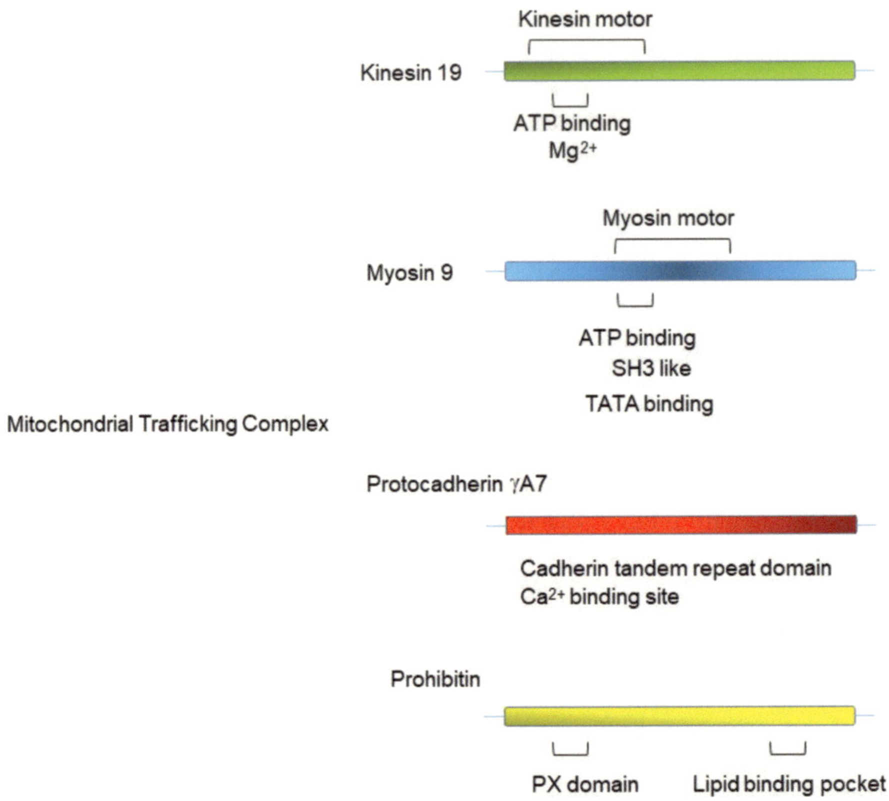

Figure 5. Domain analysis of mitochondrial trafficking complex: ATP, Ca^{2+}, and lipid-dependent signaling. Prohibitin binding proteins were analyzed using bioinformatics software and databases, including iHOP, InterPro (https://www.ebi.ac.uk/interpro/), Expasy/Prosite (https://prosite.expasy.org/), conserved domain search (https://www.ncbi.nlm.nih.gov/Structure/cdd/wrpsb.cgi), Motif (https://molbiol-tools.ca/Motifs.htm) and Pfam (http://pfam.xfam.org/). Kinesin 19 contains ATP binding domain and kinesin motor domain, whereas Myosin 9 has SH3, ATP binding, TATA binding, and myosin motor domains. Protocadherin γA7 includes repeat domain and calcium binding sequences. Prohibitin contains PX domain and the second lipid binding domain.

It is proposed that specific organelles, including mitochondria, melanosome, and phagosome, may use different kinesin and myosin motors for their distribution and trafficking in the RPE [25, 31–33]. Mitochondrial trafficking could be determined by ATP, Ca^{2+}, and lipid interactions based on their domain analysis [29, 34–38] and mitochondrial trafficking is a significant determinant of RPE apoptosis [24, 37]. Altered concentrations of mitochondrial complex, phosphoproteins, and ATP/ADP may lead to premature senescence in RPE cells [27]. Our enriched phosphoproteins and phosphopeptides analysis demonstrated that altered inositol triphosphate receptor, ankyrin, NADP reactions exist in AMD (**Figure 6**). Regulation of mitochondrial complex/lipid ratio and the energy producing machinery may enable enhanced longevity of RPE cells.

Next, a 3D surface model was used to analyze mitochondrial nodes, edges, branches, and tubular filaments (**Figure 7**). Cellular distribution and the total volume were affected by microtubules, intermediate filaments and cardiolipin. A 3D model showed that mitochondrial contact sites with endoplasmic reticulum (ER) and/or the nucleus were opened irreversibly under extended stress (24 h).

http://dx.doi.org/10.5772/intechopen.75994

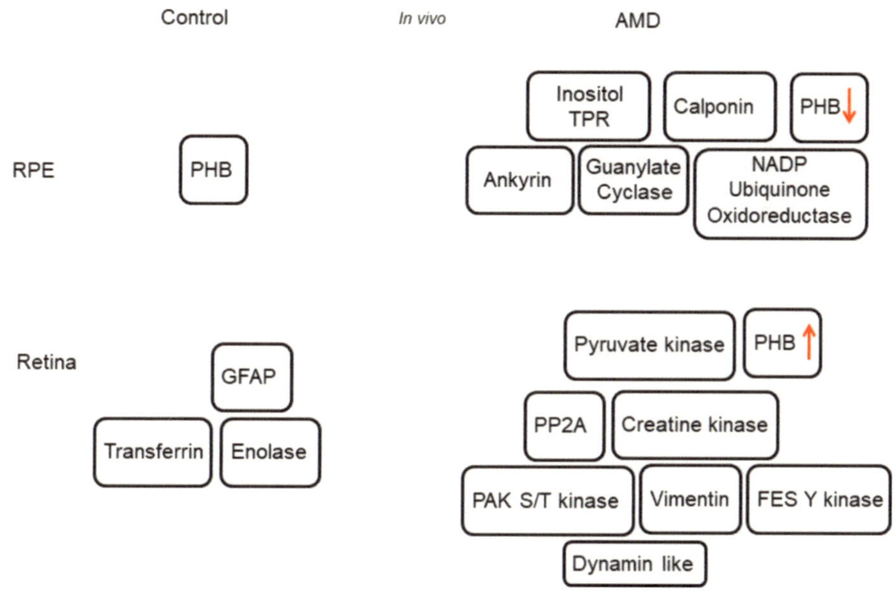

Figure 6. Mitochondrial signaling in the retina and RPE *in vivo* using human AMD eyes: mitochondrial trafficking is a significant determinant of RPE apoptosis. RPE and retina tissues (central vs. peripheral) from AMD eyes and age-matching control eyes were analyzed using phosphoproteomics and mass spectrometry analysis. We observed different expressions of inositol receptor, calponin, ankyrin, guanylate cyclase, and NADP ubiquinone oxidoreductase in the RPE and pyruvate kinase, PP2A, creatine kinase, PAK S/T kinase, vimentin, FES tyrosine kinase and dynamin like protein in the retina from AMD samples compared to control. Altered concentrations of mitochondrial complex, phosphoproteins, and ATP/ADP may lead to premature senescence in RPE cells.

In order to understand AMD protein network, the new AMD interactome with oxidative biomarkers was established using phosphoproteomics data and a computational model. The current AMD interactome demonstrated that several earlier unrelated to AMD proteins, including ubiquitin, peroxiredoxin, MAP kinase, BUB 1/3, vimentin and crystalline could be involved in AMD progression, suggesting that cytoskeletal protein phosphorylation, crystalline aggregation, and mitochondrial signaling may contribute to RPE apoptosis (**Figure 8**). To confirm oxidative stress biomarkers, specific cytoskeletal protein changes were determined *in vivo* using animal model previously (C3H female mice, 7 weeks old) [25, 30, 38]. Neurofilament, vimentin, and tubulin were upregulated under 24 h constant light compared to 12 h dark/12 h light condition [38].

3.1. Discussion

The current study determined the mitochondrial morphology quantitatively using a mathematic model and mitochondrial trafficking complex under stress conditions. Our data suggest that the kinesin-myosin-cadherin-prohibitin complex could be involved in anterograde mitochondrial trafficking, whereas PKUb S/T kinase-myosin-PI3K-lamin B2 bindings may regulate an energy demanding retrograde transport of mitochondria [25, 39–43]. Prohibitin binding with a trafficking protein complex may regulate the bidirectional transport of mitochondria along actin microfilaments, intermediate filaments, and microtubules. The mitochondrial trafficking complex implies that a specific mechanism of communication may exist in the ATP

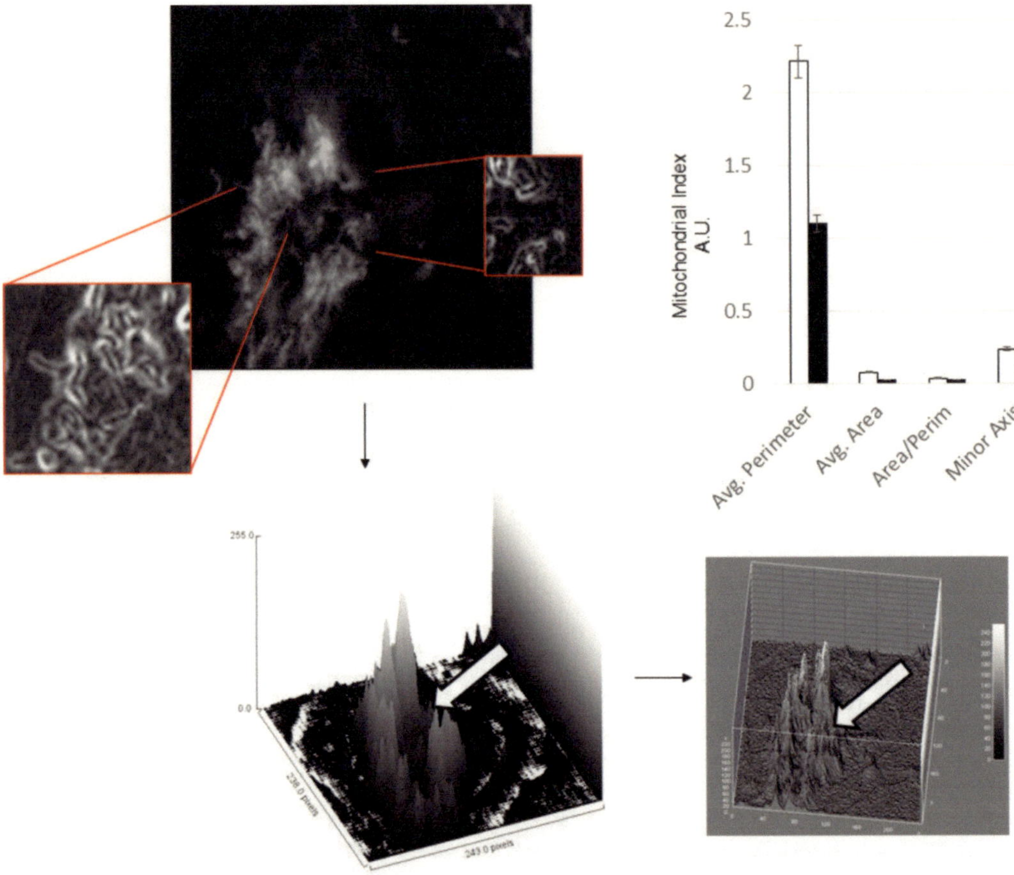

Figure 7. A 3D surface model and a graph representation by nodes, edges, branches, and tubular filaments: Mitochondrial filaments in three dimensions in RPE cells were calculated quantitatively. The connectivity, the number of mitochondrial branch points, and the interactive 3D visualization of isosurfaces were examined to identify the contact point between mitochondria and other organelles, including ER and the nucleus (white arrow). Mitochondria under oxidative stress (24 hrs) decreased their average perimeter (49%), average area (28%), area/perimeter (56%), and minor axis (32%).

and Ca^{2+} demanding regions. Mitochondrial dysfunction, altered dynamics, impaired transport, and turnover perturbation are associated with AMD.

Oxidative stress-induced apoptosis is the final cell death pathway in many irreversible ocular diseases that include AMD. While the end point of apoptosis is well established, the knowledge of early biochemical reactions and specific molecular players has been elusive. We have examined early biosignatures and mechanisms of retinal and RPE cell death under oxidative stress [44]. Our previous studies demonstrated that not only intense light but also constant moderate light and mild oxidative stress may trigger induction of anti-apoptotic Bcl-xL and erythropoietin (EPO) as well as pro-apoptotic caspases [24, 25, 27–29, 37, 38, 45–47]. We determined that protein modifications, including nitration and phosphorylation, were altered under oxidative stress possibly due to excess of NO production [26, 48–50].

The analysis of AMD interactome using proteome-genome-metabolome network suggests that there is a positive correlation between mitochondrial retrograde signaling and AMD progression. The AMD interactome suggests: (1) network-based interactions among AMD-related

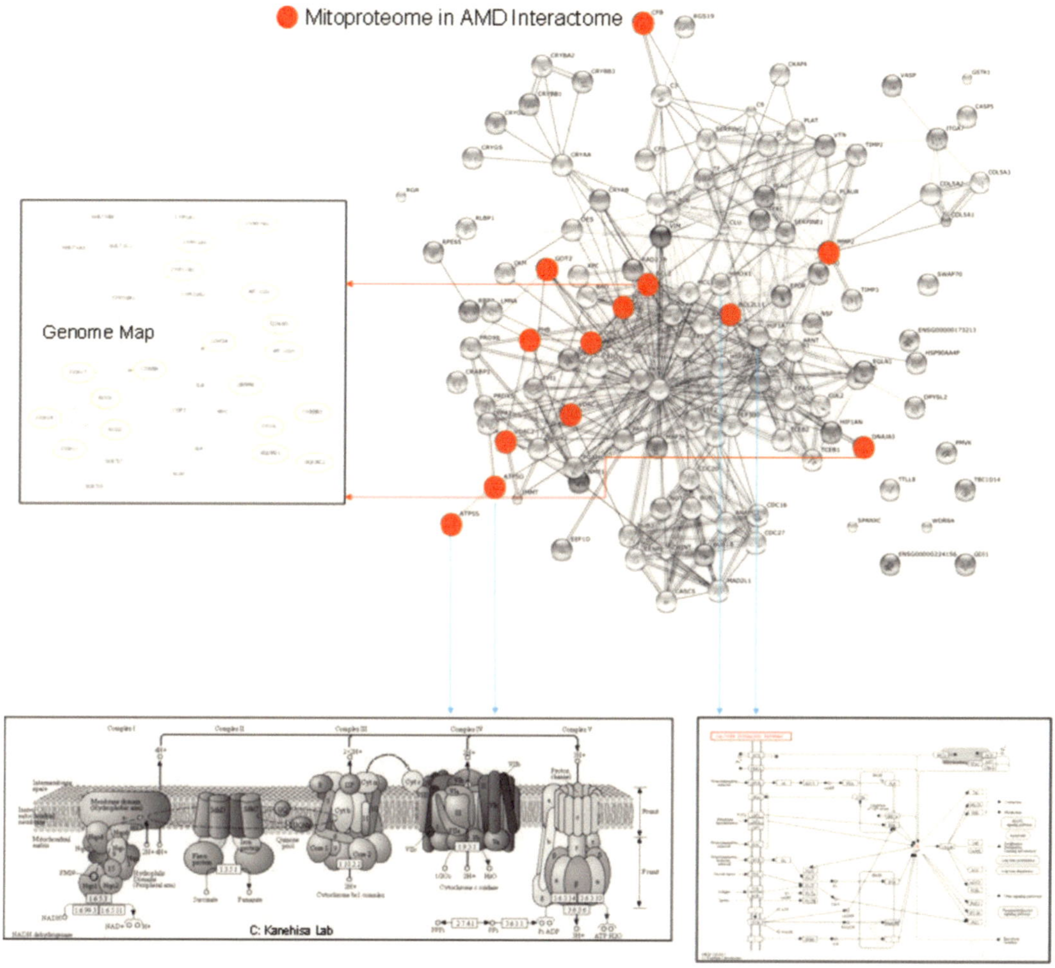

Figure 8. Genome-proteome-metabolome mapping in AMD: retrograde mitochondrial signaling. The protein interactome was established using STRING software and our proteomics data. The genome regulatory network was connected to the proteome network using Uniprobe and JASPAR. Protein phosphorylations were examined by phosphoprotein/peptide enrichment, followed by mass spectrometry analysis. Phosphorylations were compared to Phospho.ELM, and PhosphoSite. The metabolome mapping was established using KEGG and BIGG databases. Based on our proteomics and the interactome data that identified altered signaling of apoptosis in the retina and RPE both *in vitro and in vivo*, the pathological pathway determined by the AMD interactome could yield suitable targets for anti-apoptotic and anti-angiogenic therapy: (1) mitochondrial dysfunction in the peripheral RPE (prohibitin, ATP synthase); (2) oxidative stress including intense and constant light (peroxiredoxin, thioredoxin, glutathione S-transferase); (3) cytoskeletal remodeling by microtubule, actin filament, and intermediate filament (vimentin, actin, tubulin); (4) high concentration of nitric oxide (nitric oxide synthase), (5) hypoxia (HIF1, erythropoietin, VEGF); (6) disrupted circadian clock (melatonin); (7) apoptotic downstream (pJAK2, pSTAT3, Bclxl, caspases); (8) altered lipid concentrations (cardiolipin, cholesterol); (9) altered visual cycle (CRABP, CRALBP, RPE65); (10) altered energy metabolism (S/T vs. Y kinases, carnitine, pyruvate, ATP synthase); (11) aggregation of heat shock proteins and crystallins; and (12) inflammation (CFH, C3, collagen, vitronectin).

hub proteins that include UBC, MMP2, BCL, PRDX, ATP5O, C3, TF, and CRYAB, (2) increased local interactions between oxidative stress, complement activation, transcription, metabolism, (3) AMD module as a cluster in the same network neighborhood, (4) potential causal molecules including Ca^{2+}, Fe^{2+}, ATP/ADP, OPO_4^{2-}, lipids, (5) altered cytoskeleton, microtubule, abnormal mitochondrial signaling.

The mitochondrial interactome provides a base for better understanding of oxidative stress-induced apoptosis and the mechanism of age-related diseases, including AMD. As a consequence, an effective treatment of neurodegenerative diseases based on the modulation of mitochondrial network is expected to result.

Author details

Srinivas R. Sripathi[1], Weilue He[2], Johnpaul Offor[3], Diana R. Gutsaeva[4] and Wan Jin Jahng[5]*

*Address all correspondence to: wan.jahng@aun.edu.ng

1 Department of Ophthalmology, Wilmer Eye Institute, The Johns Hopkins University School of Medicine, Baltimore, USA

2 Department of Biomedical Engineering, Michigan Technological University, Houghton, USA

3 Department of Natural and Environmental Sciences, American University of Nigeria, Yola, Nigeria

4 Department of Ophthalmology, Augusta University, Augusta, USA

5 Retina Proteomics Laboratory, Department of Petroleum Chemistry, American University of Nigeria, Yola, Nigeria

References

[1] Chen H, Chan DC. Mitochondrial dynamics in mammals. Current Topics in Developmental Biology. 2004;**59**:119-144. DOI: 10.1016/S0070-2153(04)59005-1

[2] Castegna A, Iacobazzi V, Infantino V. The mitochondrial side of epigenetics. Physiological Genomics. 2015;**47**:299-307. DOI: 10.1152/physiolgenomics.00096.2014

[3] Hailey DW, Rambold AS, Satpute-Krishnan P, Mitra K, Sougrat R, Kim PK, Lippincott-Schwartz J. Mitochondria supply membranes for autophagosome biogenesis during starvation. Cell. 2010;**141**:656-667. DOI: 10.1016/j.cell.2010.04.009

[4] Chen H, McCaffery JM, Chan DC. Mitochondrial fusion protects against neurodegeneration in the cerebellum. Cell. 2007;**130**:548-562. DOI: 10.1016/j.cell.2007.06.026

[5] Gomes LC, Di Benedetto G, Scorrano L. During autophagy mitochondria elongate, are spared from degradation and sustain cell viability. Nature Cell Biology. 2011;**13**:589-598. DOI: 10.1038/ncb2220

[6] Gerhold JM, Cansiz-Arda Ş, Lõhmus M, Engberg O, Reyes A, Rennes H Van, Sanz A, Holt IJ, Cooper HM, Spelbrink JN. Human mitochondrial DNA-protein complexes attach to a cholesterol- rich membrane structure. Scientific Reports. 2015;**5**:1-14. DOI: 10.1038/srep15292

[7] Schrier SA, Falk MJ. Mitochondrial disorders and the eye. Current Opinion in Ophthalmology. 2011;**22**:325-331. DOI: 10.1097/ICU.0b013e328349419d

[8] Mikhed Y, Daiber A, Steven S. Mitochondrial oxidative stress, mitochondrial DNA damage and their role in age-related vascular dysfunction. International Journal of Molecular Sciences. 2015;**16**:15918-15953. DOI: 10.3390/ijms160715918

[9] Liang P, MacRae TH. Molecular chaperones and the cytoskeleton. Journal of Cell Science. 1997;**110**(Pt 1):1431-1440

[10] Rambold AS, Kostelecky B, Elia N, Lippincott-Schwartz J. Tubular network formation protects mitochondria from autophagosomal degradation during nutrient starvation. Proceedings of the National Academy of Sciences of the United States of America. 2011;**108**:10190-10195. DOI: 10.1073/pnas.1107402108

[11] Vilalta PM, Zhang L, Hamm-Alvarez SF. A novel taxol-induced vimentin phosphorylation and stabilization revealed by studies on stable microtubules and vimentin intermediate filaments. Journal of Cell Science. 1998;**111**(Pt 1):1841-1852 Available from: http://www.ncbi.nlm.nih.gov/pubmed/9625747

[12] Legros F, Malka F, Frachon P, Lombès A, Rojo M. Organization and dynamics of human mitochondrial DNA. Journal of Cell Science. 2004;**117**:2653-2662. DOI: 10.1242/jcs.01134

[13] Hoye AT, Davoren JE, Wipf P, Fink MP, Kagan VE. Targeting mitochondria. Accounts of Chemical Research. 2008;**41**:87-97. DOI: 10.1021/ar700135m

[14] Dai Z, Yin J, He H, Li W, Hou C, Qian X, Mao N, Pan L. Mitochondrial comparative proteomics of human ovarian cancer cells and their platinum-resistant sublines. Proteomics. 2010;**10**:3789-3799. DOI: 10.1002/pmic.200900685

[15] Lee J, Giordano S, Zhang J. Autophagy, mitochondria and oxidative stress: Cross-talk and redox signalling. The Biochemical Journal. 2012;**441**:523-540. DOI: 10.1042/bj20111451

[16] Terluk MR, Kapphahn RJ, Soukup LM, Gong H, Gallardo C, Montezuma SR, Ferrington DA. Investigating mitochondria as a target for treating age-related macular degeneration. The Journal of Neuroscience. 2015;**35**:7304-7311. DOI: 10.1523/JNEUROSCI.0190-15.2015

[17] Feher J, Kovacs I, Artico M, Cavallotti C, Papale A, Balacco Gabrieli C. Mitochondrial alterations of retinal pigment epithelium in age-related macular degeneration. Neurobiology of Aging. 2006;**27**:983-993. DOI: 10.1016/j.neurobiolaging.2005.05.012

[18] Suter M, Remé C, Grimm C, Wenzel A, Jäättela M, Esser P, Kociok N, Leist M, Richter C. Age-related macular degeneration: The lipofuscin component N-retinyl-N-retinylidene ethanolamine detaches proapoptotic proteins from mitochondria and induces apoptosis in mammalian retinal pigment epithelial cells. The Journal of Biological Chemistry. 2000;**275**:39625-39630. DOI: 10.1074/jbc.M007049200

[19] Beal MF. Mitochondria take center stage in aging and neurodegeneration. Annals of Neurology. 2005;**58**:495-505. DOI: 10.1002/ana.20624

[20] Liu Z, Butow RA. Mitochondrial retrograde signaling. Annual Review of Genetics. 2006;**40**:159-185. DOI: 10.1146/annurev.genet.40.110405.090613

[21] Brown K, Liu Y, Chen D. Aging: The mitochondrial connection. Journal of Clinical and Experimental Pathology. 2012;**S4**:003. DOI: 10.4172/2161-0681.S4-003

[22] Ambati J, Anand A, Fernandez S, Sakurai E, Lynn BC, Kuziel WA, Rollins BJ, Ambati BK. An animal model of age-related macular degeneration in senescent Ccl-2- or Ccr-2-deficient mice. Nature Medicine. 2003;**9**:1390-1397. DOI: 10.1038/nm950

[23] Kenney MC, Atilano SR, Boyer D, Chwa M, Chak G, Chinichian S, Coskun P, Wallace DC, Nesburn AB, Udar NS. Characterization of retinal and blood mitochondrial DNA from age-related macular degeneration patients. Investigative Ophthalmology and Visual Science. 2010;**51**:4289-4297. DOI: 10.1167/iovs.09-4778

[24] Sripathi SR, He W, Atkinson CL, Smith JJ, Liu Z, Elledge BM, Jahng WJ. Mitochondrial-nuclear communication by prohibitin shuttling under oxidative stress. Biochemistry. 2011;**50**:8342-8351. DOI: 10.1021/bi2008933

[25] Sripathi SR, He W, Sylvester O, Neksumi M, Um J-Y, Dluya T, Bernstein PS, Jahng WJ. Altered cytoskeleton as a mitochondrial decay signature in the retinal pigment epithelium. The Protein Journal. 2016;**35**:179-192. DOI: 10.1007/s10930-016-9659-9

[26] Sripathi SR, He W, Um J, Moser T, Dehnbostel S, Kindt K, Goldman J, Frost MC, Jahng WJ. Nitric oxide leads to cytoskeletal reorganization in the retinal pigment epithelium under oxidative stress. Advances in Bioscience and Biotechnology. 2012;**03**:1167-1178. DOI: 10.4236/abb.2012.38143

[27] Sripathi S, He W, Prigge CL, Sylvester O, Um J-Y, Powell FL, Neksumi M, Bernstein PS, Choo D-W, Bartoli M, Gutsaeva DR, Jahng WJ. Interactome mapping guided by tissue-specific phosphorylation in age-related macular degeneration. International Journal of Scientific and Engineering Research. 2017;**8**:680-698. DOI: 10.14299/ijser.2017.02.010

[28] Lee H, Chung H, Lee SH, Jahng WJ. Light-induced phosphorylation of crystallins in the retinal pigment epithelium. International Journal of Biological Macromolecules. 2011;**48**:194-201. DOI: 10.1016/j.ijbiomac.2010.11.006

[29] Sripathi SR, Sylvester O, He W, Moser T, Um J-Y, Lamoke F, Ramakrishna W, Bernstein PS, Bartoli M, Jahng WJ. Prohibitin as the molecular binding switch in the retinal pigment epithelium. The Protein Journal. 2016;**35**:1-16. DOI: 10.1007/s10930-015-9641-y

[30] Sripathi SR, Prigge CL, Elledge B, He W, Offor J, Gutsaeva DR, Jahng WJ. Melatonin modulates prohibitin and cytoskeleton in the retinal pigment epithelium. International Journal of Scientific & Engineering Research. 2017;**8**:502-506

[31] Brickley K, Stephenson FA. Trafficking kinesin protein (TRAK)-mediated transport of mitochondria in axons of hippocampal neurons. The Journal of Biological Chemistry. 2011;**286**:18079-18092. DOI: 10.1074/jbc.M111.236018

[32] Williams DS. Transport to the photoreceptor outer segment by myosin VIIa and kinesin II. Vision Research. 2002;**42**:455-462. DOI: 10.1016/S0042-6989(01)00228-0

[33] Miki H, Setou M, Kaneshiro K, Hirokawa N. All kinesin superfamily protein, KIF, genes in mouse and human. Proceedings of the National Academy of Sciences of the United States of America. 2001;**98**:7004-7011. DOI: 10.1073/pnas.111145398

[34] Huang H, Frohman MA. Lipid signaling on the mitochondrial surface. Biochimica et Biophysica Acta, Molecular and Cell Biology of Lipids. 2009;**1791**:839-844. DOI: 10.1016/j.bbalip.2009.05.012

[35] MacAskill AF, Rinholm JE, Twelvetrees AE, Arancibia-Carcamo IL, Muir J, Fransson A, Aspenstrom P, Attwell D, Kittler JT. Miro1 is a calcium sensor for glutamate receptor-dependent localization of mitochondria at synapses. Neuron. 2009;**61**:541-555. DOI: 10.1016/j.neuron.2009.01.030

[36] Fransson Å, Ruusala A, Aspenström P. The atypical Rho GTPases Miro-1 and Miro-2 have essential roles in mitochondrial trafficking. Biochemical and Biophysical Research Communications. 2006;**344**:500-510. DOI: 10.1016/j.bbrc.2006.03.163

[37] Lee H, Arnouk H, Sripathi S, Chen P, Zhang R, Bartoli M, Hunt RC, Hrushesky WJM, Chung H, Lee SH, Jahng WJ. Prohibitin as an oxidative stress biomarker in the eye. International Journal of Biological Macromolecules. 2010;**47**:685-690. DOI: 10.1016/j.ijbiomac.2010.08.018

[38] Zhang R, Hrushesky WJM, Wood PA, Lee SH, Hunt RC, Jahng WJ. Melatonin reprogrammes proteomic profile in light-exposed retina in vivo. International Journal of Biological Macromolecules. 2010;**47**:255-260. DOI: 10.1016/j.ijbiomac.2010.04.013

[39] Mishra S, Ande SR, Nyomba BLGG. The role of prohibitin in cell signaling. The FEBS Journal. 2010;**277**:3937-3946. DOI: 10.1111/j.1742-4658.2010.07809.x

[40] Rudel T, Kepp O, Kozjak-Pavlovic V, Santhanam S, Venkatraman A, Ramakrishna BS, Tirosh O, Levy EE, Reifen R, Damiani CR, Benetton CAF, Stoffel C, Bardini KC, Cardoso VH, Di Giunta G, Pinho RA, Dal-Pizzol F, Streck EL, Restivo NL, Srivastava MD, Schafer IA, Hoppel CL, Sifroni KG, Damiani CR, Stoffel C, Cardoso MR, Ferreira GK, Jeremias IC, Rezin GT, Scaini G, Schuck PF, Dal-Pizzol F, Streck EL, D'Argenio G, Calvani M, Casamassimi A, Petillo O, Margarucci S, Rienzo M, Peluso I, Calvani R, Ciccodicola A, Caporaso N, Peluso G, Baregamian N, Song J, Bailey CE, Papaconstantinou J, Evers BM, Chung DH, Briet F, Twomey C, Jeejeebhoy KN, Demine S, Reddy N, Renard P, Raes M, Arnould T, Farhadi A, Keshavarzian A, Van De Kar LD, Jakate S, Domm A, Zhang L, Shaikh M, Banan A, Fields JZ, He D, Sougioultzis S, Hagen S, Liu J, Keates S, Keates AC, Pothoulakis C, Lamont JT, Hsieh S-Y, Shih TC, Yeh C-Y, Lin C-J, Chou Y-Y, Lee Y-S, Kamizato M, Nishida K, Masuda K, Takeo K, Yamamoto Y, Kawai T, Teshima-Kondo S, Tanahashi T, Rokutan K, Kuwano Y, Tominaga K, Kawahara T, Sasaki H, Takeo K, Nishida K, Masuda K, Kawai T, Teshima-Kondo S, Rokutan K, Montgomery MK, Turner N, Nazli A, Yang P-C, Jury J, Howe K, Watson JL, Söderholm JD, Sherman PM, Perdue MH, McKay DM, Schürmann G, Brüwer M, Klotz A, Schmid KW, Senninger N, Zimmer K-P, Vanderborght M, Nassogne MC, Hermans D, Moniotte S, Seneca S, Van Coster R, Buts JP, Sokal EM, Manuscript A, Rath E, Haller D, Han J, Yu C, Souza RF, Theiss AL, Dehghan F, Lz A, Karimian H, Yahayu M, Gc E, As F, H MA, Taha R, Seidman E, Mailhot G, Boudreau F, Gendron FP, Beaulieu JF, Ménard D, Delvin E, Amre D, Levy EE, Mayall TP, Bjarnason I, Khoo UY, Peters TJ, Macpherson AJ. Mitochondrial dysfunction and insulin resistance: An update. Journal of Pediatric Gastroenterology and Nutrition. 2014;**4**:1172-1184. DOI: 10.1007/s00535-009-0119-6

[41] Schleicher M, Shepherd BR, Suarez Y, Fernandez-Hernando C, Yu J, Pan Y, Acevedo LM, Shadel GS, Sessa WC. Prohibitin-1 maintains the angiogenic capacity of endothelial cells by regulating mitochondrial function and senescence. The Journal of Cell Biology. 2008;**180**:101-112. DOI: 10.1083/jcb.200706072

[42] Peng Y-TT, Chen P, Ouyang R-YY, Song L. Multifaceted role of prohibitin in cell survival and apoptosis. Apoptosis. 2015;**20**:1135-1149. DOI: 10.1007/s10495-015-1143-z

[43] Jiang L, Dong P, Zhang Z, Li C, Li Y, Liao Y, Li X, Wu Z, Guo S, Mai S, Xie D, Liu Z, Zhou F. Akt phosphorylates prohibitin 1 to mediate its mitochondrial localization and promote proliferation of bladder cancer cells. Cell Death & Disease. 2015;**6**:e1660. DOI: 10.1038/cddis.2015.40

[44] Jahng WJ. New biomarkers in the retina and RPE under oxidative stress. In: Adio A, editor. Ocular Diseases. InTech; 2012. DOI: 10.5772/48785

[45] Lee H, Chung H, Arnouk H, Lamoke F, Hunt RC, Hrushesky WJM, Wood PA, Lee SH, Jahng WJ. Cleavage of the retinal pigment epithelium-specific protein RPE65 under oxidative stress. International Journal of Biological Macromolecules. 2010;**47**:104-108. DOI: 10.1016/j.ijbiomac.2010.05.014

[46] Arnouk H, Lee H, Zhang R, Chung H, Hunt RC, Jahng WJ. Early biosignature of oxidative stress in the retinal pigment epithelium. Journal of Proteomics. 2011;**74**:254-261. DOI: 10.1016/j.jprot.2010.11.004

[47] Sripathi SR, He W, Um JY, Moser T. Nitric oxide leads to cytoskeletal reorganization in the retinal pigment epithelium under oxidative stress. Advances in Bioscience and Biotechnology. 2012;**03**:1167-1178. DOI: 10.4236/abb.2012.38143

[48] Lopez CJ, Qayyum I, Mishra OP, Delivoria-Papadopoulos M. Effect of nitration on protein tyrosine phosphatase and protein phosphatase activity in neuronal cell membranes of newborn piglets. Neuroscience Letters. 2005;**386**:78-81. DOI: 10.1016/j.neulet.2005.04.089

[49] Rayala SK, Martin E, Sharina IG, Molli PR, Wang X, Jacobson R, Murad F, Kumar R. Dynamic interplay between nitration and phosphorylation of tubulin cofactor B in the control of microtubule dynamics. Proceedings of the National Academy of Sciences of the United States of America. 2007;**104**:19470-19475. DOI: 10.1073/pnas.0705149104

[50] Di Stasi AM, Mallozzi C, Macchia G, Petrucci TC, Minetti M. Peroxynitrite induces tyrosine nitration and modulates tyrosine phosphorylation of synaptic proteins. Journal of Neurochemistry. 1999;**73**:727-735 Available from: http://www.ncbi.nlm.nih.gov/pubmed/10428070

18 kDa Translocator Protein in Mitochondria-Related Pathology: The Case of Traumatic Brain Injury

Nahum Rosenberg, Nasra Yasin, Leo Veenman,
Orit Rosenberg, Abraham Weizman and
Moshe Gavish

Additional information is available at the end of the chapter

http://dx.doi.org/10.5772/intechopen.74057

Abstract

Translocator protein (TSPO) takes part in mitochondrial adenine triphosphate (ATP) production and transport. Mitochondrial TSPO is a part of the apoptotic and cell necrotic mechanism. Ligands to TSPO, endogenous and synthetic, have different effects on metabolism and protein expression in human well-differentiated metabolically active cells. In general, most of the TSPO ligands affect the cellular function or metabolism in the same general direction, but different specific TSPO ligands have their own unique effects in human cells. Regulation of gene expression via the actions of TSPO ligands on the mitochondrial TSPO may form an essential mechanism for the regulation of cellular functions, especially during acute organ injury, such as acute brain damage. The exact mode of action of the specific TSPO ligands is not clear enough and should be further investigated. TSPO is a potential target for therapeutic efforts to mitigate secondary tissue injury caused by programmed cell death.

Keywords: TSPO, ligand, mitochondria, cell death

1. The structure, abundance and function of TSPO

The 18 kDa translocator protein (TSPO), previously known as a peripheral benzodiazepine receptor (PBR) [1], is a highly conserved protein with various life essential functions in eukaryotic and prokaryotic species [2]. The TSPO gene in humans is situated on the chromosome 22q13.3 [3]. The amino acid sequence of TSPO of human origin (169 amino acids): 1 mappwvpamg ftlapslgcf vgsrfvhgeg lrwyaglqkp swhpphwvlg pvwgtlysam 61 gygsylvwke lggftekavv plglytgqla lnwawppiff garqmgwalv dlllvsgaaa 121 attvawyqvs plaarllypy lawlaftttl nycvwrdnhg wrggrrlpe [4].

TSPO takes part in mitochondrial ATP production and transport, and is located on cytoplasmic and nuclear membranes and on the outer membrane of mitochondria. TSPO is abundant in metabolically active cells in different organs, such as brain, kidney, and so forth. [2]. TSPO has been also found in other organs and generally is abundant in steroid-secreting tissues. Recently, it has been detected in high abundance in osteoblasts [5]. TSPO interacts with ligands to modulate various molecular cellular activities [5–9] by affecting cell death. TSPO is thought to be involved in mitochondrial cholesterol transport and related to cell death pathways (apoptosis and necrosis) as a functional part of the mitochondrial permeability transition pore (MPTP), along with additional related receptors and protein structures, for example, voltage-dependent anion channel (VDAC) and the adenine nucleotide translocase (ANT) [1, 2]. The existence of functional interconnection between TSPO and MPTP has been challenged recently in studies showing that the MPTP can induce apoptosis and cholesterol transport without the involvement of TSPO [10]. Thus, the exact mechanism of the TSPO involvement in cell death has not been determined yet, but its functional role in this process is strongly supported [1, 2, 6–8].

2. TSPO ligands

Ligands, either endogenous or synthetic, to TSPO, such as protoporphyrin IX (PPIX), PK 11195, Ro5–4864, FGIN-1-27, induce different effects on metabolism and protein expression in human well-differentiated metabolically active cells. For example, Ro5–4864, FGIN-1-27 and PPIX cause similar effects, for example, reducing cellular [^{18}F]-fluorodeoxyglucose ([^{18}F]-FDG) incorporation and parallel decrease in ATP generation [6–8]. The cellular effects of PK 11195 show protective attempts for cellular "detoxification" by increasing the cellular mitochondrial mass (**Figure 1**) [5].

In general, most of the TSPO ligands affect the cellular function or metabolism in the same general direction, but different specific TSPO ligands have their own unique effects in human cells. Regulation of gene expression via the actions of TSPO ligands on the mitochondrial TSPO may form an essential mechanism for the regulation of cellular functions.

The exact mode of action of the specific TSPO ligands is not clear enough and should be further investigated. Due to the evidence of the nonuniform response of cells to the different specific ligands, an attempt to elucidate the role of the TSPO in cellular metabolism and modulation of cell phenotype should be promoted.

3. TSPO role in organ pathology and injury

Changes in TSPO expression have been linked to several pathological conditions, including cancer, endocrine diseases, and neurological diseases [2]. For example, in the normal brain,

A:

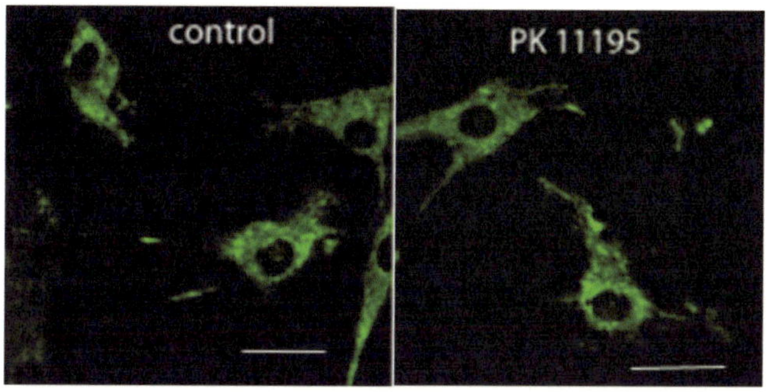

B:

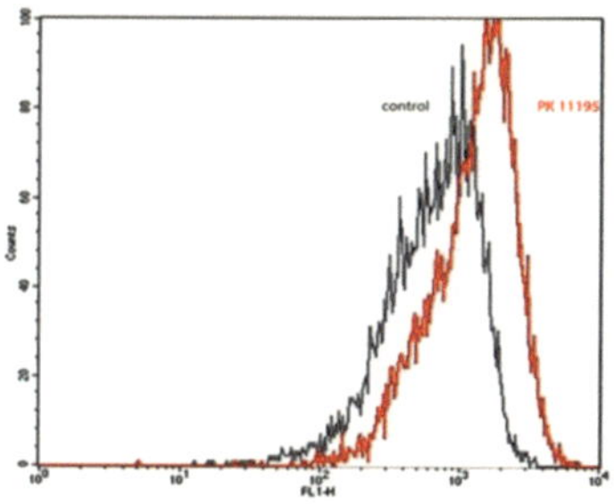

Figure 1. A: Microscopic image of cells stained by Mitotracker green stain (MTG). Strings of green stained mitochondria are apparent. Confocal microscopy, scale – 20 μ. B: Flow cytometry of cells stained by MTG. The histogram of the mitochondrial mass is shifted showing when exposed to PK 11195 (10^{-5} M) indicating on increase in the mitochondrial mass in comparison with the unexposed control.

overall TSPO expression is low, and TSPO is mainly found in glia and at very low levels in neurons [9]. But in the abnormal brain, TSPO is mainly expressed in glia, some hypertrophic astrocytes, infiltrating macrophages, and at low levels in neurons.

TSPO expression is upregulated in the injured brain and topographically localized in the inflamed areas. Additionally, in various neuropathologies, that is, gliomas, ischemia, viral encephalitis, neurodegenerative disorders (Parkinson's disease, Huntington's disease, Alzheimer's disease, and amyotrophic lateral sclerosis), local high expression of TSPO is evident [9–11, 12].

Mitochondria are the key regulators of cell survival and death. Mitochondria interact with numerous specific proteins, which are involved in genetic forms of neurodegenerative diseases [5, 9, 11]. When TSPO is a mitochondrial protein, it plays an important role in various cellular pathways related to brain damage and neurodegenerative disease [12].

The potential intracellular mechanisms related to TSPO include Ca^{++} release, ATP production, reactive oxygen species (ROS) generation, and cytochrome C release from the mitochondria in relation to programmed cell death [7, 13, 14].

4. TSPO role in cell death: the case of neural injury

Regulation of programmed cell death is not sufficient to establish tissue repair. In brain pathologies, when the TSPO is upregulated, there is a typical association with microglial activation and inflammation. High level of TSPO expression in glia, as well as the increased proliferation of microglia in gliosis, suggests that TSPO could serve as an index of the state and progression of traumatic brain injury (TBI) [3]. These studies suggest that TSPO expression measurement can be used as a biomarker of active brain disease. The precise etiology of differences in TSPO expression and its relation to injury to neural tissue, while TBI or in neurodegenerative conditions, have not been resolved yet [14].

It is possible that high TSPO local brain tissue concentration might be an etiologic factor in progressive tissue damage in TBI. This theory is based on the revealed TSPO role in the cholesterol transport via inner mitochondrial membrane that accelerates cell proliferation during reactive gliosis, which is an essential part in the pathogenesis following TBI [10].

Secondary injury has the most important effect in brain damage related to TBI. This process is caused predominantly by mitochondrial shutdown. Mitochondrial dysfunction progresses to apoptosis by the increase in oxidative stress due to depleted ATP synthesis. The final result is a local to the injured site brain tissue damage that is clinically expressed by a spectrum of cognitive or motoric impairments. Therefore, it might be logical to suggest that therapeutic efforts in TBI should address cellular pathways connected to TSPO. But there is no current therapeutic evidence that can support this hypothesis, and therefore this is a highly appealing area for further research. There is an ongoing research on novel methods to prevent, diagnose, and treat TBI focusing on maintaining mitochondrial function [15, 16].

TBI is still the leading cause of disability in young adults worldwide. Its major mechanisms are diffuse axonal injury, cerebral contusion, ischemic neurological damage, and intracranial hematomas. All these pathologies are associated to some extent with mitochondrial dysfunction [15].

Significant necrosis of the brain cortical tissue occurs rapidly upon experimental TBI. Exacerbation of the primary lesion occurs during the hours after the brain injury and leads consequently to significant neurological dysfunction. Cyclosporine A (CsA, an immunosuppressant) has shown a neuroprotective role in TBI. CsA inhibits the opening of the MPTP, which in turn maintains the mitochondrial membrane potential, and calcium homeostasis of mitochondria. These results demonstrate that MPTP modulation and mitochondrial homeostasis maintenance are related to the neuroprotective role of CsA. The CsA neuroprotective effect following brain injury indicated that pharmacological therapies can be designed to greatly affect the mitochondria and neurological outcome following a brain injury [15]. Since TSPO has been suggested to be functionally related to the MPTP, it might be involved in these cellular pathways and might be targeted in the future research of TBI treatment.

One of the cellular pathways following TBI at the cellular level is related to energetic shutdown, with subsequential interference with Ca^{2+} homeostasis. This process starts following initial brain injury by an "ischemia-like" pattern, after direct impact to the brain tissue. Additionally, this process causes impairment in the cerebral blood flow, with further local ischemic process. As the result of this initial impact, the cellular ATP synthesis decreases, and mitochondrial membrane potential collapses. As a result, the nerve terminal membrane is depolarized, glutamate and aspartate (excitatory neurotransmitters) are released and voltage-dependent Ca^{2+} and Na^{+} channels are activated. By the self-accelerating process, additional Ca^{2+} is recruited causing its pathologically increased concentration. The Ca^{2+} overload causes increased catabolic effect due to enhanced release of free radicals, with eventual cell death via cellular membrane damage [16].

ATP production via oxidative phosphorylation is the primary function of mitochondria, and Ca^{2+} is the characteristic stimulatory signal for the activation of numerous mitochondrial enzymes [16]. Mitochondria play a pivotal role in cell survival. Mitochondrial dysfunction is an early event in the CNS injury that progresses to cell necrosis.

Thus, the cell death, neural and glial, following TBI is the pathophysiological cause for overall brain damage. Cell death occurs by apoptosis, autophagy, and necrosis [17, 18]. A programmed cell necrosis (necroptosis) has a distinct and characteristic morphology due to autophagy [19]. Mitochondria are the source to cell death propagation, in addition to the extrinsic pathway and caspase-12-mediated endoplasmic reticulum (ER) apoptotic pathway. The extrinsic pathway is amplificated by mitochondria and causes apoptosis. The BH3-only protein Bid links the extrinsic and mitochondrial apoptosis. The mitochondrial apoptosis can be caspase-dependent or independent. If caspase-dependent, it involves cytochrome C, otherwise apoptosis inducing factor (AIF) governs the caspase-independent pathway.

Therefore, it may be deduced, according to the abovementioned studies, that mitochondrial membrane, Ca^{2+} and reactive oxygen species (ROS) are shown to mediate synergistically the process of cell damage induced by TBI. Mitochondrial outer membrane permeabilization (MOMP) and mitochondrial permeability transition (MPT), which are part of apoptotic pathway, are the suggested mechanisms of the pores' formation in the mitochondrial membranes. An additional important factor, the Bcl-2 family, is regulatory in apoptosis and cell necrosis as well. There are also numerous other proapoptotic factors that might be interconnected with the mentioned pathways, but their role is not clear. These factors coordinate the apoptotic activity and related to mitochondria, ER, and lysosome.

The regulation of Ca^{2+} flux between mitochondria and ER is a control point during apoptosis, along with mitochondria-associated membranes. It is important to mention that the cathepsin proteases that are released from lysosome enhance the mitochondria-mediated cell death. These cellular events are related to secondary brain damage and other pathological processes involving programmed cell death.

Additional cellular pathways, not directly related to mitochondria, such as neuron cells death by excitotoxicity, due to elevated levels of synaptic neurotransmitters, also occur during TBI. Excitotoxicity is mediated by glutamate and involves several synaptic receptors, for example, AMPA, NMDA, voltage-dependent Ca^{2+} channels (VDCC) and metabotropic glutamate (mGlu) receptors [13, 20, 21]. The Na^{+}- and Cl^{-}-dependent influx is associated with immediate cell swelling [22–25]. Extra-synaptic NMDA receptor activation can activate a cAMP response element binding (CREB) protein shut-off which, in turn, causes loss of $\Delta\Psi m$ and apoptosis [26]. Stress-activated protein kinases (SAPKs) are another class of signaling molecules that are part of NMDA receptor-dependent cell death [27].

Eventually, the mitochondrial membrane is one of the last barriers to cell death. Different receptors related to the mitochondrial membrane, including TSPO, have a crucial role in protection from or propagation to cell death. In the case of the secondary damage following TBI, the possibility of therapeutic targeting of this receptor has been raised [28].

The preservation of energy supply alone is not enough for mitochondria protection. The ongoing research on TSPO might also lead to the finding of protective pathways that will avoid the cell death cascades during the brain or other tissue injury. In the series of four papers, it was found that from all studied, only one type of synthetic TSPO ligand, PK 11195 (10^{-5} M), evolves a protective cellular response by elevating the cellular mitochondrial mass [6]. PK 11195 is unsuitable for clinical use because of its overall toxic effects *in vivo*, but it is clear that its interaction with TSPO evolves a protective anti-necrotic effect in cells. Therefore, TSPO is a good candidate for future research of mitigation of secondary tissue damage which is currently irreversible.

In conclusion, mitochondria play a pivotal role in the secondary cellular insult such as in the TBI and other types of tissue necrotic damage. The mitochondrial malfunction that occurs during such pathological effects results in cellular energy loss, with the activation of cell death pathways, which involve the interrelated actions of excitotoxicity, ROS, caspases, the Bcl-2 family and apoptosis inducing factor (AIF). In this process, the role of TSPO is still elusive but with a strong indication of a possible regulatory involvement [5]. With the clarification of the function and structure of TSPO on mitochondria, mitochondrial-targeted multipotential therapeutic strategies via TSPO might provide new hope for the treatment of cellular death, such as in TBI or in other acute injury states in other organs, with high energy demanding cellular content.

Author details

Nahum Rosenberg[1,2†], Nasra Yasin[3†], Leo Veenman[3], Orit Rosenberg[4], Abraham Weizman[5] and Moshe Gavish[3]

Address all correspondence to: mgavish@technion.ac.il

1 Musculoskeletal Research Laboratory, Rambam Health Care Campus, Haifa, Israel

2 The Ruth and Bruce Rappaport Faculty of Medicine, Technion – Israel Institute of Technology, Haifa, Israel

3 Department of Neuroscience, The Ruth and Bruce Rappaport Faculty of Medicine, Technion – Israel Institute of Technology, Haifa, Israel

4 Sheltagen Medical Ltd, Matam Park, Haifa, Israel

5 Research Unit, Geha Mental Health Center and the Laboratory of Biological Psychiatry, Felsenstein Medical Research Center, Sackler Faculty of Medicine, Tel Aviv University, Tel Aviv, Israel

† Both the authors contributed equally.

References

[1] Papadopoulos V, Baraldi M, Guilarte TR, Knudsen TB, Lacapère JJ, Lindemann P, Norenberg MD, Nutt D, Weizman A, Zhang MR, Gavish M. Translocator protein (18kDa): New nomenclature for the peripheral-type benzodiazepine receptor based on its structure and molecular function. Trends in Pharmacological Sciences. 2006;**27**(8):402-409

[2] Gavish M, Bachman I, Shoukrun R, Katz Y, Veenman L, Weisinger G, Weizman A. Enigma of the peripheral benzodiazepine receptor. Pharmacological Reviews. 1999;**51**(4):629-650

[3] Liu GJ, Middleton RJ, Hatty CR, Wai-Ying Kam W, Chan R, Pham T, Harrison-Brown M, Dodson E, Veale V, Banati RB. The 18 kDa translocator protein, microglia and neuroinflammation. Brain Pathology. 2014;**24**:631-653

[4] Owen DR, Fan J, Campioli E, Venugopal S, Midzak A, Daly E, Harlay A, Issop L, Libri V, Kalogiannopoulou D, Oliver E, Gallego-Colon E, Colasanti A, Huson L, Rabiner EA, Suppiah P, Essagian C, Matthews PM, Papadopoulos V. TSPO mutations in rats and a human polymorphism impair the rate of steroid synthesis. The Biochemical Journal. 2017; **474**(23):3985-3999

[5] Bernardi P, Rasola A, Forte M, Lippe G. The mitochondrial permeability transition pore: Channel formation by F-ATP synthase, integration in signal transduction, and role in pathophysiology. Physiological Reviews. 2015;**95**(4):1111-1155

[6] Rosenberg N, Rosenberg O, Weizman A, Veenman L, Gavish M. *In vitro* effects of the specific mitochondrial TSPO ligand Ro5 4864 in cultured human osteoblasts. Journal of Experimental and Clinical Endocrinology & Diabetes. 2018;**126**(2):77-84

[7] Rosenberg N, Rosenberg O, Weizman A, Veenman L, Gavish M. *In vitro* effect of FGIN-1-27, a ligand to 18 kDa mitochondrial translocator protein, in human osteoblast-like cells. Journal of Bioenergetics and Biomembranes. 2014;**46**:197-204

[8] Rosenberg N, Rosenberg O, Weizman A, Veenman L, Gavish M. *In vitro* catabolic effect of protoporphyrin IX in human osteoblast-like cells: Possible role of the 18 kDa mitochondrial translocator protein. Journal of Bioenergetics and Biomembranes. 2013;**45**:333-341

[9] Rosenberg N, Rosenberg O, Weizman A, Leschiner S, Sakoury J, Fares F, Soudry M, Weisinger G, Veenman L, Gavish M. *In vitro* mitochondrial effects of PK 11195, a synthetic translocator protein 18 kDa (TSPO) ligand in human osteoblast-like cells. Journal of Bioenergetics and Biomembranes. 2011;**43**:739-746

[10] Veenman L, Gavish M. Peripheral-type benzodiazepine receptors: Their implication in brain disease. Drug Development Research. 2000;**50**:355-370

[11] Papadopoulos V, Lecanu L. Translocator protein (18 kDa) TSPO: An emerging therapeutic target in neurotrauma. Experimental Neurology. 2009;**19**:53-57

[12] Veenman L, Vainshtein A, Gavish M. TSPO as a target for treatments of diseases, including neuropathological disorders. Cell Death & Disease. 2015;**6**(10):e1911

[13] Kugler W, Veenman L, Shandalov Y, Leschiner S, Spanier I, Lakomek M, Gavish M. Ligands of the mitochondrial 18 kDa translocator protein attenuate apoptosis of human glioblastoma cells exposed to erucylphosphohomocholine. Cellular Oncology. 2008;**30**: 435-450

[14] Yasin N, Veenman L, Singh S, Azrad M, Bode J, Vainshtein A, Caballero B, Marek I, Gavish M. Classical and novel TSPO ligands for the mitochondrial TSPO can modulate nuclear gene expression: Implications for mitochondrial retrograde signaling. International Journal of Molecular Sciences. 2017;**18**(4)

[15] Werner C, Engelhard K. Pathophysiology of traumatic brain injury. British Journal of Anaesthesia. 2007;**99**(1):4-9

[16] Graier WF, Frieden M, Malli R. Mitochondria and Ca(2+) signaling: Old guests, new functions. Pflügers Archiv. 2007;**455**(3):375-396

[17] Kroemer G, Galluzzi L, Vandenabeele P, Abrams J, Alnemri ES, Baehrecke EH, Blagosklonny MV, El-Deiry WS, Golstein P, Green DR, Hengartner M, Knight RA, Kumar S, Lipton SA, Malorni W, Nuñez G, Peter ME, Tschopp J, Yuan J, Piacentini M, Zhivotovsky B, Melino G. Nomenclature committee on cell death 2009. Classification of cell death: Recommendations of the nomenclature committee on cell death 2009. Cell Death and Differentiation. 2009;**16**(1):3-11

[18] Caballero B, Veenman L, Gavish M. Role of mitochondrial translocator protein (18 kDa) on mitochondrial-related cell death processes. Recent Patents on Endocrine, Metabolic & Immune Drug Discovery. 2013;**7**(2):86-101

[19] Li F, Wang L, Burgess RJ, Weinshilboum RM. Thiopurine S-methyltransferase pharmacogenetics: Autophagy as a mechanism for variant allozyme degradation. Pharmacogenetics and Genomics. 2008;**18**(12):1083-1094

[20] Palmer AM, Marion DW, Botscheller ML, Swedlow PE, Styren SD, DeKosky ST. Traumatic brain injury-induced excitotoxicity assessed in a controlled cortical impact model. Journal of Neurochemistry. 1993;**61**(6):2015-2024

[21] Ertel EA, Campbell KP, Harpold MM, Hofmann F, Mori Y, Perez-Reyes E, Schwartz A, Snutch TP, Tanabe T, Birnbaumer L, Tsien RW, Catterall WA. Nomenclature of voltage-gated calcium channels. Neuron. 2000;**25**(3):533-535

[22] Hossmann KA. Viability thresholds and the penumbra of focal ischemia. Annals of Neurology. 1994;**36**(4):557-565

[23] Siesjö BK, Katsura K, Zhao Q, Folbergrová J, Pahlmark K, Siesjö P, Smith ML. Mechanisms of secondary brain damage in global and focal ischemia: A speculative synthesis. Journal of Neurotrauma. 1995;**12**(5):943-956

[24] Brennan C, Momota H, Hambardzumyan D, Ozawa T, Tandon A, Pedraza A, Holland E. Glioblastoma subclasses can be defined by activity among signal transduction pathways and associated genomic alterations. PLoS One. 2009;**4**(11):e7752

[25] Forder JP, Tymianski M. Postsynaptic mechanisms of excitotoxicity: Involvement of postsynaptic density proteins, radicals, and oxidant molecules. Neuroscience. 2009;**158**(1): 293-300

[26] Hardingham GE, Bading H. Coupling of extrasynaptic NMDA receptors to a CREB shut-off pathway is developmentally regulated. Biochimica et Biophysica Acta. 2002;**1600**(1–2): 148-153

[27] Legos JJ, McLaughlin B, Skaper SD, Strijbos PJ, Parsons AA, Aizenman E, Herin GA, Barone FC, Erhardt JA. The selective p38 inhibitor SB-239063 protects primary neurons from mild to moderate excitotoxic injury. European Journal of Pharmacology. 2002;**447**(1): 37-42

[28] Saatman KE, Duhaime AC, Bullock R, Maas AI, Valadka A, Manley GT; Workshop Scientific Team and Advisory Panel Members. Classification of traumatic brain injury for targeted therapies. Journal of Neurotrauma 2008;**25**(7):719-738

Chapter 10

Hereditary Disorders and Human Mutations of Iron-Sulfur Assembly Genes

Namik Kaya, Zuhair Al-Hassnan, Maha Abdulrahim,
Mazhor Aldosary and Dilek Colak

Additional information is available at the end of the chapter

http://dx.doi.org/10.5772/intechopen.78006

Abstract

Multiple mitochondrial dysfunctions syndrome (MMDS) is a group of autosomal recessive mitochondrial disorders that is associated with deficiencies related to nuclear genes: *ISCA2*, *ISCA1*, *NFU1*, *IBA57*, and *BOLA3*. The syndromes are relatively new and recently discovered. Individuals with MMDS have reduced function of energy production stages in mitochondria. The dysfunctions are mostly related to iron-sulfur (Fe-S) clustering system (ISC) and its biogenesis. The signs and symptoms of the patients may begin early in life, and can be quite severe leading to death more or less during infancy. Affected individuals have various symptoms including brain dysfunction (encephalopathy), hypotonia, seizures, delayed developmental milestones, and cognition and psychomotor impairments. These individuals often have difficulty growing and gaining weight at the expected rate. Diagnosis of the disease can be challenging as in the case with most of the mitochondrial disorders. However, since the genetic causes of the MMDS are known, a laboratory test focusing on the causative genes will be helpful to determine the pathogenic mutations. This in turn would facilitate reducing the number of the diseases through carrier testing and genetic counseling and utilization of preimplantation genetic diagnosis in populations, especially those that display high rate of consanguinity, which are prone to have such autosomal recessive disorders.

Keywords: *BOLA3*, *IBA57*, *ISCA1*, *ISCA2*, *NFU1*, iron-sulfur (Fe-S) cluster (ISC), multiple mitochondrial dysfunction syndromes

1. Introduction

Mitochondria are double membrane-bound cellular organelles surrounded by outer and inner membranes [1, 2]. The organelle is considered cell's powerhouse generating adenosine triphosphate (ATP) during cellular respiration; hence, facilitating energy conversion in eukaryotes. Uniquely, each mitochondrion has its own DNA and encodes mitochondrial genes; hence, contributing the cell's proteome independently. The inheritance of the mitochondrial genome differs from nuclear genome since the donor of mitochondrial DNA (mtDNA) is the egg rather than sperm whose mitochondria are marked for obliteration upon entering the egg [3]. Hence, the organelle's DNA is inherited through females known as "maternal inheritance." Since these organelles generate energy, most biochemical reactions in the eukaryotic cells occur in the mitochondria. These reactions include pyruvate oxidation, citric acid cycle, electron transport, and oxidative phosphorylation (OXPHOS) all needed for energy production. Mitochondria also have an important role in calcium signaling, regulation of cellular metabolism, heme synthesis, steroid synthesis, apoptosis, and the biosynthesis of iron-sulfur (IS) clusters (ISC). The high number of human diseases caused by the malfunction of the mitochondrial proteins—encoded by nuclear or mtDNA—drew attention to the importance of this organelle.

2. Mitochondria

Mitochondria are genetically controlled by both nuclear DNA and the mitochondrial genome [1, 4]. A wide range of molecular defects have been identified in the human mitochondrial genome [4–9]. Diseases due to mutations in the mitochondrial genome are clinically, genetically, and biochemically diverse [1, 2, 4, 6, 10]. Similarly, deficiencies in mitochondrial genes encoded by nuclear genome can also lead various mitochondrial disorders and a wide range of cellular perturbations such as undue reactive oxygen species and distracted apoptosis, aberrant calcium homeostasis, and deficient energy production. This in turn leads failure to meet the requirements of numerous organs, especially those with high energy needs. Hence, various pathological conditions appears due to impaired mitochondrial function in human body involving different cell types, tissues, and organs including heart and brain. Such multi-organ manifestations are all mitochondria related and these diseases varies from epilepsy to cardiac myopathies.

3. Mitochondria and genetics of mitochondria-related diseases

The mitochondrial genome is a multicopy, double-stranded circular DNA molecule, which is 16.6 kb in human [11]. This genome encodes 13 essential proteins for the OXPHOS system and 24 components of the RNA machinery: 2 rRNAs and 22 tRNAs [11]. It is intronless and the only noncoding region is the displacement region (D-Loop), a region of 1.1 kb. It contains both the replication origins and the transcriptional promoters. Although mitochondria are genetically controlled by both mitochondrial and nuclear genomes, mtDNA is only maternally inherited [3]. Mitochondrial genetics differ greatly from Mendelian genetics in size, number of encoded genes, number of DNA molecules per cell, lack of introns, gene density, replication, transcription, recombination, and mode of inheritance. The 13 proteins include 7 subunits of NADH

Dehydrogenase (complex I: ND1, ND2, ND3, ND4, ND4L, ND5 and ND6), Cytochrome b (subunit of complex III), 3 subunits of Cytochrome c oxidase or complex IV (COI, COII and COIII), and 2 subunits of F0F1 ATPase (ATPase 6 and ATPase 8). They are all encoded by mtDNA and synthesized in the organelle. While, complex II (Succinate Dehydrogenase) and the remaining subunits of complexes I, III, IV, and V are entirely encoded by the nuclear genome. These nuclear-encoded proteins are synthesized on cytosolic ribosomes and subsequently transported into the mitochondria.

4. Fe-S clusters (ISCs)

ISCs are evolutionarily ancient cofactors consisting of Fe (iron) and S (sulfur) associated to the cysteine sulfurs of proteins. The clusters are found in variety of organisms including archaea, protists, prokaryotes, and eukaryotes. In a eukaryotic cell, they can be found in the mitochondria, cytosol, and nucleus where they perform diverse functions [12]. ISCs play a critical role in many fundamental molecular processes and have roles in electron transfer, structural stabilization, gene regulation, enzymatic catalysis, metabolic regulation, and sensing environmental signals [13]. Almost 30 proteins in the mitochondria and the cytosol are involved in synthesizing and assembling these clusters. ISC have two most common forms [2Fe-2S] and [4Fe-4S] clusters. ISC-related proteins of the electron transport chain in the mitochondrion are mainly located in the inner membrane. Moreover, some of these proteins are also found in the mitochondrial matrix in the organelles. For the cluster assembly, two machineries are required, the mitochondrial ISC assembly machinery and the cytosolic IS protein assembly machinery [12].

Eukaryotic IS proteins are located in mitochondria, cytosol, and nucleus, where they perform diverse functions in cellular metabolism and regulation. The mitochondrial ISC assembly machinery matures all organellar IS proteins, and additionally contributes to the biogenesis of cytosolic and nuclear IS proteins by producing an unknown sulfur-containing compound (X-S) that is exported to the cytosol and used by the cytosolic IS protein assembly machinery. Hence, mitochondria are directly responsible for the essential functions (e.g., of nuclear IS proteins involved in DNA metabolism and genome maintenance).

Mitochondria forms iron-sulfur clusters of significant proteins such as DNA polymerase and DNA helicases, and, therefore, plays a significant role in survival. There are 17 different proteins forming iron-sulfur cluster machinery that places the clusters into the Apo proteins. The mechanism of formation of iron-sulfur clusters can be divided into three steps. First, it is synthesized on a scaffold protein. Second, it is bound to transfer protein after dislocation from scaffold protein. Third, the transfer protein, the cluster and the specific ISC targeting factor place the cluster into the Apo protein. The changes in the first two steps inhibit the maturation of extra mitochondrial Fe/S proteins and disturb the iron homeostasis [14]. Assembly of Fe-S cluster also takes place by NIF, SUF, and CIA machineries. Cysteine desulfurase is an enzyme that unites Fe-S assembly machineries. It is encoded by NFS 1 which functions to deliver sulfur to ISCU [15]. ISCU is an iron-sulfur cluster assembly enzyme; encodes component of iron-sulfur scaffold protein. The changes in this gene result in severe myopathy and lactic acidosis ("ISCU Fe-S Cluster Assembly Enzyme [*Homo sapiens* (Human)] - Gene - NCBI") Complexes 1, 2, and 3 contain Fe-S clusters. They function in electron transport by transfer of one electron in redox processes [16]. The assembly of the clusters is recently studied in Yeast. In photosynthetic organisms, the iron-sulfur clusters play role in chloroplast processes and are important for plastid functioning [17].

Yeast frataxin, Isu1, and Nfs1 (cysteine desulfurase) take part in *de novo* synthesis of ISC. Many genes encode ISC assembly factors such as *BOLA3, NFU1, GLRX5, NUBPL, LYRM4, IBA57, ISCA1*, and *ISCA2*. These molecules have significant role in mitochondria. They are essential cofactors in the assembly of cluster. Deficiency of these genes leads to different diseases, for instance, GLRX5 deficiency causes sideroblastic anemia, whereas NUBPL mutations lead to respiratory chain complex 1 deficiency. On the other hand, some of these deficiencies are classified under a unique category such as MMDS.

5. Genetic factors of mitochondrial dysfunction syndromes

As the names imply, multiple mitochondrial dysfunction syndromes are disease conditions affecting mitochondria and usually lead to reduced function of more than one stages of energy production in the organelle [18]. The genetic factors causing these disorders are associated with the biogenesis of cellular ISC and currently these are the following genes: *ISCA2, NFU1, IBA57*, and *BOLA3*. More recently, *ISCA1* is also reported to lead a disease resembling MMDS and suggested to be a member of the group [19]. Interestingly, MMDS members appear to be inherited in autosomal recessive mode of inheritance (**Table 1**).

5.1. ISCA1

Iron-sulfur cluster assembly 1 (ISCA1) is one of the mitochondrial proteins required for the biogenesis and assembly of ISC [20]. This protein functions in the late stages of the ISC biogenesis and act as an iron binding molecule that may serve as a chaperone for biogenesis of Fe-S clusters [21]. It is believed that the molecule plays its pivotal role through its interaction with IOP1 (iron-only hydrogenase-like protein)/NARFL (nuclear prelamin A recognition factor-like). Knockdown of *Isca1* causes reduced activity of succinate dehydrogenase, mitochondrial aconitase, and cytosolic aconitase; hence, involving in both cytosolic and mitochondrial Fe-S protein biogenesis [22].

According to GenAtlas [23, 24], the gene has four exons and produces 14 kDa protein with 129 amino acids, which is known as mitochondrial Fe-S cluster assembly 1 homolog or otherwise HESB like domain containing 2. The gene is mapped to chromosome 9q21.33, and sits on genomic coordinates: 88.879.463–88.897.490. It is 2012 base pair long, generates four transcripts (splice variants) and highly expressed heart, esophagus, bladder, uterus, and cervix. Moreover, ISCA1 is a member of consensus coding sequence (CCDS:35056.1) which are manually checked protein annotations on the reference mouse and human genomes that ensures

Gene	Cytoband	NCBI	Genomic location	MMDS-related phenotype	MIM PT#	IM	MIM LN
NFU1	2p13.3	27247	2:69,396,112-69,438,122	Multiple mitochondrial dysfunctions syndrome 1	605711	AR	608100
BOLA3	2p13.1	388962	2:74,135,400-74,147,911	Multiple mitochondrial dysfunctions syndrome 2 with hyperglycinemia	614299	AR	613183
IBA57	1q42.13	200205	1:228,165,807-228,182,256	Multiple mitochondrial dysfunctions syndrome 3	615330	AR	615316
ISCA2	14q24.3	122961	14:74,493,719-74,495,567	Multiple mitochondrial dysfunctions syndrome 4	616370	AR	615317
ISCA1	9q21.33	81689	9:86,264,545-86,282,574	Multiple mitochondrial dysfunctions syndrome 5	617613	AR	611006

AR: autosomal recessive; IM: inheritance mode; LN: locus number; MIM: Mendelian inheritance in man; MMDS: mitochondrial dysfunction syndromes; PT#: phenotype number.

Table 1. Genes and related mitochondrial dysfunction syndromes.

consistent representation of the tracks of NCBI, Ensembl, and UCSC Genome Browsers. The gene has several synonyms such as hIsca, HBLD2, and ISA1, and localizes to mitochondria as well as cytoplasm.

Effect of depletion of ISC-related proteins on the maturation of cytosolic 4Fe-4S proteins showed that some mitochondrial Fe/S proteins such as mitochondrial aconitase, SDH, several proteins of complex I, and Rieske Fe/S protein were decreased with the deficiency of ISCA1. On the other hand, cellular heme content and mitochondrial 2Fe-2S ferrochelatase were unaffected by the depletion. This implies that ISCA1 is crucial in the maturation of mitochondrial 4Fe-4S proteins [25]. In another study, *ISCA1* was found to be associated with multiple mitochondrial dysfunctions syndrome-5. A homozygous missense mutation at a conserved residue in the Fe-S biogenesis domain (c.259G>A, p.Glu87Lys) was identified in two unrelated Indian families. This mutation destabilizes the protein subsequently causing the syndrome [19].

5.2. ISCA2

ISCA2 stands for iron-sulfur cluster assembly 2 protein and the gene encodes for A-type iron-sulfur cluster protein. Fe-S clusters are inorganic cofactors, mostly found in metalloproteins. The gene is located on chromosome 14 and expressed from the plus strand. According to Ensembl, this gene generates 4 different transcripts and has 96 orthologues. ISCA2 is a regulatory protein found in mitochondria as well as extra mitochondrial sites such as cytosol and nucleus. The protein takes part in assembly of Fe-S clusters in mitochondria which further take part in oxidation reduction (especially in complex 1 and 2), substrate activation, iron/sulfur storage, regulation of gene expression, and enzyme activity. Alternative name for ISCA2 is "HESB-like-domain-containing protein 1" for humans. First human mutation of *ISCA2* (c.229G>A; p.Glu77Ser) identified in the patients from five consanguineous families was a homozygous ancestral founder mutation that leaded to neurodegeneration, developmental, failure to thrive, quadriplegia, truncal hypotonia, optic atrophy, and leukoencephalopathy [26]. Later, additional 10 cases with the same founder mutation were also described [27]. Recently, two other patients with the same mutation were also studied with detailed functional experiments revealing complex 2 and 4 deficiencies [28]. Interestingly these patients were all Arab descent. Most recently, a second mutation, a compound heterozygous variant (a single basepair deletion causing frameshift with a premature stop codon: mutation: c.295delT; p.Phe99Leufs*18 and a missense mutation c.334A>G; p.Ser112Gly) in *ISCA2* was reported in a 2-month-old girl from Italy [29]. These mutations causes disorder of energy metabolism which results in respiratory failure, severe hypotonia, nystagmus, lactic acidosis, poor neurologic development, hyperglycemia, leukodystrophy of the brainstem with longitudinally extensive spinal cord involvement, and mtDNA deficiency ultimately leading to death [26].

5.3. NFU1

NFU1 is one of the human mitochondrial components that is involved in the assembly of the Fe-S protein cluster. It helps in the transfer of [4Fe-4S] clusters to specific protein targets and facilitates their maturation [30]. *NFU1* is mapped on the 2p13-p15 chromosomal region and codes for the NFU1 protein. During Fe-S assembly, two NFU1 monomers are needed to assemble one 4Fe-4S. Complex I, II, and III of oxidative phosphorylation have multiple Fe-S clusters. Therefore, any deficiency in these clusters causes dysfunctions of respiratory chain complexes [31]. Previous studies showed that the function of the NFU1 has been associated by the fatal mitochondrial disease, multiple mitochondrial dysfunctions syndrome 1 (MMDS1) [30]. Patients with NFU1 mutations usually manifest feeding difficulty, weakness, lethargy, and decreasing responsiveness within a few days after birth and a few had epileptic seizures [31]. It has been shown that the patients with mutations in the NFU1 gene have similar biochemical features to that seen in patients with lipoic acid defects. Thus, NFU1 mutation appears to have some effect on Fe-S enzyme lipoic acid synthase (LAS). In conclusion, NFU1 is an ISC assembly protein, and there is strong evidence that LAS deficiency is important in NFU1 mutation-related disease [31].

5.4. IBA57

IBA57 is a member of the Fe-S cluster assembly group. It is known as putative transferase CAF17 and Fe-S cluster assembly factor homolog. *IBA57* is located on 1q42.13 and codes for the IBA57 protein that is located in the mitochondrion. This protein functions in the late stages of the biosynthesis of mitochondrial 4Fe-4S proteins. Any deficiency in *IBA57* can cause an autosomal recessive spastic paraplegia-74 or multiple mitochondrial dysfunctions syndrome 3. In a previous study, it was found that the depletion of IBA57 in cell culture caused striking alterations in mitochondrial morphology, including a vast enlargement of the organelles and a loss of cristae membranes. It is also found that the function of IBA57 protein is conserved from bacteria to human, according to a study that provides an evidence for the requirement of bacterial and yeast relatives of human IBA57 for efficient maturation of [4Fe-4S] proteins. Moreover, potential diseases caused by mutations in these genes are expected to cause defects in mitochondrial respiration and in lipoic acid-dependent proteins [25]. Another study reported two siblings from consanguineous parents died with a condition characterized by generalized hypotonia, respiratory insufficiency, arthrogryposis, microcephaly, congenital brain malformations, and hyperglycinemia. Catalytic activities of the mitochondrial respiratory complexes I and II were deficient in skeletal muscle, a finding suggestive of an inborn error in mitochondrial biogenesis. Homozygosity mapping identified IBA57 located in the largest homozygous region on chromosome 1 as a culprit candidate gene. Their analysis of IBA57 revealed the homozygous mutation c.941A>C, p.Gln314Pro in those two patients [15].

5.5. BOLA3

BOLA3 is another essential protein in the Fe-S clusters production and involves in the normal maturation of lipoate-containing 2-oxoacid dehydrogenases. Another critical role of the molecule is to facilitate the assembly of the respiratory chain complexes. *BOLA3* was identified in the year 2008 during a search for similar sequences for bacterial BolA and cloned together with *BOL1* and *BOL2* [32]. According to Ensembl, the gene has five different transcripts and two isoforms. The main isoform is longer and localizes to mitochondria while the shorter isoform lacking exon 2 is restrained in the cytosplasm [18, 33]. The main transcript (ENST00000327428.9) has four exons comprising 68 variations [33]. The mRNA is nearly ubiquitously expressed in human tissues. The protein has seven domains including two low complexity segments. The main BolA domain consists of a helix-turn-helix structure close to its C terminus. The gene has three published mutations (c.123dupA; p.Glu42Argfs; c.200T>A, p.Ile67Asn; c.136C>T, p.Arg46Ter) [18, 34–36] in addition to a 5 bp deletion [37] and a single basepair insertion [18]. These mutations were identified in ethnically different families. The first patients were initially described in 2001 in a mapping study [38] that included a singleton from a consanguineous family as well as three siblings from a nonconsanguineous family. Since all the patients from two different families had similar metabolic abnormalities, a mapping strategy was employed to identify the genetic interval for the causative gene. This approach located the gene on chromosome 2. Further positional cloning studies on the subjects yielded a single significant interval on p arm extending ~5 centiMorgan region and excluding the region positioned on the q arm. Interestingly, both of these families were utilized in a follow-up study that yielded deficiencies of two ISC-related genes in each family. While the larger family with three siblings were identified to harbor splice site mutation in *NFU1* (c.545G>A) [18], the singleton had a single nucleotide duplication leading to a frame shift and eventually a premature stop codon (p.Glu42Argfs*13) in *BOL3* [18]. Later on, a few more follow-up studies revealed additional mutations in the gene. The first follow-up study focused on two patients (male and female) with quite similar clinical course appeared with hypotonia, severe neonatal lactic acidosis, and intractable cardiomyopathy [35]. A missense mutation (c.200T>A, p.Ile67Asn) was identified in the patients' DNA using exome sequencing. The other studies [34, 37] provided two additional missense mutations in *BOLA3*. Interestingly, while c.287A>G (p.His96Arg) causes a lethal infantile mitochondrial disorder [37], c.136C>T (p.Arg46*), a severe truncation mutation, leads to nonketotic hyperglycinemia [34] in the affected individuals.

Table 2 consists of previously published mutations in some Fe-S cluster genes.

Gene	Mutation type	Mutation	Disease and phenotype	References
BOLA3	Missense	c.200T>A; p.Ile67Asn	Multiple mitochondrial dysfunctions syndrome	Haack et al. [35]
BOLA3	Missense	c.287A>G p.His96Arg	Lethal infantile mitochondrial disorder	Kohda et al. [37]
BOLA3	Nonsense	c.136C>T; p.Arg46*	Nonketotic hyperglycinemia,	Baker et al. [34]
BOLA3	Microdeletion	c.225_229delGAGAA; p. Lys75*	Lethal infantile mitochondrial disorder	Kohda et al. [37]
BOLA3	Microduplication	c.123dupA	Combined respiratory chain and 2-oxoacid dehydrogenase deficiency	Cameron et al. [18]
IBA57	Missense	c.313C>T; p.Arg105Trp	Leukodystrophy with acute psychomotor regression	Torraco et al. [39]
IBA57	Missense	c.316A>G; p.Thr106Ala	Leukodystrophy with acute psychomotor regression	Torraco et al. [39]
IBA57	Missense	c.436C>T; p.Arg146Thr	Leukodystrophy, fatal infantile	Debray et al. [40]
IBA57	Missense	c.586T>G; p.Trp196Gly	Leukodystrophy, developmental delay, feeding problems and recurrent vomiting	Torraco et al. [39]
IBA57	Missense	c.686C>T; p.Pro229Leu	Leukodystrophy, developmental delay, feeding problems and recurrent vomiting	Torraco et al. [39]
IBA57	Missense	c.706C>T; p.Pro236Ser	Leukodystrophy with acute psychomotor regression and feeding difficulties	Torraco et al. [39]
IBA57	Missense	c.757G>C; p.Val253Leu	Leukodystrophy with acute psychomotor regression	Torraco et al. [39]
IBA57	Missense	c.941A>C; p.Gln314Pro	Myopathy and encephalopathy	Ajit Bolar et al. [15]
IBA57	Splice	IVS2 ds A-G-2; c.678A>G	Spastic paraplegia	Lossos et al. [41]
IBA57	Small insertion	c.87_88ins11	Leukodystrophy with acute psychomotor regression	Torraco et al. [39]
NFU1	Missense	c.62G>C; p.Arg21Pro	NFU1 deficiency	Ahting et al. [42]
NFU1	Missense	c.544C>T; p.Arg182Trp	NFU1 deficiency	Ahting et al. [42]
NFU1	Missense	c.565G>A; p.Gly189Arg	Leukoencephalopathy with cysts and hyperglycinaemia	Nizon et al. [43–45]

Gene	Mutation type	Mutation	Disease and phenotype	References
NFU1	Missense	c.568G>A; p.Gly190Arg	NFU1 deficiency	Ahting et al. [42]
NFU1	Missense	c.572A>T; p.Asp191Val	Multiple mitochondrial dysfunctions syndrome	Bai et al. [46]
NFU1	Missense	c.622G>T; p.Gly208Cys	Fatal infantile encephalopathy and/or pulmonary hypertension	Navarro-Sastre et al. [47]
NFU1	Missense	c.629G>T; p.Cys210Phe	Leukoencephalopathy	Invernizzi et al. [44]
NFU1	Splice	c.302+3A>G; p.Val56Glyfs*	NFU1 deficiency	Ahting et al. [42]
NFU1	Splice	c.545G>A; Skipping exon 6	Deficiency of the 2-oxoacid dehydrogenases accompanied by respiratory chain defects	Cameron et al. [18]
NFU1	Splice	c.545+5G>A; Skipping exon 6	Fatal infantile encephalopathy, pulmonary hypertension	Navarro-Sastre et al. [47]
NFU1	Microdeletion	c.90delC; p. Tyr30*	Multiple mitochondrial dysfunctions syndrome	Bai et al. [46]
NFU1	Microdeletion	c.146delC; p.Pro49LeufsX8	Spastic paraplegia	Tonduti et al. [45]
NFU1	Large deletion	55.6 kb region covering exons: 4–8	NFU1 deficiency	Ahting et al. [42]
ISCA1	Missense	c.259G>A; p. Glu87Lys	Multiple mitochondrial dysfunctions syndrome	Shukla et al. [19]
ISCA2	Missense	c.229G>A; p.Glu77Ser	Multiple mitochondrial dysfunctions syndrome	Al-Hassnan et al. [26] and others [27, 28]
ISCA2	Deletion and Missense	c.295delT and c.334A>G; p.Phe99Leufs*18 and p.Ser112Gly	Multiple mitochondrial dysfunctions syndrome	Toldo et al. [29]

Table 2. Published mutations in some Fe-S cluster genes.

6. Conclusion

Iron-sulfur clusters are indispensable inorganic cofactors for biological function and involve in numerous cellular processes such as respiration and DNA repair. The cluster's assembly is complex and requires sophisticated protein machinery for its maturation and insertion into apoproteins. Since mitochondria is the main site for ISC biogenesis in human, any defect disturbing the biogenesis leads to a pathological outcome mostly appears as an mitochondrial entity in human. Currently, genetic alterations in several genes involving in ISC assembly and maturation have been linked to autosomal recessive mitochondrial human diseases known as multiple mitochondrial dysfunction syndromes. It is expected that more genes and alterations will appear in the literature related to ISC pathways. Moreover, there is still need to fully elucidate the phenotypic consequences of these genetic alterations and alteration of ISC pathways during the ISC related pathogenesis in human.

Acknowledgements

This study was supported by King Abdulaziz City for Science and Technology grant 11-BIO2221-20 (NK) and King Salman Center for Disability Research grant: 2180 004 (NK).

Author details

Namik Kaya[1*], Zuhair Al-Hassnan[2], Maha Abdulrahim[1], Mazhor Aldosary[1] and Dilek Colak[3]

*Address all correspondence to: nkaya@kfshrc.edu.sa

1 Department of Genetics, King Faisal Specialist Hospital and Research Center, Riyadh, Saudi Arabia

2 Department of Medical Genetics, King Faisal Specialist Hospital and Research Center, Riyadh, Saudi Arabia

3 Department of Biostatistics and Scientific Computing, King Faisal Specialist Hospital and Research Center, Riyadh, Saudi Arabia

References

[1] Taylor RW, Turnbull DM. Mitochondrial DNA mutations in human disease. Nature Reviews. 2005;**6**:389-402

[2] Tuppen HA, Blakely EL, Turnbull DM, Taylor RW. Mitochondrial DNA mutations and human disease. Biochimica et Biophysica Acta. 2010;**1797**:113-128

[3] Cree LM, Samuels DC, Chinnery PF. The inheritance of pathogenic mitochondrial DNA mutations. Biochimica et Biophysica Acta. 2009;**1792**:1097-1102

[4] Lightowlers RN, Taylor RW, Turnbull DM. Mutations causing mitochondrial disease: What is new and what challenges remain? Science. 2015;**349**:1494-1499

[5] McFarland R, Taylor RW, Turnbull DM. Mitochondrial disease—Its impact, etiology, and pathology. Current Topics in Developmental Biology. 2007;**77**:113-155

[6] Yarham JW, Elson JL, Blakely EL, McFarland R, Taylor RW. Mitochondrial tRNA mutations and disease. Wiley Interdisciplinary Reviews. 2010;**1**:304-324

[7] Bates MG, Bourke JP, Giordano C, d'Amati G, Turnbull DM, Taylor RW. Cardiac involvement in mitochondrial DNA disease: Clinical spectrum, diagnosis, and management. European Heart Journal. 2012;**33**:3023-3033

[8] Schaefer AM, Walker M, Turnbull DM, Taylor RW. Endocrine disorders in mitochondrial disease. Molecular and Cellular Endocrinology. 2013;**379**:2-11

[9] Alston CL, Rocha MC, Lax NZ, Turnbull DM, Taylor RW. The genetics and pathology of mitochondrial disease. The Journal of Pathology. 2017;**241**:236-250

[10] Krishnan KJ, Reeve AK, Samuels DC, Chinnery PF, Blackwood JK, Taylor RW, Wanrooij S, Spelbrink JN, Lightowlers RN, Turnbull DM. What causes mitochondrial DNA deletions in human cells? Nature Genetics. 2008;**40**:275-279

[11] Taanman JW. The mitochondrial genome: Structure, transcription, translation and replication. Biochimica et Biophysica Acta. 1999;**1410**:103-123

[12] Lill R, Hoffmann B, Molik S, Pierik AJ, Rietzschel N, Stehling O, Uzarska MA, Webert H, Wilbrecht C, Muhlenhoff U. The role of mitochondria in cellular iron-sulfur protein biogenesis and iron metabolism. Biochimica et Biophysica Acta. 2012;**1823**:1491-1508

[13] van der Giezen M, Tovar J. Degenerate mitochondria. EMBO Reports. 2005;**6**:525-530

[14] Stehling O, Wilbrecht C, Lill R. Mitochondrial iron-sulfur protein biogenesis and human disease. Biochimie. 2014;**100**:61-77

[15] Ajit Bolar N, Vanlander AV, Wilbrecht C, Van der Aa N, Smet J, De Paepe B, Vandeweyer G, Kooy F, Eyskens F, De Latter E, et al. Mutation of the iron-sulfur cluster assembly gene IBA57 causes severe myopathy and encephalopathy. Human Molecular Genetics. 2013;**22**:2590-2602

[16] Brzoska K, Meczynska S, Kruszewski M. Iron-sulfur cluster proteins: Electron transfer and beyond. Acta Biochimica Polonica. 2006;**53**:685-691

[17] Kessler D, Papenbrock J. Iron-sulfur cluster biosynthesis in photosynthetic organisms. Photosynthesis Research. 2005;**86**:391-407

[18] Cameron JM, Janer A, Levandovskiy V, Mackay N, Rouault TA, Tong WH, Ogilvie I, Shoubridge EA, Robinson BH. Mutations in iron-sulfur cluster scaffold genes NFU1 and BOLA3 cause a fatal deficiency of multiple respiratory chain and 2-oxoacid dehydrogenase enzymes. American Journal of Human Genetics. 2011;**89**:486-495

[19] Shukla A, Hebbar M, Srivastava A, Kadavigere R, Upadhyai P, Kanthi A, Brandau O, Bielas S, Girisha KM. Homozygous p.(Glu87Lys) variant in ISCA1 is associated with a multiple mitochondrial dysfunctions syndrome. Journal of Human Genetics. 2017;**62**:723-727

[20] Cozar-Castellano I, del Valle Machargo M, Trujillo E, Arteaga MF, Gonzalez T, Martin-Vasallo P, Avila J. hIscA: A protein implicated in the biogenesis of iron-sulfur clusters. Biochimica et Biophysica Acta. 2004;**1700**:179-188

[21] Yang J, Tan G, Zhang T, White RH, Lu J, Ding H. Deletion of the proposed iron chaperones IscA/SufA results in accumulation of a red intermediate cysteine Desulfurase IscS in *Escherichia coli*. The Journal of Biological Chemistry. 2015;**290**:14226-14234

[22] Song D, Tu Z, Lee FS. Human ISCA1 interacts with IOP1/NARFL and functions in both cytosolic and mitochondrial iron-sulfur protein biogenesis. The Journal of Biological Chemistry. 2009;**284**:35297-35307

[23] Roux-Rouquie M, Chauvet ML, Munnich A, Frezal J. Human genes involved in chromatin remodeling in transcription initiation, and associated diseases: An overview using the GENATLAS database. Molecular Genetics and Metabolism. 1999;**67**:261-277

[24] Frezal J. Genatlas database, genes and development defects. Comptes Rendus de l'Academie des Sciences. Serie III, Sciences de la Vie. 1998;**321**:805-817

[25] Sheftel AD, Wilbrecht C, Stehling O, Niggemeyer B, Elsasser HP, Muhlenhoff U, Lill R. The human mitochondrial ISCA1, ISCA2, and IBA57 proteins are required for [4Fe-4S] protein maturation. Molecular Biology of the Cell. 2012;**23**:1157-1166

[26] Al-Hassnan ZN, Al-Dosary M, Alfadhel M, Faqeih EA, Alsagob M, Kenana R, Almass R, Al-Harazi OS, Al-Hindi H, Malibari OI, et al. ISCA2 mutation causes infantile neurodegenerative mitochondrial disorder. Journal of Medical Genetics. 2015;**52**:186-194

[27] Alfadhel M, Nashabat M, Alrifai MT, Alshaalan H, Al Mutairi F, Al-Shahrani SA, Plecko B, Almass R, Alsagob M, Almutairi FB, et al. Further delineation of the phenotypic spectrum of ISCA2 defect: A report of ten new cases. European Journal of Paediatric Neurology: EJPN: Official Journal of the European Paediatric Neurology Society. 2018;**22**:46-55

[28] Alaimo JT, Besse A, Alston CL, Pang K, Appadurai V, Samanta M, Smpokou P, McFarland R, Taylor RW, Bonnen PE. Loss-of-function mutations in ISCA2 disrupt 4Fe-4S cluster machinery and cause a fatal leukodystrophy with hyperglycinemia and mtDNA depletion. Human Mutation. 2018

[29] Toldo I, Nosadini M, Boscardin C, Talenti G, Manara R, Lamantea E, Legati A, Ghezzi D, Perilongo G, Sartori S. Neonatal mitochondrial leukoencephalopathy with brain and spinal involvement and high lactate: Expanding the phenotype of ISCA2 gene mutations. Metabolic Brain Disease. 2018

[30] Cai K, Liu G, Frederick RO, Xiao R, Montelione GT, Markley JL. Structural/functional properties of human NFU1, an intermediate [4Fe-4S] carrier in human mitochondrial iron-sulfur cluster biogenesis. Structure. 2016;**24**:2080-2091

[31] Kurt YG, Kurt B, Aydin I, Agilli M, Aydin FN. NFU1 gene mutation and mitochondrial disorders. Neurology India. 2016;**64**:630-632

[32] Zhou YB, Cao JB, Wan BB, Wang XR, Ding GH, Zhu H, Yang HM, Wang KS, Zhang X, Han ZG. hBolA, novel non-classical secreted proteins, belonging to different BolA family with functional divergence. Molecular and Cellular Biochemistry. 2008;**317**:61-68

[33] Ruffier M, Kahari A, Komorowska M, Keenan S, Laird M, Longden I, Proctor G, Searle S, Staines D, Taylor K, et al. Ensembl core software resources: Storage and programmatic

access for DNA sequence and genome annotation. Database: The Journal of Biological Databases and Curation. 2017

[34] Baker PR 2nd, Friederich MW, Swanson MA, Shaikh T, Bhattacharya K, Scharer GH, Aicher J, Creadon-Swindell G, Geiger E, MacLean KN, et al. Variant non ketotic hyperglycinemia is caused by mutations in LIAS, BOLA3 and the novel gene GLRX5. Brain. 2014;**137**:366-379

[35] Haack TB, Rolinski B, Haberberger B, Zimmermann F, Schum J, Strecker V, Graf E, Athing U, Hoppen T, Wittig I, et al. Homozygous missense mutation in BOLA3 causes multiple mitochondrial dysfunctions syndrome in two siblings. Journal of Inherited Metabolic Disease. 2013;**36**:55-62

[36] Landrum MJ, Lee JM, Benson M, Brown G, Chao C, Chitipiralla S, Gu B, Hart J, Hoffman D, Hoover J, et al. ClinVar: Public archive of interpretations of clinically relevant variants. Nucleic Acids Research. 2016;**44**:D862-D868

[37] Kohda M, Tokuzawa Y, Kishita Y, Nyuzuki H, Moriyama Y, Mizuno Y, Hirata T, Yatsuka Y, Yamashita-Sugahara Y, Nakachi Y, et al. A comprehensive genomic analysis reveals the genetic landscape of mitochondrial respiratory chain complex deficiencies. PLoS Genetics. 2016;**12**:e1005679

[38] Seyda A, Newbold RF, Hudson TJ, Verner A, MacKay N, Winter S, Feigenbaum A, Malaney S, Gonzalez-Halphen D, Cuthbert AP, et al. A novel syndrome affecting multiple mitochondrial functions, located by microcell-mediated transfer to chromosome 2p14-2p13. American Journal of Human Genetics. 2001;**68**:386-396

[39] Torraco A, Ardissone A, Invernizzi F, Rizza T, Fiermonte G, Niceta M, Zanetti N, Martinelli D, Vozza A, Verrigni D, et al. Novel mutations in IBA57 are associated with leukodystrophy and variable clinical phenotypes. Journal of Neurology. 2017;**264**:102-111

[40] Debray FG, Stumpfig C, Vanlander AV, Dideberg V, Josse C, Caberg JH, Boemer F, Bours V, Stevens R, Seneca S, et al. Mutation of the iron-sulfur cluster assembly gene IBA57 causes fatal infantile leukodystrophy. Journal of Inherited Metabolic Disease. 2015;**38**:1147-1153

[41] Lossos A, Stumpfig C, Stevanin G, Gaussen M, Zimmerman BE, Mundwiller E, Asulin M, Chamma L, Sheffer R, Misk A, et al. Fe/S protein assembly gene IBA57 mutation causes hereditary spastic paraplegia. Neurology. 2015;**84**:659-667

[42] Ahting U, Mayr JA, Vanlander AV, Hardy SA, Santra S, Makowski C, Alston CL, Zimmermann FA, Abela L, Plecko B, et al. Clinical, biochemical, and genetic spectrum of seven patients with NFU1 deficiency. Frontiers in Genetics. 2015;**6**:123

[43] Nizon M, Boutron A, Boddaert N, Slama A, Delpech H, Sardet C, Brassier A, Habarou F, Delahodde A, Correia I, et al. Leukoencephalopathy with cysts and hyperglycinemia may result from NFU1 deficiency. Mitochondrion. 2014;**15**:59-64

[44] Invernizzi F, Ardissone A, Lamantea E, Garavaglia B, Zeviani M, Farina L, Ghezzi D, Moroni I. Cavitating leukoencephalopathy with multiple mitochondrial dysfunction syndrome and NFU1 mutations. Frontiers in Genetics. 2014;**5**:412

[45] Tonduti D, Dorboz I, Imbard A, Slama A, Boutron A, Pichard S, Elmaleh M, Vallee L, Benoist JF, Ogier H, et al. New spastic paraplegia phenotype associated to mutation of NFU1. Orphanet Journal of Rare Diseases. 2015;**10**:13

[46] Bai Y, Kong X. Analysis of NFU1 gene mutation in a Chinese family affected with multiple mitochondrial dysfunction syndrome. Zhonghua yi Xue yi Chuan xue za Zhi [Chinese Journal of Medical Genetics]. 2017;**34**:26-29

[47] Navarro-Sastre A, Tort F, Stehling O, Uzarska MA, Arranz JA, Del Toro M, Labayru MT, Landa J, Font A, Garcia-Villoria J, et al. A fatal mitochondrial disease is associated with defective NFU1 function in the maturation of a subset of mitochondrial Fe-S proteins. American Journal of Human Genetics. 2011;**89**:656-667

Chapter 11

Nuclear Encoded Mitochondrial Proteins in Metabolite Transport and Oxidation Pathway Connecting Metabolism of Nutrients

Janka Vašková, Jozef Firment and Ladislav Vaško

Additional information is available at the end of the chapter

http://dx.doi.org/10.5772/intechopen.72937

Abstract

In the mitochondria, there are ongoing processes essential to the survival of cells associated with the production of energy ending in the oxidative phosphorylation and the formation of ATP, constituting a form of energy for majority of metabolic processes. Except for nutrient oxidation in the citric acid cycle interfacing with the process of oxidative phosphorylation, mitochondria are linked to a number of metabolic pathways ongoing directly in mitochondria or indirectly in cell compartments by serving substrates. Mitochondrial activities maintenance requires continual draw of intermediates from cytosol through the double mitochondrial membrane as well as transport in the reverse direction. Interconnection and regulation of all the processes are mediated by transporters and carriers, activities of which are affected by cell and body requirements. In the chapter, the main transport systems localized in membranes of mitochondria, their regulation, affection, and disorders in the background of mitochondria aberrant functions are described. Voltage-dependent anion channels, translocase of mitochondrial outer membrane, deoxynucleotide carrier, ADP/ATP nucleotide translocase, and phosphate carrier in mitochondrial inner membrane are among them. In more detail, the pyruvate carrier and its abnormal activity, but also others as di- and tri-carboxylate, glutamate, and ornithine carriers, are characterized. The uncoupling protein, as solute carrier family members, involvement is also mentioned.

Keywords: carrier, mitochondria, mitochondrial inner membrane, mitochondrial outer membrane, transporter

1. Introduction

Mitochondria are two membrane organelles present in all cells that have a nucleus. They are the energy center of the cells. Their primary role is the production of ATP in oxidative phosphorylation, and the basis of the aerobic oxidation is the citric acid cycle interconnection representing the final metabolic pathway of oxidation of all major nutrients to the respiratory chain where oxidation of reduced coenzymes results in ATP formation. The nutrient to be oxidized must transfer the mitochondria by means of the transporters, as pyruvate produced in glycolysis in the cytosol. After fatty acids released by hydrolysis of lipoproteins or triacylglycerols transport across the mitochondrial membranes, acetyl-CoA arising from β-oxidation enters the citric acid cycle. Similarly, amino acids or their catalytic products enter the citric acid cycle at different sites. The production of energy in mitochondria from various nutrients is controlled by the availability of the individual nutrients that a given organ or tissue can use. For example, in excess of carbohydrates, the energy is obtained from glycolysis rather than from fatty acids and amino acids. The needs for ATP produced in oxidative phosphorylation vary in different cell compartments, and therefore it is efficiently transported out of mitochondria. Through the activity of uncoupler proteins, mitochondria also regulate energy production in the form of heat. In addition to providing different forms of energy, mitochondria are involved in other important metabolic processes. In the excess of saccharides, the acetyl-CoA resulting from pyruvate is not used in the citric acid cycle but is transported to the cytosol for the synthesis of more energy-efficient reserve, triacylglycerols. When there is a lack of glucose, mitochondria provide the intermediates for gluconeogenesis, but also participate in the synthesis of various substances, such as urea, heme, and polyamines. Reactive oxygen and nitrogen species production and triggering the intrinsic apoptotic pathway are other significant functions. They synthesize proteins from their own DNA, but most mitochondrial proteins are encoded by nuclear genes. Mitochondria are the sole site for Fe-S cluster biogenesis, which is also the only fully conservative function. The diversity and importance of biochemical pathways taking place in the mitochondria require the access of substrates and transport products generated outside the mitochondria. In terms of ensuring the normal physiological functions of the mitochondria, it is therefore crucial to ensure the transfer of the substances through the mitochondrial membranes separating the organelle from the cytoplasm, thus allowing the course of these specialized metabolic processes. Therefore, the chapter is focused on the mitochondrial transport proteins, transporters of citric acid cycle intermediates, localized in mitochondrial outer and inner membrane, since their activities significantly affect the functions of mitochondria and subsequently functions of the given organ, tissues, and the whole organism.

2. Mitochondrial outer membrane transport proteins

The mitochondrial outer membrane (MOM) is characterized by higher lipid content than inner membrane and is permeable to small molecules such as sucrose, salts, adenine nucleotides, coenzyme A, and tRNA. It is not permeable to larger molecules such as inulin, polyglucose, cytochrome c, or albumin [1]. The outer mitochondrial membrane contains three integral membrane protein families. The entire translocation and insertion of nearly all newly synthesized proteins destined to the mitochondrial organelle is mediated through channels as part of larger protein complexes, translocase of the outer membrane (TOM complex), the sorting and assembly machinery (SAM) complex (followed by translocase of the inner membrane of mitochondria (TIM)) [2]. Channels, generally, are used to conduct ions and cycle between open and closed states, with some also exhibiting an inactivation step forming a completely continuous tunnel through a bilayer that allows for rapid conductance of many ions [3]. The third protein family are voltage-dependent anion channels (VDAC), which are permanently open under physiological conditions with some evidence-based regulations [4]. VDAC is the most abundant protein of outer mitochondrial membrane (~ 10 thousand copies per mitochondrion), whose functions in permeability of compounds between cytosol and mitochondria have been shown to be related either to physiological or pathological states [5–7]. Many cases of abnormal manifestations of mitochondria are the consequence of this type of regulation of the mitochondrial outer membrane permeability [8].

2.1. Voltage-dependent anion channel

The functions of VDAC related to four main aspects are controlling of transport of metabolites and ATP transport between mitochondria and cytoplasm, forming part of mitochondrial permeability transition pore; modulation of inner mitochondrial Ca^{2+} level through connection to endoplasmic reticulum calcium release channel IP3R with glucose-related protein 75 and through phosphorylation cluster sorting protein 2 (PACS2), regulating Bid of Bcl2 pro-apoptotic factor family-mediated apoptotic pathways; and regulation of intracellular redox substances [9]. VDAC is a way of transiting reactive oxygen species (ROS) from mitochondria to cytoplasm, though it reacts directly with the NO leading to decrease in permeability and inhibition of mitochondrial transition pore [10].

VDAC, mitochondrial porin, forms a barrel comprised of a transmembrane alpha helix and 13- and more transmembrane beta strands. Beta barrel encloses a channel large in diameter (~3 nm), which is permeable to molecules up to ~5 kDa in the open configuration [11]. *In vitro* studies have shown a conserved property of eukaryotic VDAC channels to adopt multiple conductance states [12]. In humans, three isoforms of VDAC (VDAC 1–3) located on chromosome 5, each of 30 kDa, are known [13]. VDAC1 and 2 have prototypic voltage gating, but VDAC2 also has a second discrete lower conductance and ion selective state. VDAC3 is not fully voltage-dependent [14], and unlike the previous two types, VDAC3 is evenly distributed [15].

The role of membrane potentials (Ψ) in the physiological regulation of VDAC conductance is considered with regard to appearance of Donnan potential across the outer membrane [16]. However, ambiguity is not confirmed due to the presence of charged macromolecules on both sides of outer membrane, and high ionic strength of intracellular environment decreasing Donnan potentials and causing closure of channels. Differences in pH across the outer membrane indicate the presence of Donnan potential of ~−40 mV, close to a gating potential for VDAC [17]. Positive and negative ΔΨ close VDAC symmetrically with half maximal closure at ±50 mV. In the open state, anions are favored over cations, but the selectivity is weak. In the closed state, VDAC becomes a cation selective pore of 1.8 nm in diameter that still conducts small cations, such as K^+, Na^+, and Ca^{2+}, as well as Cl^-, whose movement through VDAC collapses electrical potentials [16]. In most conductive, open state, VDAC shows significant preference especially for metabolic anions. The states of lower conductance reduce permeability to metabolic anions, thus greatly diminishing metabolite flux across the outer mitochondrial membrane [18]. The flux of charged metabolites does not significantly contribute to the membrane potential because it is confined by the internal mitochondrial membrane transport, which is even 2 orders of magnitude less than the flux of small ions through VDAC in the closed state. However, when VDAC closes, the transition of major anionic metabolites (as creatine phosphate, ATP, ADP, Pi, and respiratory substrates) is prevented [19]. A number of papers have been published that confirm the VDAC conductance regulation by several factors contributing to the explanation of mitochondria dysfunction and affection by the energy metabolism of cells.

3. Physiological implication of VDAC affection by membrane bound proteins

It has been shown that the disruption of mitochondrial functions is linked to the occurrence of mutations in genes encoding various types of intermediate filament proteins. In humans, the different morphology, distribution, and function of mitochondria in patients with neurological disorder [20, 21], types of myopathies [22, 23], or epidermolysis bullosa simplex [24] were documented. The cytoskeleton proteins as tubulin, desmin, vimentin, and plectin have been found to interact with mitochondrial outer membrane, where they are involved in the ATP/ADP transmission control through VDAC, thus mediating or influencing mitochondrial functions.

3.1. Tubulin

Tubulin binds with high affinity to cellular membranes, and bound to mitochondrial membranes represent ~ 2% of total cellular tubulin [25]. It is important for ensuring intracellular transport and DNA segregation in cell division. Rostovtseva et al. [19] have found induction of fast, reversible blockade of VDAC conductance by tubulin at nanomolar concentration in 1–100 ms range. Closing occurs in concentration-dependent manner and negative potential as low as 5 mV. The type of VDAC, phosphorylation level, and membrane lipid composition have an impact on VDAC blocking. Change in channel selectivity in blocked state results in impermeability to ATP [26]. The restriction of ATP/ADP and other respiratory substrates fluxes leads to reduction of oxidative phosphorylation and promotion of apoptosis. Therefore, signals that enhance VDAC-tubulin binding by kinase-regulated phosphorylating VDAC or by increasing the concentration of available free tubulin in the cytosol would reduce mitochondrial respiration [27].

3.2. Desmin

One other regulating mitochondria affinity to ADP and oxygen consumption through direct binding to VDAC is the muscle-specific intermediate filament protein, desmin. The function of desmin is to form a three-dimensional scaffold that interconnects the contractile apparatus to the nucleus, cellular organelles, and the sarcolemma [28]. Proximity of sarcoplasmic reticulum and mitochondria by desmin scaffold allows facilitation of direct protein and metabolite targeting to mitochondria [29–31]. Interaction of desmin with contact sites (VDAC, adenine nucleotide translocator (ANT) and mitochondrial contact site complex) affects mitochondrial permeability transition pore (mtPTP) behavior and respiratory function [32, 33]. Studies on mice have shown that desmin deficiency leads to development of skeletal and myocardial defects associated with a deteriorated structure and function of mitochondria [22, 34].

Mitochondrial abnormalities cause cardiomyocyte death and myocardial degeneration, accompanied by inflammation and fibrosis, resulting in dilated cardiomyopathy and heart failure [35–38]. The cardiac-specific small heat-shock protein, αB-crystallin, was proven to rescue desmin-deficient heart failure and maintain mitochondrial functions through inhibition of mtPTP. In addition, similarly as tubulin, desmin affects mitochondrial bioenergetics through interaction with VDAC and ATP synthase [39].

3.3. Vimentin and plectin

Association of vimentin with mitochondria increases mitochondrial membrane potential and has an important function in controlling the production of ATP to various sites in the cytoplasm [40]. As a possible mechanism of action, the similarity of the mitochondrial binding site on vimentin with the domains targeting outer mitochondrial membrane is reported. The domains interact with the VDAC, increasing its permeability for several negatively charged compounds (such as pyruvate, succinate, ADP, etc.), thus compensating decreasing membrane potential effects of hexokinase [41], or tubulin. A study by Winter et al. [42] suggests that plectin 1b also plays an important role in regulating mitochondrial outer membrane permeability to ADP and ATP through VDAC.

4. VDAC regulation by mitochondrial kinases

4.1. Hexokinases

Mitochondrial localized kinases, hexokinase, and creatine kinase have been shown to regulate outer VDAC conductance [43–45]. There are three isoforms of hexokinases (fourth is glucokinase) known to mammals, whose role is to retain glucose in the cell by phosphorylation at position 6, thereby subsequently metabolizing in glycolysis and pentose phosphate pathways. Isoenzymes are of different subcellular localization: I and II are localized in the outer mitochondrial membrane reflecting controlling glycolysis, and III and IV in the nuclei and cytoplasm more reflecting the synthesis of glycogen and the pentose-phosphate pathway. Along with highly elevated levels of aerobic glycolysis (and suppression of mitochondrial respiration, Warburg effect) when compared to healthy tissue, high expression of hexokinase and more than doubled activity concurrently with VDAC closure were found in cancer cells [8, 46–48].

Both glucose phosphorylation reaction and hexokinase binding to VDAC have been found to pronounce protective effects against cell death [49]. A study by Azouylay-Zohar et al. [41] shows hexokinase-I acting through its N-terminal mitochondrial binding domain block conductance of rat liver mitochondrial VDAC and block opening of mtPTPs. An outer membrane potential generation (OMP) by hexokinase bound to VDAC allows electrical suppression of mitochondria and calcium extrusion from mitochondrial intermembrane space (IMS). Interestingly, a significant limitation on the permeability of the MOM is the reaction velocity of hexokinase binding to VDAC that is only mild per se but the OMP becomes high enough to prevent release of ADP from mitochondrial inner membrane (MIM), which should lead to inhibition of the hexokinase reaction. Yet, OMP values directly depend on percentage bounds formed, glucose concentration, metabolic conditions, and the presence of tubulin-like effectors increasing VDAC voltage sensitivity [4]. Prevention of ATP production together with higher hexokinase activity favors glycolysis. Research has shown that cancer cells respire in the absence of glucose, suggesting that VDAC blocking is not absolute, and the respiration increases with the addition of glucose. Increase in respiration is attributed to the formation of ADP in the hexokinase-catalyzed reaction and subsequent stimulation of oxidative phosphorylation. Since not all VDACs are closed, preferential access to mitochondrial ATP may be allowed for the hexokinase reaction [8]. Another principle applies if ATP from cytosol is readily available for hexokinase, leading to so-called turbo effect of uncontrolled glycolysis activation and development of metabolic burst [4].

The product hexokinase-catalyzed reaction, glucose-6-phosphate, was found to potentiate ATP release from mitochondria with the recovery of normal metabolism, and substrate replacement, even increased by induction of release of hexokinase and glucokinase from bound to VDAC [4, 41, 50]. Therefore, the effect of hexokinase dissociation from VDAC is the subject of many studies dealing with the development of potent chemotherapy of cancer diseases.

Most interestingly, there is a view of influencing metabolism of the mitochondria by blocking VDAC after binding of glucokinase in pancreatic beta cells. The glucokinase acts as a glucose sensor to maintain glucose homeostasis also in neurons, pituitary, and endocrine K and L cells [51], as its K_m of approximately 5 mM matches the set point of blood glucose [52]. An alternatively spliced glucokinase with an additional N-terminal sequence that promotes glucokinase binding to both mitochondria and secretory granules is expressed in pancreatic beta cells [53]. Glucose-6-phosphate formed after glucose enters beta cells acts to dissociate glucokinase from mitochondria and open VDAC permitting mitochondrial uptake of ADP, Pi and respiratory substrates, formation of ATP, and release of ATP into the cytosol. Increased cytosolic ATP/ADP then inhibits K_{ATP} channels, which causes plasmalemmal depolarization, activation of Ca^{2+} channels, and Ca^{2+}-dependent exocytosis of insulin granules [8]. Then, respiratory substrates that require the passage through VDAC, such as pyruvate, lactate, and long-chain fatty acids, do not trigger insulin synthesis directly. But their permeable substrates without the need for VDAC transport such as short-chain fatty acids or methylpyruvate are capable of insulin synthesis induction [54]. Ahmed et al. [55] found that under glucotoxic conditions upregulation of VDAC1 expression occurs initiating a mitochondrial death cascade and beta cell dysfunction.

4.2. Creatine kinases

Two creatine kinase (CK) isoforms are expressed in vertebrate tissues, namely dimeric cytosolic and octameric mitochondrial located in the peripheral intermembrane space and the cristae MIM (MtCK) [56]. In addition, there are tissue-specific mitochondrial isoforms in the sarcomers of striated muscles (sMtCK), and in most other tissues, they are present as ubiquitous MtCK (uMtCK) [57]. Similar to hexokinase, creatine kinase acts as energy sensor and mediates antiapoptotic effect through VDAC-ANT complexes with preferential use of mitochondrial ATP [41, 58].

Isoenzymes are associated to subcellular structures, forming microcompartments that facilitate a functional coupling, e.g., a direct exchange of ADP and ATP between the association partners

http://dx.doi.org/10.5772/intechopen.72937

without mixing with bulk [59]. In IMS, MtCK renders a high affinity to cardiolipin and other anionic phospholipids forming a cross-link of two peripheral mitochondrial membranes [60] and to ANT, thus forming a complex of MtCK-VDAC-ANT and cardiolipin. The MtCK-VDAC association is enhanced at physiological calcium concentrations [61]. MtCK associates only with inner membrane and ANT in the cristae space. MtCK preferentially uses mitochondrial ATP that is exported via ANT to phosphorylate creatine, which has a higher diffusion rate in comparison to ATP, thus providing spatial energy shuttle. The locally produced ADP is immediately reimported into the mitochondrial matrix space via ANT, and phosphocreatine is then released into the cytosol via VDAC [62]. It keeps maintaining a relatively low [ATP]/[ADP] ratio in the mitochondrial matrix to stimulate oxidative phosphorylation. The degree of such metabolite channeling varies among different tissues, species, and developmental states [63].

Changed functionality of the CK essentially leads to changes in energy flows as well as calcium homeostasis, leading in particular to changes in muscle activity. Up to 40% of the cellular volume of the heart consists of mitochondria, with sMtCK activity being the highest among all tissues and representing up to 25% of CK activities [64]. Reducing its activity is the cause of congestive heart failure [65]. As is well reviewed in Schlattner et al. [62] with impairment of the CK system, dilated cardiomyopathy, hypertrophy, and heart failure were found in animal models. In addition, the protective effect of creatine supplementation and hence the enhancement of the CK system have been found to be beneficial in human Duchenne muscular dystrophy, mitochondrial cytopathies, and phosphorylase deficiency and in animal models of amyotrophic lateral sclerosis, Huntington's disease, Parkinsonism, and brain ischemia. However, as found in the study by Qian et al. [66], overexpression of uMtCK increased survival ability of cancer cells and downregulation of mitochondrial apoptotic pathway proteins.

5. Some other factors affecting VDAC conductance

Besides the aforementioned intermediate filament proteins and mitochondrial kinases, the conductivity of VDAC as described by Lemasters et al. [67] is regulated by a number of other factors, for example, Bcl-2 family members, protein kinase A, glycogen synthase 3β, protein C kinase ε, NADH, Ca^{2+}, ATP, and glutamate [68].

Protein kinase A phosphorylates VDAC and thus increases its sensitivity to tubulin and decreases VDAC conductance [69]. Glycogen synthase 3β–mediated VDAC phosphorylation promotes VDAC opening [70].

The Bcl-2 protein family belongs to the key factors in the regulation of apoptosis , modulation of Ca^{2+} and signal transduction pathway. The Bcl-2 protein as anti-apoptotic protein prevents the release of cytochrome c and the activity of caspase. Bax, the main regulator of Bcl-2 activity, can interact with VDAC to increase VDAC aperture and increases mitochondrial permeability, promoting apoptosis [71]. The proper proportion of Bax and Bcl-2 maintains the cell homeostasis to ensure cell survival [72].

Lemasters et al. [67] introduced a concept of aldehyde-dependent VDAC closure, mitochondrial uncoupling, and disruption of normal mitochondria functioning resulting from ethanol metabolism effects. Aldehydes derivation during lipid peroxidation, VDAC closure is probably a common feature leading to liver pathologies as was pointed out on almost indistinguishable histopathological manifestations in alcoholic liver disease, nonalcoholic fatty liver disease, nonalcoholic steatohepatitis, and toxicant-associated steatohepatitis. Ethanol is metabolized predominantly by the liver in two-step oxidation: first to acetaldehyde (AcAld) by catalytic action of alcohol dehydrogenase (ALD) followed by oxidation to acetate by aldehyde dehydrogenase (ALDH). The first step undergoes in cytosol and peroxisomes by effect of cytochrome P4502E1 and catalase. Although the oxidation is prevalent over ALD, the consequence of cytochrome P450 metabolism is overwhelmingly negative due to the formation of ROS, e.g., hydroxyethyl radicals. Of the 19 known mammalian ALDH genes, mitochondrial ALDH2 with high affinity for AcAld ($K_m < 1$ μM) is the most important for AcAld oxidation (and detoxification) to acetate [73]. In both reactions, by oxidation of 1 mole of ethanol, 2 moles of NADH are formed, further requiring oxidation in the respiratory chain. As little as 2.5 h after a single bolus dose of ethanol ingestion a swift increase of alcohol metabolism (SIAM), an adaptive increase of hepatic ethanol metabolism occurs [74]. Mitochondrial respiration causing NADH oxidation nearly doubles, but it does not lead to increased ATP generation. To the contrary, hepatic ATP decreases, glycolysis is stimulated, and glycogen stores are depleted. Furthermore, mitochondrial β-oxidation of fatty acids becomes inhibited, promoting fat accumulation within hepatocytes (steatosis) [75]. This is probably the result of decrease in MOM permeability most likely by VDAC closure, promoting selective oxidation of AcAld, since VDAC closure blocks mitochondrial ATP release, respiratory substrates uptake, and uptake of fatty acids for β-oxidation [67]. Adrenergic hormones release free fatty acids from adipose tissue, which serve as substrates for long-chain fatty acid peroxisomal β-oxidation. The ensuing peroxisomal H_2O_2 formation then can promote catalase-dependent alcohol metabolism [67]. AcAld is toxic to mitochondria and aggravates oxidative stress by binding to GSH and promoting GSH leakage [76]. Moreover, as mentioned before, ethanol metabolism and also NADH overproduction cause formation of ROS, lipid peroxidation, onset of the mitochondrial permeability transition, and apoptosis [77]. However, as has been showed, short- and medium-chain fatty acids can cross mitochondrial membrane freely using carnitine shuttle or other transport system [78] and therefore are presented in diet capable to prevent steatosis development.

5.1. Translocase of the MOM

The endosymbiotic relationship of α-proteobacteria and archaic eukaryotic cell results in massive loss and transfer of coding sequences from mtDNA to the nucleus and only less than 1% is retained in today's mtDNA. Thus, most mitochondrial proteins (1000–1500) undergo cytosol translation and are subsequently transferred to mitochondria, requiring membrane complexes of protein translocators, translocases, or translocons. They include TOM and TIM for large conductance channels with almost identical properties [79]. In addition, other mitochondria protein translocators like TOB/SAM complex in MOM and Mia40/Tim401-Erv1 redox translocator in MIM have been identified [80, 81].

The general entry gate for mitochondrial proteins is thought to be TOM40 complex in MOM consisting of core sequence Tom40, Tom22, Tom7, Tom6, Tom5, peripheral associated receptors Tom20, Tom70, and a minor component Tom71. Among them, only Tom40, Tom22, and

Tom7 commonly occur in eukaryotic organisms [82]. To prevent misfolding and aggregation, hydrophobic segments of mitochondrial precursor proteins are shielded in cytosol by chaperones that escort them to the mitochondria surface [83]. These chaperones are Hsp70 (and its partner J proteins), Hsp90, and mitochondrial import stimulation factor (MSF) [84]. MSF with precursor proteins loaded was suggested to bind to Tom70 and forward proteins to Tom20, with ATP consumption, while Hsp70 transfers proteins to Tom70 without ATP hydrolysis [85]. In addition, it was found that mitochondrial proteins are also allowed to bind Tom20 directly without Hsp70 [86]. Except for some α-helical outer membrane proteins, virtually all precursors initially enter mitochondria by passing a TOM complex. As also discussed by Dudek et al. [2], many IMS proteins are imported by the mitochondrial intermembrane space import and assembly (MIA) machinery, which couples sorting of client proteins to their oxidative folding through a disulfide bridge formation. Small Tim chaperones of IMS bound to outer membrane β-barrel proteins transfer preproteins to the sorting and assembly machinery (SAM), allowing their integration into the MOM. Tim chaperones also convoy mitochondrial metabolite carrier proteins through the IMS, which are then integrated into the MIM by translocase of the inner membrane 22 (TIM22) complex in a membrane potential–driven manner. Preproteins of matrix-targeted proteins are directly transferred from TOM to TIM23 (presequence translocase) without IMS chaperones, ensuring their translocation into the matrix or later sorting into the MIM. The only source of energy for lateral membrane integration is membrane potential. Complete import of preproteins into the matrix requires the ATP-dependent presequence translocase-associated import motor (PAM).

Affection by the TOM40 complex functions leads to dysfunction of mitochondria and oxidative damage and is in the background of misfolding protein diseases. Bender et al. [87] found a significantly reduced TOM40 in the brain of Parkinson's disease patients in connection with increased mtDNA damage and α-synuclein transgenic mice together with altered levels of complex I proteins. The stable complexes of accumulated truncated amyloid precursor protein and TOM40 cause mitochondrial dysfunction in brains of Alzheimer disease patients [88]. Other diseases in humans associated with abnormal mitochondrial transport of proteins, as reviewed in MacKenzie and Payne [89], are primary hyperoxaluria type I (caused by alanine/glyoxylate aminotransferase 1 deficiency), pyruvate dehydrogenase deficiency, susceptibility to severe alcoholic liver disease (caused by increased Ala-MnSOD activity due to inability to transfer Val-MnSOD through MIM), deafness dystonia syndrome (caused by mutations in IMS protein deafness dystonia peptide 1), dilated cardiomyopathy with ataxia (caused by dysfunctional import of matrix proteins through the TIM23 complex), spastic paraplegia (dysfunction of Hsp60), and atypical mitochondria disease involving multisystem failure (deficiency in Hsp60 causing decrease in mitochondrial metabolic pathways).

6. Mitochondrial inner membrane carriers

The inner mitochondrial membrane is relatively low permeable to ions in order to minimize energy dissipation formed on complexes through generation of electrochemical proton gradient, in its direct link with ADP phosphorylation. Random flow of charged metabolites via MIM would lead to a reduction in the membrane potential and ATP formation [1]. The relative impermeability of the MIM is the basis of chemiosmotic hypothesis proposed by Mitchell. As discussed in O'Rourke [90], Mitchell recognized three modes of ion transport. Symporters cotransport multiple ions (or an ion and a metabolite) in the same direction across the membrane often utilizing the asymmetric electrochemical ion gradient to drive the transport in a thermodynamically favorable direction, as for example mitochondrial P_i/H^+carrier. Antiporters exchange ions on different sides of the membrane. Antiporters can be electroneutral (the Na^+/H^+ antiporter of the mitochondrial or plasma membrane) or electrogenic. For electrogenic transporters, ion flux is driven by both the electrochemical gradients of the transported ions and the membrane potential. For uniporters, the transport rates are in the range of 10^4–10^6 ions s^{-1}, based on ions flowing down their electrochemical gradient.

Mitchell and Moyle [91] reported that anions, including P_i, succinate, and malonate, accelerated the rate of decay of the pH gradient induced by a pulse of oxygen. This suggested the presence of anion transport systems coupled to proton movement, leading to the identification of the anion/metabolite-coupled cotransporter family. Inner membrane anion uniporters have been less well studied, but in the 1980s, an inner membrane anion channel was postulated to account for anion-selective mitochondrial swelling responses [92]. Moreover, some mitochondrial membrane proteins (e.g., mitochondrial uncoupling protein) were identified to display anion channel activity [90]. Based on the research, seven metabolite-specific mitochondrial transporters or carriers were proposed. Studies of amino acid sequence composition showed that the carriers form a well-defined family (in humans known as the solute carrier 25 family (SLC25)), with the one defining feature, a tripartite structure of three homologous sequence repeats of about 100 amino acid residues each, which was first noted in the published sequence of the bovine ADP/ATP carrier [93]. A signature motif containing P-X-[D/E]-X-X-[R/K] sequence is conserved in all members and in all three sequence repeats [94]. According to typical sequence repeats and signature motif, eukaryotic mitochondria were found to contain 35–55 different carriers when compared to genomic DNA database [95]. The human genome encodes 48 members of the SLC25 family, of which 30 are identified [96]. The isoforms of carrier members are encoded by different genes, and only the phosphate carrier has two alternatively spliced isoforms [97].

6.1. Mitochondrial nucleotide transporter

Several proteins have been identified as carriers for purine nucleotides, their analogues, as well as pyrimidine nucleotides. The ANT was identified by Kramer and Klingenberg [98]. Other specific proteins as GTP/GDP carriers, peroxisomal adenine nucleotide transporter, CoA and S-adenosylmethionine transporters belong in [99–102].

6.1.1. ADP/ATP translocase

Deoxynucleotide carrier ((DNC) SLC25A19) transports all dNDPs in exchange for ATP or ADP [103]. The protein was later identified as thiamine pyrophosphate carrier (TPC) [104], transporting thiamine pyrophosphate, thiamine monophosphate, and deoxynucleotides in descending order of potency dNDP > dNTP > dNMP. The protein is also capable of nucleotide transport, though less efficiently. The protein in ubiquitously expressed within tissues, with the highest levels in the kidney and lung [103].

The mutation in gene-encoded DNC (chromosomal localization 17q25.1) is known to be associated with Amish microcephaly. Amish microcephaly has only been observed in Old Order Amish community in Pennsylvania, U.S.A, with a high prevalence of about 1:500. The disease is characterized by severe congenital microcephaly, elevated levels of α-ketoglutarate in urine, and premature death. The only non-CNS physical anomaly is moderate micrognathia. Patients manifest no orientation to sight or sound and no fine or gross motor development and have metabolic acidosis enhanced by episodic viral illnesses, and in some cases patients have mild hepatomegaly and difficulty maintaining normal body temperature and develop increasing irritability [97]. Study on SLC25A19 knock-out mice has shown that metabolic abnormalities in humans are due to absent TPC activity [104].

6.1.2. Deoxynucleotide carrier

Four ANT isoforms are encoded in human genome on the chromosome X. ANT1–3 are structurally similar and proteins are about 90% identical, and ANT4 only shares 66–68% consistency in the amino acid composition with other isoforms. Isoforms are specifically expressed in different types of cells and tissues. ANT1 (SLC25A4) is expressed in the skeletal muscle, brain, and heart. ANT2 (SLC25A5) is expressed in the liver and proliferating cells and is overexpressed in various types of cancer cell lines. ANT3 (SLC25A6) is ubiquitous in all tissues, and ANT4 (SLC25A31) is specific to the testis and germ cells [105]. The translocase is highly selective of the adenine nucleotide and provides a continuous shift of ADP to the mitochondria required to maintain oxidative phosphorylation and membrane potential. ANT is also implicated in leakage of protons and inducible proton leakage [106, 107].

Impaired translocase activity affects the energy metabolism of the cell by decreasing mitochondrial ATP synthesis and increasing mitochondrial membrane potential [108], thus contributing to the promotion of apoptosis. The rate-limiting factor of apoptosis is mtPTP formation, which is actually increased permeabilization of the mitochondrial membrane for all the solvents up to 1.5 kDa. It is a nonspecific pore, where ANT, VDAC, cyclophilin D, hexokinase, creatine kinase, and peripheral benzodiazepine receptor are effective but not as direct components or core structures. Moreover, there is an evidence for apoptosis regulators of the Bcl-2 family, Bak and Bax, requirement for mtPTP-dependent MOM permeabilization [109]. PTP opening is linked to mitochondrial dysfunction because its occurrence leads to the set of consequences that will arise, as mitochondrial depolarization, cessation of ATP synthesis, Ca^{2+} release, pyridine nucleotide depletion, inhibition of respiration and matrix swelling, MOM rupture, and release of pro-apoptotic proteins such as cytochrome c, endonuclease G, and AIF [110, 111]. Detrimental effects are seen for long-lasting mtPTP opening, while short-term effects are involved in physiological regulation of Ca^{2+} and ROS homeostasis [112, 113].

Cancer cells are able to survive suppression of mitochondrial oxidative phosphorylation under hypoxic conditions through higher rate of glycolysis; however, it depends on ATP uptake especially for mitochondrial potential generation and Ca^{2+} exchange [114]. The expression of ANT isoforms is related to the adaptation of metabolic properties of cancer cells. ANT2 is overexpressed in various types of human cancer cells and in several hormone-dependent cancers [115, 116]. It was found that ANT2 proves properties allowing the import of ATP into mitochondria (in coexpression with hexokinase II and a subunit of mitochondrial F0F1-ATPase, ATPsynβ), increased glycolysis, maintaining mitochondrial membrane potential, and finally prevention of apoptosis [115]. The effect of hexokinase has been described in Section 4.1. Similarly, the ATP synthasome, a complex of ANT, F0F1-ATPase, and phosphate carrier (PiC), facilitates a mechanism for adenine nucleotide and pyrophosphate release. Under pathological conditions, the imported ATP may also be hydrolyzed by F0F1-ATPase to maintain mitochondrial membrane potential [115]. This type of hydrolysis has also been reported in order to prevent neurodegeneration [117] and in activated macrophages [118].

Roussel et al. [119] found isoforms ANT1 and 2 to mediate uncoupling by fatty acids and to lower mitochondrial membrane potential in heart and skeletal muscle in rats. ANT is inhibited by competitive displacement of the nucleotide by long-chain acyl-carnitines (LCAC) [120]. LCAC may accumulate under pathological conditions with excess lipid supply, obesity, and mitochondrial β-oxidation defects [121]. ANT inhibition is thought to contribute to mitochondrial defects in metabolic syndrome [122].

The ANT function in subcellular compartment energy supply is important and therefore it is not surprising that the altered structure and subsequently properties of this solute carrier protein associated with DNA mutations are also associated with serious clinical conditions. Mutations linked to mitochondrial disorders with autosomal recessive inheritance cause mitochondrial myopathy and cardiomyopathy presented in childhood or early adulthood. It is characterized by lactic acidosis, fatigue, proximal muscle weakness, and exercise intolerance [123, 124]. Several different autosomal-dominant mutations in ANT1 gene have been associated with an adulthood-onset disorder, autosomal-dominant progressive external ophthalmoplegia, characterized by ptosis, restriction of eye movement, and accumulation of clonally expanded mtDNA deletions in postmitotic tissues [125, 126]. Thompson et al. [127] have recently described recurrent *de novo*–dominant mutation with severe early-onset of mitochondrial disease. Mutations in the gene encoding ANT1 are associated with the presence of mtDNA deletions. The most likely mechanism of how the defective carrier affects the appearance of mtDNA mutations is the unsufficient adenine nucleotide availability for dATP synthesis and consequent imbalance in dNTP pools [127].

6.2. Mitochondrial phosphate carrier

The role of mitochondrial phosphate carrier (PiC, SLC25A3) is importing inorganic phosphate into the mitochondrial matrix. A part of ATP synthasome enables efficient energy production, since Pi is essential for F_1F_0-ATP synthase to catalyze formation of ATP from ADP. For PiC, two isoforms differing in alternative splicing of mutually exclusive exon are documented in tissue-specific expression pattern. PiC-A is expressed in heart and skeletal muscle, while PiC-B is expressed in liver, kidney, and other tissues [128]. The PiC gene is located on chromosome 12q23.1. In 2007, the presence of a homozygous mutation in PiC-A was found in two siblings of nonconsanguineous Turkish parents. Given the role of PiC in energy production, the clinical manifestation of PiC deficiency is associated with multisystemic disorder characterized by muscle hypotonia, lactic acidosis, severe hypertrophic cardiomyopathy, and shortened lifespan [129, 130]. Besides that, PiC has been suggested to impact mtPTP opening [131].

6.3. Mitochondrial pyruvate carrier

Important one is another of the mentioned carriers. Pyruvate is the end product of glycolysis in the cytosol. In mitochondria, pyruvate entering the tricarboxylic acid cycle supports the ATP generation but also serves as a link to anabolic pathways for lipid, amino acid biosynthesis, and gluconeogenesis. The main sources of pyruvate in the cytoplasm are reactions catalyzed by pyruvate kinase. Two more sources are lactate dehydrogenase (LDH) and alanine aminotransferase (ALT), which are important to mention in terms of linking metabolic pathways between tissues. Reversible transamination of pyruvate and glutamate to alanine and α-ketoglutarate catalyzed by ALT converts the pyruvate from muscles into a transport form, alanine, which is reused in the liver for gluconeogenesis. LDH reversibly catalyzes reduction of pyruvate to lactate concurrently with oxidation of NADH to NAD^+. Enzyme gains importance especially in muscle tissue in conditions requiring excessive energy production and in cancer cells. During increased need for ATP for muscle activity, the energy requirements to support continued muscle activity exceed mitochondrial capacity for ATP production. As glycolysis requires NAD^+, ATP production is limited when NAD^+ depletes and NADH accumulates. In this case, LDH ensures ATP production in glycolysis by regenerating NAD^+. With a steady supply of NAD^+, and until acidosis becomes limiting, glycolysis can produce ATP to support work rates exceeding those that could be supported by oxidative phosphorylation alone [132]. The lactate is transported to the circulatory system from where it is taken up by the liver and converted back into pyruvate.

The cross-connection of pyruvate with catabolic and anabolic pathway in mitochondria depends on its passage through mitochondrial membranes. Pyruvates cross MOM through VDAC; however, transport through MIM requires specific carrier. Although the existence of carrier was known earlier, the existence of genes on chromosome 6q27 encoding of mitochondrial pyruvate carrier (MPC) formed by hetero-oligomeric complex of two proteins, MPC1 and MPC2, has been revealed recently. Both proteins are needed for sufficient activity [133, 134]. Proteins do not contain any sequence homology to other mitochondrial carriers. Instead, they have been proposed to belong to the PQ-loop/MtN3/MPC superfamily [135]. Members of PQ-loop family are located in a variety of organelles performing diverse functions. They combine common characteristic features that are seven transmembrane domains and two conserved glutamine motifs. Subunits MPC1 and 2 contain three of seven transmembrane domains and are only half size of other PQ-loop family members [136]. Pyruvate uptake has been proposed to be coupled with the electrochemical gradient, occurring with the symport of one proton, or exchange with one hydroxide ion [137].

MPC activity increases in response to glucagon and decreases in response to insulin. Adrenaline and cortisol also have been found to increase pyruvate carboxylation by increasing mitochondrial pyruvate import [138]. The MPC2 transcript levels have been found to increase up to 1.5-fold under fasting conditions. In a physiological response to fasting (e.g., excessive exercise or prolonged food deprivation), hepatic mitochondrial ketone export and pyruvate import through MPC allows to enhance hepatic gluconeogenesis and maintains membrane potential [132]. Conversely, unregulated rate of gluconeogenesis contributes to chronic hyperglycemia in diabetes. Except for some substances (e.g., α-cyano-4-hydroxy cinnamate, UK-5099, and several thiazolidinediones) acting as specific MPC inhibitors, inhibitory effects of α-ketoacids and phenylpyruvate were found [139, 140]. The accumulation of phenylpyruvate in phenylketonuria prevents pyruvate transfer to mitochondria. Malate was shown to significantly increase mitochondrial pyruvate uptake while not affecting affinity. A genetic background of diminished pyruvate utilization due to pyruvate transport deficiency accompanied by lactic acidosis resulting also from the described metabolic possibilities of pyruvate are the mutations in MPC1 and/or MPC2 genomic loci [133, 141].

A ^{13}C metabolic flux analysis of cells after transcriptional or pharmacological inhibition of MPC, published by Vacanti et al. [142], revealed that inhibition of MPC activity leads to shift from glucose to amino acid and fatty acid oxidation. Citric acid cycle and fatty acid synthesis were maintained due to malic enzyme flux, glutaminolysis, fatty acid, and branched chain amino acid oxidation. Alternatively, pyruvate interconversion into gluconeogenic substrates (e.g., alanine) that can enter mitochondria independently of the MPC could compensate for loss of the MPC [143].

7. Aberrant pyruvate transfer

Altered metabolism of pyruvate resulting from the inability to transfer pyruvate is present in cancer and other metabolic diseases. Pyruvate metabolism and carbon flux are altered in many cancer cells. Metabolic switch to enhanced glycolysis and decreased oxidative phosphorylation (Warburg effect) leads to elevated lactate production, which is advantageous for cancer cells. The first advantage is regeneration of NAD^+ for the continuation of glycolysis. Another is proton-linked transport of lactate out of the cell, increasing the acidity of the extracellular space. Acidification of the extracellular environment provides protection from the immune system [144]. Furthermore, lactic acid appears to influence the activity of matrix metalloproteinases breaking down the extracellular matrix aiding in tumor proliferation and metastasis [145] and can be utilized as fuel source by cancer cells located at the surface of the tumor [146]. Schell et al. [147] found *MPC1* genomic locus as the most frequently deleted region across cancer cells, while *MPC2* locus does not appear to be frequently lost. MPC1 underexpression correlates with poor survival in almost all cancers examined, including colon, kidney, lung, bladder, and brain [147]. The correlation of survival with *MPC2* expression is more variable, but associated with poor prognosis in kidney and colon cancer [147].

Increased pyruvate levels in cerebrospinal fluid reflecting an impaired metabolism of pyruvate have been detected in neurodegenerative disorders including Leigh's syndrome, Alzheimer's disease, and Parkinson's disease [148, 149]. Neuronal metabolism depends upon the uptake of lactate produced by astrocytes (astrocyte-neuron lactate shuttle), its conversion to pyruvate by LDH, and subsequent oxidation in mitochondria to form energy. Glucose is shifted into the pentose phosphate pathway for the NADPH generation to maintain reduced glutathione levels [150]. Due to the lack of pyruvate metabolism in neurodegenerative diseases, synthesis of acetylcholine is also insufficient because it requires acetyl-CoA [143]. To the present, there are not many findings available about MPC inhibition in neuronal cells except for α-cyano-4-hydroxy cinnamate or phenylpyruvate effects. Most likely, MPC efficacy and susceptibility to disease progression are also related to genetic predisposition. Mitochondrial pyruvate supply restriction can also display a neuroprotective effect by increase in glutamate oxidation. Maintaining the levels of synaptic glutamate during glutamatergic neurotransmission comes at energetic cost leading to periods of increased levels of glutamate. High levels of glutamate cause complex I inhibition through receptor-stimulated Ca^{2+} overload, which is an attribute of acute neuropathologies [151].

MPC1 and MPC2 are highly expressed in brown adipose tissue compared with other tissues [152]. Brown adipocytes use predominantly fatty acids as an energy source for uncoupled respiration and thermogenesis, which requires replenishment of oxaloacetate through pyruvate carboxylation to enter citric acid cycle. MPC is supposed to be important in shifting between formation and oxidation of fatty acids in fat cell metabolism.

Alteration in pyruvate metabolism plays a conspicuous role in heart disease. Heart muscle predominantly metabolizes fatty acids, ketone bodies, lactate, and glucose depending on their availability and neurohormonal signaling. Up to 95% of the heart's ATP generation comes from mitochondrial oxidation, and typically approximately 60–90% of this mitochondrial ATP production comes from fatty acids, whereas 10–40% is from pyruvate oxidation. The myocardium is a significant consumer of lactate even at the maximum load, because of specific expression of LDH-B isoform preferring reaction catalysis toward pyruvate [153]. It was found that acute stress (such as ischemia) and chronic stress (hypertrophy and heart failure) change substrate availability and metabolism [143]. Reduction in pyruvate oxidation leads to increased anaerobic glycolysis and lactate formation. However, age-related decrease in MPC activity was observed [154]. Shift in substrate utilization in order to maintain citric acid cycle can lead to serious states of energy deficiency called "starved heart." The effect was observed in cancer treatment with doxorubicin reducing carnitine transport followed by reduced fatty acid oxidation [155].

7.1. Mitochondrial di- and tricarboxylic acid transport

7.1.1. Tricarboxylate carrier

The tricarboxylate carrier (SLC25A1) catalyzes an electroneutral exchange of the dibasic form of a tricarboxylic acid (citrate, isocitrate, and cis-aconitate) with proton for another tricarboxylate-H^+, dicarboxylate (malate and succinate), or phosphoenolpyruvate [156]. An importance of the citrate carrier (CiC) results from formation of a link between carbohydrate catabolism and lipogenesis. The CiC overlaps with oxoglutarate carrier ((OGC) SLC25A11) by transporting the 2-oxoglutarate in exchange for malate and malonate [157]. CiC facilitates transport of citrate across MIM, followed by passive diffusion through VDAC in MOM into the cytosol. In the cytosol, fatty acids and cholesterol are synthesized from citrate. Citrate also acts as inhibitor of phosphofructokinase 1, thus affecting the rate of glycolysis, positive allosteric modulator of acetyl-CoA carboxylase in fatty acid synthesis pathway, and serves as a substrate for the formation of malate, the conversion of which into pyruvate facilitates NADPH production necessary for lipogenesis [158]. High CiC mRNA levels in liver, kidney, and pancreas; lower levels in heart, skeletal muscle, and placenta; and no detectable mRNA in brain and lung were detected [128]. High liver and kidney CiC mRNA levels are supposed to be due to gluconeogenesis and lipogenesis. Moreover, CiC plays a role in gluconeogenesis from lactate where phosphoenolpyruvate carboxykinase is located in mitochondria. Similarly as in other animals, mitochondrial phosphoenolpyruvate isoforms are present mainly in the liver, kidney, and adipose tissue [159]. The relatively high CiC mRNA level in pancreas could be explained with the role of CiC in regulation of insulin secretion. On the other hand, the low CiC mRNA level in skeletal muscle correlates to the very low activity of gluconeogenesis and fatty acid synthesis [160].

Except for decisive interconnection between lipogenesis, gluconeogenesis, and glycolysis, CiC has been proposed to play a role in the maintenance of chromosome integrity and in the regulation of autophagy [161]. A particularly important role played by the CiC is in the regulation of insulin secretion by providing isocitrate for NADP-dependent isocitrate dehydrogenase [162].

The studies have shown that the CiC activity and properties could be changed under specific conditions: starvation-induced decrease of CiC activity and considerable reduction of CiC mRNA in starved rats. The reduced CiC mRNA levels were ascribed to shortened half-life and accelerated degradation of CiC mRNA. Refeeding, however, leads to renewal of mRNA and increased activity of CiC [163]. The polyunsaturated fatty acid (PUFA) administration also dramatically affects CiC gene expression by transcriptional and posttranscriptional mechanisms. Rat liver mitochondria showed more decreased CiC activity and reduced transcriptional rate of CiC mRNA when affected by n-3 PUFA than by n-6 [164]. During the inflammation, CiC gene expression is activated by NF-κB, which causes an increased availability of cytosolic acetyl-CoA and NADPH + H+ for synthesis and activity of compounds and enzymes involved in inflammatory response (e.g., COX2, iNOS, and NADPH oxidase) [156].

The human SLC25A1 gene is localized on chromosome 22, within the region associated with allelic losses in DiGeorge/22q11 syndrome, velo-cardio-facial syndrome, and a subtype of schizofrenia [165]. To date, recessive mutations of CiC gene in 20 persons with combined D,L-hydroxyglutaric aciduria were described. The clinical phenotype of disorder is characterized by severe developmental delay, hypotonia, seizures, secondary microcephaly, hypoplasia or agenesis of the corpus callosum, optic nerve hypoplasia, dysmorphic feature, lactic acidosis, and recurrent apneic crises [166]. CIC has also been reported to be upregulated in ovarian and colon cancer [167].

7.2. Dicarboxylate carrier

Dicarboxylate carrier protein ((DIC) SLC25A10) transporting malate and succinate out of mitochondria in exchange for P_i is ubiquitously expressed in mammalian mitochondria. The carrier is inhibited by P_i and other phosphate and substrate analogues. Malate exchange for P_i provides a cytosolic source of malate for CiC and therefore plays a significant role in fatty acid synthesis [168]. DIC interacts with malate dehydrogenase by acting as an oxaloacetate shuttle, thus improving functional coupling of citric acid cycle with shuttle. In the cytosol, malate is converted into oxaloacetate following conversion into phosphoenolpyruvate by carboxykinase-catalyzed reaction. The reaction is rate-limiting for gluconeogenesis. No less important role of the carrier is the transport of reduced glutathione into the mitochondria shared with OGC. Therefore, limiting protein expression results in significantly reduced levels of glutathione in the mitochondria and subsequent altered redox conditions [169]. It was found that the activity of DIC is increased in type I diabetes, in contrast to decreased activities of CiC [170].

8. Oxoglutarate carrier

The OGC mediates transfer of oxoglutarate across MIM in exchange for dicarboxylate. OGC is a component of malate-aspartate shuttle; thus, dicarboxylate is usually malate. After export, malate is converted into oxaloacetate, which is in transamination reaction with glutamate converted into oxoglutarate and aspartate. The oxoglutarate is then transported by OGC. Binding the succinate to the matrix side of the carrier increases the affinity for malate, while phenylsuccinate, pyridoxalphosphate, retinoic acid, or alcohol was found to inhibit OGC [171, 172]. The OGC inhibition causes a decrease in mitochondrial reduced glutathione levels by 40–50% [138]. The carrier has also been proposed as a porphyrin transporter, and its inhibition blocks porphyrin conversion to heme in mitochondria. The downregulation of OGC has been reported in horse muscle with recurrent exertional rhabdomyolysis [173].

8.1. Mitochondrial glutamate carriers

8.1.1. Glutamate carrier

Another one from SLC25 family is a glutamate carrier. Two glutamate-transfer isoforms are known for the glutamate carrier: GC1 (SLC25A22) and GC2 (SLC25A18). They transport glutamate across the MIM in symport with a proton or in exchange for hydroxyl ions. In mitochondria, glutamate is converted by glutamate dehydrogenase into α-ketoglutarate while reducing NAD $(P)^+$. Ammonia is released and reduced coenzyme enters the complex I of respiratory chain. The mRNAs of GC1 have been found to be highly expressed than that of GC2 in liver, pancreas, and kidney but are similar in the brain. Moreover, the K_m and V_{max} values are higher than those of GC2 (5.2 vs. 0.26 mM; 12.2 vs. 3.9 μmol/min/g of proteins). Therefore, an acceptable explanation, for the expression pattern is that GC2 is responsible for the basic function, whereas GC1 functions in tissues with increased demands [174].

GC1 has been demonstrated to have an important physiological function in the control of glucose-stimulated insulin secretion in pancreatic β cells [96]. The signaling mechanism leads to adjustment of insulin release to levels greater than the sole contribution of Ca^{2+}-induced triggering pathway in rats. Stimulation of β cells with high glucose might result in rapid saturation of the respiratory chain [175], favored by glucokinase properties (as mentioned in Section 4.1.) and low lactate release. Saturated electron transport chain would then promote export of metabolites (GTP, citrate, NADH, and glutamate) out of the mitochondria compensated by activity of anaplerotic pathways [176]. Energetic sufficiency favors the glutamate dehydrogenase reaction from α-ketoglutarate toward glutamate formation. Glutamate is taken up by secretory granules, which are consistent with the expression of vesicular glutamate transporters (VGLUT1 and 2) in insulin-secreting cells [177]. Inside the secretory granule, glutamate could induce pH changes and activate metabotropic receptors mGlu5, thereby mediating insulin release [178]. Alternative mechanisms include activation of acetyl-CoA carboxylase and inhibition of phosphatase activities involved in insulin exocytosis [179].

GC1 is highly expressed in astrocytes from different structures (retina, spinal cord, and cortex) [180] and represents the principal gate for glutamate entry into the mitochondria of astrocytes. Restricting glutamate access to mitochondria results in reduced ATP and NAD(P)H formation. A defective glutamate carrier may lead to glutamate accumulation in the astrocytes cytosol and then to glutamate liberation in the synaptic cleft. The release could result in neuronal synchronicity, which may contribute to the generation of epileptic-like discharges in the brain [181]. Mutations in the human *GC1* gene (localized on chromosome 11p15.5) are responsible for the autosomal recessive form of early infantile epileptic encephalopathy caused by complete loss of transport and uniport activity of the protein [182–184]. Clinical manifestations are similar to epileptic spasms and focal seizures associated with suppression bursts beginning in the first days of life, microcephaly, hypotonia, abnormal retinogram recording, and psychomotor retardation [183].

9. Aspartate/glutamate carrier

Glutamate can also enter mitochondria through aspartate/glutamate carrier (AGC1 and 2 isoforms, known as aralar and citrin) combining the input of glutamate to the release of aspartate [185]. The export of aspartate is favored in energized mitochondria. Moreover, in increased cytosolic calcium concentration, respiration is strongly increased associated with the reduction of mitochondrial membrane potential [185]. A decrease in ROS production could be expected given the opposite relationship between the mitochondrial membrane potential and ROS production [186]. Another attribute contributing to this effect is glutamate entry through AGC1 (SLC25A12) in cotransport with proton. The loss of membrane potential is compensated by the extrusion of four protons by the respiratory chain when one molecule of glutamate is processed through the citric acid cycle generating two molecules of NADH [187]. AGC together with the OGC plays a crucial role in the transport of NADH from cytosol to the mitochondria as a part of malate-aspartate shuttle [188]. Therefore, AGC1 and AGC2 (SLC25A13) are expressed in tissues differently according to their demands for maintenance of the redox balance between anaerobic and aerobic glycolysis. An interesting finding is that expression of AGC1 and AGC2 is almost completely restricted to neurons and photoreceptor cells [180, 189], in contrast to GC1 expressed in astrocytes. Cytosolic Ca^{2+} has a direct role in the regulation of *AGC1* gene expression via cAMP response element-binding protein in neuronal cells, underlining the key role of AGC1 in the central nervous system by upregulation in neuronal differentiation and downregulation in neuroinflammation [190]. AGC1 is also highly expressed in skeletal and heart muscle [191]. Upregulation of both isoforms was found in several cancers, which is also related to the change in glycolytic metabolism [187].

9.1. Ornithine carriers

Translocation of the ornithine and related substrates is mediated by mitochondrial ornithine carrier (ORC). The physiological importance of this carrier reclines on urea production, delivery-rate control of arginine, and interferential formation of NO, agmatine, creatine, glutamine, glutamate polyamines, and proline [192]. The human isoforms ORC1 (SLC25A15), ORC2 (SLC25A2), and ORC3 (SLC25A29) [193, 194] provide transport by exchange or by exchange for H^+ but differ in substrate transport rates, substrate specificity, and tissue expression. They all facilitate passage of L-ornithine, L-lysine, and L-arginine. The ORC1 prefers transport of amino acid substrates with shorter and noncyclized side chains. It does not enable transport of L-homoarginine, D-ornithine, D-histidine, and D-arginine. The ORC2 transports all substrates with the same efficiency (L,D-forms of ornithine, lysine, histidine, arginine, and L-citrulline, L-homoarginine). The ORC3 enables transport of L-forms with longer side chains across MIM, e.g., lysine, arginine, and histidine [192]. The isoform expresses lower affinity to ornithine and does not transport citrulline [194].

Activity of ORC1 and 2 is enhanced by P_i, malate, and dicarboxylates and inhibited by pyridoxal 5′-phosphate (PLP), mercurials, spermine, and spermidine. The affinity of ORC2 to lysine and arginine is lower and to ornithine and citrulline is higher in comparison to ORC1. Moreover, ORC2 has been reported to be about three times less active than ORC1. The dispositions are also related to protein expression. The ORC1 is expressed in most tissues, with the highest levels in the liver, pancreas, lungs, kidney, and testis, unlike the ORC2 being more restricted to these organs [193]. ORC3 is expressed in heart, brain, liver, and kidney and is induced after partial hepatectomy or fasting [195, 196]. The import of arginine, lysine, and histidine allows for protein synthesis in mitochondria and that for ornithine enables degradation of arginine surplus. Transfer of ornithine out of the mitochondria allows for synthesis of polyamines reversibly inhibiting ORC activity. Ornithine is synthesized in mitochondria from glutamate in tissues with low arginase activity (except for the liver), from glutamine in intestinal mitochondria or when deficient in the diet [193]. Considering ornithine and citrulline transport efficiency and level of protein expression in the liver, the ORC1 isoform is of highest importance in urea cycle continuance [193].

Mutation in the gene encoding ORC1 isoform (localized on 13q14.1 chromosome) causes hyperornithinemia-hyperammonemia-homocitrullinuria (HHH syndrome), characterized by early-onset neurological deficits. Hyperammonemia results from impaired urea cycle due to ORC1 malfunction. Ornithine accumulates in the cytosol leading to hyperornithinemia and increases polyamine synthesis. Carbamoyl phosphate condensates with lysine in the absence of ornithine inside the mitochondria, leading to homocitrullinuria, or enters pyrimidine synthesis, thus increasing excretion of orotic acid and uracil [97, 197]. Overexpression of ORC2 might only partially compensate defective function of ORC1 due to lower affinity for ornithine and citrulline [196, 198]. ORC3 has not been found to compensate lack of ORC1 function but is probably responsible for lysine transport in patients with HHH syndrome [194].

9.2. Mitochondrial uncoupling proteins

Uncoupling proteins (UCP) sharing the same tripartite structure belongs to the family of the mitochondrial anion carriers. Six families of UCP members encoding by 45 genes have been described [199]. In mammals, UCPs consist of five homologs: UCP1 (SLC25A7), UCP2 (SLC25A8), UCP3 (SLC25A9), UCP4 (SLC25A27), and UCP5 (SLC25A14, BMCP1). *UCP1* genes are localized on human chromosome 4. The human and mouse *UCP2* genes are located 7–20 kb downstream of the *UCP3* stop codon, as the result of a duplication; the *UCP3-UCP2* locus is located on human chromosome 11q13 (between the genetic markers D11S916 and D11S911). The UCP5 homolog *Bmcp1* is located on Xq25–26 chromosome (between the markers DXS1206 and DXS1047), and *UCP4* on 6p11.2-q12 (close to the genetic marker SHGC-34952) [200].

UCPs are ubiquitous, except for UCP2 [201], however, exhibiting tissue-specific expression pattern. As reviewed in Gutérrez-Aquilar and Baines [202], UCP1 is unique to brown adipose tissue, UCP3 to heart and skeletal muscle, and UCP4 and 5 are typical to the brain. The general designation of this carrier family is derived from observed function of the first member, UCP1 in brown fat tissue—the heat production in the nonshivering thermogenesis [199]. According to Mitchell's theory, any proton leak not coupled with ATP synthesis would provoke uncoupling of respiration and thermogenesis. The discharge of proton gradient formed in respiratory chain causes dissipation of energy of oxidation as heat. Besides adaptive thermogenesis, uncoupling of respiration allows continuous reoxidation of coenzymes that are essential to metabolic pathways [203], prevents inhibition of mitochondrial respiration from excessive ATP production, and decreases ROS formation [204].

The activity of UCPs requires ubiquinone as a cofactor [205] and is regulated by two ligands. UCP1 is activated by fatty acids and inhibited by purine nucleoside di- and triphosphates. UCP2 and 3 can be activated by fatty acid and are less sensitive to purine inhibition. There are not many findings about UCP4 and 5 regulation; however, they were reported to be GDP-sensitive [206]. The mechanism of proton transport is still controversial. The UCP is referred to act as a pure proton transporter activated by fatty acids, while by other mechanism, UCP facilitates protonated fatty acid transbilayer movements, flip-flop, to the matrix where they release the proton and are then transported back to the IMS by UCP [199, 206]. Consistently with transport of fatty acid anion, UCP1 was shown to transport a variety of ions, suggesting that UCP1 is a hydroxyl anion transporter rather than a proton carrier [207].

As has already been mentioned, the physiological function of UCP1 is the production of heat in brown adipocytes. The UCP1 induction is influenced by thyroid hormones and sympathetic nerves and therefore also by drugs activating adrenoceptors [203]. Capsaicin was found to increase levels of all UCPs [206]. A mutation in gene encoding UCP1 is associated to diabetic retinopathy [208].

Although, UCP2 and 3 are not involved in thermogenesis, polymorphisms in the coding region of the *UCP2* gene are associated with the level of energy expenditure during sleep [209]. These two members reduce ROS formation by mild uncoupling [208] and related to function to decrease mitochondrial oxidative stress load and transport fatty acid peroxides to MOM [210]. Cytokines and thyroid hormone upregulate UCP2 and UCP3 [211]. Thus, physiological response of macrophages is lowering the UCP levels and enhancing the ROS production. Moreover, UCP2 was proposed to act as carrier for the superoxide anion [205]. The expression of UCP2 is induced under starvation when there are elevated levels of fatty acid in the circulation. The expression of UCP3 increases during fasting [212]. In leptin-induced lipolysis, fatty acids are not exported to the liver but are oxidized in adipocytes, where UCP2 initiates fat oxidation that is not associated with energy-requiring processes [213]. Pharmacological inhibition and genetic mutations in UCP2 and UCP3 have been shown to reverse damaging consequences of obesity and diabetes-induced pancreatic β-cell dysfunction [214, 215].

UCP4 and 5 have been shown to be upregulated by oxidative stress, while insulin downregulates their levels [216]. Mutations in *UCP4* gene have been linked to schizophrenia [217]. For all UCPs, a continuity of upregulation of the expression and incidence of tumor diseases has been described [202].

10. Conclusion

As it follows from this review, the proper course of metabolic processes in the mitochondria requires direction of transport systems to the needs of the organism. The activities of transporters can be regulated differently by hormones, phosphorylation and dephosphorylation, cytokines, concentration of metabolites, and individual nutrition components, which can alter their amount and activity. Most metabolites or their precursors can be mutually transported by different transport systems to provide the desired concentrations on both sides of the mitochondrial membranes. The specificity of transport and regulation of compounds in different organs and tissues provide various isoforms encoded by different nuclear genes. More detailed knowledge of transport mechanisms can contribute to better diagnosis and treatment of metabolic disorders.

Acknowledgements

This work was supported by Slovak Grant Agency for Science VEGA 1/0782/15.

Author details

Janka Vašková[1]*, Jozef Firment[2] and Ladislav Vaško[1]

*Address all correspondence to: janka.vaskova@upjs.sk

1 Department of Medical and Clinical Biochemistry, Faculty of Medicine, Pavol Jozef Šafárik University in Košice, Košice, Slovak Republic

2 1st Clinic of Anaesthesiology and Instensive Medicine, Faculty of Medicine, Louis Pasteur University Hospital, Pavol Jozef Šafárik University in Košice, Košice, Slovak Republic

References

[1] Wohlrab H. Transport proteins (carriers) of mitochondria. IUBMB Life. 2009;**61**(1):40-46. DOI: 10.1002/iub.139

[2] Dudek J, Rehling P, van der Laan M. Mitochondrial protein import: Common principles and physiological networks. Biochimica et Biophysica Acta. 2013;**1833**(22):274-285. DOI: 10.1016/j.bbamcr.2012.05.028

[3] Schell JC, Rutter J. The long and winding road to the mitochondrial pyruvate carrier. Cancer & Metabolism. 2013;**1**(1):6. DOI: 10.1186/2049-3002-1-6

[4] Lemeshko VV. VDAC electronics: 1. VDAC-hexo(gluco)kinase generator of the mitochondrial outer membrane potential. Biochimica et Biophysica Acta. 2014;**1838**(5):1362-1371. DOI: 10.1016/j.bbamem.2014.01.001

[5] Colombini M. VDAC structure, selectivity, and dynamics. Biochimica et Biophysica Acta. 2012;**1818**(6):1457-1465. DOI: 10.1016/j.bbamem.2011.12.026

[6] Colombini M, Mannella CA. VDAC, the early days. Biochimica et Biophysica Acta. 2012;**1818**(6):1438-1443. DOI: 10.1016/j.bbamem.2011.11.014

[7] Fulda S, Galluzzi L, Kroemer G. Targeting mitochondria for cancer therapy. Nature Reviews Drug Discovery. 2010;**9**(6):447-464. DOI: 10.1038/nrd3137

[8] Lemasters JJ, Holmuhamedov E. Voltage-dependent anion channel (VDAC) as mitochondrial governator—Thinking outside the box. Biochimica et Biophysica Acta. 2006;**1762**(2):181-190. DOI: 10.1016/j.bbadis.2005.10.006

[9] Li H, Zheng L, Mo Y, Gong Q, Jiang A, Zhao J. Voltage-dependent anion channel 1(VDAC1) participates the apoptosis of the mitochondrial dysfunction in desminopathy. PLoS One. 2016;**11**(12):e0167908. DOI: 10.1371/journal.pone.0167908

[10] Cheng Q, Sedlic F, Pravdic D, Bosnjak ZJ, Kwok WM. Biphasic effect of nitric oxide on the cardiac voltage-dependent anion channel. FEBS Letters. 2011;**585**(2):328-334. DOI: 10.1016/j.febslet.2010.12.008

[11] Vander Heiden MG, Chandel NS, Li XX, Schumacker PT, Colombini M, Thompson CB. Outer mitochondrial membrane permeability can regulate coupled respiration and cell survival. Proceedings of the National Academy of Sciences of the United States of America. 2000;**97**(9):4666-4671. DOI: 10.1073/pnas.090082297

[12] Mannella CA. The 'ins' and 'outs' of mitochondrial membrane channel. Trends in Biochemical Sciences. 1992;**17**(8):315-320. DOI: 10.1016/0968-0004(92)90444-E

[13] Colombini M. VDAC: The channel at the interface between mitochondria and the cytosol. Molecular and Cellular Biochemistry. 2004;**256-257**(1-2):107-15. DOI: 10.1023/B:MCBI.0000009862.17396.8d

[14] Craigen WJ, Graham BH. Genetic strategies for dissecting mammalian and drosophila voltage-dependent anion channel functions. Journal of Bioenergetics and Biomembranes. 2008;**40**(3):207-212. DOI: 10.1007/s10863-008-9146-x

[15] Neumann D, Bückers J, Kastrup L, Hell SW, Jakobs S. Two-color STED microscopy reveals different degrees of colocalization between hexokinase-I and the three human VDAC isoforms. PMC Biophysics. 2010;**3**(1):4. DOI: 10.1186/1757-5036-3-4

[16] Tan W, Colombini M. VDAC closure increases calcium ion flux. Biochimica et Biophysica Acta. 2007;**1768**(10):2510-2515. DOI: 10.1016/j.bbamem.2007.06.002

[17] Porcelli AM, Ghelli A, Zanna C, Pinton P, Rizzuto R, Rugolo M. pH difference across the outer mitochondrial membrane measured with a green fluorescent protein mutant. Biochemical and Biophysical Research Communications. 2005;**326**(4):799-804. DOI: 10.1016/j.bbrc.2004.11.105

[18] Rostovtseva TK, Tan W, Colombini M. On the role of VDAC in apoptosis: Fact and fiction. Journal of Bioenergetics and Biomembranes. 2005;**37**(3):129-142. DOI: 10.1007/s10863-005-6566-8

[19] Rostovtseva TK, Sheldon KL, Hassanzadeh E, Monge C, Saks V, Bezrukov SM, Sackett DL. Tubulin binding blocks mitochondrial voltage-dependent anion channel and regulates respiration. Proceedings of the National Academy of Sciences of the United States of America. 2008;**105**(48):18746-18751. DOI: 10.1073/pnas.0806303105

[20] Brownlees J, Ackerley S, Grierson AJ, Jacobsen NJ, Shea K, Anderton BH, Leigh PN, Shaw CE, Miller CC. Charcot-Marie-tooth disease neurofilament mutations disrupt neurofilament assembly and axonal transport. Human Molecular Genetics. 2002;**11**(23):2837-2844. DOI: 10.1093/hmg/11.23.2837

[21] Pérez-Ollé R, López-Toledano MA, Goryunov D, Cabrera-Poch N, Stefanis L, Brown K, Liem RK. Mutations in the neurofilament light gene linked to Charcot-Marie-tooth disease cause defects in transport. Journal of Neurochemistry. 2005;**93**(4):861-874. DOI: 10.1111/j.1471-4159.2005.03095.x

[22] Milner DJ, Mavroidis M, Weisleder N, Capetanaki Y. Desmin cytoskeleton linked to muscle mitochondrial distribution and respiratory function. The Journal of Cell Biology. 2000;**150**(6):1283-1298. DOI: 10.1083/jcb.150.6.1283

[23] Capetanaki Y. Desmin cytoskeleton: A potential regulator of muscle mitochondrial behavior and function. Trends in Cardiovascular Medicine. 2002;**12**(8):339-348. DOI: 10.1016/S1050-1738(02)00184-6

[24] Uttam J, Hutton E, Coulombe PA, Anton-Lamprecht I, Yu QC, Gedde-Dahl T Jr, Fine JD, Fuchs E. The genetic basis of epidermolysis bullosa simplex with mottled pigmentation. Proceedings of the National Academy of Sciences of the United States of America. 1996;**93**(17):9079-9084. DOI: http://www.jstor.org/stable/40005

[25] Carré M, André N, Carles G, Borghi H, Brichese L, Briand C, Braguer D. Tubulin is an inherent component of mitochondrial membranes that interacts with the voltage-dependent anion channel. The Journal of Biological Chemistry. 2002;**277**(37):33664-33669. DOI: 10.1074/jbc.M203834200

[26] Gurnev PA, Rostovtseva TK, Bezrukov SM. Tubulin-blocked state of VDAC studied by polymer and ATP partitioning. FEBS Letters. 2011;**585**(14):2363-2366. DOI: 10.1016/j.febslet.2011.06.008

[27] Rostovtseva TK, Bezrukov SM. VDAC inhibition by tubulin and its physiological implications. Biochimica et Biophysica Acta. 2012;**1818**(6):1526-1535. DOI: 10.1016/j.bbamem.2011.11.004

[28] Capetanaki Y, Bloch RJ, Kouloumenta A, Mavroidis M, Psarras S. Muscle intermediate filaments and their links to membranes and membranous organelles. Experimental Cell Research. 2007;**313**(10):2063-2076. DOI: 10.1016/j.yexcr.2007.03.033

[29] Fountoulakis M, Soumaka E, Rapti K, Mavroidis M, Tsangaris G, Maris A, Weisleder N, Capetanaki Y. Alterations in the heart mitochondrial proteome in a desmin null heart failure model. Journal of Molecular and Cellular Cardiology. 2005;**38**(3):461-474. DOI: 10.1016/j.yjmcc.2004.12.008

[30] Martindale JJ, Wall JA, Martinez-Longoria DM, Aryal P, Rockman HA, Guo Y, Bolli R, Glembotski CC. Overexpression of mitogen-activated protein kinase kinase 6 in the heart improves functional recovery from ischemia in vitro and protects against myocardial infarction in vivo. The Journal of Biological Chemistry. 2005;**280**(1):669-676. DOI: 10.1074/jbc.M406690200

[31] Maloyan A, Sanbe A, Osinska H, Westfall M, Robinson D, Imahashi K, Murphy E, Robbins J. Mitochondrial dysfunction and apoptosis underlie the pathogenic process in alpha-B-crystallin desmin-related cardiomyopathy. Circulation. 2005;**112**(22):3451-3461. DOI: 10.1161/CIRCULATIONAHA.105.572552

[32] Harner M, Körner C, Walther D, Mokranjac D, Kaesmacher J, Welsch U, Griffith J, Mann M, Reggiori F, Neupert W. The mitochondrial contact site complex, a determinant of mitochondrial architecture. The EMBO Journal. 2011;**30**(21):4356-4370. DOI: 10.1038/emboj.2011.379

[33] Strauss M, Hofhaus G, Schröder RR, Kühlbrandt W. Dimer ribbons of ATP synthase shape the inner mitochondrial membrane. The EMBO Journal. 2008;**27**(7):1154-1160. DOI: 10.1038/emboj.2008.35

[34] Papathanasiou S, Rickelt S, Soriano ME, Schips TG, Maier HJ, Davos CH, Varela A, Kaklamanis L, Mann DL, Capetanaki Y. Tumor necrosis factor-α confers cardioprotection through ectopic expression of keratins K8 and K18. Nature Medicine. 2015;**21**(9):1076-1084. DOI: 10.1038/nm.3925

[35] Psarras S, Mavroidis M, Sanoudou D, Davos CH, Xanthou G, Varela AE, Panoutsakopoulou V, Capetanaki Y. Regulation of adverse remodelling by osteopontin in a genetic heart failure model. European Heart Journal. 2012;**33**(15):1954-1963. DOI: 10.1093/eurheartj/ehr119

[36] Mavroidis M, Davos CH, Psarras S, Varela A, C Athanasiadis N, Katsimpoulas M, Kostavasili I, Maasch C, Vater A, van Tintelen JP, Capetanaki Y. Complement system modulation as a target for treatment of arrhythmogenic cardiomyopathy. Basic Research in Cardiology 2015;**110**(3):27. DOI: 10.1007/s00395-015-0485-6

[37] Capetanaki Y, Papathanasiou S, Diokmetzidou A, Vatsellas G, Tsikitis M. Desmin related disease: A matter of cell survival failure. Current Opinion in Cell Biology. 2015;**32**:113-120. DOI: 10.1016/j.ceb.2015.01.004

[38] van Spaendonck-Zwarts KY, van Hessem L, Jongbloed JD, de Walle HE, Capetanaki Y, van der Kooi AJ, van Langen IM, van den Berg MP, van Tintelen JP. Desmin-related myopathy. Clinical Genetics. 2011;**80**(4):354-366. DOI: 10.1111/j.1399-0004.2010.01512.x

[39] Diokmetzidou A, Soumaka E, Kloukina I, Tsikitis M, Makridakis M, Varela A, Davos CH, Georgopoulos S, Anesti V, Vlahou A, Capetanaki Y. Desmin and αB-crystallin interplay in the maintenance of mitochondrial homeostasis and cardiomyocyte survival. Journal of Cell Science. 2016;**129**(20):3705-3720. DOI: 10.1242/jcs.192203

[40] Chernoivanenko IS, Matveeva EA, Gelfand VI, Goldman RD, Minin AA. Mitochondrial membrane potential is regulated by vimentin intermediate filaments. The FASEB Journal. 2015;**29**(3):820-827. DOI: 10.1096/fj.14-259903

[41] Azoulay-Zohar H, Israelson A, Abu-Hamad S, Shoshan-Barmatz V. In self-defence: Hexokinase promotes voltage-dependent anion channel closure and prevents mitochondria-mediated apoptotic cell death. The Biochemical Journal. 2004;**377**(Pt 2):347-355. DOI: 10.1042/BJ20031465

[42] Winter L, Abrahamsberg C, Wiche G. Plectin isoform 1b mediates mitochondrion-intermediate filament network linkage and controls organelle shape. The Journal of Cell Biology. 2008;**181**(6):903-911. DOI: 10.1083/jcb.200710151

[43] Guzun R, Gonzalez-Granillo M, Karu-Varikmaa M, Grichine A, Usson Y, Kaambre T, Guerrero-Roesch K, Kuznetsov A, Schlattner U, Saks V. Regulation of respiration in muscle cells in vivo by VDAC through interaction with the cytoskeleton and MtCK within mitochondrial Interactosome. Biochimica et Biophysica Acta. 2012;**1818**(6):1545-1554. DOI: 10.1016/j.bbamem.2011.12.034

[44] Mathupala SP, Ko YH, Pedersen PL. Hexokinase-2 bound to mitochondria: cancer's stygian link to the "Warburg effect" and a pivotal target for effective therapy. Seminars in Cancer Biology. 2009;**19**(1):17-24. DOI: 10.1016/j.semcancer.2008.11.006

[45] Pastorino JG, Hoek JB. Regulation of hexokinase binding to VDAC. Journal of Bioenergetics and Biomembranes. 2008;**40**(3):171-182. DOI: 10.1007/s10863-008-9148-8

[46] Gatenby RA, Gillies RJ. Why do cancers have high aerobic glycolysis? Nature Reviews. Cancer. 2004;**4**(11):891-899. DOI: 10.1038/nrc1478

[47] Marín-Hernández A, Rodríguez-Enríquez S, Vital-González PA, Flores-Rodríguez FL, Macías-Silva M, Sosa-Garrocho M, Moreno-Sánchez R. Determining and understanding the control of glycolysis in fast-growth tumor cells. Flux control by an over-expressed but strongly product-inhibited hexokinase. The FEBS Journal. 2006;**273**(9):1975-1988. DOI: 10.1111/j.1742-4658.2006.05214.x

[48] Maldonado EN, Patnaik J, Mullins MR, Lemasters JJ. Free tubulin modulates mitochondrial membrane potential in cancer cells. Cancer Research. 2010;**70**(24):10192-201. DOI: 10.1158/0008-5472.CAN-10-2429

[49] Sun L, Shukair S, Naik TJ, Moazed F, Ardehali H. Glucose phosphorylation and mitochondrial binding are required for the protective effects of hexokinases I and II. Molecular and Cellular Biology. 2008;**28**(3):1007-1017. DOI: 10.1128/MCB.00224-07

[50] Shoshan-Barmatz V, Mizrachi D. VDAC1: From structure to cancer therapy. Frontiers in Oncology. 2012;**2**:164. DOI: 10.3389/fonc.2012.00164

[51] Magnuson MA, Matschinsky FM. Glucokinase as a glucose sensor: Past, present and future. In: Matschinsky FM, Magnuson MA, editors. Glucokinase and Glycemic Disease: From Basics to Novel Therapeutics. Basel: Karger; 2004. pp. 1-17. DOI: 10.1159/000079003

[52] Matschinsky FM. Regulation of pancreatic beta-cell glucokinase: From basics to therapeutics. Diabetes. 2002;**51**(Suppl 3):S394-S404. DOI: 10.2337/diabetes.51.2007.S394

[53] Arden C, Harbottle A, Baltrusch S, Tiedge M, Agius L. Glucokinase is an integral component of the insulin granules in glucose-responsive insulin secretory cells and does not translocate during glucose stimulation. Diabetes. 2004;**53**(9):2346-2352. DOI: 10.2337/diabetes.53.9.2346

[54] Leclercq-Meyer V, Garcia-Martinez JA, Villanueva-Peñacarrillo ML, Valverde I, Malaisse WJ. In vitro and in vivo insulinotropic action of methyl pyruvate. Hormone and Metabolic Research. 1995;**27**(11):477-481. DOI: 10.1055/s-2007-980006

[55] Ahmed M, Muhammed SJ, Kessler B, Salehi A. Mitochondrial proteome analysis reveals altered expression of voltage dependent anion channels in pancreatic β-cells exposed to high glucose. Islets. 2010;**2**(5):283-292. DOI: 10.4161/isl.2.5.12639

[56] Schlattner U, Forstner M, Eder M, Stachowiak O, Fritz-Wolf K, Wallimann T. Functional aspects of the X-ray structure of mitochondrial creatine kinase: A molecular physiology approach. Molecular and Cellular Biochemistry. 1998;**184**(1-2):125-140. DOI: 10.1023/A:1006851330913

[57] Boero J, Qin W, Cheng J, Woolsey TA, Strauss AW, Khuchua Z. Restricted neuronal expression of ubiquitous mitochondrial creatine kinase: Changing patterns in development and with increased activity. Molecular and Cellular Biochemistry. 2003;**244**(1-2): 69-76. DOI: 10.1023/A:1022409101641

[58] Majewski N, Nogueira V, Robey RB, Hay N. Akt inhibits apoptosis downstream of BID cleavage via a glucose-dependent mechanism involving mitochondrial hexokinases. Molecular and Cellular Biology. 2004;**24**(2):730-740. DOI: 10.1128/MCB.24.2.730-740.2004

[59] Vendelin M, Lemba M, Saks VA. Analysis of functional coupling: Mitochondrial creatine kinase and adenine nucleotide translocase. Biophysical Journal. 2004;**87**(1):696-713. DOI: 10.1529/biophysj.103.036210

[60] Rojo M, Hovius R, Demel RA, Nicolay K, Wallimann T. Mitochondrial creatine kinase mediates contact formation between mitochondrial membranes. The Journal of Biological Chemistry. 1991;**266**(30):20290-20295

[61] Schlattner U, Dolder M, Wallimann T, Tokarska-Schlattner M. Mitochondrial creatine kinase and mitochondrial outer membrane porin show a direct interaction that is modulated by calcium. The Journal of Biological Chemistry. 2001;**276**(51):48027-30. DOI: 48027-30

[62] Schlattner U, Tokarska-Schlattner M, Wallimann T. Mitochondrial creatine kinase in human health and disease. Biochimica et Biophysica Acta. 2006;**1762**(2):164-180. DOI: 10.1016/j.bbadis.2005.09.004

[63] Tiivel T, Kadaya L, Kuznetsov A, Käämbre T, Peet N, Sikk P, Braun U, Ventura-Clapier R, Saks V, Seppet EK. Developmental changes in regulation of mitochondrial respiration by ADP and creatine in rat heart in vivo. Molecular and Cellular Biochemistry. 2000;**208**(1-2): 119-128. DOI: 10.1023/A:1007002323492

[64] Wyss M, Smeitink J, Wevers RA, Wallimann T. Mitochondrial creatine kinase: A key enzyme of aerobic energy metabolism. Biochimica et Biophysica Acta. 1992;**1102**(2):119-166. DOI: 10.1016/0005-2728(92)90096-K

[65] Zhang J. Myocardial energetics in cardiac hypertrophy. Clinical and Experimental Pharmacology & Physiology. 2002;**29**(4):351-359. DOI: 10.1046/j.1440-1681.2002.03657.x

[66] Qian XL, Li YQ, Gu F, Liu FF, Li WD, Zhang XM, Fu L. Overexpression of ubiquitous mitochondrial creatine kinase (uMtCK) accelerates tumor growth by inhibiting apoptosis of breast cancer cells and is associated with a poor prognosis in breast cancer patients. Biochemical and Biophysical Research Communications. 2012;**427**(1):60-66. DOI: 10.1016/j.bbrc.2012.08.147

[67] Lemasters JJ, Holmuhamedov EL, Czerny C, Zhong Z, Maldonado EN. Regulation of mitochondrial function by voltage dependent anion channels in ethanol metabolism and the Warburg effect. Biochimica et Biophysica Acta. 2012;**1818**(6):1536-1544. DOI: 10.1016/j.bbamem.2011.11.034

[68] Shoshan-Barmatz V, De Pinto V, Zweckstetter M, Raviv Z, Keinan N, Arbel N. VDAC, a multi-functional mitochondrial protein regulating cell life and death. Molecular Aspects of Medicine. 2010;**31**(3):227-285. DOI: 10.1016/j.mam.2010.03.002

[69] Sheldon KL, Maldonado EN, Lemasters JJ, Rostovtseva TK, Bezrukov SM. Phosphorylation of voltage-dependent anion channel by serine/threonine kinases governs its interaction with tubulin. PLoS One. 2011;**6**(10):e25539. DOI: 10.1371/journal.pone.0025539

[70] Das S, Wong R, Rajapakse N, Murphy E, Steenbergen C. Glycogen synthase kinase 3 inhibition slows mitochondrial adenine nucleotide transport and regulates voltage-dependent anion channel phosphorylation. Circulation Research. 2008;**103**(9):983-991. DOI: 10.1161/CIRCRESAHA.108.178970

[71] Banerjee J, Ghosh S. Bax increases the pore size of rat brain mitochondrial voltage-dependent anion channel in the presence of tBid. Biochemical and Biophysical Research Communications. 2004;**323**(1):310-314. DOI: 10.1016/j.bbrc.2004.08.094

[72] Wang T, Li Y, Wang Y, Zhou R, Ma L, Hao Y, Jin S, Du J, Zhao C, Sun T, Yu J. Lycium barbarum polysaccharide prevents focal cerebral ischemic injury by inhibiting neuronal apoptosis in mice. PLoS One. 2014;**9**(3):e90780. DOI: 10.1371/journal.pone.0090780

[73] Marchitti SA, Brocker C, Stagos D, Vasiliou V. Non-P450 aldehyde oxidizing enzymes: The aldehyde dehydrogenase superfamily. Expert Opinion on Drug Metabolism & Toxicology. 2008;**4**(6):697-720. DOI: 10.1517/17425255.4.6.697

[74] Yuki T, Thurman RG. The swift increase in alcohol metabolism. Time course for the increase in hepatic oxygen uptake and the involvement of glycolysis. The Biochemical Journal. 1980;**186**(1):119-126

[75] Bradford BU, Rusyn I. Swift increase in alcohol metabolism (SIAM): Understanding the phenomenon of hypermetabolism in liver. Alcohol. 2005;**35**(1):13-17. DOI: 10.1016/j.alcohol.2004.12.001

[76] Lieber CS. Alcoholic fatty liver: Its pathogenesis and mechanism of progression to inflammation and fibrosis. Alcohol. 2004;**34**(1):9-19. DOI: 10.1016/j.alcohol.2004.07.008

[77] Adachi M, Ishii H. Role of mitochondria in alcoholic liver injury. Free Radical Biology & Medicine. 2002;**32**(6):487-491. DOI: 10.1016/S0891-5849(02)00740-2

[78] Bartlett K, Eaton S. Mitochondrial beta-oxidation. European Journal of Biochemistry. 2004;**271**(3):462-469. DOI: 10.1046/j.1432-1033.2003.03947.x

[79] Grigoriev SM, Muro C, Dejean LM, Campo ML, Martinez-Caballero S, Kinnally KW. Electrophysiological approaches to the study of protein translocation in mitochondria. International Review of Cytology. 2004;**238**:227-274. DOI: 10.1016/S0074-7696(04)38005-8

[80] Endo T, Yamano K. Multiple pathways for mitochondrial protein traffic. Biological Chemistry. 2009;**390**(8):723-730. DOI: 10.1515/BC.2009.087

[81] Chacinska A, Koehler CM, Milenkovic D, Lithgow T, Pfanner N. Importing mitochondrial proteins: Machineries and mechanisms. Cell. 2009;**138**(4):628-644. DOI: 10.1016/j.cell.2009.08.005

[82] Maćasev D, Whelan J, Newbigin E, Silva-Filho MC, Mulhern TD, Lithgow T. Tom22', an 8-kDa trans-site receptor in plants and protozoans, is a conserved feature of the TOM complex that appeared early in the evolution of eukaryotes. Molecular Biology and Evolution. 2007;**21**(8):1557-1564. DOI: 10.1093/molbev/msh166

[83] Bhangoo MK, Tzankov S, Fan AC, Dejgaard K, Thomas DY, Young JC. Multiple 40-kDa heat-shock protein chaperones function in Tom70-dependent mitochondrial import. Molecular Biology of the Cell. 2007;**18**(9):3414-3428. DOI: 10.1091/mbc.E07-01-0088

[84] Murakami H, Pain D, Blobel G. 70-kD heat shock-related protein is one of at least two distinct cytosolic factors stimulating protein import into mitochondria. The Journal of Cell Biology. 1988;**107**(6 Pt 1):2051-2057

[85] Komiya T, Sakaguchi M, Mihara K. Cytoplasmic chaperones determine the targeting pathway of precursor proteins to mitochondria. The EMBO Journal. 1996;**15**(2):399-407

[86] Endo T, Yamano K. Transport of proteins across or into the mitochondrial outer membrane. Biochimica et Biophysica Acta. 2010;**1806**(6):706-714. DOI: 10.1016/j.bbamcr.2009.11.007

[87] Bender A, Desplats P, Spencer B, Rockenstein E, Adame A, Elstner M, Laub C, Mueller S, Koob AO, Mante M, Pham E, Klopstock T, Masliah E. TOM40 mediates mitochondrial dysfunction induced by α-synuclein accumulation in Parkinson's disease. PLoS One. 2013;**8**(4):e62277. DOI: 10.1371/journal.pone.0062277

[88] Devi L, Prabhu BM, Galati DF, Avadhani NG, Anandatheerthavarada HK. Accumulation of amyloid precursor protein in the mitochondrial import channels of human Alzheimer's disease brain is associated with mitochondrial dysfunction. The Journal of Neuroscience. 2006;**26**(35):9057-9068. DOI: 10.1523/JNEUROSCI.1469-06.2006

[89] MacKenzie JA, Payne RM. Mitochondrial protein import and human health and disease. Biochimica et Biophysica Acta. 2007;**1772**(5):509-523. DOI: 10.1016/j.bbadis.2006.12.002

[90] O'Rourke B. Mitochondrial ion channels. Annual Review of Physiology. 2007;**69**:19-49. DOI: 10.1146/annurev.physiol.69.031905.163804

[91] Mitchell P, Moyle J. Respiration-driven proton translocation in rat liver mitochondria. The Biochemical Journal. 1967;**105**(3):1147-1162

[92] Garlid KD. Cation transport in mitochondria—The potassium cycle. Biochimica et Biophysica Acta. 1996;**1275**(1-2):123-126

[93] Saraste M, Walker JE. Internal sequence repeats and the path of polypeptide in mitochondrial ADP/ATP translocase. FEBS Letters. 1982;**144**(2):250-254

[94] Nelson DR, Felix CM, Swanson JM. Highly conserved charge-pair networks in the mitochondrial carrier family. Journal of Molecular Biology. 1998;**277**(2):285-308. DOI: 10.1006/jmbi.1997.1594

[95] Kunji ER. The role and structure of mitochondrial carriers. FEBS Letters. 2004;**564**(3):239-244. DOI: 10.1016/S0014-5793(04)00242-X

[96] Casimir M, Lasorsa FM, Rubi B, Caille D, Palmieri F, Meda P, Maechler P. Mitochondrial glutamate carrier GC1 as a newly identified player in the control of glucose-stimulated insulin secretion. The Journal of Biological Chemistry. 2009;**284**(37):25004-25014. DOI: 10.1074/jbc.M109.015495

[97] Palmieri F. Diseases caused by defects of mitochondrial carriers: A review. Biochimica et Biophysica Acta. 2008;**1777**(7-8):564-578. DOI: 10.1016/j.bbabio.2008.03.008

[98] Krämer R, Klingenberg M. Reconstitution of adenine nucleotide transport with purified ADP, ATP-carrier protein. FEBS Letters. 1977;**82**(2):363-367

[99] Prohl C, Pelzer W, Diekert K, Kmita H, Bedekovics T, Kispal G, Lill R. The yeast mitochondrial carrier Leu5p and its human homologue Graves' disease protein are required for accumulation of coenzyme A in the matrix. Molecular and Cellular Biology. 2001;**21**(4):1089-1097. DOI: 10.1128/MCB.21.4.1089-1097.2001

[100] Vozza A, Blanco E, Palmieri L, Palmieri F. Identification of the mitochondrial GTP/GDP transporter in Saccharomyces cerevisiae. The Journal of Biological Chemistry. 2004;**279**(20):20850-20857. DOI: 10.1074/jbc.M313610200

[101] Marobbio CM, Agrimi G, Lasorsa FM, Palmieri F. Identification and functional reconstitution of yeast mitochondrial carrier for S-adenosylmethionine. The EMBO Journal. 2003;**22**(22):5975-5982. DOI: 10.1093/emboj/cdg574

[102] Marobbio CM, Di Noia MA, Palmieri F. Identification of a mitochondrial transporter for pyrimidine nucleotides in *Saccharomyces cerevisiae*: Bacterial expression, reconstitution and functional characterization. The Biochemical Journal. 2006;**393**(Pt 2):441-446. DOI: 10.1042/BJ20051284

[103] Dolce V, Fiermonte G, Runswick MJ, Palmieri F, Walker JE. The human mitochondrial deoxynucleotide carrier and its role in the toxicity of nucleoside antivirals. Proceedings of the National Academy of Sciences of the United States of America. 2001;**98**(5):2284-2288. DOI: 10.1073/pnas.031430998

[104] Lindhurst MJ, Fiermonte G, Song S, Struys E, De Leonardis F, Schwartzberg PL, Chen A, Castegna A, Verhoeven N, Mathews CK, Palmieri F, Biesecker LG. Knockout of Slc25a19 causes mitochondrial thiamine pyrophosphate depletion, embryonic lethality, CNS malformations, and anemia. Proceedings of the National Academy of Sciences of the United States of America. 2006;**103**(43):15927-15932. DOI: 10.1073/pnas.0607661103

[105] Dolce V, Scarcia P, Iacopetta D, Palmieri F. A fourth ADP/ATP carrier isoform in man: Identification, bacterial expression, functional characterization and tissue distribution. FEBS Letters. 2005;**579**(3):633-637. DOI: 10.1016/j.febslet.2004.12.034

[106] Brand MD, Pakay JL, Ocloo A, Kokoszka J, Wallace DC, Brookes PS, Cornwall EJ. The basal proton conductance of mitochondria depends on adenine nucleotide translocase content. The Biochemical Journal. 2005;**392**(Pt 2):353-362. DOI: 10.1042/BJ20050890

[107] Samartsev VN, Mokhova EN, Skulachev VP. The pH-dependent reciprocal changes in contributions of ADP/ATP antiporter and aspartate/glutamate antiporter to the fatty acid-induced uncoupling. FEBS Letters. 1997;**412**(1):179-182

[108] Vander Heiden MG, Chandel NS, Schumacker PT, Thompson CB. Bcl-xL prevents cell death following growth factor withdrawal by facilitating mitochondrial ATP/ADP exchange. Molecular Cell. 1999;**3**(2):159-167

[109] Bernardi P, Rasola A, Forte M, Lippe G. The mitochondrial permeability transition pore: Channel formation by F-ATP synthase, integration in signal transduction, and role in pathophysiology. Physiological Reviews. 2015;**95**(4):1111-1155. DOI: 10.1152/physrev.00001.2015

[110] Bernardi P, Krauskopf A, Basso E, Petronilli V, Blachly-Dyson E, Di Lisa F, Forte MA. The mitochondrial permeability transition from in vitro artifact to disease target. The FEBS Journal. 2006;**273**(10):2077-2099. DOI: 10.1111/j.1742-4658.2006.05213.x

[111] Rasola A, Bernardi P. Mitochondrial permeability transition in Ca^{2+}-dependent apoptosis and necrosis. Cell Calcium. 2011;**50**(3):222-233. DOI: 10.1016/j.ceca.2011.04.007

[112] Petronilli V, Penzo D, Scorrano L, Bernardi P, Di Lisa F. The mitochondrial permeability transition, release of cytochrome c and cell death. Correlation with the duration of pore openings in situ. The Journal of Biological Chemistry. 2001;**276**(15):12030-12034. DOI: 10.1074/jbc.M010604200

[113] Zorov DB, Juhaszova M, Sollott SJ. Mitochondrial reactive oxygen species (ROS) and ROS-induced ROS release. Physiological Reviews. 2014;**94**(3):909-950. DOI: 10.1152/physrev.00026.2013

[114] Hao W, Chang CP, Tsao CC, Xu J. Oligomycin-induced bioenergetic adaptation in cancer cells with heterogeneous bioenergetic organization. The Journal of Biological Chemistry. 2010;**285**(17):12647-12654. DOI: 10.1074/jbc.M109.084194

[115] Chevrollier A, Loiseau D, Chabi B, Renier G, Douay O, Malthièry Y, Stepien G. ANT2 isoform required for cancer cell glycolysis. Journal of Bioenergetics and Biomembranes. 2005;**37**(5):307-316. DOI: 10.1007/s10863-005-8642-5

[116] Le Bras M, Borgne-Sanchez A, Touat Z, El Dein OS, Deniaud A, Maillier E, Lecellier G, Rebouillat D, Lemaire C, Kroemer G, Jacotot E, Brenner C. Chemosensitization by knockdown of adenine nucleotide translocase-2. Cancer Research. 2006;**66**(18):9143-9152. DOI: 10.1158/0008-5472.CAN-05-4407

[117] Chinopoulos C, Adam-Vizi V. Mitochondria as ATP consumers in cellular pathology. Biochimica et Biophysica Acta. 2010;**1802**(1):221-227. DOI: 10.1016/j.bbadis.2009.08.008

[118] Garedew A, Henderson SO, Moncada S. Activated macrophages utilize glycolytic ATP to maintain mitochondrial membrane potential and prevent apoptotic cell death. Cell Death and Differentiation. 2017;**242**(6):1132. DOI: 10.1038/cdd.2010.27

[119] Roussel D, Chainier F, Rouanet J, Barré H. Increase in the adenine nucleotide translocase content of duckling subsarcolemmal mitochondria during cold acclimation. FEBS Letters. 2000;**477**(1-2):141-144. DOI: 10.1016/S0014-5793(00)01790-7

[120] Woldegiorgis G, Yousufzai SY, Shrago E. Studies on the interaction of palmitoyl coenzyme A with the adenine nucleotide translocase. The Journal of Biological Chemistry. 1982;**257**(24):14783-14787

[121] Franch J, Knudsen J, Ellis BA, Pedersen PK, Cooney GJ, Jensen J. Acyl-CoA binding protein expression is fiber type-specific and elevated in muscles from the obese insulin-resistant Zucker rat. Diabetes. 2002;**51**(2):449-454. DOI: 10.2337/diabetes.51.2.449

[122] Ciapaite J, Bakker SJ, Diamant M, van Eikenhorst G, Heine RJ, Westerhoff HV, Krab K. Metabolic control of mitochondrial properties by adenine nucleotide translocator determines palmitoyl-CoA effects. Implications for a mechanism linking obesity and type 2 diabetes. The FEBS Journal. 2006;**273**(23):5288-5302. DOI: 10.1111/j.1742-4658.2006.05523.x

[123] Echaniz-Laguna A, Chassagne M, Ceresuela J, Rouvet I, Padet S, Acquaviva C, Nataf S, Vinzio S, Bozon D, Mousson de Camaret B. Complete loss of expression of the ANT1 gene causing cardiomyopathy and myopathy. Journal of Medical Genetics. 2012;**49**(2):146-150. DOI: 10.1136/jmedgenet-2011-100504

[124] Körver-Keularts IM, de Visser M, Bakker HD, Wanders RJ, Vansenne F, Scholte HR, Dorland L, Nicolaes GA, Spaapen LM, Smeets HJ, Hendrickx AT, van den Bosch BJ. Two novel mutations in the SLC25A4 gene in a patient with mitochondrial myopathy. JIMD Reports. 2015;**22**:39-45. DOI: 10.1007/8904_2015_409

[125] Siciliano G, Tessa A, Petrini S, Mancuso M, Bruno C, Grieco GS, Malandrini A, DeFlorio L, Martini B, Federico A, Nappi G, Santorelli FM, Murri L. Autosomal dominant external ophthalmoplegia and bipolar affective disorder associated with a mutation in the ANT1 gene. Neuromuscular Disorders. 2003;**13**(2):162-165. DOI: 10.1016/S0960-8966(02)00221-3

[126] Deschauer M, Hudson G, Müller T, Taylor RW, Chinnery PF, Zierz S. A novel ANT1 gene mutation with probable germline mosaicism in autosomal dominant progressive external ophthalmoplegia. Neuromuscular Disorders. 2005;**15**(4):311-315. DOI: 10.1016/j.nmd.2004.12.004

[127] Thompson K, Majd H, Dallabona C, Reinson K, King MS, Alston CL, He L, Lodi T, Jones SA, Fattal-Valevski A, Fraenkel ND, Saada A, Haham A, Isohanni P, Vara R, Barbosa IA, Simpson MA, Deshpande C, Puusepp S, Bonnen PE, Rodenburg RJ, Suomalainen A, Õunap K, Elpeleg O, Ferrero I, McFarland R, Kunji ER, Taylor RW. Recurrent de novo

dominant mutations in SLC25A4 cause severe early-onset mitochondrial disease and loss of mitochondrial DNA copy number. American Journal of Human Genetics. 2016;**99**(4):860-876. DOI: 10.1016/j.ajhg.2016.08.014

[128] Huizing M, Ruitenbeek W, van den Heuvel LP, Dolce V, Iacobazzi V, Smeitink JA, Palmieri F, Trijbels JM. Human mitochondrial transmembrane metabolite carriers: Tissue distribution and its implication for mitochondrial disorders. Journal of Bioenergetics and Biomembranes. 1998;**30**(3):277-284

[129] Mayr JA, Zimmermann FA, Horváth R, Schneider HC, Schoser B, Holinski-Feder E, Czermin B, Freisinger P, Sperl W. Deficiency of the mitochondrial phosphate carrier presenting as myopathy and cardiomyopathy in a family with three affected children. Neuromuscular Disorders. 2011;**21**(11):803-808. DOI: 10.1016/j.nmd.2011.06.005

[130] Mayr JA, Merkel O, Kohlwein SD, Gebhardt BR, Böhles H, Fötschl U, Koch J, Jaksch M, Lochmüller H, Horváth R, Freisinger P, Sperl W. Mitochondrial phosphate-carrier deficiency: A novel disorder of oxidative phosphorylation. American Journal of Human Genetics. 2007;**80**(3):478-484. DOI: 10.1086/511788

[131] Varanyuwatana P, Halestrap AP. The roles of phosphate and the phosphate carrier in the mitochondrial permeability transition pore. Mitochondrion. 2012;**12**(1):120-125. DOI: 10.1016/j.mito.2011.04.006

[132] Quistorff B, Grunnet N. The isoenzyme pattern of LDH does not play a physiological role; except perhaps during fast transitions in energy metabolism. Aging (Albany NY). 2011;**3**(5):457-460. DOI: 10.18632/aging.100329

[133] Bricker DK, Taylor EB, Schell JC, Orsak T, Boutron A, Chen YC, Cox JE, Cardon CM, Van Vranken JG, Dephoure N, Redin C, Boudina S, Gygi SP, Brivet M, Thummel CS, Rutter J. A mitochondrial pyruvate carrier required for pyruvate uptake in yeast, drosophila, and humans. Science. 2012;**337**(6090):96-100. DOI: 10.1126/science.1218099

[134] Herzig S, Raemy E, Montessuit S, Veuthey JL, Zamboni N, Westermann B, Kunji ER, Martinou JC. Identification and functional expression of the mitochondrial pyruvate carrier. Science. 2012;**337**(6090):93-96. DOI: 10.1126/science.1218530

[135] Jézégou A, Llinares E, Anne C, Kieffer-Jaquinod S, O'Regan S, Aupetit J, Chabli A, Sagné C, Debacker C, Chadefaux-Vekemans B, Journet A, André B, Gasnier B. Heptahelical protein PQLC2 is a lysosomal cationic amino acid exporter underlying the action of cysteamine in cystinosis therapy. Proceedings of the National Academy of Sciences of the United States of America. 2012;**109**(50):E3434-E3443. DOI: 10.1073/pnas.1211198109

[136] Saudek V. Cystinosin, MPDU1, SWEETs and KDELR belong to a well-defined protein family with putative function of cargo receptors involved in vesicle trafficking. PLoS One. 2012;**7**(2):e30876. DOI: 10.1371/journal.pone.0030876

[137] Halestrap AP. Pyruvate and ketone-body transport across the mitochondrial membrane. Exchange properties, pH-dependence and mechanism of the carrier. The Biochemical Journal. 1978;**172**(3):377-387

[138] Patel MS, Korotchkina LG, Sidhu S. Interaction of E1 and E3 components with the core proteins of the human pyruvate dehydrogenase complex. Journal of Molecular Catalysis B: Enzymatic. 2009;**61**(1-2):2-6. DOI: 10.1016/j.molcatb.2009.05.001

[139] Halestrap AP, Denton RM. The specificity and metabolic implications of the inhibition of pyruvate transport in isolated mitochondria and intact tissue preparations by alpha-cyano-4-hydroxycinnamate and related compounds. The Biochemical Journal. 1975;**148**(1):97-106

[140] Halestrap AP, Brand MD, Denton RM. Inhibition of mitochondrial pyruvate transport by phenylpyruvate and alpha-ketoisocaproate. Biochimica et Biophysica Acta. 1974;**367**(1):102-108

[141] Deng WJ, Nie S, Dai J, JR W, Zeng R. Proteome, phosphoproteome, and hydroxyproteome of liver mitochondria in diabetic rats at early pathogenic stages. Molecular & Cellular Proteomics. 2010;**9**(1):100-116. DOI: 10.1074/mcp.M900020-MCP200

[142] Vacanti NM, Divakaruni AS, Green CR, Parker SJ, Henry RR, Ciaraldi TP, Murphy AN, Metallo CM. Regulation of substrate utilization by the mitochondrial pyruvate carrier. Molecular Cell. 2014;**56**(3):425-435. DOI: 10.1016/j.molcel.2014.09.024

[143] McCommis KS, Finck BN. Mitochondrial pyruvate transport: A historical perspective and future research directions. The Biochemical Journal. 2015;**466**(3):443-454. DOI: 10.1042/BJ20141171

[144] Upadhyay M, Samal J, Kandpal M, Singh OV, Vivekanandan P. The Warburg effect: Insights from the past decade. Pharmacology & Therapeutics. 2013;**137**(3):318-330. DOI: 10.1016/j.pharmthera.2012.11.003

[145] Tsai YP, Wu KJ. Hypoxia-regulated target genes implicated in tumor metastasis. Journal of Biomedical Science. 2012;**19**:102. DOI: 10.1186/1423-0127-19-102

[146] Boidot R, Végran F, Meulle A, Le Breton A, Dessy C, Sonveaux P, Lizard-Nacol S, Feron O. Regulation of monocarboxylate transporter MCT1 expression by p53 mediates inward and outward lactate fluxes in tumors. Cancer Research. 2012;**72**(4):939-948. DOI: 10.1158/0008-5472.CAN-11-2474

[147] Schell JC, Olson KA, Jiang L, Hawkins AJ, Van Vranken JG, Xie J, Egnatchik RA, Earl EG, DeBerardinis RJ, Rutter J. A role for the mitochondrial pyruvate carrier as a repressor of the Warburg effect and colon cancer cell growth. Molecular Cell. 2014;**56**(3):400-413. DOI: 10.1016/j.molcel.2014.09.026

[148] Ahmed SS, Santosh W, Kumar S, Christlet HT. Metabolic profiling of Parkinson's disease: Evidence of biomarker from gene expression analysis and rapid neural network detection. Journal of Biomedical Science. 2009;**16**:63. DOI: 10.1186/1423-0127-16-63

[149] Martin E, Rosenthal RE, Fiskum G. Pyruvate dehydrogenase complex: Metabolic link to ischemic brain injury and target of oxidative stress. Journal of Neuroscience Research. 2005;**79**(1-2):240-247. DOI: 10.1002/jnr.20293

[150] Bolaños JP, Almeida A, Moncada S. Glycolysis: A bioenergetic or a survival pathway? Trends in Biochemical Sciences. 2010;**35**(3):145-149. DOI: 10.1016/j.tibs.2009.10.006

[151] Divakaruni AS, Wallace M, Buren C, Martyniuk K, Andreyev AY, Li E, Fields JA, Cordes T, Reynolds IJ, Bloodgood BL, Raymond LA, Metallo CM, Murphy AN. Inhibition of the mitochondrial pyruvate carrier protects from excitotoxic neuronal death. The Journal of Cell Biology. 2017;**216**(4):1091-1105. DOI: 10.1083/jcb.201612067

[152] Vigueira PA, McCommis KS, Schweitzer GG, Remedi MS, Chambers KT, Fu X, McDonald WG, Cole SL, Colca JR, Kletzien RF, Burgess SC, Finck BN. Mitochondrial pyruvate carrier 2 hypomorphism in mice leads to defects in glucose-stimulated insulin secretion. Cell Reports. 2014;**7**(6):2042-2053. DOI: 10.1016/j.celrep.2014.05.017

[153] Stanley WC, Recchia FA, Lopaschuk GD. Myocardial substrate metabolism in the normal and failing heart. Physiological Reviews. 2005;**85**(3):1093-1129. DOI: 10.1152/physrev.00006.2004

[154] Paradies G, Petrosillo G, Gadaleta MN, Ruggiero FM. The effect of aging and acetyl-L-carnitine on the pyruvate transport and oxidation in rat heart mitochondria. FEBS Letters. 1999;**454**(3):207-209. DOI: 10.1016/S0014-5793(99)00809-1

[155] Abdel-Aleem S, El-Merzabani MM, Sayed-Ahmed M, Taylor DA, Lowe JE. Acute and chronic effects of adriamycin on fatty acid oxidation in isolated cardiac myocytes. Journal of Molecular and Cellular Cardiology. 1997;**29**(2):789-797. DOI: 10.1006/jmcc.1996.0323

[156] Huypens P, Pillai R, Sheinin T, Schaefer S, Huang M, Odegaard ML, Ronnebaum SM, Wettig SD, Joseph JW. The dicarboxylate carrier plays a role in mitochondrial malate transport and in the regulation of glucose-stimulated insulin secretion from rat pancreatic beta cells. Diabetologia. 2011;**54**(1):135-145. DOI: 10.1007/s00125-010-1923-5

[157] Monné M, Miniero DV, Iacobazzi V, Bisaccia F, Fiermonte G. The mitochondrial oxoglutarate carrier: From identification to mechanism. Journal of Bioenergetics and Biomembranes. 2013;**45**(1-2):1-13. DOI: 10.1007/s10863-012-9475-7

[158] Gnoni GV, Priore P, Geelen MJ, Siculella L. The mitochondrial citrate carrier: Metabolic role and regulation of its activity and expression. IUBMB Life. 2009;**61**(10):987-994. DOI: 10.1002/iub.249

[159] Chakravarty K, Cassuto H, Reshef L, Hanson RW. Factors that control the tissue-specific transcription of the gene for phosphoenolpyruvate carboxykinase-C. Critical Reviews in Biochemistry and Molecular Biology. 2005;**40**(3):129-154. DOI: 10.1080/10409230590935479

[160] Dolce V, Cappello AR, Capobianco L. Mitochondrial tricarboxylate and dicarboxylate-tricarboxylate carriers: From animals to plants. IUBMB Life. 2014;**66**(7):462-471. DOI: 10.1002/iub.1290

[161] Morciano P, Carrisi C, Capobianco L, Mannini L, Burgio G, Cestra G, De Benedetto GE, Corona DF, Musio A, Cenci G. A conserved role for the mitochondrial citrate transporter Sea/SLC25A1 in the maintenance of chromosome integrity. Human Molecular Genetics. 2009;**18**(21):4180-4188. DOI: 10.1093/hmg/ddp370

[162] Joseph JW, Jensen MV, Ilkayeva O, Palmieri F, Alárcon C, Rhodes CJ, Newgard CB. The mitochondrial citrate/isocitrate carrier plays a regulatory role in glucose-stimulated insulin secretion. The Journal of Biological Chemistry. 2006;**281**(47):35624-35632. DOI: 10.1074/jbc.M602606200

[163] Siculella L, Sabetta S, di Summa R, Leo M, Giudetti AM, Palmieri F, Gnoni GV. Starvation-induced posttranscriptional control of rat liver mitochondrial citrate carrier expression. Biochemical and Biophysical Research Communications. 2002;**299**(3):418-423. DOI: 10.1016/S0006-291X(02)02666-9

[164] Siculella L, Sabetta S, Damiano F, Giudetti AM, Gnoni GV. Different dietary fatty acids have dissimilar effects on activity and gene expression of mitochondrial tricarboxylate carrier in rat liver. FEBS Letters. 2004;**578**(3):280-284. DOI: 10.1016/j.febslet.2004.11.014

[165] Stoffel M, Karayiorgou M, Espinosa R 3rd, Beau MM. The human mitochondrial citrate transporter gene (SLC20A3) maps to chromosome band 22q11 within a region implicated in DiGeorge syndrome, velo-cardio-facial syndrome and schizophrenia. Human Genetics. 1996;**98**(1):113-115

[166] Smith A, McBride S, Marcadier JL, Michaud J, Al-Dirbashi OY, Schwartzentruber J, Beaulieu CL, Katz SL, FORGE Canada Consortium, Majewski J, Bulman DE, Geraghty MT, Harper ME, Chakraborty P, Lines MA. Severe neonatal presentation of mitochondrial citrate carrier (SLC25A1) deficiency. JIMD Reports. 2016;**30**:73-79. DOI: 10.1007/8904_2016_536

[167] Cheng L, Lu W, Kulkarni B, Pejovic T, Yan X, Chiang JH, Hood L, Odunsi K, Lin B. Analysis of chemotherapy response programs in ovarian cancers by the next-generation sequencing technologies. Gynecologic Oncology. 2010;**117**(2):159-169. DOI: 10.1016/j.ygyno.2010.01.041

[168] Mizuarai S, Miki S, Araki H, Takahashi K, Kotani H. Identification of dicarboxylate carrier Slc25a10 as malate transporter in de novo fatty acid synthesis. The Journal of Biological Chemistry. 2005;**280**(37):32434-32441. DOI: 10.1074/jbc.M503152200

[169] Kamga CK, Zhang SX, Wang Y. Dicarboxylate carrier-mediated glutathione transport is essential for reactive oxygen species homeostasis and normal respiration in rat brain mitochondria. American Journal of Physiology. Cell Physiology. 2010;**299**(2):C497-C505. DOI: 10.1152/ajpcell.00058.2010

[170] Kaplan RS, Mayor JA, Blackwell R, Wilson GL, Schaffer SW. Functional levels of mitochondrial anion transport proteins in non-insulin-dependent diabetes mellitus. Molecular and Cellular Biochemistry. 1991;**107**(1):79-86

[171] Cione E, Pingitore A, Perri M, Genchi G. Influence of all-trans-retinoic acid on oxoglutarate carrier via retinoylation reaction. Biochimica et Biophysica Acta. 2009;**1791**(1):3-7. DOI: 10.1016/j.bbalip.2008.09.004

[172] Coll O, Colell A, García-Ruiz C, Kaplowitz N, Fernández-Checa JC. Sensitivity of the 2-oxoglutarate carrier to alcohol intake contributes to mitochondrial glutathione depletion. Hepatology. 2003;**38**(3):692-702. DOI: 10.1053/jhep.2003.50351

[173] Barrey E, Jayr L, Mucher E, Gospodnetic S, Joly F, Benech P, Alibert O, Gidrol X, Mata X, Vaiman A, Guérin G. Transcriptome analysis of muscle in horses suffering from recurrent exertional rhabdomyolysis revealed energetic pathway alterations and disruption in the cytosolic calcium regulation. Animal Genetics. 2012;**43**(3):271-281. DOI: 10.1111/j.1365-2052.2011.02246.x

[174] Fiermonte G, Palmieri L, Todisco S, Agrimi G, Palmieri F, Walker JE. Identification of the mitochondrial glutamate transporter. Bacterial expression, reconstitution, functional characterization, and tissue distribution of two human isoforms. The Journal of Biological Chemistry. 2002;**277**(22):19289-19294. DOI: 10.1074/jbc.M201572200

[175] Antinozzi PA, Ishihara H, Newgard CB, Wollheim CB. Mitochondrial metabolism sets the maximal limit of fuel-stimulated insulin secretion in a model pancreatic beta cell: A survey of four fuel secretagogues. The Journal of Biological Chemistry. 2002;**277**(14):11746-11755. DOI: 10.1074/jbc.M108462200

[176] Frigerio F, Casimir M, Carobbio S, Maechler P. Tissue specificity of mitochondrial glutamate pathways and the control of metabolic homeostasis. Biochimica et Biophysica Acta. 2008;**1777**(7-8):965-972. DOI: 10.1016/j.bbabio.2008.04.031

[177] Bai L, Zhang X, Ghishan FK. Characterization of vesicular glutamate transporter in pancreatic alpha- and beta-cells and its regulation by glucose. American Journal of Physiology. Gastrointestinal and Liver Physiology. 2003;**284**(5):G808-G814. DOI: 10.1152/ajpgi.00333.2002

[178] Storto M, Capobianco L, Battaglia G, Molinaro G, Gradini R, Riozzi B, Di Mambro A, Mitchell KJ, Bruno V, Vairetti MP, Rutter GA, Nicoletti F. Insulin secretion is controlled by mGlu5 metabotropic glutamate receptors. Molecular Pharmacology. 2006;**69**(4):1234-1241. DOI: 10.1124/mol.105.018390

[179] Kowluru A, Chen HQ, Modrick LM, Stefanelli C. Activation of acetyl-CoA carboxylase by a glutamate- and magnesium-sensitive protein phosphatase in the islet beta-cell. Diabetes. 2001;**50**(7):1580-1587. DOI: 10.2337/diabetes.50.7.1580

[180] Berkich DA, Ola MS, Cole J, Sweatt AJ, Hutson SM, LaNoue KF. Mitochondrial transport proteins of the brain. Journal of Neuroscience Research. 2007;**85**(15):3367-3377. DOI: 10.1002/jnr.21500

[181] Goubert E, Mircheva Y, Lasorsa FM, Melon C, Profilo E, Sutera J, Becq H, Palmieri F, Palmieri L, Aniksztejn L, Molinari F. Inhibition of the mitochondrial glutamate carrier SLC25A22 in astrocytes leads to intracellular glutamate accumulation. Frontiers in Cellular Neuroscience. 2017;**11**:149. DOI: 10.3389/fncel.2017.00149

[182] Molinari F, Kaminska A, Fiermonte G, Boddaert N, Raas-Rothschild A, Plouin P, Palmieri L, Brunelle F, Palmieri F, Dulac O, Munnich A, Colleaux L. Mutations in the mitochondrial glutamate carrier SLC25A22 in neonatal epileptic encephalopathy with suppression bursts. Clinical Genetics. 2009;**76**(2):188-194. DOI: 10.1111/j.1399-0004.2009.01236.x

[183] Molinari F, Raas-Rothschild A, Rio M, Fiermonte G, Encha-Razavi F, Palmieri L, Palmieri F, Ben-Neriah Z, Kadhom N, Vekemans M, Attie-Bitach T, Munnich A, Rustin P,

Colleaux L. Impaired mitochondrial glutamate transport in autosomal recessive neonatal myoclonic epilepsy. American Journal of Human Genetics. 2005;**76**(2):334-339. DOI: 10.1086/427564

[184] Poduri A, Heinzen EL, Chitsazzadeh V, Lasorsa FM, Elhosary PC, LaCoursiere CM, Martin E, Yuskaitis CJ, Hill RS, Atabay KD, Barry B, Partlow JN, Bashiri FA, Zeidan RM, Elmalik SA, Kabiraj MM, Kothare S, Stödberg T, McTague A, Kurian MA, Scheffer IE, Barkovich AJ, Palmieri F, Salih MA, Walsh CA. SLC25A22 is a novel gene for migrating partial seizures in infancy. Annals of Neurology. 2013;**74**(6):873-882. DOI: 10.1002/ana.23998

[185] Lasorsa FM, Pinton P, Palmieri L, Fiermonte G, Rizzuto R, Palmieri F. Recombinant expression of the Ca^{2+}-sensitive aspartate/glutamate carrier increases mitochondrial ATP production in agonist-stimulated Chinese hamster ovary cells. The Journal of Biological Chemistry. 2003;**278**(40):38686-38692. DOI: 10.1074/jbc.M304988200

[186] Quinlan CL, Treberg JR, Perevoshchikova IV, Orr AL, Brand MD. Native rates of superoxide production from multiple sites in isolated mitochondria measured using endogenous reporters. Free Radical Biology & Medicine. 2012;**53**(9):1807-1817. DOI: 10.1016/j.freeradbiomed.2012.08.015

[187] Amoedo ND, Punzi G, Obre E, Lacombe D, De Grassi A, Pierri CL, Rossignol R. AGC1/2, the mitochondrial aspartate-glutamate carriers. Biochimica et Biophysica Acta. 2016;**1863**(10):2394-2412. DOI: 10.1016/j.bbamcr.2016.04.011

[188] Palmieri F. The mitochondrial transporter family SLC25: Identification, properties and physiopathology. Molecular Aspects of Medicine. 2013;**34**(2-3):465-484. DOI: 10.1016/j.mam.2012.05.005

[189] Xu Y, Ola MS, Berkich DA, Gardner TW, Barber AJ, Palmieri F, Hutson SM, LaNoue KF. Energy sources for glutamate neurotransmission in the retina: Absence of the aspartate/glutamate carrier produces reliance on glycolysis in glia. Journal of Neurochemistry. 2007;**101**(1):120-131. DOI: 10.1111/j.1471-4159.2006.04349.x

[190] Menga A, Iacobazzi V, Infantino V, Avantaggiati ML, Palmieri F. The mitochondrial aspartate/glutamate carrier isoform 1 gene expression is regulated by CREB in neuronal cells. The International Journal of Biochemistry & Cell Biology. 2015;**60**:157-166. DOI: 10.1016/j.biocel.2015.01.004

[191] Iijima M, Jalil A, Begum L, Yasuda T, Yamaguchi N, Xian Li M, Kawada N, Endou H, Kobayashi K, Saheki T. Pathogenesis of adult-onset type II citrullinemia caused by deficiency of citrin, a mitochondrial solute carrier protein: Tissue and subcellular localization of citrin. Advances in Enzyme Regulation. 2001;**41**:325-342. DOI: https://doi.org/10.1016/S0065-2571(00)00022-4

[192] Monné M, Miniero DV, Daddabbo L, Palmieri L, Porcelli V, Palmieri F. Mitochondrial transporters for ornithine and related amino acids: A review. Amino Acids. 2015;**47**(9):1763-1777. DOI: 10.1007/s00726-015-1990-5

[193] Fiermonte G, Dolce V, David L, Santorelli FM, Dionisi-Vici C, Palmieri F, Walker JE The mitochondrial ornithine transporter. Bacterial expression, reconstitution, functional

characterization, and tissue distribution of two human isoforms. The Journal of Biological Chemistry. 2003;**278**(35):32778-32783. DOI: 10.1074/jbc.M302317200

[194] Porcelli V, Fiermonte G, Longo A, Palmieri F. The human gene SLC25A29, of solute carrier family 25, encodes a mitochondrial transporter of basic amino acids. The Journal of Biological Chemistry. 2014;**289**(19):13374-13384. DOI: 10.1074/jbc.M114.547448

[195] Sekoguchi E, Sato N, Yasui A, Fukada S, Nimura Y, Aburatani H, Ikeda K, Matsuura A. A novel mitochondrial carnitine-acylcarnitine translocase induced by partial hepatectomy and fasting. The Journal of Biological Chemistry. 2003;**278**(40):38796-38802. DOI: 10.1074/jbc.M306372200

[196] Camacho JA, Rioseco-Camacho N. The human and mouse SLC25A29 mitochondrial transporters rescue the deficient ornithine metabolism in fibroblasts of patients with the hyperornithinemia-hyperammonemia-homocitrullinuria (HHH) syndrome. Pediatric Research. 2009;**66**(1):35-41. DOI: 10.1203/PDR.0b013e3181a283c1

[197] Salvi S, Santorelli FM, Bertini E, Boldrini R, Meli C, Donati A, Burlina AB, Rizzo C, Di Capua M, Fariello G, Dionisi-Vici C. Clinical and molecular findings in hyperornithinemia-hyperammonemia-homocitrullinuria syndrome. Neurology. 2001;**57**(5):911-914. DOI: 10.1212/WNL.57.5.911

[198] Camacho JA, Rioseco-Camacho N, Andrade D, Porter J, Kong J. Cloning and characterization of human ORNT2: A second mitochondrial ornithine transporter that can rescue a defective ORNT1 in patients with the hyperornithinemia-hyperammonemia-homocitrullinuria syndrome, a urea cycle disorder. Molecular Genetics and Metabolism. 2003;**79**(4):257-271. DOI: 10.1016/S1096-7192(03)00105-7

[199] Ledesma A, de Lacoba MG, Rial E. The mitochondrial uncoupling proteins. Genome Bio logy. 2002;**3**(12):REVIEWS3015. DOI: http://genomebiology.com/2002/3/12/reviews/3015

[200] Ricquier D, Bouillaud F. The uncoupling protein homologues: UCP1, UCP2, UCP3, StUCP and AtUCP. The Biochemical Journal. 2000;**345**(Pt 2):161-179. DOI: 10.1042/bj3450161

[201] Fleury C, Neverova M, Collins S, Raimbault S, Champigny O, Levi-Meyrueis C, Bouillaud F, Seldin MF, Surwit RS, Ricquier D, Warden CH. Uncoupling protein-2: A novel gene linked to obesity and hyperinsulinemia. Nature Genetics. 1997;**15**(3):269-272. DOI: 10.1038/ng0397-269

[202] Gutiérrez-Aguilar M, Baines CP. Physiological and pathological roles of mitochondrial SLC25 carriers. The Biochemical Journal. 2013;**454**(3):371-386. DOI: 10.1042/BJ20121753

[203] Rousset S, Alves-Guerra MC, Mozo J, Miroux B, Cassard-Doulcier AM, Bouillaud F, Ricquier D. The biology of mitochondrial uncoupling proteins. Diabetes. 2004;**53**(Suppl 1): S130-S135. DOI: 10.2337/diabetes.53.2007.S130

[204] Cannon B, Shabalina IG, Kramarova TV, Petrovic N, Nedergaard J. Uncoupling proteins: A role in protection against reactive oxygen species—Or not? Biochimica et Biophysica Acta. 2006;**1757**(5-6):449-458. DOI: 10.1016/j.bbabio.2006.05.016

[205] Echtay KS, Winkler E, Klingenberg M, Coenzyme Q. Is an obligatory cofactor for uncoupling protein function. Nature. 2000;**408**(6812):609-613. DOI: 10.1038/35046114

[206] Divakaruni AS, Brand MD. The regulation and physiology of mitochondrial proton leak. Physiology (Bethesda, Md.). 2011;**26**(3):192-205. DOI: 10.1152/physiol.00046.2010

[207] Garlid KD, Jaburek M, Jezek P. Mechanism of uncoupling protein action. Biochemical Society Transactions. 2001;**29**(Pt 6):803-806. DOI: 10.1042/bst0290803

[208] Brondani LA, de Souza BM, Duarte GC, Kliemann LM, Esteves JF, Marcon AS, Gross JL, Canani LH, Crispim D. The UCP1 −3826A/G polymorphism is associated with diabetic retinopathy and increased UCP1 and MnSOD2 gene expression in human retina. Investigative Ophthalmology & Visual Science. 2012;**53**(12):7449-7457. DOI: 10.1167/iovs.12-10660

[209] Walder K, Norman RA, Hanson RL, Schrauwen P, Neverova M, Jenkinson CP, Easlick J, Warden CH, Pecqueur C, Raimbault S, Ricquier D, Silver MH, Shuldiner AR, Solanes G, Lowell BB, Chung WK, Leibel RL, Pratley R, Ravussin E. Association between uncoupling protein polymorphisms (UCP2-UCP3) and energy metabolism/obesity in pima indians. Human Molecular Genetics. 1998;**7**(9):1431-1435

[210] Goglia F, Skulachev VP. A function for novel uncoupling proteins: Antioxidant defense of mitochondrial matrix by translocating fatty acid peroxides from the inner to the outer membrane leaflet. The FASEB Journal. 2003;**17**(12):1585-1591. DOI: 10.1096/fj.03-0159hyp

[211] Lanni A, Moreno M, Goglia F. Mitochondrial actions of thyroid hormone. Comprehensive Physiology. 2016;**6**(4):1591-1607. DOI: 10.1002/cphy.c150019

[212] Weigle DS, Selfridge LE, Schwartz MW, Seeley RJ, Cummings DE, Havel PJ, Kuijper JL, BeltrandelRio H. Elevated free fatty acids induce uncoupling protein 3 expression in muscle: A potential explanation for the effect of fasting. Diabetes. 1998;**47**(2):298-302. DOI: 10.2337/diab.47.2.298

[213] Wang MY, Lee Y, Unger RH. Novel form of lipolysis induced by leptin. The Journal of Biological Chemistry. 1999;**274**(25):17541-17544. DOI: 10.1074/jbc.274.25.17541

[214] Zhang CY, Baffy G, Perret P, Krauss S, Peroni O, Grujic D, Hagen T, Vidal-Puig AJ, Boss O, Kim YB, Zheng XX, Wheeler MB, Shulman GI, Chan CB, Lowell BB. Uncoupling protein-2 negatively regulates insulin secretion and is a major link between obesity, beta cell dysfunction, and type 2 diabetes. Cell. 2001;**105**(6):745-755. DOI: 10.1016/S0092-8674(01)00378-6

[215] de Luis DA, Aller R, Izaola O, Sagrado MG, Conde R, Primo D, de la Fuente B, Ovalle HF, Mambrilla MR. Relationship of -55C/T polymorphism of uncoupling protein 3 (UCP3) gene with metabolic syndrome by ATP III classification. Journal of Clinical Laboratory Analysis. 2012;**26**(4):272-278. DOI: 10.1002/jcla.21517

[216] Yonezawa T, Haga S, Kobayashi Y, Katoh K, Obara Y. Saturated fatty acids stimulate and insulin suppresses BMCP1 expression in bovine mammary epithelial cells. Biochemical and Biophysical Research Communications. 2009;**390**(3):915-919. DOI: 10.1016/j.bbrc.2009.10.077

[217] Mouaffak F, Kebir O, Bellon A, Gourevitch R, Tordjman S, Viala A, Millet B, Jaafari N, Olié JP, Krebs MO. Association of an UCP4 (SLC25A27) haplotype with ultra-resistant schizophrenia. Pharmacogenomics. 2011;**12**(2):185-193. DOI: 10.2217/pgs.10.179

Section 5

Chemicals as Mitochondrial Dysfunction Inducers

Chapter 12

Pyrethroid Insecticides as the Mitochondrial Dysfunction Inducers

Celal Guven, Yusuf Sevgiler and Eylem Taskin

Additional information is available at the end of the chapter

http://dx.doi.org/10.5772/intechopen.80283

Abstract

Pyrethroids are used to decrease vector-based health concerns and to increase field yield against agricultural pests. Their metabolism is a concern to disrupt a cell's homeostatic machinery via reactive oxygen species (ROS) production. They interact with lipid membranes to damage the fine balance between membrane lipids and membrane proteins, especially mitochondrial substrate transporters and electron carriers. Pyrethroids cause a shift in the metabolic energy production strategy, resulting in ROS production and intracellular lipid deposition. The change of open/closed conformation of some mitochondrial membrane proteins increases the vulnerability of mitochondria to Ca^{2+} ions. Membrane lipid fluidity change is also a concern because of permeability to the substrates and ions to produce energy and other substrates necessary for the cell. Pyrethroids can change the Ca^{2+} signaling and its interaction with ROS signals via disruption of the fine balance between endoplasmic reticulum and mitochondria. They can disrupt the mitochondrial DNA (mtDNA) via their hydrophobic nature or their ROS production capacity. In conclusion, mitochondria are the center of pyrethroid toxicity, and dysfunction of this organelle via pyrethroid toxicity plays an important role in the fate of cell. Their lipophilic and pro-oxidative nature together with Ca^{2+} homeostasis plays a synergistic role in this mitochondrial effect.

Keywords: pyrethroids, insecticides, mitochondria, calcium, reactive oxygen species, mtDNA

1. Introduction

A pesticide has been described as an agent applied to kill, repel, or mitigate industry-, public health- and/or agriculture-related pests. They can also be used as plant growth regulator or nitrogen stabilizer. We use them to reduce the risk of decreased agricultural and industrial yield and prevent public health concerns such as vector-borne diseases, asthma and allergies, and microbial contamination (for more information: https://www.epa.gov/pesticides). Pesticides have entered into our lives more than 3000 years ago [1] and dried, ground Dalmatian pyrethrum flowers (contain natural pyrethrins) have been used against insect pests since ancient China. It has also been used in Europe more than 200 years ago against cockroaches, bedbugs, flies, and mosquitoes [2]. A pyrethrin-derived synthetic pyrethroid allethrin has been synthesized in 1949 and entered the market in 1952 to use against household pests [3]. To date, there are over 3500 pyrethroid-containing products registered [4].

The primary toxic effect of pyrethroids is on the voltage-gated sodium channels (VGSCs) like organochlorines such as DDT. The opening of these channels is extended by pyrethroid action and this causes the altered nerve function. According to their effect and chemical structure, pyrethroids divided into two types. Type I chemicals (allethrin, bifenthrin, bioresmethrin, permethrin, phenothrin, resmethrin, tefluthrin, and tetramethrin) do not contain a cyano group and they cause slowing in the closure of VGSCs. Therefore, the observed symptoms are tremors and seizures. On the contrary, Type II chemicals (cyfluthrin, cyhalothrin, cypermethrin, cyphenothrin, deltamethrin, fenpropathrin, fenvalerate, flucythrinate, flumethrin, fluvalinate, and tralomethrin) are the ones that are predominantly alpha-cyano-3-phenoxybenzyl alcohol esters and they cause a longer duration in the sodium current. The observed symptom is choreoathetosis accompanied by profuse salivation [5, 6]. Permethrin, a Type I pyrethroid, has not a disordering effect on polar head groups of phospholipids while it localizes within the hydrocarbon core [7]. Because of its cyano group, cypermethrin, a Type II, localizes preferentially in the hydrophilic/hydrophobic region of the lipid plasma membrane, shows greater permanence and more fluidic effect on the membrane compared to permethrin [8]. Therefore, the permanence of cypermethrin can be connected to the prolonged opening of sodium channels. This interaction could also be related to the more reduction of lipid-lipid interactions compared to Type Is; therefore, it decreases plasma membrane fluidity that is linked to the affected Na^+-K^+ ATPase activity to become the plasma membrane more permeable to the Na^+ cations [8]. Type I pyrethroids have a higher binding affinity to the protein of VGSCs [9] while they penetrate more easily into the cell. Although this is another issue for a review, the mutations observed on the VGSCs' protein produce more resistant individuals against pyrethroid intoxication (for more information, see Silva et al. [10]). There is also a discrimination between these types according to their effects on calcium and chloride channels [11]. **Table 1** shows the chemical structures of pyrethroids that are mostly discussed in the current chapter.

Long-term health effects of pesticides such as their developmental and reproductory, endocrine disruption, neurobehavioral, carcinogenic, and immunological ones besides their acute impact have been considered by many scientists and regulatory services such as WHO, FAO, USEPA, and ECHA for many years. Currently, we experience the pesticides via drinking water, soil, food, and air. Directly ingesting of pesticide products can be assessed as a suicide action, but millions of acute poisoning cases occur in every year worldwide [12]. Although

http://dx.doi.org/10.5772/intechopen.80283

the pyrethroid insecticides are less persistent in the environment compared to organochlorines, they are highly lipophilic with their high octanol/water partition coefficient (K_{ow}) [13]. Therefore, dietary exposure to these compounds trigger the safety concerns [14]. Indoor application to control household pests is also another path for human exposure.

Significant pyrethroid residues have been found in drinking water, human breast milk, and cow milk in a sample location of South Africa where indoor residual spraying was applied for malaria control compared to a mountain population [15]. Malaria control or agricultural applications have caused pyrethroid accumulation such as cypermethrin, lambda-cyhalothrin, esfenvalerate/fenvalerate, and permethrin in breast milk from Brazil, Colombia, and Spain mothers [16]. However, the residues never exceeded the maximum daily intake levels. Babina et al. reported that more than one chemical and simultaneous exposure to organophosphate and pyrethroids was common in South Australian preschool children [17]. Barr et al. surveyed the U.S. population with 5046 samples between the period of 1999 and 2002 to detect pyrethroid residues in urine samples, and they concluded that pyrethroid exposure is widespread in the U.S. population and children probably have higher exposure risk compared to adolescents and adults [18]. Exposure to pyrethroids in the levels common in Canadian children's urine has been associated with parent-reported behavioral anomalies [19]. A sex-dependent attention-deficit/hyperactivity disorder has been found in U.S.

Allethrin[1]

(Type I)

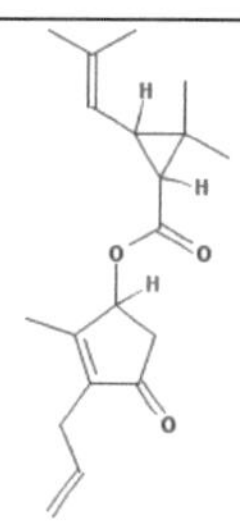

IUPAC name: (2-methyl-4-oxo-3-prop-2-enylcyclopent-2-en-1-yl) 2,2-dimethyl-3-(2-methylprop-1-enyl) cyclopropane-1-carboxylate

CAS No: 584-79-2

Metofluthrin[2]

(Type I)

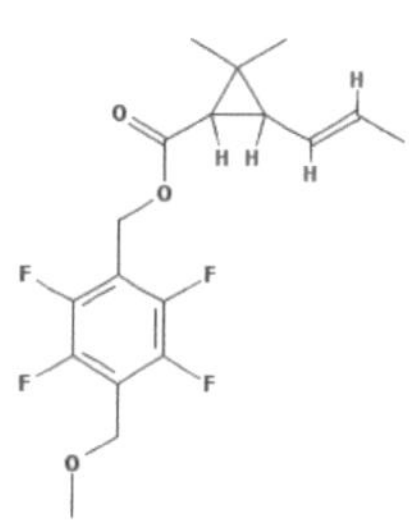

IUPAC name: [2,3,5,6-tetrafluoro-4-(methoxymethyl) phenyl] methyl 2,2-dimethyl-3-[(E)-prop-1-enyl] cyclopropane-1-carboxylate

CAS No: 240494-70-6

Permethrin[3]

(Type I)

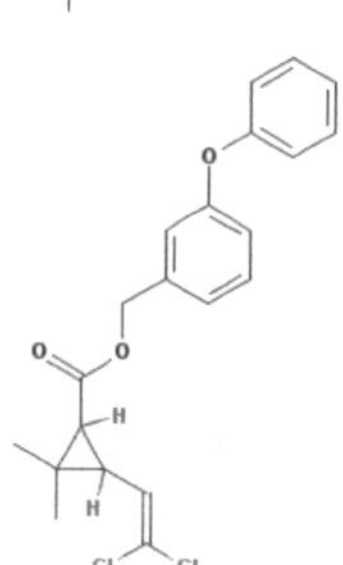

IUPAC name: (3-phenoxyphenyl) methyl 3-(2,2-dichloroethenyl)-2,2-dimethylcyclopropane-1-carboxylate

CAS No: 52645-53-1

Cypermethrin[4] (Type II)	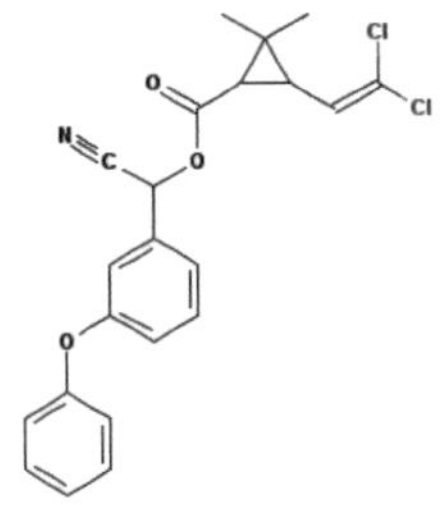	IUPAC name: [cyano-(3-phenoxyphenyl) methyl] 3-(2,2-dichloroethenyl)-2,2-dimethylcyclopropane-1-carboxylate CAS No: 52315-07-8
Deltamethrin[5] (Type II)	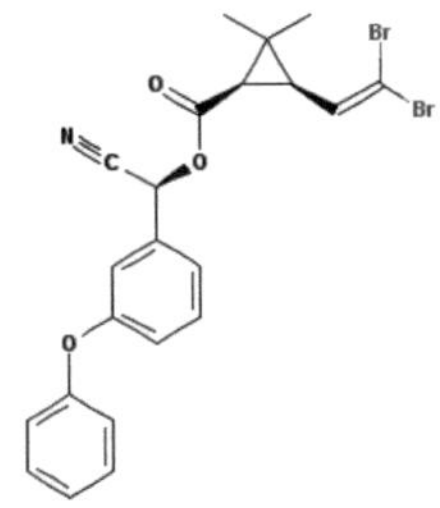	IUPAC name: [(S)-cyano-(3-phenoxyphenyl) methyl] (1R,3R)-3-(2,2-dibromoethenyl)-2,2-dimethylcyclopropane-1-carboxylate CAS No: 52918-63-5

[1]National Center for Biotechnology Information. PubChem Compound Database; CID = 11,442, https://pubchem.ncbi.nlm.nih.gov/compound/11442 (accessed June 18, 2018).

[2]National Center for Biotechnology Information. PubChem Compound Database; CID = 5,282,227, https://pubchem.ncbi.nlm.nih.gov/compound/5282227 (accessed June 18, 2018).

[3]National Center for Biotechnology Information. PubChem Compound Database; CID = 40,326, https://pubchem.ncbi.nlm.nih.gov/compound/40326 (accessed June 18, 2018).

[4]National Center for Biotechnology Information. PubChem Compound Database; CID = 2912, https://pubchem.ncbi.nlm.nih.gov/compound/2912 (accessed June 18, 2018).

[5]National Center for Biotechnology Information. PubChem Compound Database; CID = 40,585, https://pubchem.ncbi.nlm.nih.gov/compound/40585 (accessed June 18, 2018).

Table 1. Chemical structures of the pyrethroids that are mostly discussed in the current chapter.

children associated with detectable levels of pyrethroid metabolites in the urine; therefore, abnormalities in the dopamine system that is more threatening for boys may be a result of growing use of pesticides, especially pyrethroids [20]. Urinary pyrethroid residues have been correlated with increased chronic heart disease in nonoccupational exposed Chinese people [21]. Occupational exposure to pyrethroids, for example, in the textile industry, is also an important issue throughout the world [22].

2. Reactive oxygen formation and its relation to the biotransformation of pyrethroids

Pyrethroids are the esters of acids like chrysanthemic acid, halo-substituted chrysanthemic acid, and 2-(4-chlorophenyl)-3-methyl butyric acid and alcohols like allethrolone and 3-phenoxybenzyl alcohol and they mostly contain more than one asymmetric carbon atom [3]. The stereoisomeric nature plays a significant role in the biotransformation of some pyrethroids like fenvalerate [23]. This can also contribute to their toxic effect. For example, different stereoisomeric forms of permethrin have caused the increase in intracellular reactive oxygen species (ROS) and lipid peroxidation levels and decrease in superoxide dismutase (SOD) and catalase (CAT) activities in rat pheochromocytoma cells (PC12); but this effect is enantioselective, and the most effective stereoisomer is 1*R*-*trans*-permethrin [24].

Pyrethroid biotransformation in mammals including human consists oxidation, ester hydrolysis (both are called as Phase I reactions), and conjugation with endogenous molecules (Phase II reactions) [3, 25, 26]. Oxidation reactions are catalyzed by isoforms of cytochrome P450s (CYP450s), and ester bonds are hydrolyzed by carboxylesterase(s) [26].

The produced metabolites can be more potent endocrine disruptors than parent compound for humans [27]. Romero et al. found that CYP450-mediated oxidation products of deltamethrin (2′-OH and 4′-OH deltamethrin) are more toxic than the parent compound measured with cell viability, lipid peroxidation, and nitric oxide formation on human dopaminergic neuroblastoma SH-SY5Y cells [28]. Moreover, abnormal locomotor activity observed in prenatal deltamethrin exposure has been associated with increased expression of CYP450 enzymes in the offsprings of rats [29]. However, the pyrethroids are commonly used as a replacement of organophosphate and organochlorine insecticides because of their low mammalian toxicity at the first time of their popularity. The low toxicity has been attributed to their rapid metabolism in mammals [18]. For this reason, their metabolism considered as a detoxification because of rapid clearance from the body [25, 30]. Most of the metabolites are highly hydrophilic, and then rapidly excreted via urine and feces. Some of the metabolites from *R*-cyano-3-phenoxybenzyl alcohol derivative pyrethroids, however, shows incomplete excretion and have longer bioretention in skin and stomach [25, 26]. Moreover, some of the conjugation metabolites are lipophilic and participate in toxicity reactions [25]. The biotransformation to hydrophilic compounds may also be a source of their toxicity in mammals as described below.

A single dose of cypermethrin and/or fenvalerate has caused the increase in SOD and CAT activities and in lipid peroxidation levels in the erythrocytes of rats [31]. As specified, non-cyano (Type I)—cyano (Type II) discrimination can also be observed in oxidative stress-inducing potential of these chemicals. For example, permethrin (a Type I) disturbed the antioxidant defense more than cypermethrin (a Type II) in the erythrocytes of treated rats [8]. Because of its cyano group, cypermethrin shows longer permanence in the membrane, while permethrin can pass easily from this lipid bilayer with its lipophilic nature to reach more readily to cellular subcompartments such as endoplasmic reticulum (ER) membranes that contain CYP450s. Although the presence of α-cyano group decreases the hydrolysis rate of ester bond [32], this group decomposes to cyanides and aldehydes to produce free radicals [33]. Endogenously formed superoxide anion radical is dismutated to hydrogen peroxide (H_2O_2) spontaneously or a SOD-catalyzed reaction. The formed H_2O_2 is degraded to water via CAT in peroxisomes and/or glutathione peroxidases (GPx) in the cytosol, mitochondria, nucleus, and also in peroxisomes [34, 35]. Although the H_2O_2 is not assessed as a ROS, it can act as a substrate for hydroxyl radical formation via a metal (it is mostly iron) catalyzed reaction if it cannot convert to water efficiently. Hydroxyl radical is the strongest radical capable of oxidizing DNA, cellular membrane lipids, and proteins, and there is no effective agent to escape them in the cell [35]. The most important intracellular iron source is the active site of CYP450s because of their iron content in the catalytically active center [36–40].

Pro-oxidant nature of CYP450-mediated pyrethroid metabolism needs further clarification because of superoxide and H_2O_2 release from CYP450 enzymatic complex by CYP450-inducers [35–40]. Pro-oxidative toxicity of pyrethroids has been reported in mammalian studies. Raina et al. suggest that the induction of oxidative stress in dermal cypermethrin exposed rats should be related to its biotransformation via CYP450-catalysis [41]. Metofluthrin, a known carcinogenic agent at high doses, induces mainly CYP2B isoforms and increases oxidative stress via the increase of reduced glutathione (GSH) levels (a well-known cellular antioxidant molecule) in rats [42]. Without an induction of apoptosis, the authors conclude that the metofluthrin has reversible effects, and it may be noncarcinogenic for a human. On the contrary, deltamethrin and permethrin exposure has caused the induction of caspase 3/7 activities; therefore, it has been concluded that oxidative potentials of pyrethroids can trigger the apoptosis in human HepG2 cells and primary hepatocytes [43]. Deltamethrin and permethrin have also caused the stimulation of mRNA transcripts of CYP1A1, CYP3A4, and CYP2B6 isoforms and CYP3A4 protein levels. NADPH-dependent microsomal ROS formation has been observed in the liver of etofenprox exposed rats, and it has been concluded that observed lipid peroxidation and DNA oxidation in the liver should be related with CYP2B-induction by etofenprox exposure [34]. CYP450-mediated cytosolic and/or mitochondrial ROS formation [44, 45] might cause cell death [46], and we conclude that CYP450 activation via pyrethroid exposure might cause mitochondrial damage and cell death. Therefore, CYP450 inducers should be evaluated with this type of side effect.

Deltamethrin exposure has caused early ROS formation and subsequent decrease in GSH levels, Bcl-2 protein expression, and mitochondrial membrane potential and increase in Bax, p38 MAPK expressions, and caspase-3 activity in isolated splenocytes from mice [47]. Similar results have also been found in the brain of deltamethrin exposed rats [48]. The number of apoptotic cells has been decreased by *N*-acetylcysteine, a well-known antioxidant agent, while buthionine sulfoximine, a GSH depleting agent, worsened the effects [47]. Therefore, when redox balance favors the ROS formation, it could be the main curator of mitochondrial dysfunction and related cell death. Not only synthetic ones but also natural pyrethrins can cause ROS formation and related mitochondrial dysfunction and apoptosis in human hepatocarcinoma cell line HepG2 [49].

In fact, cells can die because of the ER stress-dependent pathways in pyrethroid intoxication. For example, Zhao et al. have suggested nonmitochondrial apoptotic pathway with an extracellular route [50]. According to their model, fenvalerate acts as an endocrine disruptor through the induction of apoptosis of mice germ cells. Fas/FasL-directed caspase-8 activation has caused the germ cell apoptosis without the change in Bcl-2, Bax, mitochondrial and cytosolic cytochrome c, and cleaved procaspase-9 levels.

Interestingly, ER and mitochondria have multiple contact sites called mitochondria-ER associated membranes with a characteristic set of proteins. From these domains, not only Ca^{2+} but also ROS-mediated signals may be transmitted to the mitochondria after ROS-based ER stress (for more details, see [51]). On these domains, inositol-1,4,5-triphosphate receptors interact with voltage-dependent anion channels (VDACs) on the outer membrane of mitochondria to transfer Ca^{2+}. As an important second messenger, Ca^{2+} interacts with other signaling systems such as subtoxic levels of ROS. There is a fine balance between these two signaling systems and dysfunction in either of these systems can affect another one. Therefore, this situation is harmful or a signal for defense for a cell [52]. As stated in the review of Chirumbolo and Bjørklund [53], we believed that pyrethroids can exert their toxicity via the induction of ROS on ER membranes via CYP450 activity and uncontrolled Ca^{2+} release from ER stores (and/or intracellular flux), which are used to conduct a fine balance between the ER and mitochondria deciding the autophagy or apoptosis. In this sense, we try to explain the mitochondrial effects of pyrethroids considering their oxidative stress-inducing potential and Ca^{2+} homeostasis of the cell.

3. Cellular Ca^{2+} stores and pyrethroids

Cellular Ca^{2+} stores can be a target for pyrethroid action and pyrethroid-mediated intracellular Ca^{2+} load could be related to mitochondrial changes. For example, early life exposure to permethrin increased the intracellular Ca^{2+} influx in the heart of permethrin exposed rats [54]. Pyrethroids can activate the dose-dependent Ca^{2+}-influx in the tetrodotoxin-sensitive pathway (a specific inhibitor of VGSCs) with different potencies and efficacies in mouse primary cortical neurons [55]. However, the changes in Ca^{2+} dynamics could not always be dependent on VGSCs, at least for bifenthrin at nanomolar concentrations in mouse primary cortical neurons [56]. In fact, pyrethroids can modify voltage-gated Ca^{2+} channels at concentrations similar to VGSCs, and Type IIs are more potent to induce Ca^{2+} influx according to voltage- and patch-clamp electrophysiological and *in situ* functional studies [57]. High intracellular Ca^{2+} levels can cause damage to mitochondria [58, 59], and changes in intracellular Ca^{2+} levels via release from ER stores or via Ca^{2+} influx triggers the ROS formation and cell death [58, 60].

Deltamethrin can inactivate the VGSCs. Downregulation of gene transcripts of these proteins in deltamethrin exposed human SK-N-AS neuroblastoma cells has also been observed with an intracellular Ca^{2+} elevation and calpain activation-mediated pathway [61]. Therefore, this situation causes the ER stress-related nonmitochondrial apoptotic pathway in human SK-N-AS neuroblastoma cells by deltamethrin [62]. According to this model, deltamethrin-induced VGSC opening has been caused Ca^{2+} overload and activation of ER stress pathway engaging calpain and caspase-12 without an increase in cytosolic cytochrome c levels (an indicator for mitochondrial apoptotic pathway). In this way, resultant sodium influx via opening the VGSCs can activate the phosphatidylinositol turnover; the intermediates formed via this turnover will activate protein kinase C and the Ca^{2+} release from internal stores [63]. Deltamethrin can activate directly the protein kinase C enzyme at its very low dose [64]. According to the authors, "*deltamethrin has a direct-action site likely to be on protein kinase C, an inositol polyphosphates-independent Ca^{2+} triggering site (e.g., ryanodine receptor and ER stores), and/or phosphoprotein phosphatase.*" Interestingly, deltamethrin was able to increase the inositol 1,4,5-triphosphate levels in rat brain slices in the presence of neomycin or LiCl [64].

Cypermethrin and fenvalerate have rescued the tsBN7 (a temperature sensitive cell type) cells from apoptotic death with elevated temperature compared to cyclosporine A, a mitochondrial membrane permeability transition pore (mtPTP) inhibitor [65]. According to the authors, elevation in cytosolic Ca^{2+} is at the core of the formation of mtPTP, and these pyrethroids could be effective via their disruptive effect on Ca^{2+} balance. Ca^{2+} overload only can contribute to the formation of mtPTP; however, oxidative stress measured with excessive ROS formation and Ca^{2+} overload has a synergistic role in the formation of this pore to stimulate mitochondrial apoptosis [66].

Voltage-gated Ca^{2+}-channel activation by allethrin has caused the mitochondrial cell death in rat Leydig cell tumor derived LC540 cells [67]. Allethrin exposure in these cell lines have resulted in the elevation of ROS, lipid peroxidation, intracellular Ca^{2+}, cleaved PARP levels (executed by caspase-1), increased p53 gene expression, fluctuated SOD, CAT, GPx enzyme activities, and decreased mitochondrial membrane potential, Bcl-2, and pro-caspase-3 protein levels. It has been concluded that mitochondrial apoptosis by allethrin could be an important factor in decreased male fertility [67]. Similarly, allethrin exposure has caused the significant decrease in mitochondrial membrane potential and subsequent release of cytochrome c to the cytosol in the human corneal epithelial cell line [68]. Pro-apoptotic Bax expression has been increased, while anti-apoptotic Bcl-2 decreased, resulting in caspase-3 activation. Therefore, allethrin can trigger the mitochondrial apoptotic pathway in human corneal epithelial cells; although, they have not correlated their results with Ca^{2+} signaling.

An interesting support to these findings has been obtained with an estrogen receptor α and β binding studies of pyrethroids [69]. The studied chemicals have weak (fenvalerate) or no (permethrin, deltamethrin, and bifenthrin) binding capacity to estrogen receptor α, while permethrin has shown high affinity binding to estrogen receptor β. Lower but still strong binding to this protein has been observed with deltamethrin and fenvalerate, while bifenthrin has no binding capacity to this receptor. In another study, cypermethrin and permethrin exposure have increased the estrogen receptor α and β mRNA levels in TM4 mouse Sertoli cells to adapt decreased spermatogenic potential under pyrethroid toxicity [70]. Estrogen receptor β plays a role in preventing the mitochondrial apoptotic pathway and its suppression causes Bax activation, cytochrome c release, caspase 3 activation, and PARP cleavage [71].

Dissipation of mitochondrial membrane potential is an important event of apoptotic and necrotic cell deaths. It was observed in deltamethrin exposed rat primary hepatocytes with subsequent elevation of ROS, while programmed necrosis has been measured in these cells [72]. A common cell death sign or toxic insult starts a common cell death progression; but the ATP presence determines the type of cell death, apoptosis or necrosis [66]. Pro-apoptotic potential via the mitochondrial pathway of pyrethroids has been reported in many studies [47, 49, 73]; however, necrosis can also be occurred because of the ATP demand as was seen in the kidney of permethrin exposed rats [74] or in the heart of cypermethrin exposed frogs (*Rana cameroni*) [75].

Anti-apoptotic protein Bcl-xL interacts with VDACs to transfer Ca^{2+} into the mitochondria [76]. A continuous supply of Ca^{2+} into mitochondria via this way is necessary to maintain mitochondrial bioenergetics because of pyruvate, 2-oxoglutarate, and the NAD^+-dependent isocitrate dehydrogenases, and three intramitochondrial tricarboxylic acid cycle (TCA) enzymes are stimulated by Ca^{2+} [77]. Anti-apoptotic members of Bcl-2 proteins (Bcl-2 itself, Bcl-xL, and Mcl-1) localized on the mitochondrial outer membrane and interact with the inositol-1,4,5-triphosphate receptors on the ER membrane to arrange the mitochondrial Ca^{2+} load during apoptotic signals and/or to enhance the mitochondrial metabolism for cellular resistance [76, 78].

Endoplasmic reticulum-mediated Ca^{2+} to mitochondria is necessary to adequate supply of reducing equivalents for oxidative phosphorylation because of enhanced phosphorylation of pyruvate dehydrogenase complex and activated AMPK (AMP-activated protein kinase) in the absence of this supply [79]. Giacomello et al. proposed a schema for anti- or pro-apoptotic proteins in ER-mediated Ca^{2+} supply to mitochondria [80]. Namely, Bax and other pro-apoptotic members of Bcl-2 family proteins enhance the ER Ca^{2+} load, and then mitochondria expose higher Ca^{2+} concentrations, mtPTP opens; while anti-apoptotic members of Bcl-2 cause the balanced Ca^{2+} concentration from ER stores; then apoptosis is inhibited, and the needed ATP levels are supplied enhancing the mitochondrial metabolism. According to Distelhorst and Bootman, under autophagy-promoting conditions, a mitochondrial Ca^{2+} transfer from ER protects the cells from death via adequate elimination of energy demands, while the excessive accumulation of Ca^{2+} via apoptosis-inducing chemicals and/or ROS triggers the irreversible apoptosis progression [81]. In fact, differential stimulation pathway of protein kinase C may result in the desensitization of inositol-1,4,5-triphosphate receptors via their phosphorylation by protein kinase C, which translocates to ER membranes in G-protein coupled protein subunit alpha s-cAMP pathway. In this way, desensitization of receptor to its ligand, inositol 1,4,5-triphosphate results in limited Ca^{2+} release from ER stores [82]. Enan and Matsumura have observed the translocation of protein kinase C from the cytosol to the membrane fraction in pyrethroid exposed rat brain synaptosomes [64]. Deltamethrin has caused the intracellular Ca^{2+} elevation, ROS formation, and mitochondrial apoptosis in HGB human glioblastoma cells; while these effects have been reversed by protein kinase C, ER Ca^{2+} pump, and inositol 1,4,5 formation inhibitors [83]. On the contrary, increased intracellular Ca^{2+} levels were not dependent on the phosphoinositide pathway in the effects of different pyrethroids in mouse primary neocortical neuron culture [55]. Therefore, tissue specificity and the dose-response curve of pyrethroid action on mitochondrial Ca^{2+} supply from ER and apoptosis induction should be further investigated.

4. Mitochondrial electron transport chain and energy production are affected by pyrethroid intoxication

Type I and type II pyrethroids could also be separated according to their toxic effects on different parts of the cell including mitochondria. Noncyano pyrethroid pyrethrin and permethrin increased the mitochondrial metabolic enzyme activities measured with the WST-1 method at low doses probably to support the bioenergetics needs of the cell in SH-SY5Y cells [84] while there is no or little effect on total ATP content. Mitochondrial enzyme activities and total ATP content have been decreased at higher doses. However, the most pronounced effect has been seen with an α-cyano compound cypermethrin starting with the low doses [84]. The same distinction could be done by their effect on human estrogen regulated breast cancer cell line (MCF-7). Coadministration of oestradiol has been potentiated the effects of these pyrethroids measured with total ATP and mitochondrial metabolic enzyme activities; but, the most pronounced effect has been observed in cypermethrin exposure, also [85].

According to the study of Gassner et al., permethrin and cyhalothrin caused the inhibition of complex I of electron transport chain in isolated rat liver mitochondria, and there are more than

40 regions of complex I as potential binding sites for pyrethroids because of their hydrophobic nature [86]. Inhibition of complex I may be related to ROS formation; but, it should be noted that complex I inhibitors can be divided into two groups as ROS producers and ROS production inhibitors [87]. Inhibition of complex I activity by permethrin has been caused a reduction in superoxide radical formation in striatum submitochondrial particles of rats [88]. Inhibition of succinate dehydrogenase activity, which has a role in TCA and in complex II, has been decreased after acute and subacute bifenthrin exposure in rat brain [89]. Deltamethrin has a major inhibition site between complexes II and III because of unaffected NADH dehydrogenase (complex I) and cytochrome c oxidase (complex IV) activities in the isolated rat liver mitochondrial preparation [90]. In this mitochondrial preparation, NADH oxidase, succinate oxidase, succinate dehydrogenase (complex II), NADH-cytochrome c reductase, and succinate cytochrome c reductase activities have been inhibited. Deltamethrin has also caused an inhibition of ADP-stimulated oxygen consumption and impaired the mitochondrial membrane potential [90].

A discrepancy has been found compared to the results presented by Braguini et al. [90]. Cytochrome c oxidase activity has decreased within different time series in deltamethrin-exposed rat brains *in vivo* [91]. In these *in vivo* mitochondrial preparations, deltamethrin has caused a decrease in mitochondrial cytochrome c levels, mitochondrial membrane permeability transition, and mitochondrial membrane potential. These changes can result in a mitochondrial apoptosis and may reveal the neurotoxic action of pyrethroids. However, succinate cytochrome c reductase activity has not changed, while cytochrome c oxidase activity increased in the liver of deltamethrin-intoxicated rats *in vivo* [92]. In these liver preparations, biotransformation enzymes of pyrethroids have also not changed. In addition to their ROS inducing by ER-bound CYP450 activities, pyrethroids can disturb the electron transfer on the transport chain and can cause the altered ATP levels and ROS formation to induce mitochondrial dysfunction and sequential death.

Metabolic shift determined by increased lactate levels are observed in tumor cells although they are grown in oxygenic cultures, and this can be a strategy to avoid oxidative stress and apoptosis induction [93]. Pyrethroid intoxication causes a metabolic shift through the oxidative phosphorylation to anaerobic glycolysis and altered lipid and protein metabolism *in vivo*. Several pyrethroids have decreased the hepatic protein levels, increased hepatic lactate dehydrogenase, blood and plasma urea levels in rats [94, 95]. Authors have concluded that pyrethroids are able to stimulate metabolic shift from oxidative phosphorylation to anaerobic glycolysis. A support for these observations has been obtained in the muscle and heart of cypermethrin exposed rats [96]. It has caused the decreased succinate dehydrogenase while increased glucose-6-phosphate dehydrogenase and lactate dehydrogenase activities reflecting the anaerobiosis. Decreased succinate dehydrogenase activity indicates the inadequate substrate supply for TCA [96]. A similar metabolic shift due to succinate dehydrogenase and malate dehydrogenase inhibition with increased lactate formation and lactate dehydrogenase activity has also been observed in cypermethrin-intoxicated fish *Labeo rohita* [97] or in fenvalerate-intoxicated fish *Oreochromis niloticus* [98].

Hepatic aspartate aminotransferase, alanine aminotransferase, lactate dehydrogenase activities, total lipids, phospholipids, free fatty acids, and cholesterol levels have increased, while glycogen and total protein levels decreased in beta-cyfluthrin exposed rats [95]. Aminotransferases produce oxaloacetate and pyruvate intermediates that are transported into the mitochondrial matrix to maintain TCA or fatty acid production, and accumulation of oxaloacetate has caused the inhibition of malate dehydrogenase activity, a part of TCA of mitochondria in cypermethrin exposed rats [89].

Metabolomics approach is very effective to understand pyrethroid-induced metabolic changes. Reports show the metabolic shift to anaerobic fuel consumption and elevated fuel supply via gluconeogenesis to maintain energy levels in pyrethroid-induced stress conditions. For example, permethrin exposure increased urine lactate, acetate, 3-D-hydroxybutyrate, creatine, glycine, and formate while decreased citrate and 2-oxoglutarate levels in rats [99]. Elevated levels of urinary acetate and decreased TCA intermediates show the energy metabolism disorders. Similarly, Liang et al. reported that permethrin and deltamethrin exposure can cause the disturbance in energy metabolism via the enhanced rate of anaerobic glycolysis and fatty acid β-oxidation, and ketogenesis [100]. They found that these pyrethroids reduced the excretion of TCA intermediates and increased lactate, acetate, 3-D-hydroxybutyrate levels in treated rats. In another study, serum and urine metabolites levels have been changed by deltamethrin exposure, and then it was suggested that decreased utilization of pyruvate in TCA and consecutive anaerobiosis in exposed rats [101]. While a shift from aerobic respiration to anaerobiosis was also found in the brain of lambda-cyhalothrin exposed goldfish (*Carassius auratus*), a marked decrease has been observed in brain *N*-acetyl-aspartate levels, because of neuronal mitochondrial membrane damage via the ROS formation [102]. *N*-acetyl-aspartate is considered as a marker for mitochondrial dysfunction in neurons [103]. Higher levels of malate and alanine in cypermethrin exposed earthworms provide an argument for the increased gluconeogenesis and fueling the TCA for energy [104]. These effects have also been observed in the former studies [100–102]. However, as an opposite of these results, permethrin exposure has caused an increase in TCA intermediates and cellular fatty acids and a decrease in glutamate levels in rat neuroblastoma cell line B50 [105]. Increased fatty acid β-oxidation should be a response to permethrin toxicity in these cells.

Voltage-dependent anion channels located in the mitochondrial outer membrane is the only way to supply TCA intermediates from cytosol to mitochondria, and its closure causes a metabolic shift [106]. However, urea generation is also operated in the mitochondrial matrix, and it requires a bulk of substrates such as ornithine, citrulline, adenine nucleotides, respiratory substrates, and other metabolites across the mitochondrial outer membrane in/out of mitochondria, possibly via VDACs [107]. The mitochondrial outer membrane is rich in VDACs that opens in normal operated mitochondria and mitochondrial hexokinase bounds to VDAC to orchestrate respiration, glycolytic pathway, and other metabolic pathways such as the pentose phosphate shunt [108]. We think that pyrethroids can be effective on these mitochondrial membrane proteins via their substrate and/or membrane docking interaction(s), finally causing a metabolic shift in exposed cells together with their electron transfer disorder effect on transport chain.

5. Lipid metabolism is a target for pyrethroid-induced mitochondrial dysfunction

Reactive oxygen species reduces the oxygen consumption and decreases the fatty acid oxidation in adipocytes causing the lipid accumulation [109]. According to Chirumbolo and

Bjorklund, mitochondrial ROS formation and dysfunction could play a central role in the machinery of lipid accumulation via the interaction with AMPK and peroxisome proliferator-activated receptor (PPAR) pathways [110]. Stressed cells accumulate lipids and enhance the hypoxic stimulus, and this occurs via AMPK-signaling pathways.

Cypermethrin induces the *pyruvate kinase, glucose transporter, stearoyl-CoA desaturase-1, acyl-CoA oxidase,* and *carnitine palmitoyltransferase 1-α* mRNA levels in the liver of mice [111]. *PPAR-α* have also increased with increased pyruvate levels. In this study, hepatic free fatty acid transport genes have also been upregulated; then, cypermethrin is able to defect lipid metabolism and can cause the lipid accumulation (evidenced by increased lipid droplets in histologic sections) in this organ. An interesting situation is the overexpression of *stearoyl-CoA desaturase-1* gene because its activation is related to mitochondrial ROS generation, caspase-3 activation, and apoptotic cell death in the heart of rats fed with saturated fatty acid rich diet [112]. In this study, AMPK phosphorylation has been decreased with the overexpression of *stearoyl-CoA desaturase-1* gene. AMPK inactivation results in the activation of acetyl-CoA carboxylase. It increases malonyl CoA synthesis, and malonyl CoA reduces carnitine palmitoyltransferase activity to transport fatty acids into mitochondria for oxidation. Therefore, fatty acid oxidation is decelerated. It is known that mitochondrial fatty acid oxidation is an important ROS source [113]. However, mitochondria need fatty acids to maintain AMP/ATP ratio and to maintain its functions in physiological levels. Therefore, a subtle balance of fatty acid oxidation must be conducted. In this sense, PPAR (including all three forms) agonists upregulate the AMPK activity to mediate many physiological functions to protect cells from mitochondrial membrane potential change and ROS formation [114].

Carnitine palmitoyltransferase-1 and PPAR-α gene expressions have been upregulated by cypermethrin exposure in the liver of zebrafish (*Danio rerio*) with ROS activation [115]. The results reveal the importance of cypermethrin-induced oxidative stress on impaired fatty acid β-oxidation and mitochondrial dysfunction. PPAR-α is the most significant orchestrator of altered fatty acid metabolism in this process. Relation of pyrethroid-induced lipid accumulation and mitochondrial dysfunction has been conducted with some newer research. While Jin et al. [111] has not been found up or downregulated mRNA expression of *ppar-γ* with cypermethrin intoxication, Moustafa and Hussein [116] reported that lambda-cyhalothrin intoxication caused upregulation of *ppar-α* and *ppar-γ* transcripts in the liver of rats. Hepatic fat infiltration and periportal fatty changes have also been observed with an elevated ROS formation.

Cobalt chloride, a hypoxia mimetic agent, has caused downregulation of PPAR-γ, increased lipid accumulation, mitochondrial ROS production, and autophagy in mouse pre-adipocyte cells [117]. It is known that elevated levels of TNF-α can be found in dysfunctional neuronal cells. The high level exposure of TNF-α to mimic these cells has caused decreased PPAR-γ and AMPK proteins, ATP levels, and mitochondrial mass, while ROS levels and caspase-3 (an apoptotic executioner enzyme) increased in human neuronal stem cells [118]. Rosiglitazone, a PPAR-γ agonist, protected the cells from these adverse effects of TNF-α. Mitochondrial complex I activity has decreased in deltamethrin treated human dopaminergic neuroblastoma SH-SY5Y cells [73]. These cells had typical mitochondrial apoptotic signals. The authors revealed that the mitochondrial apoptosis was antagonized by PPARγ agonist rosiglitazone resulting in the inhibited translocation of PTEN-induced putative kinase 1 (PINK1) to defend cells against ROS formation by dysfunctional mitochondria. In mitochondrial damage conditions, PINK1 accumulation in outer membrane results with a selective autophagy [119]. Therefore, PINK1-dependent mitophagy is responsible for maintaining a healthy mitochondrial population for undesired excessive ROS formation [120, 121]. Exposure to deltamethrin has caused the apoptotic and autophagic death in rat pheochromocytoma cell line PC12 [122]. Although the autophagy inhibitor, 3-methyladenine exacerbated the deltamethrin toxicity, pre-treatment with autophagy inducer rapamycin and antioxidant *N*-acetylcysteine have increased the cell viability via the prevention of apoptosis progression.

However, autophagy itself can be responsible for the ROS formation [123, 124]; therefore complex I-inhibition related cell death could be derived from PINK1-mediated mitophagy because of the inhibition of ROS formation and apoptosis via an antioxidant or PPAR-γ agonist treatment during mitochondrial autophagosome formation [124, 125]. Mitochondrial fusion can constitute a link between ROS formation and lipid accumulation. Downregulation of Mfn2 gene in human embryonic kidney cells 293 with siRNA caused triglyceride and ROS accumulation and decreased oxygen consumption [126]. Interestingly, impaired mitochondrial dynamics and dysfunctional autophagy can also be a cause *in vivo* triglyceride accumulation in aged rat tissues [126].

Shen et al. [127] reported that mouse pre-adipocyte cells showed increased fat accumulation via AMPK/PPAR-γ intersection by deltamethrin exposure. Phosphorylated AMPK/AMPK (pAMPK/AMPK) ratio has been decreased, while PPAR-γ protein levels increased in these deltamethrin exposed cells. Permethrin has also caused similar changes in these cells with the elevation of triglyceride levels and decrement of *carnitine palmitoyltransferase 1-α* mRNA levels [128]. In this study, permethrin exposure decreased protein kinase B (Akt) and increased its activated phosphorylated forms (at Ser473 and Thr308) in C2C12 myotubes in the presence of insulin. Therefore, permethrin alters lipid metabolism in adipocytes and impaired glucose metabolism in myotubes and then increases the obesity and type-2 diabetes progression risks in exposed individuals. Authors discussed that these changes are related to mitochondrial Ca^{2+} and ROS formation. In another study, pAMPK levels have been increased with increased autophagosome formation and abnormal autophagy in cypermethrin treated rats and SH-SY5Y neuroblastoma cells [129]. Authors indicated that increased phosphorylation of AMPK shows the decreased AMP/ATP ratio via mitochondrial dysfunction. Although the above authors revealed the mitochondrial dysfunction-related adipogenesis, Xiao et al. [130] have defined an intracellular Ca^{2+}- and ER stress-related adipogenesis in permethrin exposed mouse pre-adipocyte cells.

Solute carrier family 25 member 25 (Slc25a25) and *solute carrier family 2 member 1 (Slc2a1)* gene expressions have been affected by deltamethrin and cyfluthrin exposure in the cortical samples of rat brain *in vivo* with many other membrane proteins [131]. Slc25a25 serves as a solute carrier for adenine nucleotides in and from the mitochondrial inner membrane, while Slc2a1 is a major glucose transporter in the blood-brain barrier. These pyrethroids have also affected *pyruvate dehydrogenase kinase 4 (pdk4)* gene expression, which plays a role in glucose metabolism via inhibition of pyruvate dehydrogenase complex by phosphorylation.

Therefore, pyrethroids can be effective on cells at different levels of metabolism. In a similar manner, permethrin caused a significant elevation of *pdk4* and *phosphoenolpyruvate carboxylase (pepck)* gene transcripts in the muscle and liver of mice, respectively [132]. Permethrin exposure displayed similar results [133] that were seen in the study of Kim et al. [128]. In addition, phosphorylated Akt at Thr308 and glucose transporter 4 (glut4) protein levels have been decreased in the muscle; therefore, authors concluded that permethrin can alter the glucose and lipid metabolism via an AMPK-dependent pathway and produce insulin resistance and obesity risk in exposed groups. In contrast, insulin-stimulated Akt phosphorylation has been decreased by permethrin in pAMPK-independent and the ERK-dependent manner in C2C12 myotubes, and this mechanism could be a reason for insulin resistance development [134]. Therefore, the exact mechanism of lipid accumulation in different cell types may use different pathways; however, we believed that ER-mitochondria axis and their relation in Ca^{2+} and ROS signaling are the main curators of these effects of pyrethroids.

Affected lipid metabolism by pyrethroids has also been observed in other studies including fish and mammals [135, 136].

6. Mitochondrial membrane structures and dynamics in pyrethroid intoxication

Another effect of pyrethroids is on the structural integrity and dynamics of mitochondria observed in histopathological studies. *cis*-Permethrin has caused inner membrane disruption, and the cristae have been replaced with a denser matrix in Leydig cells of mice testis [137]. Therefore, hitching of cholesterol delivery diminished the pregnenolone formation, contributing to the endocrine disrupting function of pyrethroids. Mitochondrial swelling associated with ER cisternae has been observed in the liver of cypermethrin exposed rats [138]. Dilated round or ovoid mitochondria with short cristae and clear matrix have also been noticed while small damaged mitochondria containing electron dense inclusions occurred in different time series. A similar result has also been found from an amphibian study. According to Yilmaz et al. [139], severely damaged cristae and loss of mitochondrial matrix have been found in the cypermethrin exposed sciatic nerves of *Rana ridibunda*. Typical tubular appearance loss, perturbed fusion/fission equilibrium favoring the fission, and decreased mitochondrial membrane potential have been observed in tefluthrin, deltamethrin, bifenthrin, and α-cypermethrin exposed rat cerebral astrocytoma C6 cells with an increase in cell death ratio [140]. Obvious mitochondrial hypertrophy with distended membranes has been found in the liver of deltamethrin exposed rats [92]. Deltamethrin exposure resulted in irregular contours of mitochondria, tiny and few cristae, and cloudy matrix. Mitochondrial morphometry has also been affected by deltamethrin exposure. Therefore, mitochondria may be the most vulnerable organelle with its structure-function relationship for pyrethroids toxicity.

Pyrethroids can pass and interact with biological membranes because of their lipophilic nature [84]. As mitochondrion stand its membranous structures, mitochondrial membranes and other proteins in addition to the electron transport proteins are candidate structures for pyrethroid action. For example, fenvalerate has not interacted with mitochondrial membrane proteins measured with intrinsic protein fluorescence, mainly by tryptophan fluorescence quenching in the isolated mitochondria from *Helicoverpa armigera* larvae (cotton bollworm) [141]. Because of its hydrophobic nature, deltamethrin has increased the mitochondrial membrane rigidity in the isolated rat liver mitochondrial preparation and this can cause the impaired transport of different ions between cytosol and mitochondrial matrix [90]. Permethrin has caused a decrease in mitochondrial membrane fluidity and this could be a reason for a bioenergetic crisis in the cell because of irregular energy transduction in striatum submitochondrial particles of rats [88]. Mitochondrial membrane fluidity at the hydrophilic-hydrophobic region of the bilayer has decreased, while fluidity in the hydrophobic core increased in the heart of 300-day old rats exposed the permethrin between 6 and 21 days of their life [142]. Moreover, decreased cholesterol levels in mitochondrial membranes have been observed while it increased in the plasma membrane of heart cells. Therefore, these observations and pro-oxidative properties of permethrin could cause the altered cardiac ultrastructure and function. This effect of permethrin has also been found in Leydig cells of mice testis as discussed above [137]. As an integral membrane protein, VDAC interacts with membrane cholesterol [143] and ATP synthesis, ATP/ADP exchange by adenine nucleotide translocator (ANT) at the inner membrane, ATP/ADP and metabolite exchange by VDAC can be affected by associated membrane composition [93].

Effects of pyrethroids are not limited to mitochondrial membranes because of fluidity decline in the hydrophobic core of cypermethrin exposed rat erythrocyte plasma membrane [144]. Similar fluidity decline has been observed in deltamethrin exposed common carp (*Cyprinus carpio*) erythrocyte plasma membranes [145]. Phosphatidylethanolamine, phosphoglyceride, phosphatidic acids, and cardiolipin levels were decreased, making the membrane more rigid and less permeable. Decreasing these components can cause oxidative stress and cell membrane ageing. Interestingly, cardiolipin is an exclusive component of the inner mitochondrial membrane, and it plays a significant role in governing the mitochondrial bioenergetics processes (interaction with respiratory chain proteins and substrate carriers) and dynamics [146]. Cardiolipin reduction has been observed via ROS-induced lipid peroxidation in nerve growth factor-deprived rat sympathetic neurons and this has caused the loss of mitochondrial density [147]. As a membranous structure, the same finding may be observed with mitochondrial preparations, but it is an issue for further studies. It has been concluded that high lipophilicity and pro-oxidative potential of pyrethroids can affect the biological membranes with their functional proteins to mediate the dysfunctional mitochondria.

While 18 kDa translocator protein (TSPO; formerly known as peripheral benzodiazepine receptor) ligands PK 11195 and Ro5-4864 are anti-apoptotic in the concentrations close to their TSPO affinity, they can also be pro-apoptotic agents at higher levels [148, 149]. It has been evidenced that pyrethroids can bind and interact with TSPO [150, 151], located on the mitochondrial outer membrane and participates to cholesterol transport as a cholesterol channel into mitochondria collectively with VDAC and ANT [152, 153]. Many type I and type II pyrethroids can bind this protein on rat brain membranes, while fluvalinate and fenvalerate have poor potency [154]. Furthermore, *cis*-permethrin has decreased the mRNA levels of *tspo* in mice testis [137]. In the study of Vadhana et al. [142], mitochondrial cholesterol levels have been decreased, while cellular and plasma cholesterol levels increased in the heart of permethrin exposed rats. The pyrethroids may interact with TSPO protein with high affinity to affect its interaction with VDAC [93] to decrease cholesterol levels in mitochondria. Because mitochondrial function mostly depends on its membranous structures, a decrease in membranous and inner mitochondrial cholesterol levels could be effective on ROS production and abnormal autophagy as is exemplified above sections. Increased TSPO to VDAC ratio has been correlated with increased ROS production, decreased mitophagy, and accumulation of damaged mitochondria [155, 156]. Therefore, oxidative-stress inducing and apoptotic potential of pyrethroids could also be originated with this capability. TSPO attends to the ROS formation via mitochondrial membrane potential transition [148]. Produced ROS affect the bonding form of cytochrome c to cardiolipin through the tightly to loosely conformation and results in the release of it [157] to induce mitochondrial apoptotic pathway. Interestingly, in the events of VDAC closure and blockage of TSPO function cause a permeability increase of VDAC to Ca^{2+} and this can accelerate the mtPTP opening [158].

7. Mitochondrial DNA and pyrethroids

There are very few studies on the mitochondrial DNA (mtDNA) alterations induced by pyrethroids in vertebrates. According to the results of Wang and Zhao [159] study, mtDNA somatic mutation frequency has been increased in the lung tissue of pesticide exposed (including pyrethroids) fruit growers. They have concluded that the increased frequency of mtDNA mutations may result from ROS formation, and the frequency has somewhat like cancer patients' tissues. Because of the adjacency of mtDNA to possible ROS formation centers in mitochondria [160], pyrethroid-induced mtDNA mutations could be linked to their ROS inducing potentials. In cypermethrin exposed zebrafish larvae, ROS induction has been augmented, while *ogg1* (8-oxoguanine DNA glycosylase) mRNA levels decreased [161]. This gene is responsible for the excision of 8-oxoguanine bases occurred via ROS action on DNA. This enzyme has many alternative splicing variants, all of them are targeted to the mitochondria for localization (PUBMED Gene ID:4968; https://www.ncbi.nlm.nih.gov/gene/4968, last access: January 7, 2018). According to the study of Sampath et al. [162], $Ogg^{-/-}$ mice exhibited a preference to carbohydrate metabolism over fatty acid oxidation via downregulated key fatty acid oxidation genes' and TCA genes' mRNAs. Then, they are susceptible to adiposity and hepatic steatosis. Therefore, pyrethroids might able to change the cellular substrate metabolism, and mtDNA mutations are probably involved in this process.

Pyrethroids bifenthrin, cypermethrin, and deltamethrin have increased ϱ-mutation frequency in *Saccharomyces cerevisiae* culture in a dose-dependent manner [163]. This type of mutation occurs mainly on mtDNA by large deletions [164], and mitochondrial protein synthesis and electron transport are blocked [163–165]. Interestingly, there are some studies related to the binding of pyrethroids to DNA macromolecule via different bonding mechanisms [166–169]. For example, permethrin can intercalate with DNA, and it is prone to bind G-C base pairs [167]. On the other hand, a complexation driven mechanism mainly by hydrogen-bond and van der Waals forces has been observed between DNA and tau-fluvalinate and fluvalinate molecules [169]. AT-rich sequences are more susceptible sites for this complexation.

We believed that pyrethroids can interact with mtDNA as seen in their electron transport complex bonding potential; therefore, can create mutations on mtDNA. However, further mechanistic research is needed.

8. Conclusion

In conclusion, pyrethroids can perform their toxic action via their oxidative potentials including unbalanced Ca^{2+} flux in/out of the organelles and cells. Mitochondria might be the most vulnerable organelle for pyrethroid toxicity. Pyrethroids probably can change the interaction of mitochondrion and ER to create an imbalance between the fine equilibrium of ROS and Ca^{2+} signals. This affects the form of cellular metabolic energy production, accumulation of lipids and other metabolites, and cell death type. Pyrethroids can also change the mitochondrial membrane structures to affect their ability for metabolism and ROS production capacity. These effects may be related to the endocrine disruption, diabetic, dopaminergic, and obesity-induction potential of pyrethroids that are observed in exposed individuals as exemplified in the above sections such as altered lipid metabolism and cholesterol delivery into the mitochondria. However, there are many gaps that must be solved, such as, interaction with mitochondrial membrane proteins, specific mutagenesis caused by pyrethroid molecule and mtDNA interaction, etc.

Author details

Celal Guven[1], Yusuf Sevgiler[2] and Eylem Taskin[3]*

*Address all correspondence to: eylemtaskin@yahoo.com

1 Department of Biophysics, Faculty of Medicine, Nigde Omer Halisdemir University, Nigde, Turkey

2 Department of Biology, Faculty of Science and Letters, Adiyaman University, Adiyaman, Turkey

3 Department of Physiology, Faculty of Medicine, Nigde Omer Halisdemir University, Nigde, Turkey

References

[1] Oberemok VV, Laikova KV, Gninenko YI, Zaitsev AS, Nyadar PM, Adeyemi TA. A short history of insecticides. Journal of Plant Protection Research. 2015;**55**(3):221-226. Available from: https://www.degruyter.com/view/j/jppr.2015.55.issue-3/jppr-2015-0033/jppr-2015-0033.xml

[2] Davies TGE, Field LM, Usherwood PNR, Williamson MS. DDT, pyrethrins, pyrethroids and insect sodium channels. IUBMB Life. 2007;**59**(3):151-162

[3] WHO. Allethrins [Internet]. EHC 87. Geneva: World Health Organization; 1989. Available from: http://www.inchem.org/documents/ehc/ehc/ehc87.htm [Accessed: Jan 6, 2018]

[4] USEPA. Pyrethrins and Pyrethroids [Internet]. 2018. Available from: https://www.epa.gov/ingredients-used-pesticide-products/pyrethrins-and-pyrethroids [Accessed: Jan 7, 2018]

[5] Soderlund DM, Bloomquist JR. Neurotoxic actions of pyrethroid insecticides. Annual Review of Entomology. 1989;**34**(1):77-96. Available from: http://www.annualreviews.org/doi/10.1146/annurev.en.34.010189.000453

[6] Wismer T, Means C. Toxicology of newer insecticides in small animals. Veterinary Clinics of North America—Small Animal Practice. 2012;**42**:335-347

[7] Stelzer KJ, Gordon MA. Interactions of pyrethroids with phosphatidylcholine liposomal membranes. Biochimica et Biophysica Acta (BBA)—Biomembranes. 1985;**812**(2):361-368

[8] Nasuti C, Cantalamessa F, Falcioni G, Gabbianelli R. Different effects of type I and type II pyrethroids on erythrocyte plasma membrane properties and enzymatic activity in rats. Toxicology. 2003;**191**:233-244

[9] Motomura H, Narahashi T. Interaction of tetramethrin and deltamethrin at the single sodium channel in rat hippocampal neurons. Neurotoxicology. 2001;**22**:329-339

[10] Silva APB, Santos JMM, Martins AJ. Mutations in the voltage-gated sodium channel gene of anophelines and their association with resistance to pyrethroids—A review. Parasites & Vectors. 2014;**7**:450

[11] Breckenridge CB, Holden L, Sturgess N, Weiner M, Sheets L, Sargent D, et al. Evidence for a separate mechanism of toxicity for the Type I and the Type II pyrethroid insecticides. Neurotoxicology. 2009;**30**:S17-S31

[12] Goldmann L. Childhood Pesticide Poisoning. The Chemicals Programme of the United Nations Environment Programme UNEP Chemicals, International Environment House, Châtelaine, Switzerland; 2004. pp. 1-37

[13] Laskowski DA. Physical and chemical properties of pyrethroids. Reviews of Environmental Contamination and Toxicology. 2002;**174**:49-170

[14] Petrarca MH, Ccanccapa-Cartagena A, Masiá A, Godoy HT, Picó Y. Comparison of green sample preparation techniques in the analysis of pyrethrins and pyrethroids in baby food by liquid chromatography–tandem mass spectrometry. Journal of Chromatography. A. 2017;**1497**:28-37

[15] Sereda B, Bouwman H, Kylin H. Comparing water, bovine milk, and indoor residual spraying as possible sources of ddt and pyrethroid residues in breast milk. Journal of Toxicology and Environmental Health, Part A. 2009;**72**(13):842-851

[16] Corcellas C, Feo ML, Torres JP, Malm O, Ocampo-Duque W, Eljarrat E, et al. Pyrethroids in human breast milk: Occurrence and nursing daily intake estimation. Environment International. 2012;**47**:17-22

[17] Babina K, Dollard M, Pilotto L, Edwards JW. Environmental exposure to organophosphorus and pyrethroid pesticides in South Australian preschool children: A cross sectional study. Environment International. 2012;**48**:109-120

[18] Barr DB, Olsson AO, Wong LY, Udunka S, Baker SE, Whitehead RD, et al. Urinary concentrations of metabolites of pyrethroid insecticides in the general U.S. population: National health and nutrition examination survey 1999-2002. Environmental Health Perspectives. 2010;**118**(6):742-748

[19] Oulhote Y, Bouchard MF. Urinary metabolites of organophosphate and pyrethroid pesticides and behavioral problems in Canadian children. Environmental Health Perspectives. 2013;**121**(11-12):1378-1384

[20] Wagner-Schuman M, Richardson JR, Auinger P, Braun JM, Lanphear BP, Epstein JN, et al. Association of pyrethroid pesticide exposure with attention-deficit/hyperactivity disorder in a nationally representative sample of U.S. children. Environmental Health. 2015;**14**:44

[21] Han J, Zhou L, Luo M, Liang Y, Zhao W, Wang P, et al. Nonoccupational exposure to pyrethroids and risk of coronary heart disease in the Chinese population. Environmental Science & Technology. 2017;**51**(1):664-670. Available from: http://pubs.acs.org/doi/abs/10.1021/acs.est.6b05639

[22] Lu D, Wang D, Feng C, Jin Y, Zhou Z, Wu C, et al. Urinary concentrations of metabolites of pyrethroid insecticides in textile workers. Environment International. 2013;**60**:137-144

[23] Miyamoto J, Kaneko H, Takamatsu Y. Stereoselective formation of a cholesterol ester conjugate from fenvalerate by mouse microsomal carboxyesterase(s). Journal of Biochemical Toxicology. 1986;**1**(2):79-93

[24] Hu F, Li L, Wang C, Zhang Q, Zhang X, Zhao M. Enantioselective induction of oxidative stress by permethrin in rat adrenal pheochromocytoma (PC12) cells. Environmental Toxicology and Chemistry. 2010;**29**(3):683-690

[25] Kaneko H. Pyrethroids: Mammalian metabolism and toxicity. Journal of Agricultural and Food Chemistry. 2011;**59**(7):2786-2791

[26] Mikata K, Isobe N, Kaneko H. Biotransformation and enzymatic reactions of synthetic pyrethroids in mammals. Topics in Current Chemistry. 2012;**314**:113-135

[27] Tyler CR, Beresford N, van der Woning M, Sumpter JP, Tchorpe K. Metabolism and environmental degradation of pyrethroid insecticides produce compounds with endocrine activities. Environmental Toxicology and Chemistry. 2000;**19**(4):801-809. Available from: http://doi.wiley.com/10.1002/etc.5620190404

[28] Romero A, Ramos E, Castellano V, Martínez MA, Ares I, Martínez M, et al. Cytotoxicity induced by deltamethrin and its metabolites in SH-SY5Y cells can be differentially prevented by selected antioxidants. Toxicology in Vitro. 2012;**26**(6):823-830

[29] Johri A, Yadav S, Singh RL, Dhawan A, Ali M, Parmar D. Long lasting effects of prenatal exposure to deltamethrin on cerebral and hepatic cytochrome P450s and behavioral activity in rat offspring. European Journal of Pharmacology. 2006;**544**(1-3):58-68

[30] Wakeling EN, Atchison WD, Neal AP. Pyrethroids and their effects on ion channels. In: Pesticides—Advances in Chemical and Botanical Pesticides, InTech, London, United Kingdom. 2012. pp. 39-66

[31] Kale M, Rathore N, John S, Bhatnagar D. Lipid peroxidative damage on pyrethroid exposure and alterations in antioxidant status in rat erythrocytes: A possible involvement of reactive oxygen species. Toxicology Letters. 1999;**105**(3):197-205

[32] Anadón A, Arés I, Martínez MA, Martínez-Larrañaga MR. Pyrethrins and synthetic pyrethroids: Use in veterinary medicine. In: Ramawat KG, Mérillon JM, editors. Natural Products: Phytochemistry, Botany and Metabolism of Alkaloids, Phenolics and Terpenes. Berlin Heidelberg: Springer-Verlag Berlin Heidelberg; 2013. pp. 4061-4086

[33] Kakko I. Toxic Mechanisms of Pyrethroids Studied in Vitro [Internet]. University of Tampere; 2004. Available from: http://tampub.uta.fi/bitstream/handle/10024/67410/951-44-6005-7.pdf;sequence=1

[34] Muse KE, Oberley TD, Sempf JM, Oberley LW. Immunolocalization of antioxidant enzymes in adult hamster kidney. The Histochemical Journal. 1994;**26**(9):734-753

[35] Halliwell B, Gutteridge JMC. Free Radicals in Biology and Medicine. 3 ed. Oxford University Press; 936 p. ISBN: 9780198500452

[36] Klimek J. Cytochrome P-450 involvement in the NADPH-dependent lipid peroxidation in human placental mitochondria. Biochimica et Biophysica Acta (BBA)—Lipids and Lipid Metabolism. 1990;**1044**(1):158-164

[37] Baliga R, Zhang Z, Shah SV. Role of cytochrome P-450 in hydrogen peroxide-induced cytotoxicity to LLC-PK1 cells. Kidney International. 1996;**50**:1118-1124

[38] Baliga R, Zhang Z, Baliga M, Ueda N, Shah SV. Role of cytochrome P-450 as a source of catalytic iron in cisplatin-induced nephrotoxicity. Kidney International. 1998;**54**(5):1562-1569. Available from: http://www.ncbi.nlm.nih.gov/pubmed/9844132

[39] Baliga R, Zhang Z, Baliga M, Ueda N, Shah SV. In vitro and in vivo evidence suggesting a role for iron in cisplatin-induced nephrotoxicity. Kidney International. 1998;**53**(2):394-401. Available from: http://www.ncbi.nlm.nih.gov/pubmed/9461098

[40] Hojo Y, Shiraki A, Tsuchiya T, Shimamoto K, Ishii Y, Suzuki K, Shibutani M, Mitsumori K. Liver tumor promoting effect of etofenprox in rats and its possible mechanism of action. The Journal of Toxicological Sciences. 2012;**37**(2):297-306

[41] Raina R, Verma PK, Pankaj NK, Prawez S. Induction of oxidative stress and lipid peroxidation in rats chronically exposed to cypermethrin through dermal application. Journal of Veterinary Science. 2009;**10**(3):257-259

[42] Deguchi Y, Yamada T, Hirose Y, Nagahori H, Kushida M, Sumida K, et al. Mode of action analysis for the synthetic pyrethroid metofluthrin-induced rat liver tumors: Evidence

for hepatic CYP2B induction and hepatocyte proliferation. Toxicological Sciences. 2009; **108**(1):69-80

[43] Das PC, Streit TM, Cao Y, Rose RL, Cherrington N, Ross MK, et al. Pyrethroids: Cytotoxicity and induction of CYP isoforms in human hepatocytes. Drug Metabolism and Drug Interactions. 2008;**23**(3-4):211-236 Available from: http://www.ncbi.nlm.nih.gov/pubmed/19326768

[44] Chen Q, Cederbaum AI. Cytotoxicity and apoptosis produced by cytochrome P450 2E1 in Hep G2 cells. Molecular Pharmacology. 1998;**53**(4):638-648. Available from: http://www.ncbi.nlm.nih.gov/pubmed/9547353%5Cnhttp://molpharm.aspetjournals.org/content/53/4/638.full.pdf

[45] Shah A, Kumar S, Simon SD, Singh DP, Kumar A. HIV gp120- and methamphetamine-mediated oxidative stress induces astrocyte apoptosis via cytochrome P450 2E1. Cell Death & Disease. 2013;**4**:e850

[46] Gil J, Almeida S, Oliveira CR, Rego AC. Cytosolic and mitochondrial ROS in staurosporine-induced retinal cell apoptosis. Free Radical Biology & Medicine. 2003;**35**(11):1500-1514

[47] Kumar A, Sasmal D, Bhaskar A, Mukhopadhyay K, Thakur A, Sharma N. Deltamethrin-induced oxidative stress and mitochondrial caspase-dependent signaling pathways in murine splenocytes. Environmental Toxicology. 2016;**31**(7):808-819

[48] Wu A, Ren T, Hu Q, Liu Y. Deltamethrin induces altered expression of P53, Bax and Bcl-2 in rat brain. Neuroscience Letters. 2000;**284**(1-2):29-32

[49] Yang Y, Zong M, Xu W, Zhang Y, Wang B, Yang M, et al. Natural pyrethrins induces apoptosis in human hepatocyte cells via Bax- and Bcl-2-mediated mitochondrial pathway. Chemico-Biological Interactions. 2017;**262**:38-45

[50] Zhao XF, Wang Q, Ji YL, Wang H, Liu P, Zhang C, et al. Fenvalerate induces germ cell apoptosis in mouse testes through the Fas/FasL signaling pathway. Archives of Toxicology. 2011;**85**(9):1101-1108

[51] Marchi S, Patergnani S, Pinton P. The endoplasmic reticulum-mitochondria connection: One touch, multiple functions. Biochimica et Biophysica Acta—Bioenergetics. 2014; **1837**(4):461-469

[52] Görlach A, Bertram K, Hudecova S, Krizanova O. Calcium and ROS: A mutual interplay. Redox Biology. 2015;**6**:260-271

[53] Chirumbolo S, Bjørklund G. PERM hypothesis: The fundamental machinery able to elucidate the role of xenobiotics and hormesis in cell survival and homeostasis. International Journal of Molecular Sciences. 2017;**18**:165

[54] Dhivya Vadhana MS, Siva Arumugam S, Carloni M, Nasuti C, Gabbianelli R. Early life permethrin treatment leads to long-term cardiotoxicity. Chemosphere. 2013;**93**(6):1029-1034

[55] Cao Z, Shafer TJ, Murray TF. Mechanisms of pyrethroid insecticide-induced stimulation of calcium influx in neocortical neurons. The Journal of Pharmacology and Experimental Therapeutics. 2011;**336**(1):197-205. Available from: http://jpet.aspetjournals.org/content/336/1/197.full

[56] Cao Z, Cui Y, Nguyen HM, Jenkins DP, Wulff H, Pessah IN. Nanomolar bifenthrin alters synchronous Ca^{2+} oscillations and cortical neuron development independent of sodium channel activity. Molecular Pharmacology. 2014;**85**(4):630-639. Available from: http://molpharm.aspetjournals.org/cgi/doi/10.1124/mol.113.090076

[57] Marshall J, Steven BS. Advances in the mode of action of pyrethroids. In: Matsuo N, Mori T, editors. Pyrethroids: From Chrysanthemum to Modern Industrial Insecticide (Part of the Topics in Current Chemistry book series. Vol. 314). Heidelberg, Berlin: Springer-Verlag Berlin Heidelberg; 2012. pp. 49-72

[58] Paschen W. Role of calcium in neuronal cell injury: Which subcellular compartment is involved? Brain Research Bulletin. 2000:**53**(4);409-413

[59] Milatovic D, Gupta RC, Aschner M. Anticholinesterase toxicity and oxidative stress. Scientific World Journal. 2006;**6**:295-310. Available from: http://www.hindawi.com/journals/tswj/2006/683173/abs/

[60] Bondy SC, LeBel CP. The relationship between excitotoxicity and oxidative stress in the central nervous system. Free Radical Biology & Medicine. 1993;**14**(6):633-642

[61] Magby JP, Richardson JR. Role of calcium and calpain in the downregulation of voltage-gated sodium channel expression by the pyrethroid pesticide deltamethrin. Journal of Biochemical and Molecular Toxicology. 2015;**29**(3):129-134

[62] Hossain MM, Richardson JR. Mechanism of pyrethroid pesticide-induced apoptosis: Role of calpain and the ER stress pathway. Toxicological Sciences. 2011;**122**(2):512-525

[63] Gusovsky F, Hollingsworth EB, Daly JW. Regulation of phosphatidylinositol turnover in brain synaptoneurosomes: Stimulatory effects of agents that enhance influx of sodium ions. Proceedings of the National Academy of Sciences of the United States of America. 1986;**83**(9):3003-3007

[64] Enan E, Matsumura F. Activation of phosphoinositide/protein kinase C pathway in rat brain tissue by pyrethroids. Biochemical Pharmacology. 1993;**45**(3):703-710

[65] Niederer KE, Morrow DK, Gettings JL, Irick M, Krawiecki A, Brewster JL. Cypermethrin blocks a mitochondria-dependent apoptotic signal initiated by deficient N-linked glycosylation within the endoplasmic reticulum. Cellular Signalling. 2005;**17**(2):177-186

[66] Lemasters J, Theruvath T, Zhong Z, Nieminen A. Mitochondrial calcium and the permeability transition in cell death. Biochimica et Biophysica Acta. 2010;**1787**(11):1395-1401

[67] Madhubabu G, Yenugu S. Allethrin induces oxidative stress, apoptosis and calcium release in rat testicular carcinoma cells (LC540). Toxicology in Vitro. 2014;**28**(8):1386-1395. Available from: http://www.ncbi.nlm.nih.gov/pubmed/25072698%5Cnhttp://www.sciencedirect.com/science/article/pii/S0887233314001404

[68] Gupta G, Chaitanya RK, Golla M, Karnati R. Allethrin toxicity on human corneal epithelial cells involves mitochondrial pathway mediated apoptosis. Toxicology in Vitro. 2013;**27**(8):2242-2248

[69] Luft S, Milki EA, Glustrom E, Ampiah-Bonney R, O'Hara P. Binding of organochloride and pyrethroid pesticides to estrogen receptors α and β: A fluorescence polarization assay. Biophysical Journal. 2009;**96**(3, Suppl. 1):444a

[70] Taylor JS, Thomson BM, Lang CN, Sin FYT, Podivinsky E. Estrogenic pyrethroid pesticides regulate expression of estrogen receptor transcripts in mouse sertoli cells differently from 17-estradiol. Journal of Toxicology and Environmental Health, Part A. 2010;**73**(16):1075-1089

[71] Liang J, Xie Q, Li P, Zhong X, Chen Y. Mitochondrial estrogen receptor β inhibits cell apoptosis via interaction with Bad in a ligand-independent manner. Molecular and Cellular Biochemistry. 2014;**401**(1-2):71-86

[72] Arora D, Siddiqui MH, Sharma PK, Shukla Y. Deltamethrin induced RIPK3-mediated caspase-independent non-apoptotic cell death in rat primary hepatocytes. Biochemical and Biophysical Research Communications. 2016;**479**(2):217-223

[73] Ko J, Park JH, Park YS, Koh HC. PPAR-γ activation attenuates deltamethrin-induced apoptosis by regulating cytosolic PINK1 and inhibiting mitochondrial dysfunction. Toxicology Letters. 2016;**260**:8-17

[74] Guvenc D, Kabak Y, Atmaca E, Aksoy A, Guvenc T. Examination of caspase-dependent apoptotic and necrotic changes in rat kidney exposed to different doses of permethrin. Biotechnic & Histochemistry. 2013;**88**(2):76-85

[75] Coşkun B, Çömelekoğlu Ü, Polat A, Kaymaz FF. Evaluation of the toxic effects of cypermethrin inhalation on the frog heart. Ecotoxicology and Environmental Safety. 2004;**57**(2):220-225

[76] Huang H, Hu X, Eno CO, Zhao G, Li C, White C. An interaction between Bcl-xL and the voltage-dependent anion channel (VDAC) promotes mitochondrial Ca^{2+} uptake. The Journal of Biological Chemistry. 2013;**288**(27):19870-19881

[77] Rutter GA, Rizzuto R. Regulation of mitochondrial metabolism by ER Ca^{2+} release: An intimate connection. Trends in Biochemical Sciences. 2000;**25**:215-221

[78] White C, Li C, Yang J, Petrenko NB, Madesh M, Thompson CB, et al. The endoplasmic reticulum gateway to apoptosis by Bcl-X(L) modulation of the InsP3R. Nature Cell Biology. 2005;**7**(10):1021-1028. Available from: http://www.pubmedcentral.nih.gov/articlerender.fcgi?artid=2893337&tool=pmcentrez&rendertype=abstract

[79] Cárdenas C, Miller RA, Smith I, Bui T, Molgó J, Müller M, et al. Essential regulation of cell bioenergetics by constitutive InsP3 receptor Ca^{2+} transfer to mitochondria. Cell. 2010;**142**(2):270-283

[80] Giacomello M, Drago I, Pizzo P, Pozzan T. Mitochondrial Ca^{2+} as a key regulator of cell life and death. Cell Death and Differentiation. 2007;**14**:1267-1274

[81] Distelhorst CW, Bootman MD. Bcl-2 interaction with the inositol 1,4,5-trisphosphate receptor: Role in Ca^{2+} signaling and disease. Cell Calcium. 2011;**50**:234-241

[82] Hui X, Reither G, Kaestner L, Lipp P. Targeted activation of conventional and novel protein kinases C through differential translocation patterns. Molecular and Cellular Biology. 2014;**34**(13):2370-2381. Available from: http://mcb.asm.org/cgi/doi/10.1128/MCB.00040-14

[83] Hsu SS, Chou CT. Deltamethrin-induced [Ca^{2+}]i rise and death in HGB human glioblastoma cells. The Chinese Journal of Physiology. 2012;**55**(4):294-304

[84] Kakko I, Toimela T, Tähti H. The toxicity of pyrethroid compounds in neural cell cultures studied with total ATP, mitochondrial enzyme activity and microscopic photographing. Environmental Toxicology and Pharmacology. 2004;**15**(2-3):95-102

[85] Kakko I, Toimela T, Tähti H. Oestradiol potentiates the effects of certain pyrethroid compounds in the MCF7 human breast carcinoma cell line. Alternatives to Laboratory Animals. 2004

[86] Gassner B, Wüthrich A, Scholtysik G, Solioz M. The pyrethroids permethrin and cyhalothrin are potent inhibitors of the mitochondrial complex I. The Journal of Pharmacology and Experimental Therapeutics. 1997;**281**(2):855-860. Available from: http://www.ncbi.nlm.nih.gov/pubmed/9152394

[87] Fato R, Bergamini C, Bortolus M, Maniero AL, Leoni S, Ohnishi T, et al. Differential effects of mitochondrial complex I inhibitors on production of reactive oxygen species. Biochimica et Biophysica Acta. 2009;**1787**(5):384-392. Available from: http://www.sciencedirect.com/science/article/pii/S0005272808007093

[88] Falcioni ML, Nasuti C, Bergamini C, Fato R, Lenaz G, Gabbianelli R. The primary role of glutathione against nuclear DNA damage of striatum induced by permethrin in rats. Neuroscience. 2010;**168**(1):2-10

[89] Singh AK, Saxena PN, Sharma HN. Stress induced by beta-cyfluthrin, a type-2 pyrethroid, on brain biochemistry of Albino rat (*Rattus norvegicus*). Biologie et Médecine. 2009; **1**(2):74-86

[90] Braguini WL, Cadena SMSC, Carnieri EGS, Rocha MEM, De Oliveira MBM. Effects of deltamethrin on functions of rat liver mitochondria and on native and synthetic model membranes. Toxicology Letters. 2004;**152**(3):191-202

[91] Chen D, Huang X, Liu L, Shi N. Deltamethrin induces mitochondrial membrane permeability and altered expression of cytochrome C in rat brain. Journal of Applied Toxicology. 2007;**27**(4):368-372

[92] Catinot R, Hoellinger H, Pfister A, Sonnier M, Simon MT. Effects on rats of subacute intoxication with deltamethrin via an osmotic pump. Drug and Chemical Toxicology. 1989;**12**(3-4):173-196

[93] Campbell AM, Chan SHP. Mitochondrial membrane cholesterol, the voltage dependent anion channel (VDAC), and the Warburg effect. Journal of Bioenergetics and Biomembranes. 2008;**40**(3):193-197. Available from: http://www.ncbi.nlm.nih.gov/pubmed/18677555

[94] El-Demerdash FM, Yousef MI, Kedwany FS, Baghdadi HH. Role of α-tocopherol and β-carotene in ameliorating the fenvalerate-induced changes in oxidative stress, hemato-biochemical parameters, and semen quality of male rats. Journal of Environmental Science and Health, Part B. Pesticides, Food Contaminants, and Agricultural Wastes. 2004;**39**(3):443-459

[95] Bhushan B, Saxena PN, Saxena N. Biochemical and histological changes in rat liver caused by cypermethrin and beta-cyfluthrin. Arhiv za Higijenu Rada i Toksikologiju. 2013;**64**(1):57-67

[96] Ravi Sekhar P, Savithri Y, Nagarjuna A, Madhava Rao S, Pushpa Raj CJ, Jayantha RK. Effect of cypermethrin on selected dehydrogenase enzymes in muscle and heart tissues of Albino rats. Journal of Indian Society of Toxicology. 2009;**5**(1):1-5

[97] Philip GH, Reddy PM, Sridevi G. Cypermethrin-induced in vivo alterations in the carbohydrate metabolism of freshwater fish, labeo rohita. Ecotoxicology and Environmental Safety. 1995;**31**(2):173-178

[98] Radhaiah V, Jayantha RK. Toxicity of the pyrethroid insecticide fenvalerate to a fresh water fish, *Tilapia mossambica* (Peters): Changes in glycogen metabolism of muscle. Ecotoxicology and Environmental Safety. 1990;**19**(1):116-121

[99] Liang Y-J, Wang H-P, Long D-X, Wu Y-J. Applying biofluid metabonomic techniques to analyze the combined subchronic toxicity of propoxur and permethrin in rats. Bioanalysis. 2012;**4**(24):2897-2907. Available from: http://www.future-science.com/doi/10.4155/bio.12.277

[100] Liang YJ, Wang HP, Long DX, Li W, Wu YJ. A metabonomic investigation of the effects of 60 days exposure of rats to two types of pyrethroid insecticides. Chemico-Biological Interactions. 2013;**206**(2):302-308

[101] Wang HP, Liang YJ, Sun YJ, Chen JX, Hou WY, Long DX, et al. 1H NMR-based metabonomic analysis of the serum and urine of rats following subchronic exposure to dichlorvos, deltamethrin, or a combination of these two pesticides. Chemico-Biological Interactions. 2013;**203**(3):588-596

[102] Li M, Wang J, Lu Z, Wei D, Yang M, Kong L. NMR-based metabolomics approach to study the toxicity of lambda-cyhalothrin to goldfish (*Carassius auratus*). Aquatic Toxicology. 2014;**146**:82-92

[103] Signoretti S, Marmarou A, Tavazzi B, Lazzarino G, Beaumont A, Vagnozzi R. N-Acetylaspartate reduction as a measure of injury severity and mitochondrial dysfunction following diffuse traumatic brain injury. Journal of Neurotrauma. 2001;**18**(10):977-991. Available from: http://www.ncbi.nlm.nih.gov/pubmed/11686498

[104] Ch R, Singh AK, Pandey P, Saxena PN, Reddy Mudiam MK. Identifying the metabolic perturbations in earthworm induced by cypermethrin using gas chromatography-mass spectrometry based metabolomics. Scientific Reports. 2015;**5**:15674

[105] Hayton S, Maker GL, Mullaney I, Trengove RD. Untargeted metabolomics of neuronal cell culture: A model system for the toxicity testing of insecticide chemical exposure. Journal of Applied Toxicology. 2017;**37**(12):1481-1492

[106] Maldonado EN. VDAC–tubulin, an anti-Warburg pro-oxidant switch. Frontiers in Oncology. 2017;**7**:4

[107] Lemasters JJ, Holmuhamedov EL, Czerny C, Zhong Z, Maldonado EN. Regulation of mitochondrial function by voltage dependent anion channels in ethanol metabolism and the Warburg effect. Biochimica et Biophysica Acta. 2012;**1818**(6):1536-1544. Available from: http://www.pubmedcentral.nih.gov/articlerender.fcgi?artid=3422743&tool=pmcentrez&rendertype=abstract

[108] Mathupala SP, Ko YH, Pedersen PL. The pivotal roles of mitochondria in cancer: Warburg and beyond and encouraging prospects for effective therapies. Biochimica et Biophysica Acta—Bioenergetics. 2010;**1797**:1225-1230

[109] Wang T, Si Y, Shirihai OS, Si H, Schultz V, Corkey RF, et al. Respiration in adipocytes is inhibited by reactive oxygen species. Obesity. 2010;**18**(8):1493-1502

[110] Chirumbolo S, Bjørklund G. Pyrethroid pesticides in the autophagy/apoptosis balance: Role in adipocyte lipidogenesis. Food and Chemical Toxicology. 2017;**106**:568-569

[111] Jin Y, Lin X, Miao W, Wu T, Shen H, Chen S, et al. Chronic exposure of mice to environmental endocrine-disrupting chemicals disturbs their energy metabolism. Toxicology Letters. 2014;**225**(3):392-400

[112] Matsui H, Yokoyama T, Sekiguchi K, Iijima D, Sunaga H, Maniwa M, et al. Stearoyl-Coa desaturase-1 (SCD1) augments saturated fatty acid-induced lipid accumulation and inhibits apoptosis in cardiac myocytes. PLoS One. 2012;**7**(3):e33283

[113] Rosca MG, Vazquez EJ, Chen Q, Kerner J, Kern TS, Hoppel CL. Oxidation of fatty acids is the source of increased mitochondrial reactive oxygen species production in kidney cortical tubules in early diabetes. Diabetes. 2012;**61**(8):2074-2083

[114] Lee WH, Kim SG. AMPK-Dependent metabolic regulation by PPAR agonists. PPAR Research. 2010; Article ID: 549101. 10 pages

[115] Jin Y, Zheng S, Pu Y, Shu L, Sun L, Liu W, et al. Cypermethrin has the potential to induce hepatic oxidative stress, DNA damage and apoptosis in adult zebrafish (*Danio rerio*). Chemosphere. 2011;**82**(3):398-404

[116] Moustafa GG, Hussein MMA. Lambda cyhalothrin toxicity induces alterations in lipogenic genes and inflammatory factors in rat liver. The Japanese Journal of Veterinary Research. 2016;**64**(1):25-38

[117] Marques AP, Rosmaninho-Salgado J, Estrada M, Cortez V, Nobre RJ, Cavadas C. Hypoxia mimetic induces lipid accumulation through mitochondrial dysfunction and stimulates autophagy in murine preadipocyte cell line. Biochimica et Biophysica Acta, General Subjects. 2017;**1861**(3):673-682

[118] Chiang M-C, Cheng Y-C, Lin K-H, Yen C-H. PPARγ regulates the mitochondrial dysfunction in human neural stem cells with tumor necrosis factor alpha. Neuroscience. 2013;**229**:118-129. Available from: http://linkinghub.elsevier.com/retrieve/pii/S0306452212010871

[119] Pickrell AM, Youle RJ. The roles of PINK1, Parkin, and mitochondrial fidelity in parkinson's disease. Neuron. 2015;**85**:257-273

[120] Zhang HT, Mi L, Wang T, Yuan L, Li XH, Dong LS, et al. PINK1/Parkin-mediated mitophagy play a protective role in manganese induced apoptosis in SH-SY5Y cells. Toxicology in Vitro. 2016;**34**:212-219

[121] Liu N, Wu J, Zhang L, Gao Z, Sun Y, Yu M, et al. Hydrogen sulphide modulating mitochondrial morphology to promote mitophagy in endothelial cells under high-glucose and high-palmitate. Journal of Cellular and Molecular Medicine. 2017;**21**(12):3190-3203

[122] Park YS, Park JH, Ko J, Shin IC, Koh HC. mTOR inhibition by rapamycin protects against deltamethrin-induced apoptosis in PC12 Cells. Environmental Toxicology. 2017;**32**(1):109-121

[123] Du J, Teng R-JJ, Guan T, Eis A, Kaul S, Konduri GG, et al. Role of autophagy in angiogenesis in aortic endothelial cells. American Journal of Physiology. Cell Physiology. 2011;**302**(2):C383-C391. Available from: http://www.pubmedcentral.nih.gov/articlerender.fcgi?artid=3328843&tool=pmcentrez&rendertype=abstract

[124] Basit F, van Oppen LM, Schöckel L, Bossenbroek HM, van Emst-de Vries SE, Hermeling JC, et al. Mitochondrial complex I inhibition triggers a mitophagy-dependent ROS increase leading to necroptosis and ferroptosis in melanoma cells. Cell Death & Disease. 2017;**8**(3):e2716. Available from: http://www.nature.com/doifinder/10.1038/cddis.2017.133

[125] Corona JC, de Souza SC, Duchen MR. PPARγ activation rescues mitochondrial function from inhibition of complex I and loss of PINK1. Experimental Neurology. 2014;**253**:16-27

[126] Zhao L, Zou X, Feng Z, Luo C, Liu J, Li H, et al. Evidence for association of mitochondrial metabolism alteration with lipid accumulation in aging rats. Experimental Gerontology. 2014;**56**:3-12

[127] Shen P, Hsieh TH, Yue Y, Sun Q, Clark JM, Park Y. Deltamethrin increases the fat accumulation in 3T3-L1 adipocytes and *Caenorhabditis elegans*. Food and Chemical Toxicology. 2017;**101**:149-156

[128] Kim J, Park Y, Yoon KS, Clark JM, Park Y. Permethrin alters adipogenesis in 3T3-L1 adipocytes and causes insulin resistance in C2C12 myotubes. Journal of Biochemical and Molecular Toxicology. 2014;**28**(9):418-424

[129] Mishra AK, Mishra S, Rajput C, Ur Rasheed MS, Patel DK, Singh MP. Cypermethrin activates autophagosome formation Albeit inhibits autophagy owing to poor lysosome quality: Relevance to Parkinson's disease. Neurotoxicity Research. 2018;**33**(2):377-387

[130] Xiao X, Qi W, Clark JM, Park Y. Permethrin potentiates adipogenesis via intracellular calcium and endoplasmic reticulum stress-mediated mechanisms in 3T3-L1 adipocytes. Food and Chemical Toxicology. 2017 Nov;**109**(Pt 1):123-129

[131] Harrill J. Effect of Pyrethroid Insecticides on Gene Expression in the Mammalian Central Nervous System. Chapel Hill: University of North Carolina; 2008

[132] Xiao X. Effects of Permethrin, a Pyrethroid Insecticide, on Glucose and Lipid Metabolism. Amherst: University of Massachusetts; 2017

[133] Xiao X, Kim Y, Kim D, Yoon KS, Clark JM, Park Y. Permethrin alters glucose metabolism in conjunction with high fat diet by potentiating insulin resistance and decreases voluntary activities in female C57BL/6J mice. Food and Chemical Toxicology. 2017;**108**:161-170

[134] Sun Q, Peng Y, Qi W, Kim Y, Clark JM, Kim D, et al. Permethrin decreased insulin-stimulated AKT phosphorylation dependent on extracellular signal-regulated kinase-1 (ERK), but not AMP-activated protein kinase α (AMPKα), in C2C12 myotubes. Food and Chemical Toxicology. 2017;**109**:95-101

[135] Cengiz EI, Unlu E. Sublethal effects of commercial deltamethrin on the structure of the gill, liver and gut tissues of mosquitofish, Gambusia affinis: A microscopic study. Environmental Toxicology and Pharmacology. 2006;**21**(3):246-253

[136] Hocine L, Merzouk H, Merzouk SA, Ghorzi H, Youbi M, Narce M. The effects of alpha-cypermethrin exposure on biochemical and redox parameters in pregnant rats and their newborns. Pesticide Biochemistry and Physiology. 2016;**134**:49-54

[137] Zhang S-Y, Ito Y, Yamanoshita O, Yanagiba Y, Kobayashi M, Taya K, et al. Permethrin may disrupt testosterone biosynthesis via mitochondrial membrane damage of Leyedig cells in adult male mouse. Endocrinology. 2007;**148**(8):3941-3949. Available from: http://www.ncbi.nlm.nih.gov/pubmed/17463061

[138] Aldana L, De Mejia EG, Craigmill A, Tsutsumi V, Armendariz-Borunda J, Panduro A, et al. Cypermethrin increases apo A-1 and apo B mRNA but not hyperlipidemia in rats. Toxicology Letters. 1998;**95**(1):31-39

[139] Yilmaz ŞN, Çömelekoğlu Ü, Coşkun B, Balli E, Özge A. Effects of cypermethrin on isolated frog sciatic nerve: An ultrastructural study. Turkish Journal of Medical Sciences. 2008;**38**(2):121-125

[140] Romero DM, Berardino BG, Wolansky MJ, Kotler ML. Vulnerability of C6 astrocytoma cells after single-compound and joint exposure to type I and type II pyrethroid insecticides. Toxicological Sciences. 2017;**155**(1):196-212

[141] Akbar SMD, Sreeramulu K, Sharma HC. Tryptophan fluorescence quenching as a binding assay to monitor protein conformation changes in the membrane of intact mitochondria. Journal of Bioenergetics and Biomembranes. 2016;**48**(3):241-247

[142] Vadhana MSD, Carloni M, Nasuti C, Fedeli D, Gabbianelli R. Early life permethrin insecticide treatment leads to heart damage in adult rats. Experimental Gerontology. 2011;**46**(9):731-738

[143] Weiser BP, Salari R, Eckenhoff RG, Brannigan G. Computational investigation of cholesterol binding sites on mitochondrial VDAC. The Journal of Physical Chemistry. B. 2014;**118**(33):9852-9860

[144] Gabbianelli R, Falcioni G, Nasuti C, Cantalamessa F. Cypermethrin-induced plasma membrane perturbation on erythrocytes from rats: Reduction of fluidity in the hydrophobic core and in glutathione peroxidase activity. Toxicology. 2002;**175**(1-3):91-101

[145] Kotkat HM, Rady AA, Janos N. Influence of pesticide pyrethroid deltamethrin pollution on the phospholipid composition of carp erythrocyte plasma membrane. Asian Fisheries Science. 1999;**12**:165-173

[146] Paradies G, Paradies V, De Benedictis V, Ruggiero FM, Petrosillo G. Functional role of cardiolipin in mitochondrial bioenergetics. Biochimica et Biophysica Acta—Bioenergetics. 2014;**1837**:408-417

[147] Kirkland RA, Adibhatla RM, Hatcher JF, Franklin JL. Loss of cardiolipin and mitochondria during programmed neuronal death: Evidence of a role for lipid peroxidation and autophagy. Neuroscience. 2002;**115**(2):587-602

[148] Veenman L, Shandalov Y, Gavish M. VDAC activation by the 18 kDa translocator protein (TSPO), implications for apoptosis. Journal of Bioenergetics and Biomembranes. 2008;**40**(3):199-205

[149] Papadopoulos V, Lecanu L. Translocator protein (18 kDa) TSPO: An emerging therapeutic target in neurotrauma. Experimental Neurology. 2009;**219**(1):53-57

[150] Devaud LL, Szot P, Murray TF. PK 11195 antagonism of pyrethroid-induced proconvulsant activity. European Journal of Pharmacology. 1986;**121**(2):269-273

[151] Devaud LL, Murray TF. Involvement of peripheral-type benzodiazepine receptors in the proconvulsant actions of pyrethroid insecticides. The Journal of Pharmacology and Experimental Therapeutics. 1988 Oct;**247**(1):14-22

[152] Papadopoulos V, Amri H, Boujrad N, Cascio C, Culty M, Garnier M, et al. Peripheral benzodiazepine receptor in cholesterol transport and steroidogenesis. Steroids. 1997; **62**(1):21-28

[153] Doperalski NJ, Martyniuk CJ, Prucha MS, Kroll KJ, Denslow ND, Barber DS. Cloning and expression of the translocator protein (18 kDa), voltage-dependent anion channel, and diazepam binding inhibitor in the gonad of largemouth bass (*Micropterus salmoides*) across the reproductive cycle. General and Comparative Endocrinology. 2011;**173**(1):86-95

[154] Ramadan AA, Bakry NM, Marei ASM, Eldefrawi AT, Eldefrawi ME. Action of pyrethroid on K+-stimulated calcium uptake by, and [3H]nimodipine binding to, rat brain synaptosomes. Pesticide Biochemistry and Physiology. 1988;**32**:114-122

[155] Gatliff J, East D, Crosby J, Abeti R, Harvey R, Craigen W, et al. TSPO interacts with VDAC1 and triggers a ROS-mediated inhibition of mitochondrial quality control. Autophagy. 2014;**10**(12):2279-2296

[156] Li F, Liu J, Garavito M, Ferguson-Miller S. Perspective: Evolving understanding of translocator protein 18 kD (TSPO). Pharmacological Research. 2015;**99**:404-409. Available from: http://www.ncbi.nlm.nih.gov/pmc/articles/PMC4567528/

[157] Ott M, Robertson JD, Gogvadze V, Zhivotovsky B, Orrenius S. Cytochrome c release from mitochondria proceeds by a two-step process. Proceedings of the National Academy of Sciences. 2002;**99**(3):1259-1263. Available from: http://www.pnas.org/cgi/doi/10.1073/pnas.241655498

[158] Azarashvili T, Krestinina O, Baburina Y, Odinokova I, Grachev D, Papadopoulos V, et al. Combined effect of G3139 and TSPO ligands on Ca(2+)-induced permeability transition in rat brain mitochondria. Archives of Biochemistry and Biophysics. 2015;**587**:70-77. Available from: http://www.ncbi.nlm.nih.gov/pmc/articles/PMC4882157/

[159] Wang CY, Zhao ZB. Somatic mtDNA mutations in lung tissues of pesticide-exposed fruit growers. Toxicology. 2012;**291**(1-3):51-55

[160] Bendich AJ. Mitochondrial DNA, chloroplast DNA and the origins of development in eukaryotic organisms. Biology Direct. 2010;**5**:42

[161] Shi X, Gu A, Ji G, Li Y, Di J, Jin J, et al. Developmental toxicity of cypermethrin in embryo-larval stages of zebrafish. Chemosphere. 2011;**85**(6):1010-1016

[162] Sampath H, Vartanian V, Rollins MR, Sakumi K, Nakabeppu Y, Lloyd RS. 8-Oxoguanine DNA glycosylase (OGG1) deficiency increases susceptibility to obesity and metabolic dysfunction. PLoS One. 2012;**7**(12):e51697

[163] Krzepiłko A, Świeciło A. The influence of selected pyrethroid on the growth and number of ϱ-mutants in *Saccharomyces cerevisiae* yeast. Polish Journal of Environmental Studies. 2007;**16**(3):403-406

[164] Bernardi G. The petite mutation in yeast. Trends in Biochemical Sciences. 1979;**4**:197-201

[165] Longo VD, Gralla EB, Valentine JS. Superoxide dismutase activity is essential for stationary phase survival in *Saccharomyces cerevisiae*. Biochemistry. 1996;**271**(21):12275-12280

[166] Ahmadi F, Jamali N. Study of DNA-deltamethrin binding by voltammetry, competitive fluorescence, thermal denaturation, circular dichroism, and atomic force microscopy techniques. DNA and Cell Biology. May 2012;**31**(5):811-819

[167] Zhang Y, Zhang G, Li Y, Hu Y. Probing the binding of insecticide permethrin to calf thymus DNA by spectroscopic techniques merging with chemometrics method. Journal of Agricultural and Food Chemistry. 2013;**61**(11):2638-2647

[168] Ahmadi F, Ghanbari K. Proposed model for binding of permethrin and deltamethrin insecticides with ct-DNA, a structural comparative study. Ecotoxicology and Environmental Safety. 2014;**106**:136-145

[169] Tao M, Zhang G, Pan J, Xiong C. Deciphering the groove binding modes of tau-fluvalinate and flumethrin with calf thymus DNA. Spectrochimica Acta Part A: Molecular and Biomolecular Spectroscopy. 2016;**155**:28-37

Chapter 13

Mitochondrial Dysfunction Associated with Doxorubicin

Celal Guven, Yusuf Sevgiler and Eylem Taskin

Additional information is available at the end of the chapter

http://dx.doi.org/10.5772/intechopen.80284

Abstract

Cancer prevalence is scaling up each year. Anthracycline groups are still the best chemotherapeutic agent. The most popular anticancer drug in the group is doxorubicin (DOX). Unfortunately, DOX has potent toxicity on noncancerous tissues, e.g., heart, kidneys, etc. However, it is well documented that the severest toxicity of the drug affects heart tissue. Of course, some reasons have been suggested why and/or how the heart is so vulnerable to toxicity. The primary mechanism responsible for DOX's cardiospecific toxicity remains unidentified so far; however, mitochondrial dysfunction induced by DOX is now considered one of the leading reasons for DOX's toxicities and undesired side effects. Mitochondrial reactive oxygen production in the heart is a significant contributor to developing mitochondrial dysfunction-exposed DOX based on a variety of evidence. The objective of this review chapter is to critically evaluate and highlight the role of mitochondria in the development of DOX-induced cardiotoxicity.

Keywords: doxorubicin, cardiotoxicity, bioenergy stress, heart, mitochondrial toxicity, mitochondrial membrane potential

1. Introduction

This chapter gives the state of the art on doxorubicin (DOX) toxicity in mitochondria, particularly heart tissue. It is well known that cancer is a global threat to human health. The therapeutic effect of the drug is still below expectations in satisfaction. The drug that is the subject of the current chapter is a good chemotherapeutic against various soft solid cancer types. However, its toxic effect on noncancerous tissue, especially heart tissue, has not been ruled out. Therefore, even cancer patient can accomplish to fight cancer; they have still kept going to fight various severe diseases related to chemotherapeutic agents. The clinic utilization of drug is limited due to its side effects. When the molecular mechanism of the chemotherapeutic drug's side effects is clarified, it will be possible to manage all side effects. Hopefully, DOX may be able to improve the lifespan of cancer patients, which is why the purpose of the present chapter is to summarize its toxic effects on cardiac mitochondria.

2. Cancer: a modern epidemic

Cancer has a very high mortality and morbidity rate worldwide [1, 2] and is scaling up every year. In 2012 14 million people were diagnosed with cancer and 8.2 million people died due to cancer and cancer-associated diseases [3]. It is estimated that these figures will double by the year 2030 [4]. Patients are treated with radiotherapy, chemotherapy, and combination therapy. However, radiotherapy has been reported to be toxic and chemotherapy has been suggested to partially reduce the number of side effects. So, a chemotherapeutic agent is preferred to cure cancer [2]. Chemotherapy considerably enhances the survival rate of cancer patients. But, it is recognized to lead to side effect such as cardiovascular disease after growing survival population of a cancer patient with chemotherapy [5]. Therefore, cardiovascular diseases induced by chemotherapy are associated with high morbidity and mortality. The issue of heart damage caused by chemotherapy is a top priority due to the elevated cancer population treated with chemotherapy [6]. Anthracycline antibiotic groups are one of chemotherapeutic agents that is widely used in the treatment of solid and hematological cancer [7]. It has been indicated that the 5-year survival rate of childhood cancer patients was 30% before the discovery of group agents. However, this rate is around 80% today [8]. Still, extensive studies report that the group causes cardiotoxicity [6].

3. Anthracycline chemotherapy agents

Anthracycline antibiotics include DOX, daunorubicin, epirubicin, and idarubicin (**Figure 1**) [9]. DOX and daunorubicin are natural syntheses from *Streptomyces*, although epirubicin and idarubicin are synthetic derivatives from natural products [10]. Anthracyclines have a very high survival rate (~75%) within childhood cancer patients [11]. The drugs have been well recognized as a potential treatment against hematological cancers, including leukemias, lymphomas, solid carcinomas, and sarcomas [10, 12]. All these drugs have been reported to cause cardiotoxicity, classified as an acute and chronic effect [10]. Intracellular anthracycline tends to accumulate in the nucleus at the drug-sensitive cancer cell. However, the drug-resistant cancer cells have been outlined to find the chemotherapic agent at the cytoplasm [10]. Although some mechanism is proposed to explain the molecular structure, including oxidative stress, mitochondrial DNA (mtDNA) damage, etc., the molecular base of anthracycline on noncancerous tissue is still a mystery [12]. Because DOX is the most toxic drug in its class this chapter will evaluate only DOX toxicity, in particular heart damage [10].

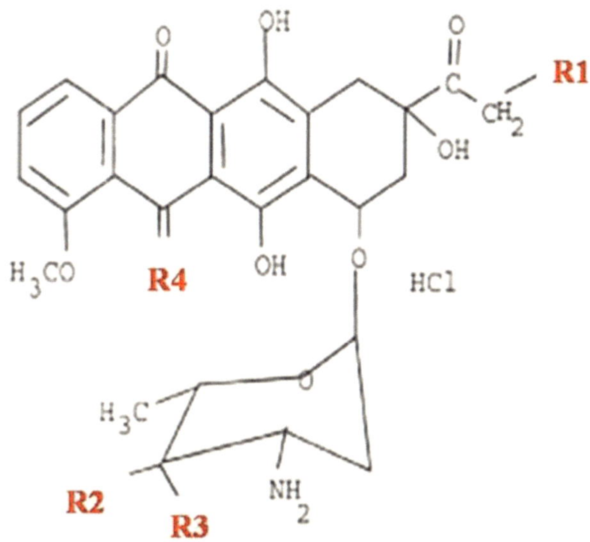

	R1	R2	R3	R4
Doxorubicin	OH	H	OH	O
Daunorubicin	H	H	OH	O
Epirubicin	OH	OH	H	O
5-Iminodaunorubicin	H	H	OH	NH

Figure 1. The chemical differences between anthracycline antibiotics. Modified from Berthiaume et al. [13].

4. Doxorubicin: anticancer antibiotics

DOX was discovered by Farmitalia Research Laboratories, and they gave it the name Adriamycin after the Adriatic Sea [14]. So, DOX is also known as Adriamycin [15], discovered from *Streptomyces peucetius* (*Streptomyces peucetius* var. *caesius*) in 1967 [16–18]; however, some studies said it was discovered in 1969 [4, 13], and its clinical utilization began in the 1970s [13] after approved in 1974 by the US Food and Drug Administration [19]. DOX is a nonselective class-I anthracyline antibiotic [20]. It has positively charged groups, mannose amine, so that the drug can efficiently bind to a negatively charged molecule, such as nucleic acid. The standard cure is in the drug range 10–50 mg/m^2 [18].

DOX has been widely used in the treatment of human and nonhuman tumors, including leukemia [15], lymphomas, soft tissue sarcomas, and solid cancer [21], e.g., breast tumors, osteosarcomas, Kaposi's sarcoma, Hodgkin's and non-Hodkin's lymphomas [14, 22], thyroid and lung carcinomas, stomach, breast, bone, and ovarian cancers [23]. DOX is used for the treatment of solid childhood tumors too, such as non-Hodgkin's lymphomas, Hodgkin's disease, and soft tissue sarcomas [22].

DOX has been administered by intravenous infusion [13]. Peak plasma concentration and half-life have been reported to be 5–15 μmol/L and 20–30 h, respectively [13]. Another study, however, stated that the peak plasma concentration of patients treated with DOX is between 2 and 6 μM after bolus injection, but typically 1–2 μM [24]. DOX is reported to be very low when bound to plasma proteins [25]. The plasma clearance of DOX is measured between 324 and 809 mL/min/m^2, dominantly by biliary excretion; the maximum volume is around 809–1214 L/m^2. Moreover, the half-life of the drug is around 5 min, which means that reuptake velocity is very high for tissues. However, elimination velocity is slow within the range 20–48 h [26]. After injection, DOX is disseminated to the heart, liver, kidneys, and intestine [25].

4.1. Doxorubicin's chemical structure

The chemical structure of DOX is {(7*S*, 9*S*)-7-[(2*R*, 4*S*, 5*S*, 6*S*)-4-amino-5-hydroxy-6-methyloxan-2-yl] oxy-6, 9, 11-trihydroxy-9-(2-hydroxyacetyl)-4-methoxy-8, 10-dihydro-7*H*-tetracene-5, 12-dione (**Figure 2**). Due to structural specifications with a tetracycline moiety containing a quinone and a conjugated amino sugar residue, DOX can undergo metabolic modification by enzymes dominantly in the liver and kidneys during the elimination process. Some oxidoreductase enzymes, especially nicotinamide adenine dinucleotide phosphate (NADPH)-dependent cytochrome P450 reductases at the endoplasmic reticulum (ER), nicotinamide adenine dinucleotide (NADH) dehydrogenase (complex I) at the electron transport chain (ETC), and cytosolic xanthine oxidase, have been suggested to play an important role in DOX elimination. The oxidoreductase enzyme can convert DOX to its semiquinone form by using molecular oxygen [13].

DOX's structure includes a glycoside group with anthraquinone moiety. The structure is responsible for its antineoplastic activity and also its toxicity [14]. DOX contains a tetracyclic ring with two quinone-hydroquinones and daunosamine. Though the tetracyclic sugar is nonsoluble in water, daunosamine sugar is soluble in water. DOX has been produced in a derivative form, e.g., daunorubicin. The difference between DOX and daunorubicin is only in the hydroxyl groups. Even though there is a slight difference between the drugs, their

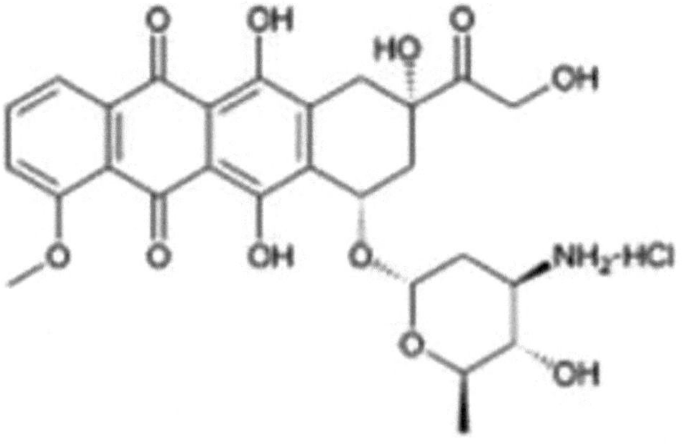

Figure 2. The chemical structure of doxorubicin antibiotics. From Imstepf et al. [27].

activities very are different to each other. How DOX intercalates DNA is related to the drug's chemical structure, including its chromophore's hydroxyl and daunosamine sugar's amino groups [22] (**Figure 2**).

4.2. The mechanism of doxorubicin's anticancer activity

It is agreed that the mechanism of its anticancer activity and its toxic impact follow different molecular mechanisms [13, 28, 29]. The anticancer activity of DOX relies on the interaction of the cell nucleus, mitochondria, and membranes. There are a number of reasons that explain the antineoplastic efficiency of the drug [17]:

1. DOX intercalates the DNA double strand, causing DNA replication and protein synthesis inhibition.
2. Reactive oxygen species (ROS) are produced, leading to the destruction of DNA and elevation of lipid peroxidation.
3. DNA is cross-linked and subject to alkylation.
4. DNA strands become obstructed and divided and there is helices activity.
5. The membrane structure is affected.
6. Prevention of topoisomerase II (TOPII) results in elevation of DNA damage [17].

The anticancer effect of DOX is associated with intercalation of the DNA strands, regulatory protein, covalent binding to DNA, and condensation of histone protein. However, its toxic impact on tissue does not rely on DNA impact [15].

The therapeutic effects of DOX have been associated with binding and intercalation of DNA strands, resulting in the destruction of replication and transcription of DNA by topoisomerase inhibition [4, 13, 30]. The reason why enzymes are so crucial is because TOPII has a role to play in modulating the DNA superhelical state [31], relaxing accumulated positive supercoils, and unlinking intertwined DNA strands. Thus, proteins are vital for complete DNA replication [22].

Also, DOX's cardiotoxicity has been related to disrupting TOPIIβ [30]. DOX selects toxic cardiac mitochondria through selective accumulation and redox cycling. However, free DOX enters the nuclei of cancer cells without entering mitochondria, which causes lack of mitochondrial pathway therapy [31]. Besides nuclear DNA, DOX intercalates with the mtDNA double helix, binds to a protein, and has a role in DNA replication and transcription as well [23].

To give more detailed knowledge on drug intercalation, DOX is one of the great anticancer drugs that kills cancerous cells by interaction with the cells' DNA; it also produces covalent adducts, resulting in inhibition of DNA synthesis by DNA polymerase blocking. DOX could also interfere with DNA and TOPIIα, finally forming a TOPIIα/DOX/DNA complex. The interruption of DNA and TOPIIα by DOX causes DNA breakage and cell death. A special situation has been reported whereby heart tissue does not contain TOPIIα, but expresses TOPIIβ [20]. So, the TOPIIβ/DOX/DNA complex could only occur in the heart tissue [20, 28]. It is strongly supported that DOX's cardiotoxicity associates with TOPIIβ based on a TOPIIβ knockout mice study. When DNA damage occurs for some reason, e.g., by using DOX, the ataxia/telangiectasia-mutated protein is activated to trigger tumor suppressor protein p53. Activation of p53 by DOX has been indicated to elevate ROS production, double-strand DNA damage, and apoptotic cell death as well. Furthermore, another effect of p53 addresses one of the cardioprotective transcription factors, known as GATA-4. AMP-activated protein kinase (AMPK) plays the role of energy sensor to maintain enough available energy levels. If energy status drops too low by enhancing ROS production, and intracellular Ca^{2+} accumulates, AMPK can be activated and/or its phosphorylation can be elevated [20].

4.3. The risk factors of doxorubicin's toxicity

DOX utilization is limited due to its toxic effect [27]. There are well-established factors that pointed to an increase in DOX-related heart damage. These factors are total cumulative dose, one course or a day's full dose, radiation, especially mediastinal, age, gender, other cardiotoxic drugs or chemicals, cardiovascular illness, and liver pathologies [17].

One of the riskiest factors for toxicity is the drug's cumulative dose [4]. Extensive reports are available in the literature. The mortality of congestive heart failure-induced DOX is around 50% at higher than a 500 mg/m^2 cumulative dose [17]. This side effect is related to its dose, which is reported to be between 75 and 1095 mg/m^2, and the median dose of its toxicity is around 390 mg/m^2 [10]. The risk of developing toxicity on noncancerous tissue has been reported to enhance the cumulative dose, e.g., at 400 mg/m^2 with 3–5% [4, 10, 20], 550 mg/m^2 with 7–26% [4, 10], 700 mg/m^2 with 18–48% [4, 10, 20], or 950 mg/m^2 with 50% [10]. Furthermore, the risk of toxicity has been reported to enhance at 550 mg/m^2 [10]. When mice are given a total of 71 mg/m^2 DOX, the risk of heart damage is almost 100% [20]. Also, cancer type determines the risk ratio. For example, around 20% of lung cancer patients treated with DOX have been reported to develop heart failure [32]. DOX, an anthracycline antibiotic, therapy has been indicated to develop side effects in almost 35% of patients [33]. Its clinical utilization is, therefore, limited because many tissues become toxic when patients are treated with a 550–600 mg/m^2 cumulative dose [15]. DOXs toxicity can reach a 50% mortality rate at the highest cumulative dose [14].

The detrimental effect of DOX is related to its dosage and treatment duration. Its utilization is recognized to develop into cachexia and cardiotoxic impact over time [4]. DOX can even cause cardiomyopathy after years of treatment [4]. Cardiomyopathy has been claimed to occur following final DOX treatment of 0–231 days (median 23 days) and final daunorubicin treatment of 9–192 days (median 60 days). Cardiotoxicity due to DOX therapy has been seen even after 20 years [10]. In other words, its toxic effect is mostly dose and time dependent [13]. DOX-induced cardiotoxicity causes death in 50% of patients within 2 years [34].

DOX is used not only for childhood cancer patient treatment, but also for adults cancer patients [35]. So, age is an important factor in the development of cardiotoxicity of DOX [9]. For example, it is reported that patients over 65 years and under 4 years treated with DOX are more susceptible to cardiomyopathy. Children, adolescents, and the elderly treated with

DOX are at high risk of developing cardiac damage. It seems that in children DOX causes some stem cells to vanish, including pluripotent, undifferentiated, and cardiac stem cells. The decreased stem cell ability in the heart by DOX results in decompensating for the decline of cardiac mass induced by the drug's treatment. However, DOX has been shown to accumulate in cardiac tissue in elderly patients, resulting in reduced blood flow in the heart [17].

Another factor associated with DOX toxicity is gender [36]. Unusually, female cancer patients treated with DOX have higher mortality vs. male cancer patients, but females develop cardiovascular disease 10 years later than males. However, after the menopause, females become more vulnerable than males at the same age [37].

4.4. Cytotoxic effect of doxorubicin on noncancerous tissues

DOX is widely used for cancer therapy [38]. However, it has been recognized to have a toxic effect on noncancerous tissue such as the heart [13, 39], liver, kidneys [22], as well as the brain [40], and its poisonous effect is related to its dose [38]. This is why the drug's use for cancer treatment is limited based on its undesired impact on healthy tissue. Unfortunately, the mechanism of its toxic effect on noncancerous tissue has been not understood so far [38, 39].

DOX side effect symptoms are nausea, vomiting, alopecia, myelosuppression, stomatitis, and gastrointestinal disturbances [14], which are typical of cytotoxic chemotherapic agents [28]. The soft side effects of drugs include nausea, fever, and vomiting. Nausea, fever, and vomiting appear after DOX therapy as soft side effects. However, hypotension, arrhythmias, tachycardia, and congestive heart failure are also described after treatment as severe undesired side effects [17].

DOX's cytotoxicity includes two molecular mechanisms: intercalation of nuclear DNA and elevation of ROS production [41]. A cancer cell's DNA replication is well known to be faster than normal cells [41]. If DOX generates normal levels of ROS, it might selectively destroy heart pump function [41]. The most accepted mechanism leading to DOX's toxicity is oxidative stress, which causes damage to membrane lipid peroxidation products and decreases antioxidants as well. The most severe ROS generation by DOX is in the heart vs. other organs or tissues, e.g., kidneys, liver, etc. [10]. Extensive research has been suggested as to why DOX's cardiotoxicity relies on oxidative stress, mitochondrial dysfunction, and mitochondrial energy-forming disruption [16]. DOX treatment after 3 h has been reported to cause oxidative stress, lipid peroxidation, as well as lipid aldehydes in cardiac tissue [42]. Selective toxicity of the heart by DOX will explain these reasons. There is strong evidence supporting a critical role of oxidative stress on DOX's toxicological effect, though the molecular mechanism of its toxicity is still a mystery. According to study results from animal and human tissue, DOX disrupts the myofibril, mitochondrial membrane [13].

DOX's anticancer activity is associated with intercalation to DNA by decreasing TOPII activity after double-strand breakage, resulting in alleviation of DNA replication and protein synthesis. However, it is accepted that DOX's toxicity and anticancer efficiency are different from each other. The cytotoxic effect of DOX is produced by a mechanism such as ceramide synthesis by CREB3L1 activation, oxidative damage to DNA, losing mitochondrial membrane potential (MMP), caspase-3 activation, and p53 and c-Jun NH2-terminal kinase (JNK) activations. Nuclear factor-kappa B (NF-κB), a proapoptotic factor, could participate in DOX's cytotoxicity [33].

The clinical utilization of DOX is limited because of its toxic impact, especially on heart tissues, e.g., heart failure, cardiomyopathy [20]. The mortality rate of congestive heart failure induced by DOX is estimated at around 20%. There is no explanation for how DOX causes its toxicity on noncancerous tissue. However, it is thought to be multiple and complex mechanisms, nitrosative and nitrative stress, DNA damage, dysregulation of metabolites, and inflammation [16] involving DOX's toxicity, eventually triggering apoptotic cell loss [43]. The dysfunction of energy production has played a critical role in the development of both acute and chronic DOX toxicity and is related to time-dependent mitochondrial dysfunction [43]. Also, there is limited knowledge of its toxic mechanism, including disruption of calcium homeostasis by activation of calcium-dependent kinases, phospholipases, proteases [15], myofibrillar disruption, apoptotic cell death, as well as mitochondrial dysfunction. The mitochondrial toxic effect of DOX relates to the generation of ROS, destroying energy production [44]. The impact on its mitochondrial toxicity is caused by blocking the ETC associated with cardiolipin, which is an inner mitochondrial membrane protein [44]. DOX's toxicity is mainly associated with enhancing mitochondrial ROS production and decreasing mitochondrial biogenesis [38].

However, its clinical utility is limited due to irreversible myocardial damage and dysfunction. Apoptosis mediated by DOX contributes to heart failure. DOX's main intracellular target is mitochondria, causing mitochondrial damage and ROS elevation, and initiating apoptosis [21]. So, DOX gives rise to degrading contractile proteins [29]. However, limited knowledge of how mitochondrial dysfunction triggers cardiac apoptotic cell death-mediated DOX is still a mystery. Therefore, further studies are needed to increase knowledge [21].

DOX has detrimental effects, classified as acute and chronic abnormalities, including arrhythmias, heart failure, and ventricular dysfunction. The primary issue for DOX therapy is to overcome and minimize its toxic effect without altering its therapeutic impact on cells with cancer. Knowledge of its detrimental effect remains a mystery. There are, however, disorders that may explain its side effect, such as mitochondrial dysfunction and ROS production. Mitochondria have an essential function, including energy metabolism, cellular apoptosis, and cell death pathways, apoptosis, and necrosis [35]. The cardiotoxicity of DOX relies on its dosage. For example, electrocardiologic abnormalities have been reported to occur at a low dose, although dilated cardiomyocytes and congestive heart failure have been reported at a high dose [13]. After left ventricular end diastolic pressure and left ventricular ejection fraction are suppressed, DOX dilates cardiomyopathy because of the decline in heart pump function. Besides cardiomyopathy, DOX also leads to the development of cardiac remodeling, including cytoplasmic vacuolization, myofibrillar clutter, or sarcoplasmic reticulum (SR) swelling. This is why further studies are required to evaluate DOX's toxic effects on noncancerous tissue [4]. There is no defined specific therapy to cope with DOX's cardiomyopathy yet, except receiving traditional treatment of congestive heart failure, e.g., angiotensin converting enzyme blockers, etc. [24].

Based on our best knowledge of the mechanisms associated with apoptosis, oxidative stress, and mitochondrial dysfunction, to avoid undesired toxicity it has been suggested to use some form of antioxidant. Unfortunately, antioxidant therapy has failed to accomplish the drug's toxicity effect in many tissues, particularly the heart and liver according to clinical data [39]. This is why any approaches to use the drug clinically may reduce its toxic effects on noncancerous mass. Therefore, further studies are needed to evaluate the molecular mechanism of DOX's toxicity [45].

5. Cardiospecific toxicity of doxorubicin

The most severe toxic effect of DOX is on the heart [17]. This toxic effect is related to mitochondria because DOX targets cellular mitochondria, resulting in mitochondrial damage and cell death [20]. Cardiomyocytes are differentiated and nondividing cells, so they would not be a direct target of the drug since it blocks DNA replication and synthesis [28]. Therefore, cardiomyocytes have an insufficient regenerative ability after significant injury [46, 47]. In case of severe damage, the majority of heart muscle functions can be terminally lost. DOX could selectively oxidize mtDNA associated with heart failure [28]. For some reasons the most severe detrimental effect of DOX is seen as heart based. These reasons are:

1. The heart contains a high volume of mitochondria per cardiomyocyte.
2. There is a high affinity for cardiolipin in the mitochondrial inner membrane of the heart.
3. Existing cardiospecific NADH dehydrogenase results in elevated ROS production.
4. There is lower antioxidant capacity in the cardiac tissue. The opening of the mitochondrial permeability transition (MPT) pore initiates apoptosis by releasing a proapoptotic factor, such as cytochrome, SMAC/DIABLO, and the apoptosis-inducing factor (AIF). MPT can form with the voltage-dependent anion channel (VDAC) and the adenine nucleotide translocase (ANT) matrix chaperon cyclophilin D (Cyp D). The open probabilities of MPT can be enhanced by DOX, so mitochondriopathy has been related to DOX's cardiotoxicity [23].

Cardiomyocytes contain high mitochondrial density, and one cardiomyocyte occupies 40–45% of mitochondria [21, 34]. The organelle has a function to maintain standard cardiac capacity due to a high-demanding, high-energy substrate for contractile function [21]. DOX accumulates in mitochondria 100 times more than plasma [34]. After binding DOX, cardiolipin loses the cofactor role in mitochondrial enzymes [34].

DOX tends to accumulate in the nucleus and mitochondria. In heart tissue, mitochondria make up around 50% of its volume [48]. DOX has a high affinity to bind the inner mitochondrial membrane and is collected on the matrix side [3]. One of DOX's similarities in the inner mitochondrial membrane is cardiolipin, which has a much higher affinity vs. other lipids in mitochondria (around 80 times). Phosphatidylethanolamine and cardiolipin are adaptors in the hexagonal (HII) phase in existent divalent cations, e.g., DOX, leading to changes in fluidity and functionality of mitochondrial membranes. DOX inactivates mitochondrial lipid-dependent enzymes, such as NADH dehydrogenase, cytochrome-*c* oxidase, and cytochrome-*c* reductase. DOX binds to cardiolipin, causing inactivation of complex I–III. DOX and NADH/NADH dehydrogenase incubations have been suggested to reduce sequestration at the SR by around 80% [48]. Also, mitochondrial TOPI is also found to relate to anthracyline-based cardiac toxicity [11].

The heart's mitochondria have two NADH dehydrogenases. One, known as cytosolic or intermembranous, is located at the outer surface of the inner mitochondrial membrane. However, the other one, known as matrix NADH dehydrogenase, is placed at the matrix surface of the inner mitochondrial membrane. Complex I relates to cytosolic NADH dehydrogenase as a function to capture the electrons from the mitochondrial cytosol to the electron transport system (ETS). Moreover, cytosolic NADH dehydrogenase probably participates in DOX-induced heart toxicity. The molecular weight of DOX is around 600 Da. So, DOX with a hydrophilic structure could smoothly transit from the outer membrane to the mitochondrial cytosol. However, it is difficult to pass through an inner mitochondrial membrane with a lipoidal structure. Therefore, DOX cannot reach the matrix NADH dehydrogenase. This is why DOX is almost impossible to convert its semiquinone form at most cell types, e.g., renal or hepatic tissues and tumor cells as well. On the other hand, heart tissue contains cytosolic NADH dehydrogenase at mitochondria. This is why DOX can be converted to its semiquinone form, leading to oxidative stress by transferring one electron to molecular oxygen [10]. Furthermore, the semiquinone form can produce dihydroquinone via itself by deletion of the sugar moiety to make its aglycone form. The primary metabolites are suggested to be of aglycone form because the form can easily pass through the inner membrane due to its lipoidal structure. In this way, the major form could substitute coenzyme-Q10 and block complex I and II as well at around a 100 μM concentration. Thus, this results in dissociation of coenzyme-Q10 from mitochondria. This is why the plasma coenzyme-Q10 level is increased in cancer patients receiving DOX therapy and decreased in heart tissue as well. The aglycone form of DOX could deliver electrons to an oxygen molecule, enhancing the superoxide radical. Superoxide dismutase at mitochondria can serve to convert hydrogen peroxide (H_2O_2) to hydroxyl radicals and water, which is why heart tissue is susceptible to oxidative stress produced by ETS and the DOX semiquinone form as well. The other detrimental effect of the aglycone form breaks energy synthesis from mitochondria due to the substitution of coenzyme-Q10 acting as a potent antioxidant. Aglycone derivatives of DOX lose the anticancer impact of the drug because it does not bind to DNA [10].

Excess electrons generated are captured by oxidizing agents, such as oxygen, and the cardiac tissue has a very high oxygen consumption rate [36]. Heart tissue needs more energy to maintain contractile function and cell survival, which is why cardiomyocytes have substantial mitochondrial volume. The mechanism of DOX's toxicity is still a mystery. However, many studies have suggested the association between ROS and reactive nitrogen species (RNS) with their side effects [20] (**Figure 3**). In other words, the heart has been extensively exposed to oxidative stress. The reason for this is due to the enormous volume of mitochondria and weak antioxidant defense in the tissue [17]. The heart contains low-level catalase enzymes; in addition, DOX immediately inactivates selenium-dependent glutathione (GSH)-peroxidase-1 and cytosolic Cu–Zn superoxide dismutase enzymes after therapy [17, 36, 42]. DOX is claimed to have a univalent redox potential of around −320 mV [17]. This fact can be combined with information that a high proton concentration might have potential to enhance mitochondrial ROS production [49]. Based on this potential, DOX is a suitable substrate for certain oxidoreductase enzymes, which are NADPH-dependent cytochrome P450 reductase, NADH dehydrogenase, and xanthine oxidase. DOX is highly reduced by complex I, resulting in semiquinone. It is well determined to have DOX affinity to cardiolipin with phospholipids. Cardiolipin acts as a cofactor for respiratory chain enzymes, e.g., cytochrome-c oxidase and NADH cytochrome-c oxidoreductase [17].

The semiquinone and molecular oxygen reaction is very fast ($k = 10^8\ M^{-1}\ s^{-1}$). Semiquinone and H_2O_2 can be catalyzed under very low oxygen conditions. Cholesterol is a crucial element to determine the localization and/or association of the drug. If cholesterol is high, DOX can

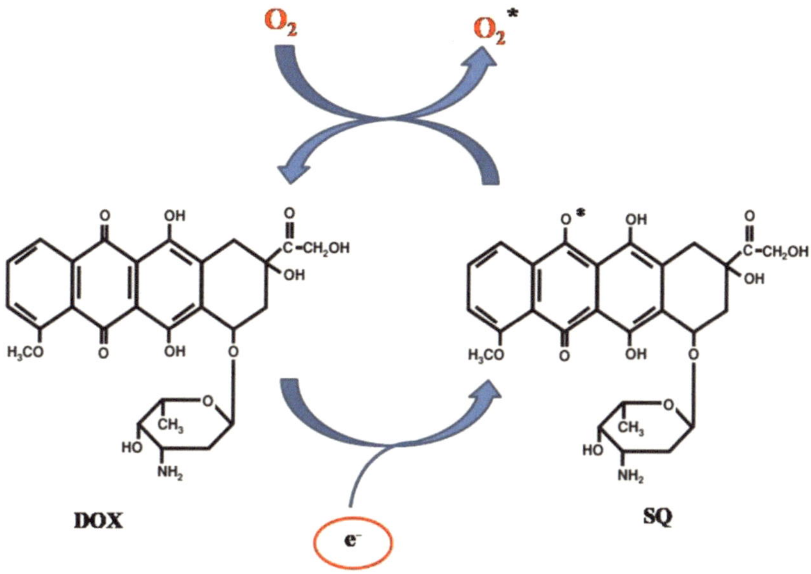

Figure 3. The formation of a semiquinone radical (SQ) from doxorubicin (DOX) by capturing one electron, which causes auto-oxidation in existing molecular oxygen, resulting in superoxide radical formation. Modified from Carvalho et al. [17].

lower its binding to the membrane. This knowledge is vital when the inner mitochondrial membrane is thought not to contain cholesterol. So, cholesterol and DOX or DOX's derivatives as semiquinone compete with binding of the hydrophobic region of the mitochondrial membrane. There are reasons why mitochondrial lipid peroxidation is high. The first reason is that the outer mitochondrial layer produces more ROS. The second reason is that the inner mitochondrial membrane is a very rich nonsaturated fatty acid. The third reason is that cardiolipin exists as 18% of total lipids in the mitochondria. So, DOX has a very high affinity for cardiolipin [48]. DOX tends to accumulate in mitochondria; therefore, mitochondrial ROS and RNS can be produced [28]. Elevation of ROS causes the enhancement of NF-κB and inducible nitric oxide synthase (iNOS) [28]. This process could trigger a positive feedback. iNOS also initiates to form ROS, which will be looked at in another section of this chapter.

5.1. The acute toxic effect of doxorubicin

It is well known that DOX's toxicity is based on its cumulative dose. It is reported that DOX could be lethal when mice are treated with DOX as a single dose of 12.5–25 mg/kg or two 15 mg/kg doses. Thus, the survival rate of drug treatment is between 40 and 0% at lower and higher doses, respectively [10]. DOX's toxicity has been classified as acute and chronic. Its acute effect occurs when patients receive drug treatment and has been reported to show transient arrhythmias, hypotension, and pericarditis. However, chronic DOX's results are evident even years after treatment and give rise to more severe damage, including congestive heart failure and dilated cardiomyopathy [43].

Acute toxicity has been seen by electrocardiographic (ECG) alternation as suppression of myocardial contractile function [10]. Another myocardial dysfunction induced by the acute DOX effect is diastolic dysfunction after therapy. Although there are no severe symptoms of diastolic dysfunction, it is becoming a very crucial issue for chronic DOX therapy due to concomitant systolic dysfunction [24]. The signs are transient electrophysiological alternations, including sinus tachycardia, supraventricular, and reversible arrhythmias, ST- and T-wave alternations, prolonged QT interval, QRS voltage decline, and flattening of the T wave, predicted at 11% within all cases [14, 17]. Some symptoms have been reported to appear rarely but are more severe, e.g., pericarditis, myocarditis, and acute left ventricular failure [17]. Also, one of the previous studies indicated that DOX led to pericardial, peritoneal, and pleural effusion [49]. The other severe side effects are hyperpigmentation of the skin veins used for drug injection, stomatitis, and myelosuppression [18]. Moreover, other acute effects cause loss of body, heart, and liver weights and also enhance lipid peroxidation [10]. Acute drug-exposure is suggested to cause ROS generation from complex I at ETC in mitochondria [13], as well as the initiation of apoptosis [50]. With this knowledge, our previous studies have shown that antioxidant supplementation might be an excellent candidate to moderate DOX's toxicity [51–56].

Interestingly, a transient DOX effect has been reported to shift mitochondrial dynamics to fission at the heart. However, acute DOX therapy at the liver tissue is reported to decrease fusion, but not alter fission. This means that a decrease in fusion leads to an increase in mitochondrial fragmentation in the liver. DOX is said to improve mitophagy at the organ. When mitochondrial fusion and mitophagy occur, mitochondrial content reduces. DOX also causes a decrease in citrate synthase. Acute DOX has been mentioned not to change proliferating cell nuclear antigen, which means that mitochondrial fission does not accompany cell proliferation [39].

However, all acute toxic effects are transient, occur within the first 24 h after drug therapy, and are spontaneously ameliorated [10]. Sometimes an acute DOX effect can transiently appear and disappear within a few minutes to a week. Acute DOX is prevalent in cancer patients receiving DOX therapy at around 20–30% [17]. The chronic toxic effects of DOX cause cardiomyopathy and congestive heart failure [10].

5.2. The chronic toxic effect of doxorubicin

The chronic toxic effect of DOX results in an irreversible defect in cardiomyopathy, congestive heart failure. A dose of DOX at 430–600 mg/m^2 given to 50–60% of patients has been reported to develop left ventricular failure. However, a cumulative dose of DOX at 300 mg/m^2 has been shown to increase heart failure by almost 2%. Moreover, causing heart failure induced by DOX is quickly enhanced after a 550 mg/m^2 dose [17], which is a limited dosage because it induces irreversible toxicity [48]. To see the chronic effects of the drug takes a year of therapy. However, rapid treatment still leads to damaged heart tissue [17]. Other toxicities of DOX have been reported to be palmar–plantar erythrodysesthesia (also known as a hand–foot syndrome) [48] and typhlitis [57]. DOX's toxic impact on tissue is associated with:

1. A high affinity to bind membrane lipid-dependent pH, resulting in membrane alternation of lipid structure by lipid peroxidation [48].
2. Production of a semiquione structure [48].

3. Bioalkylation at C7 aglycone by metabolic activation, resulting in alkylation and destruction of DNA [48].

4. A high affinity for iron (both ferric and ferrous forms) and copper so the drug can reduce activation through metal chelating effects, leading to free radical formation [48].

Chronic DOX therapy leads to heart failure; cardiomyopathy has been reported to be associated with oxidative stress and mitochondrial dysfunction [58]. Mitochondria are essential organelles that synthesize ATP with a total of four membrane-associated complexes: complex I, II, III, and IV. The amount of ATP production is related to the complexes' activities (**Figure 3**). For example, high activity produces more ATP, although low activity has the opposite effect. DOX is toxic to mitochondria; all complexes could be inhibited, leading to energy stress. A recent study result showed that cryptotanshinone treatment, which is obtained from *Salvia miltiorrhiza* root, could reverse the toxic compound effect of DOX, except complex II (succinate dehydrogenase) by elevation of MMP, resulting in enhanced ATP formation [58]. How the increase in MMP by cryptotanshinone treatment occurs can be explained by a decline in free radicals, particularly superoxide anion. Since the increase in oxidative stress destroys the reduction/oxidation balance in mitochondria, DOX has been well accepted to elevate ROS generation [58]. So, the cryptotanshinone mitigates the imbalance, eventually increasing both MMP and ATP production [58]. However, lengthy drug exposure is reported not to be related to drug interaction with ETC enzymes, but the molecular mechanism of extended DOX treatment to produce ROS is so far not well understood. So, further studies are required to evaluate the production of ROS induced by lengthy DOX treatment [13].

DOX has been reported to cause severe histological and electrophysiological (electrocardiogram) alternations of cardiac tissue related to cardiomyopathy, and also creatine phosphokinase elevation at 450 mg/m^2 cumulative dose. In contrast to acute studies, body weight gain has been reported in animal research with chronic DOX therapy. Histopathological and electrophysiological, including flattened-inverted T wave and declining QRS voltage, alternations have appeared in chronic DOX therapy [10]. Chronic DOX's toxicity led to more severe arrhythmias, including sudden death [59]. High blood pressure was reported after DOX treatment [60]. Histopathological variation of DOX's cardiotoxicity is observed as myofibrillar loss, sarcoplasmic swelling, cytoplasmic, myelin, and mitochondrial vacuolization, and crystal degeneration in mitochondria [23]. The acute and chronic toxic effects of DOX are summarized in **Table 1**.

5.3. The mechanism of reactive oxygen species production of doxorubicin

Under the standard physiologic condition, ROS can be by synthesis only 1–5% of oxygen consumption [11]. The most acceptable hypothesis of DOX's toxicity is extensive ROS production [4]. The reason for elevation by DOX is associated with its accepting and donating electrons. DOX contains a hexose sugar with tetracycline having quinone and hydroquinone moieties, which are part of the capture electron, producing semiquinone. A superoxide radical can be provided by semiquinone from an oxygen molecule. A superoxide radical does not have a

Acute DOX treatment	Chronic DOX treatment
1. Transient arrhythmias	1. More serious arrhythmias
2. Transient hypotension	2. Hypertension
3. Alternation of ECG	3. More severe ECG alternation
4. ROS production	4. High ROS production
5. Transient histopathological alternation	5. Permanent histopathological alternation
6. Induction of apoptosis	6. Induction of apoptosis
7. Alteration of mitochondrial dynamics	7. Mitochondrial dysfunction

Table 1. Comparison of some parameters of acute and chronic doxorubicin toxicities.

potentially harmful effect. However, superoxide radicals can be transformed by superoxide dismutase converting to H_2O_2; this is called a Fenton or Haber–Weiss reaction, and the highly toxic hydrogen radical can be produced from H_2O_2. DOX can be reduced in some intracellular enzymes, e.g., xanthine oxidase and microsomal NADPH-cytochrome P450 reductase that expresses in almost all cells. Mitochondrial NADH dehydrogenase, which mediates to produce ROS when DOX is present, is not present in other tissues, except cardiac tissue. This is why DOX is highly toxic to heart tissue because it causes ROS to elevate [10].

Given more detailed knowledge regarding its structure and radical formation, DOX can be reduced at the C13 position from doxorubicinol. Although DOX can be transformed to doxorubicinone at its daunosamine sugar by acid-catalyzed hydrolysis, doxorubicinol can also undergo the same acid-catalyzed hydrolysis to form doxorubicinolone. Both can then experience protonation at C7, resulting in the formation of 7-deoxydoxorubicinone and 7-deoxydoxorubicinolone, respectively, by deletion of the sugar. After double reducing DOX, a tautomer of C7 deoxyaglycone, that is, C-7-quinone-methide, is produced. C7-quinone-methide can connect to DNA and form free radicals [22].

The drug can form ROS via two pathways: the first is iron dependent, and the second is redox cycling, which is catalyzed by NADPH oxidoreductases [30]. DOX has one of the paths, which produces ROS, and is mediated by iron (Fe). According to the Haber–Weiss reaction, the superoxide radical formed by DOX could be transformed into H_2O_2, and then a hydroxyl radical can be produced by H_2O_2 in existing iron. Another way is for DOX to directly interplay, resulting in a ferro (Fe^{2+}) to ferric (Fe^{3+}) form of abundant ROS [28].

Oxidative stress produced by DOX relies on nitric oxide synthase (NOS) and nicotinamide adenine dinucleotide phosphate-oxidase (NOX). NOX and/or NOS can transform DOX to its semiquinone form, causing oxidative stress. When nitric oxide is produced by NOS, peroxynitrite, reactively oxidizing DNA, proteins, and lipids are produced as by-products. Moreover, two isoforms of NOS, namely endothelial NOS and inducible NOS (iNOS), have been reported to play a role in DOX's toxicity to produce RNS. Besides NOS, DOX can synthesize radicals by complexing with iron to produce hydroxyl radicals, which are also very dangerous for cells and can have a detrimental effect on DNA, proteins, and especially lipids [20].

DOX's ROS production effect is capable of transferring one electron to oxygen resulting in superoxide radicals. So, DOX oxidizes complex I of ETC [44]. DOX contains a quinine moiety, so it can reduce one electron catalyzed by NADPH, resulting in production of semiquinone free radicals. The semiquinone can undergo oxidation by molecular oxygen to superoxide oxygen radicals [30, 38].

The reason why mitochondrial ROS production is crucial is because it could amplify its detrimental effect by triggering intracellular signal pathways. According to one previous study, mitogen-activated kinases (MAPK) have participated in DOX's cardiotoxicity by ROS production [5]. Research has suggested that cardiotoxicity induced by DOX involves p-JNK, the p-ERK1/2 [61], as well as p38 [5]. Based on our previous studies, the renin–angiotensin system also crosstalks with DOX's toxicity [62, 63]. However, we need to investigate which intracellular signal pathways are potentially involved in DOX's toxicity.

5.4. Apoptotic cell death induced by doxorubicin

Apoptosis plays a role in developmental and homeostatic mechanisms. So, uncontrolled apoptosis relies on an illness, e.g., cancer [64]. This is why apoptosis, known as programmed cell death [65], has a role in the development of cancer and cancer treatment [2]. Apoptotic pathways start as intrinsic or mitochondrial and extrinsic stimulus stimulated by the cell death receptor [64]. There are many ways to initiate the intrinsic apoptotic path, particularly nutrient deficiency, genotoxic damage induced by cytotoxic chemotherapies, and radiation [64].

Extensive research has been conducted on DOX's apoptotic pathways. The evidence supports a significant role of oxidative stress induced by DOX. The difficulties in determining DOX's apoptotic pathways are related to the drug's dosage, route [26], and duration of treatment [9]. It is almost impossible to explain a single, unique apoptotic pathway induced by DOX [26]. However, literature data have suggested that DOX has been reported to trigger apoptosis in both pathways, intrinsic or mitochondrial and extrinsic [57, 66].

The pathways are controlled under pre- and proapoptotic factors. Apoptosis can be triggered by proapoptotic factors such as Bax or Bak activation by BH3-only protein, BIM, and also BID. When Bax and Bak become oligomerized, mitochondrial outer membrane permeabilization occurs and results in releasing cytochrome-*c* to the cytosol. Then the apoptosome can be formed by cytochrome-*c* with apoptotic protease-activating factor-1 (APAF-1), resulting in a triggering caspase cascade, including caspase-3 (**Figure 4**). In contrast to proapoptotic factors, e.g., Bcl-2, Bcl-XL can prevent apoptotic pathways maintaining monomeric Bax/Bak or BH3-only proteins [64]. Caspase-8 participates in extrinsic pathways, whereas caspase-3 and -9 have a role in the intrinsic route [2].

Bax activation releases cytochrome-*c* by the mitochondrial permeability transition pore (PMT) activation, resulting in APAF-1 activation [26]. After the apoptosome complex is formed by APAF-1, cytochrome-*c*, dATP, and caspase-9, procaspase-3 can be transformed into its activated form by the apoptosome [67]. Alternatively, DOX can facilitate apoptosis through mitochondrial p53 by depolarizing MMP. Recently published data are suggests that p53 elevation by DOX treatment influences Bcl-2 decline and Bax expression [26, 67].

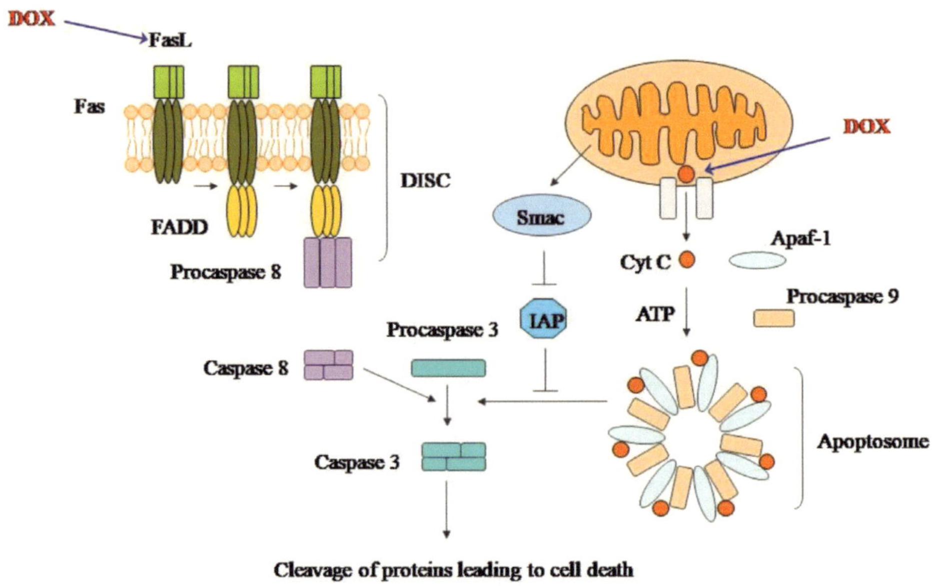

Figure 4. Apoptotic cell death by doxorubicin (DOX). Cyt C: Cytochrome-*c*. Modified from Meredith et al. [22].

DOX's toxicity is mainly thought to relate to ROS enhancement and TOPII inhibition [68]. Therefore, the therapy improves ROS production as described in the previous section. Cell death is stimulated based on transforming DOX to a semiquinone radical via complex I [15]. However, the heart has cardioselective external NADH dehydrogenase, which is a kind of alternative complex I, resulting in a long DOX redox cycle [14]. When semiquinone reverses to produce DOX, oxygen converts to a superoxide anion free radical. This superoxide radical can be scavenged by GSH, creating its oxidation form, glutathione disulfide [15]. It must be remembered that cardiac tissue has less antioxidant capacity than other tissues [14]. A decline in GSH causes oxidation of thiol groups in proteins, including MPT, resulting in depolarization of MMP. Enhancing MMP gives rise to decreased ATP production, and release of proteins from mitochondria to the cytosol, such as cytochrome-*c*. So, releasing cytochrome-*c* can trigger apoptosis and/or necrosis. Eventually, this causes cell loss [15]. DOX, therefore, leads to decreased heart muscle thickness [64] due to apoptotic cell death.

DOX's toxicity on mitochondria is dose and time dependent. The mitochondrial toxicity of DOX has been observed from 2 to 13 weeks at a low dose. Moreover, mitochondria play an essential role in the regulation of calcium homeostasis. Under the standard physiological condition, there is little impact of mitochondria on calcium homeostasis. However, the mitochondrial function of calcium homeostasis is essential under pathological circumstances to decrease cytosolic calcium. Calcium efflux into mitochondria causes MMP to depolarize. DOX's effect on calcium homeostasis in mitochondria is based on inhibition of the inward calcium flux and exaggeration of the release of calcium from mitochondria by swelling of the mitochondria–calcium-dependent pathways through MPT, resulting in enhanced calcium concentration at the cytosol [15]. Cytosolic calcium concentration at 30 nM is tightly controlled by several pumps, channels, and exchangers [69]. Besides initiating its role in apoptosis, calcium homeostasis has a crucial function for cell metabolism. Several mitochondrial dehydrogenases, e.g., pyruvate dehydrogenase, isocitrate dehydrogenase, oxoglutarate dehydrogenase, and glycerol-3-phosphate dehydrogenase, are controlled by intracellular calcium concentration. As a result, the influx of calcium to mitochondria plays a central role in the regulation of cell metabolism. Therefore, any reason for preventing calcium entering mitochondria might also cause a drop-off in bioenergy production [69]. Furthermore, DOX at a low dose gives rise to a decline in the calcium storage capacity of mitochondria. The decline in mitochondria calcium storage capacity by DOX exaggerates its dosage. Eventually, the effects of DOX lead to the dissipation of MMP [15]. The other way that DOX disrupts both intracellular calcium homeostasis and mitochondrial calcium loading is via connexin 43 (Con-43). Con-43 is one of the essential gap junction proteins, and plays a role in the regulation of mitochondrial function. So, when Con-43 is blocked by a gap junction blocker it releases cytochrome-*c* and induces apoptosis. According to a recent study, DOX treatment enhanced Con-43 from cytosol to mitochondria through heat shock protein 90 and translocase of the outer membrane 20 pathways [70].

MPT pore, one of the redox-sensitive proteins, has a function to regulate mitochondrial tasks [15]. It is thought that the pore consists of many proteins; however, this has been not fully understood yet [13]. So far, MPT is believed to contain VDAC [17], ANT [13], and Cyp D (also called Cyp F). The most crucial elements of the pore have been claimed to be Cyp D [17]. MPT is controlled by creatine kinase (CK), hexokinase, the Bcl-2 family, and peripheral-type benzodiazepine receptors [17]. DOX reduces mitochondrial calcium loading capacity based on triggering of the MPT pore [17]. So, oxidative stress through complex I [15], dissipation of MMP, and loss of mitochondrial calcium capacity trigger MPT, resulting in enhanced inner mitochondrial membrane permeability, and eventually augmentation of small molecules less than 1.5 kDa due to the opening of nonselective protein pores [13, 17]. Besides loss of MMP, opening the pore triggers apoptosis by releasing cytochrome-*c* and another apoptotic factor from mitochondria to cytosol and subsequent activation of caspase pathways [13]. This is why the opening of MPT initiates apoptosis by releasing cytochrome-*c* or SMAC/DIABLO. DOX prompts the opening of MPT through oxidation of thiol residues in mitochondrial proteins. The other way of initiating apoptosis by DOX is to delete GATA-4, which is a transcriptional factor encoding Bcl-XL antiapoptotic genes preventing mitochondrial function and integrity. Anthracycline also blocks AKT phosphorylation, resulting in GSK3β activation, leading GATA-4 suppression in the nucleus. DOX causes bioenergetic stress by reducing mitochondrial ATP production and damaging CK isoenzymes and AMPK [17]. DOX is shown to change Bax and Bcl-2 protein levels as well [13]. Moreover, MPT opening gives rise to mitochondria-related osmotic swelling and structural detriment. The MPT formation is needed to clarify, so further studies are needed to evaluate MPT structure [17].

ER and mitochondrial dysfunction have been reported to include and follow the same apoptotic pathways [67, 71]. DOX also triggers apoptosis by ER dysfunction through activation of an ER stress sensor and transcription factor 6 [21]. Moreover, a study also found that apoptosis-related ER stress by DOX is instigated to elevate Ca^{2+}, calpain-1 protein level, and caspase-12, which is a marker of ER stress [67]. Cardiac damage mediated by DOX can be merged with lysosome dysfunction causing autophagic flux as well. DOX damages mitochondria by tending to accumulate in it, triggering apoptotic cell death [21].

Extrinsic pathways involve death receptors, their ligand interaction, e.g., Fas/FasL, and then caspase-8 activation [57]. DOX also uses the extrinsic pathways for instigating apoptosis by elevation of Fas protein levels, caspase-8, and BID [67] (**Figure 4**). Even so, DOX's leading approach to initiate apoptosis is through intrinsic, called mitochondrial, pathways. The outer membrane of mitochondria has a central role in the natural apoptotic route because it has pro- and preapoptotic factors. The elevation of ROS and depolarization of MMP by DOX release proapoptotic factors to the cytosol, e.g., cytochrome-*c*. p38, p53, Bax, and caspase-3 have also been suggested to participate in the induction of apoptosis. p53 enhances the permeability of the outer membrane to release proapoptotic factors, such as Bax [57]. DOX has been reported to increase p53 in the nucleus and mitochondria from the heart. So, p53 localization is thought to associate with mtDNA. However, there is limited knowledge available of nuclear and mitochondrial p53 localization by DOX in cardiac tissue. DOX has been suggested to elevate 8-hydroxydeoxyguanosine (8-OHdG) and p53 levels in mitochondria within 3 and 24 h. Cytochrome-*c* release is an assessment of cytosolic/mitochondrial cytochrome-*c*. DOX enhances the ratio of heart tissue by around 35%. It can trigger apoptosis through p53 stabilization by MAPK [72].

The MAPK family has extracellular signal-regulated kinases (ERK), p38 MAPK, and JNK [73]. While ERK1/2 predominantly operates cell proliferation, JNK and p38 participate in cell death pathways. DOX has been shown to kill prostate cancer cells by phosphorylation of p38 and JNK [74]. One of the MAPKs is p38, which has a pivotal role in cell growth, apoptosis, and inflammation. The apoptotic role of p38 depends on cell type, stimuli, or isoform activation of p38, which has four isoforms: p38α, β, γ, and δ. One study showed that DOX triggers apoptosis at the MCF-7 breast cancer cell line by elevation of caspase-3 and caspase-9 during 24 h of treatment [65]. So, p38 is one of the intrinsic pathway activators dependent on cellular stress, mitochondrial dysfunction, and caspase activation [57]. ERK1/2 probably has a role in the activation of caspase-3, Bax, p53, and cytochrome-*c* release. Moreover, ERK1/2 could contribute external apoptotic pathways at the caspase-8 level [75]. ERK1/2 could also phosphorylate p53. So, DOX activates apoptosis by the p53-dependent activation of caspases-2, -3, -8, -9, and -12 [66]. The release of caspase-12 activates caspase-3 [66].

Through extrinsic (receptor-mediated) or intrinsic (mitochondrial) pathways. Both pathways have a role in the trigger of apoptosis as upstream (initiator) caspase, e.g., caspase-8 and -9, and downstream (effector) caspase, e.g., caspase-3, -6 and -7 [76]. When MMP is depolarized and opened, mitochondrial apoptotic factors are released such as cytochrome-*c* and AIF to the cytosol [73]. Cytochrome-*c* can contain an apoptosome formation with APAF-1, caspase-9. Caspase-3 can be activated from both pathways [73]. The human fibroblast cell was used in one of the previous studies and reported that DOX at 3 μM concentration causes apoptosis through caspase-3, -7, and -9 by ROS [76]. DOX has been said to stimulate apoptosis via caspase-3-dependent pathways. The bcl-2 protein family is shown to play a role in apoptosis in cardiomyocytes as expected. Also, Bcl-2 and Bax can affect the MPT pore [68] (**Figure 4**).

DOX also stimulates apoptosis by an AIF. There are three sides of AIF: a NAD binding, FAD binding, and C-terminal. AIF is located at the intermembrane space or weakly binded to inner mitochondrial membrane and exhibits NADH oxidase activity. AIF can be released to the cytosol via PMT and translocate to the nucleus by poly (ADP-ribose) polymerase-1, resulting in stimulation of chromatin condensation and DNA breakage, eventually triggering apoptosis by caspase-independent pathways. The other function of AIF is to repair and mature mitochondrial complex I and peroxide scavenging activities. Elevation of cytosolic AIF leads to release of cytochrome-*c*, resulting from depolarization of MMP. Why the molecular mechanism of DOX toxicity is so crucial is based on its effective utilization of therapy against cancer. This is why finding an effective therapy to counteract its toxicity, especially of the heart, will give hope to cancer patients treated with DOX to overcome nondesired effects. The other mechanism of cell death mediated with DOX decreases GATA, controlling apoptosis through antiapoptotic Bcl-X gene activation [77].

6. Mitochondrial dysfunction induced by doxorubicin

Mitochondria have a role in regulating cell death or survival under cell stress or damage. The organelle has its own genome encoding 37 genes, of which 13 are complex I, III, IV; complex II is encoded by nuclear DNA [22]. So, mitochondrial dysfunction is associated with disease and aging as well.

Besides its nuclear effect, DOX has been reported to cause mitochondrial dysfunction, energy stress via disruption of the ETC [4]. It is well recognized that mitochondrial bioenergetics mechanism disruption has been thought to play an essential role in the development of the drug's toxicity, especially its cardiotoxicity. Adequate ATP production is not just necessary to maintain contractile function, it is also crucial for protein synthesis, the protein quality control function of ER, cytoskeletal function, and clearing cellular waste from lysosomes as well [4]. Moreover, DOX's mitochondrial effect is shown to change ultrastructure, swelling, and oxidative capacity. Furthermore, DOX tends to accumulate in nuclei and mitochondria vs. plasma [43]. All this is needed to explain why or how DOX selectively targets mitochondria in noncancerous tissue rather than cancerous tissue. One reason is that cancer has been reported to alter a cell's metabolic activation. A healthy cell produces energy by oxidative phosphorylation in mitochondria. However, a cancer cell synthesizes its energy by the glycolytic pathway, known as the Warburg effect. Enhancing glycolytic activity could be multifactorial, relying on mtDNA damage, oxidative phosphorylation defect, mitochondrial dysfunction, etc. [78]. Another reason could be that DOX is more toxic to mitochondria in noncancerous cells than in cancerous cells. Moreover, DOX could alter mitochondrial function in noncancerous and cancerous cells, resulting in different apoptotic pathways [79].

6.1. The acute mitochondrial toxic effect of doxorubicin

The acute toxic effect of DOX on mitochondria has been reported to rely on its dose, especially redox cycling and ETC blocking. A low concentration of DOX treatment has been reported to have minimal alternation to ATP production and MMP, resulting from enhancing hydroxyl radical (*OH), H_2O_2, and oxygen consumption. Although up to 160 μM DOX concentration has been emphasized, redox cycling is the primary process to augment ROS production; ETC blocking is the primary source of ROS manufacture at densities higher than 160 μM. Until it reaches a threshold, which means 480 μM, mitochondrial toxicity is progressively enhanced.

Eventually, mitochondrial collapse is inevitable, resulting in MMP dissipation, improvement in ROS production, inhibition of ATP production, and also oxygen utilization. A dose of 1 mg/kg of DOX has been reported to increase superoxide radicals within 2 h, although a 37 mg/m^2 dose, which equals to 5–30 μM mitochondrial concentration, has the same effect on human beings [44].

6.2. The chronic mitochondrial toxic effect of doxorubicin

The heart, skeletal muscle, and brain are reasonably active organs [14], so energy demand is very high. This is why the majority of energy production is based on mitochondria for maintaining heart function [80]. Therefore, organ failure can develop because of damage to mitochondrial function [14].

Mitochondria have a role in regulating cell survival and death, proliferation, and calcium and redox homeostasis. It is reported that the inner mitochondrial structure is different from tissue to tissue, based on their metabolic activities; even the structure is different in the same tissue [14]. For example, heart tissue has been indicated to have two types of mitochondria. One is located near the T tubule and SR, and the other is firmly located at a contractile component of myocytes. The dynamic of the organelle is limited due to its close relation with the cytoskeleton [14]. So, these two mitochondria present different features, including dynamic organization, calcium accumulation, functional capacity, and localization. Subsarcolemmal mitochondria are situated at the plasma membrane and have a role in supplying ATP to the ion pump. However, intermyofibrillar mitochondria are situated between the myofibrillar structure and produce energy for the contraction/relaxation function of the tissue [80].

Mitochondria have two shapes or morphologies: long and filamentous (fused) and short and punctuated (fragmented). The form is vital to respond to damage. For example, fused mitochondria are suggested for counteracting apoptosis, while fragmented mitochondria are susceptible to apoptosis [81]. Mitochondria have two structures: long tubules and small round vesicles [82].

Mitochondria are dynamic organelles and perform trafficking, fusion, and fission, called mitochondrial dynamics [14, 21, 83]. The importance of mitochondrial dynamics is that mitochondria have to divide from existing organelles and proliferate via growth [83]. There is a balance between the fission and fusion processes. If the balance shifts towards fission, it causes damage, including mitochondrial fragmentation, mitophagy, a rise in oxidative stress, and cell death [21]. This equilibrium could relate to a number of factors, e.g., cell conditions such as stress, cell compartmentation such as neuronal axons or dendrites, and mitochondrial function as well. The dynamic is crucial for mitochondrial morphogenesis [82]. The importance of dynamics is to scale up because of its role in mitochondrial function, apoptosis, or aging [83]. DOX also leads to senescence of cardiomyocytes by inhibition of Akt Ser473 phosphorylation [21].

Mitochondrial morphological alternation is claimed to provide some idea about DOX's degree of toxicity. For example, the morphological shift at organelles is displayed at the beginning of DOX toxicity on heart tissue. Mitochondria have a homeostatic balance between fission (divide) and fusion. Fission could cause mitophagy, apoptosis, and cell proliferation. However, fusion provides a homogeneous network of mitochondria. Imbalance of the mitochondrial dynamic causes it to lose cell function, e.g., when the shift towards fission could initiate apoptotic cell death due to severe ROS production. In contrast, the change towards fusion would increase mitochondrial dysfunction because of extinguishment of the mitophagy mechanism. The dynamic provides healthy, functional mitochondria and cells [39].

To maintain its function the heart prefers to metabolize fatty acid in mitochondria and peroxisomes via β-oxidation due to its high demand energy [14]. Mitochondrion starts energy production by the tricarboxylic acid cycle (TCA) in the ETS. Mitochondrial ATP is synthesized by ETS steps. Although TCA elements are placed in the mitochondrial matrix, except for succinate dehydrogenase, ETS elements having a spherical shape are present at the mitochondrial inner membrane and project to the mitochondrial matrix. The space between the inner and outer layer is called the intermembrane space or mitochondrial cytosol. A molecule with hydrophilic structure can transit the inner membrane as a requirement of the transport system. The outer membrane of mitochondria can pass through almost all particles less than 10,000 Da [10]. The respiratory chain is under the control of four complexes: complex I (NADH dehydrogenase), complex II (succinate dehydrogenase), complex III (cytochrome-*c* reductase), and complex IV(cytochrome-*c* oxidase) [34] (**Figure 5**). Complex V is ATP synthase [11]. After synthesis, ATP can be transferred from the inner mitochondrial membrane to the cytosol through ANT and the outer membrane VDAC. MPT induction opens the nonselective pores permitting the diffusion of a 1.5 kDa small molecule [14]. Electrons can be relocated from complex I (NADH dehydrogenase) and II (succinate dehydrogenase) to coenzyme Q10 with a quinine structure as DOX. Then, particles are moved to complex III, cytochrome-*c*, and complex IV. Eventually, oxygen can capture the particle, resulting in water synthesis (**Figure 5**). All ETS elements associated with the enzyme are placed near the matrix surface of the inner mitochondrial membranes. It has been reported that complex I and II could not reach the particles in the mitochondrial cytosol from any organ and any cancer cells, except the heart. The mitochondria of cardiac tissue has two position on the outer surface of inner mitochondrial membrane and faces the matrix [10]. However, overexposed DOX causes mitochondrial dysfunction, consisting of decreasing state 3 respiration, complex I, and ANT activities. Moreover, lengthy DOX treatment increases susceptibility to calcium, resulting in dissipation of MMP at low and high concentrations [13].

Bioenergetics failure may be primarily a mechanism of DOX cardiotoxicity [13]. So, the other molecular base of DOX toxicity on noncancerous tissue relies on the destruction of mtDNA. Oxidative stress leads to damage to mtDNA, especially heart tissue. Additionally, DOX represents the harmful effect of mtDNA much more than nuclear DNA. If the integrated knowledge that the mtDNA repair system is fragile vs. the nuclear DNA system, DOX is understood to be highly toxic to mitochondria [10]. The mitochondrial genome has 13 subunits of ETC codes, which are almost all of the ETC complex, except complex II, a succinate dehydrogenase encoded by nuclear DNA [13]. mtDNA has also been encoded by mitochondrial ribosomal and transfer RNA [10]. DOX damages mtDNA via elevation of ROS [13]. Oxidative damage of DNA has been evaluated by using 8-OHdG formation. After DOX treatment, 8-OHdG has been reported to reach a peak value at 24 h, but a baseline value at 14 days [13]. The chronic

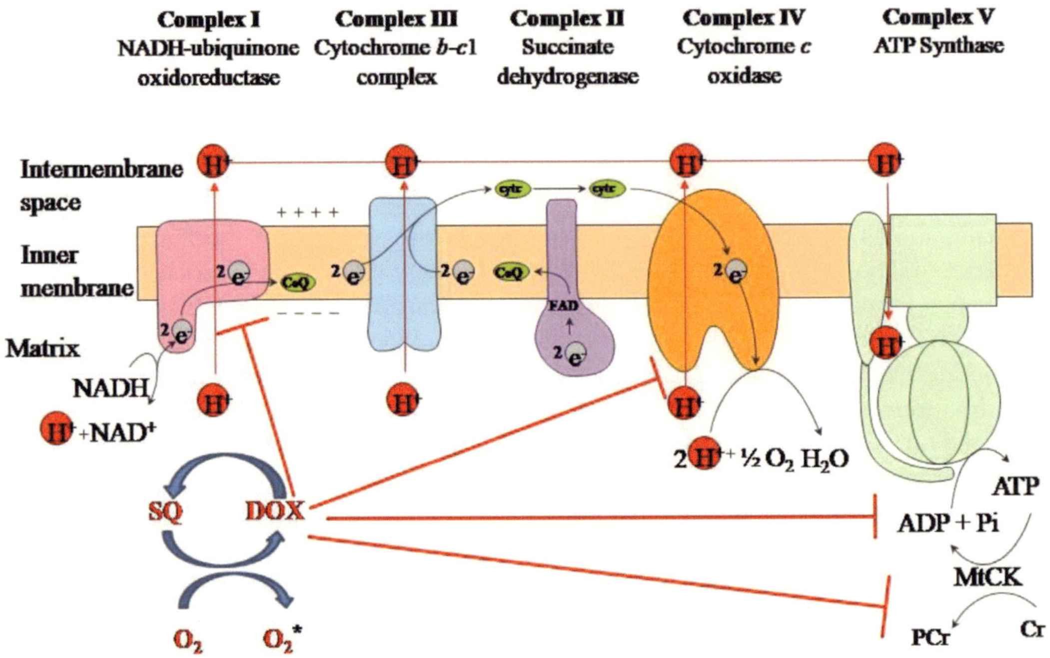

Figure 5. The effect of doxorubicin and its derivate on the electron transport system and mitochondrial energy production. Modified from Govender et al. [34].

effect of DOX on mitochondria has been reported to appear when it destroys mtDNA [44], mainly developing mtDNA deletion. The prevalence of the elimination has been reported to be between 33 and 80% at a low and high dose of DOX, respectively [10]. When DOX oxidizes mtDNA, mitochondria can no longer produce high-energy substrate, resulting from destroying to reproduce mtDNA [10]. This alternation is explained by DNA repair and elimination of damage to the genomic material, which changes or eliminates the protein function. Alternation or disappearance of mitochondrial protein function elevates ROS formation as well [13]. At this moment, we should take time to diagnose DOX's chronic cardiotoxic effect, e.g., heart failure, dilated cardiomyopathy, and congestive heart failure [10]. Moreover, mitochondrial complex I activity has been claimed to inhibit isolated mitochondria from cardiac tissue, but not hepatic tissue by chronic DOX therapy for 28 weeks. This notion has given rise to the thought that the drug's toxicity in mitochondria is cardioselective [10]. One study suggested that endurance exercises reduce DOX toxicity based on modulation of state 3 alternation at mitochondria. Also, the study reported that apoptosis induced by DOX could be counteracted by endurance exercises giving rise to a decline in apoptotic factors, such as Bax or Bax/Bcl-2 ratio. Moreover, DOX alters the ultrastructure of heart tissue by mitochondrial destruction, including damaging cristae and vacuoles, and causing distension and abnormal size and shape [80]. Mainly, the outer mitochondrial membrane plays a role in the transduction of signals, e.g., apoptotic [82]. Endurance exercises have been suggested to reverse the ultrastructural alternation, e.g., a rise in glycogen storage, and enhance cytosolic and mitochondrial sodium oxide dismutase. Due mostly to the sensitive oxidative stress of MPT, elevation of antioxidant by endurance exercises leads to decreased apoptosis induced by DOX [80].

Another chronic drug mechanism is associated with cardiolipin. DOX has high affinity for cardiolipin; therefore, DOX–cardiolipin complex formation interrupts the standard oxidative phosphorylation mechanism. DOX can be transformed into the semiquinone form by NADPH reductases in mitochondria. The opening of MTP led to swelling of mitochondria and depolarizing mitochondria membrane potential, structural and cytoskeleton disorganization, and mtDNA injury. Peroxisome proliferator-activated receptor-*c* coactivator-1α (PGC-1α) has a crucial role in mitochondrial biogenesis and oxidative metabolism [16]. Also, alternative posttranslational modification could participate in the alteration of mitochondrial function. Posttranslational modification through acetylation and deacetylation from lysine residues play a crucial role in regulating mitochondrial function. Mitochondrial proteins are modulated posttranslationally as sirtuin enzymes, sirtuin-3, -4, and -5, by deacetylation. Posttranslational modification can occur under redox stress and nutrient flux. Mitochondria express mostly sirtuin-3 and nuclear NAD^+-dependent histone deacetylase [34].

6.3. Bioenergetics dysfunction induced by doxorubicin

Mitochondria have sources of bioenergetics and ROS as well. This is why mitochondria become the target of multiple factors such as drugs, including DOX, and environmental compounds. PGC-1α plays an essential role in the regulation of mitochondrial function, including production of bioenergy and energy homeostasis. PGC-1α can regulate gene transcription, including mitochondrial services such as NRF-1, PPARa, and ERRa, which modulate and are divided into three groups of metabolic enzymes in the TCA cycle: antioxidant enzymes, other mitochondrial protein components of the ETC complexes, and mitochondrial transcription factor A (TFAM) [38].

When mitochondrial dysfunction occurs, i.e., enhancing ROS, reduction of ATP synthesis, a complex transcriptional network, including PGC-1α can be triggered to maintain cellular homeostasis. PGC-1α can transcript three groups of genes, which are mentioned above. Although PGC-1α's effect on three groups is suggested to have a minor impact at a low mitochondrial toxic concentration to alter ROS and ATP production, its effect on the groups is essential at a high level of mitochondrial toxins. It is reported that DOX's toxic effect is related to increasing mitochondrial ROS production and the most destructive impact of DOX appears in cardiac tissue due to its accumulation in cardiac cells [38].

It is well known that heart tissue contains a high cell volume of mitochondria, almost 35% due to the requirement of energy supply because of maintaining the contraction function of the tissue [15]. The heart produces energy requirement by using β-oxidation of fatty acid in mitochondria. The cardiotoxicity of DOX might be related to swelling and destroy bioenergy from the organelle and myofibril of cardiac tissue. DOX also increases oxidative stress, resulting in enhancing mitochondria dysfunction. The other mechanism of DOX on mitochondrial malfunction is reported to be associated with the dissipation of mitochondrial ETC at different levels. So, NADH and succinate oxidase in cardiac tissue have been shown to be blocked by DOX treatment. Also, DOX separates complex I from ETC, resulting in the elevation of oxidative damage by producing semiquinone free radicals. Moreover, DOX might inhibit stage-3 and stage-4 respiration. The other mechanism for blocking mitochondrial function is related to the prevention of Mg-dependent F0F1-ATPase in muscle, including heart and skeletal muscle. The other mechanism associates with DOX's structure since DOX has a high affinity to bind cardiolipin, which is one of lipids and locates at the inner mitochondrial membranes. DOX's toxicity on mitochondria is related to its dose and is time dependent. Mitochondrial toxicity of DOX has been observed from 2 to 13 weeks at a low dose. Moreover, mitochondria play an essential role in the regulation of calcium homeostasis. Under normal physiological conditions, there is little impact of mitochondria on calcium homeostasis. However, the mitochondrial function of calcium homeostasis is essential under pathological circumstances to decrease cytosolic calcium. So, calcium efflux into mitochondria depolarizes MMP. DOX's effect on calcium homeostasis at mitochondria is based on inhibition of the inward calcium flux and exaggeration of the release of calcium from mitochondria by swelling of the mitochondria–calcium-dependent pathways through MPT, resulting in enhancing calcium concentration at the cytosol. Furthermore, DOX at a low dose gives rise to a decline in the calcium storage capacity of mitochondria. DOX attenuates mitochondria calcium storage capacity exaggerated at its high dose, which means it is related to dose. Eventually, the effects of DOX lead to the dissipation of MMP. The mitochondrial permeability pore is highly sensitive to MMP and regulated by the redox status of mitochondria. DOX also opens MPT in the manufacture of ROS through complex I, which is mentioned above (**Figure 5**). Thus, DOX's MPT effect might be based on the prevention of ANT, an element of the MPT pore complex. It is interesting to note that DOX-treated cardiomyocytes have fewer ATP levels (~30%) vs. normal cardiomyocytes [15].

It is suggested that ROS produced by mitochondria has a critical role in DOX's cardiotoxicity. Hepatic tissue plays a role in detoxification by the cytochrome P450 enzyme in the ER, which also occurs in DOX's redox cycling. However, this bioreductive activation of DOX by cytochrome P450 in the heart is much less than in the liver. So, ROS production and DOX redox cycling in the ER in the heart are negligible [13]. Because it is continuously working, the heart needs ATP by β-oxidation in mitochondria. Therefore, cardiomyocytes contain tremendous mitochondrial density (around 25–30%) vs. the other cell types. This is why ROS production by mitochondria is significant compared to the other compartments of cardiomyocytes in heart tissue [13]. DOX has been reported to have high affinity to bind to cardiolipin from inner mitochondria. Also, DOX inhibits complexes II–IV from ETS [13]. Another suggestion is that DOX affects complex I, II, III, and IV [42]. DOX can also alter mitochondrial membrane organization but not physically interact with mitochondrial enzymes. According to isolated mitochondria and in vivo studies, DOX can capture an electron from complex I, resulting in a decline in oxidative phosphorylation and elevated oxygen consumption [13].

DOX elevates the nonphosphorylating rate of oxygen consumption (state 4) and decreases phosphorylation-linked oxygen consumption (state 3). Therefore, DOX triggers the manufacture of superoxide. Also, these impacts lead to declining ATP synthesis. Energy stress induced by DOX eventually prefers other pathways for producing ATP, e.g., glycolysis. However, glycolytic ATP does not have sufficient energy to maintain cell function. The metabolic switch is a requirement to make alternations such as enhancing glucose transporter type 1 (GLUT1) transportation to plasmalemma. So, glucose uptake increases by using GLUT1 within 1 h of DOX treatment [13].

Some compensating mechanism is recommended to modulate energy supply to maintain cellular function, e.g., CK or AMPK. Studies have shown how to decrease ATP and phosphocreatine (PCr). One μM DOX concentration has indicated a decline of ~50% ATP production within 24 h. Why is the reduction essential to utilize around 90% ATP synthesized by mitochondria? When mitochondrial function is destroyed, heart or tissue function is automatically affected by low energy supply. DOX's mitochondrial effect is shown to change the ultrastructure, swelling, and oxidative capacity as well. Although DOX inhibits state 3, state 4 is activated by the drug. DOX is highly bound to cardiolipin, one of the anionic phospholipids from the inner membrane of mitochondria. When DOX binds to cardiolipin, enzymes from respiration and oxidation, e.g., cytochrome-*c*, might be inactive due to the alternation of the lipid environment. After binding cardiolipin to DOX, cardiolipin-related proteins such as cytochrome-*c* and mitochondrial creatine kinase (MtCK) are released from the mitochondrial inner membrane to the cytosol. Besides the indirect effect of that enzyme, DOX also has a direct effect on these enzymes. The mitochondrial impact of DOX can amplify its toxic effect by using the target organelle's enzyme system. DOX inactivates NADH dehydrogenase, cytochrome P-450 reductase, and xanthine oxidase. Moreover, DOX tends to accumulate in nuclei and mitochondria vs. plasma. The heart mainly utilizes fatty acid to generate energy by β-oxidation. So, DOX also destroys β-oxidation by inhibiting of consumption of palmitate, a long chain fatty acid, through impairment of carnitine palmitoyltransferase I (CPTI) and/or its substrate L-carnitine. DOX elevates glycolysis as a compensatory response to a decline in fatty acid oxidation. However, some studies' results show a decrease in both fatty acid and glucose oxidation by using cell line and rat models. Why glucose utilization is decreased after DOX treatment is explained by two theories. One is that DOX might reduce glucose supply. It is reported that DOX treatment initially increases glycolysis (~50%; within 1 h of exposure to the drug), but later depresses it sharply. The second explanation is that DOX reduces phosphofructokinase (PFK) activity, one of the rate-limiting enzymes of glycolysis. So, one reason for DOX's low-energy generation is that it disrupts cell metabolism tissue. The other reason is the effects of DOX's CK system. There are two CK isoforms in the heart: cytosolic and mitochondrial (MtCK). CK can easily produce PCr from creatine. Transformation of creatine to PCr closely binds between energy generation and utilization. MtCK, an octameric, is accompanied by ANT) and VDAC (porin), so transforming energy by the generation of oxidative phosphorylation to the cytoplasm. However, cytosolic CK isoform (MM-, MB-, BBCK), a dimeric, links to both energy manufacture by glycolysis and energy consumption, including actomyosin ATPase at myofibrils, the Ca^{2+}-ATPase at the SR, Na^{+}, and K^{+}-ATPase in the sarcolemma [43]. DOX inactivates the entire CK system, especially MtCK. MtCK's effects dissociate its structure from octamer to dimer, resulting in dissociation from the mitochondrial inner membrane. Moreover, cardiac MtCK has been reported to be more sensitive to DOX than ubiquitous MtCK, leading to selective toxicity in heart tissue. The inactivation of DOX on MtCK has been indicated to be linked to the drug's dose. At a low dose below 100 μM, MtCK became inactive because of DOX's redox modification from its cysteine residues. Its high dose, however, depresses MtCK due to ROS production. Furthermore, DOX and MtCK have been indicated to have a common feature, i.e., they tend to attach to an inner mitochondrial membrane. So, the feature provides high DOX concentration around the MtCK. Additionally, when DOX is activated by peroxidase/H_2O_2, CK inhibition via DOX accelerates. The inhibition link to oxidative and nitrous stress means that CK is very vulnerable to the redox status of cells. Even a μM DOX concentration has been reported to lead to dimerization of MtCK and augments inhibition and dimerization at a 20 μM concentration. Also, it is indicated that total CK activity has been noticed to reduce (by nearly 20%) for DOX treatment compared to 20 μM concentrations. Even under this circumstance, CK can still maintain its function due to a compensatory mechanism that causes to reduce muscle-type CK (MCK) (a myofibrillar isoform) and elevate brain-type CK (BCK; a fetal isoform) that is raised by heart failure or cardiac hypertrophy. It is important to know that CK shift is reported to be within 1 h at 2 μM DOX treatment. So, CK system dysfunction might probably participate in DOX-mediated heart failure. MtCK inhibition by dimerization not only causes energy transfer from mitochondria to the cytosol but also affects the mitochondrial respiratory chain. Moreover, inhibition destroys the three-modal interaction between MtCK, ANT, and DAC, which means that MtCK plays a role in MPT. So, destruction of modal interaction could trigger apoptosis as well. Besides programmed cell death, myofibrillar CK functionally integrates with the sarcoplasmic Ca^{2+} pump (SERCA). When a CK defect occurs, cytosolic Ca^{2+} balance is destroyed, leading to defects in contraction and relaxation coupling due to Ca^{2+} accumulation. Ca^{2+}accumulation could trigger apoptosis as well. This is why dysfunction of CK causes innate apoptosis in two ways. When energy disruption occurs such as CK dysfunction, AMPK is activated to regain energy balance. AMPK is one of the sensory energy proteins that compensates for shifting from ATP to ADP and/or AMP. It means that AMPK is highly sensitive to a ratio of AMP/ATP and oxidative stress as well. Under energy stress, AMPK changes the metabolic activity of cells to increase ATP synthesis by elevation of fatty acid oxidation, glycolysis, and a decline in ATP utilization. All these processes are crucial to surviving cells to maintain protein, lipid, and carbohydrate manufacture. It is reported that DOX inhibits AMPK, resulting in energy stress. In a study by using isolated heart, DOX at 2 μM, which is the plasma peak value of the patients treated with the drug, was reported to cause to plume AMPK and acetyl-CoA carboxylase proteins after 1-h perfusion. Therefore, further study is needed to evaluate the mechanism. However, it is suggested that DOX causes energy and oxidative stress in both reactive and nitrogen stress. AMPK inhibition means that DOX leads to a change in metabolic activity of cells by a decline in fatty acid oxidant. How the fatty acid oxidant decreases relates to enhancing acetyl-CoA carboxylase, resulting in CPTI by malonyl-CoA, eventually leading to a decrease in mitochondrial fatty acid oxidation. Besides the decline of mitochondrial fatty acid oxidation, AMPK inhibition also causes to reduce glycolysis by decreasing of PFK and glucose uptake as well. Under physiological conditions, energy stress is expected to activate AMPK [43].One study showed that AMPK, glucose, and fatty acid is related to gene and protein expressions, and acetyl-CoA carboxylase have been decreased by DOX in males more than in females. AMPK is also a crucial function for cardiolipin synthesis and remodeling. By AMPK, PGC-1α/β modulates cardiolipin synthesis as well [36].

6.4. Doxorubicin's effect on myocardial energy metabolism

It is well known that heart tissue contains a high cell volume of mitochondria nearly (25–35%) [3, 15] due to the requirement of energy supply to maintain the contraction function of the tissue [84]. The heart produces an energy requirement by using the β-oxidation of fatty acid in mitochondria [15]. Adequate ATP production is not just significant to maintain contractile function, but is also crucial for protein synthesis, controlling the protein quality function of ER, cytoskeletal function, and to clear the cellular waste from lysosomes. This is why DOX destroys energy production systems and has been reported to destroy the protein degradation function, resulting in overwhelming the ER and mitochondria [4].

The impact of DOX on bioenergetics and oxidative stress might partially be associated with its structure because it has a high affinity to bind to cardiolipin, which is one of the lipids and locates at the inner mitochondrial membrane [13, 43]. ROS production by mitochondria might be a significant contributor to the drug's toxicity in heart tissue [13]. This is why mitochondria is one of the targets of multiple factors such as drugs including DOX and environmental compounds. There are defined control systems that maintain healthy, functional mitochondria. One of the systems is PGC-1α, which plays an essential role in the regulation of mitochondrial function, including production of bioenergy and energy homeostasis. PGC-1α can regulate gene transcription, including mitochondrial functions such as NRF-1, PPARa, and ERRa, which modulate and divided three groups in metabolic enzymes in the TCA cycle: antioxidant enzymes, other mitochondrial protein components of the ETC complexes, and TFAM [38]. When mitochondrial dysfunction occurs, i.e., enhancing ROS and reducing ATP synthesis, a complex transcriptional network, including PGC-1α, can be triggered to maintain cellular homeostasis. PGC-1α can transcribe three groups of genes, which are mentioned above. Although PGC-1α has an effect on three groups it is suggested to have a minor impact at a low mitochondrial toxic concentration to alter ROS and ATP production; its effect on the groups is important at high concentration of mitochondrial toxins. It is reported that DOX's toxic effect is related to increasing mitochondrial ROS production and the most destructive impact of DOX can appear in cardiac tissue due to its accumulation in cardiac cells [38]. One study has noticed that DOX led to a decrease in PGC-1α and its related genes, including NRF1, TFAM, SOD2, CS, VDAC, and COXIV. PGC-1α is phosphorylated by AMPK, and is also modulated by acetylation by SIRT1. The posttranslational modification of PGC-1α is a potent mechanism for mitochondrial function by oxidative stress and apoptosis. So, SIRT1 is suggested to decline mitochondrial dysfunction and cardiotoxicity induced by DOX [16]. The other control system is SIRT-3 which is one of NAD-dependent deacetylases and places at mitochondria. Deacetylase plays a crucial role in maintaining healthy mitochondrial function by deacetylation of metabolic, apoptotic, and ROS-production enzymes. Also, SIRT-3 has been shown to enhance Foxo-3a, which is associated with an antioxidant mechanism. Thus, SIRT-3 closes the MPT by blocking Cyp D activity. SIRT-3 has a modulating effect on cardiac hypertrophy via strengthening the LKB1 event, which is one of the upstream kinases of AMPK. One study has reported that SIRT-3 is decreased by DOX treatment due to the rise in ROS production and mitochondrial dysfunction. So, reducing SIRT-3 leads to elevation to ROS and HIF1α stabilization, which is an essential factor to shift metabolism from β-oxidation of fatty acid to glycolysis (the Warburg effect) [85]. Further, the inhibition of protein or slicing of the HIF1α gene has been suggested to decrease drug resistance against DOX [86].

It is well known that the heart can produce ATP from fatty acid. However, metabolic shift is developed from fatty acid to glucose due to a compensating energy demand under pathologic conditions. So, the expression of peroxisome proliferator-activated receptor gamma is also affected by the drug, resulting in decline in adipogenesis and destruction of glucose intake via glucose transporter type 4 (GLUT4) [34]. In contrast, according to previous study results, 1 h after 1 μM of DOX was given to cultured adult rat cardiac cells, sarcomeric titin protein was reported significantly to degrade via the calpain-dependent mechanism. DOX increases glucose uptake by GLUT1 into plasma membrane [24], which is a requirement of the metabolic switch in the first hours of treatment [13]. However, it is reported that GLUT4 was not affected by DOX [24]. Also, DOX impairs PFK, which is a rate-limiting glycolytic flux [24, 34]. Energy stress induced by DOX eventually prefers the other pathways for producing ATP, e.g., glycolysis. However, glycolytic ATP does not have sufficient energy to maintain cell function [13]. The cardiotoxicity of DOX might relate to swelling and destroy bioenergy from the organelle and myofibril of cardiac tissue. DOX also increases oxidative stress, resulting in enhancing mitochondrial dysfunction [15].

The other mechanism of DOX on mitochondrial dysfunction is reported to be associated with dissipation of mitochondrial ETC at different levels. So, NADH and succinate oxidase in cardiac tissue has been shown to be blocked by DOX treatment. Also, DOX separates complex I from ETC, resulting in elevated oxidative damage by producing semiquinone free radicals [15]. Also, DOX inhibits complexes II–IV from ETS [13]. DOX disrupts complex I, III, and IV, and is especially susceptible to complex I and IV [34]. Specifically, DOX decreases the content of the complex I NDUFB8 subunit and the ATP synthase ATP5A subunit [87]. The opinion of others is that DOX can alter mitochondrial membrane organization but not physical interaction with any mitochondrial enzymes [13]. In other words, DOX affects all complexes from I to IV [42]. There is a discrepancy between DOX's effects on the stage of respiration. One of the studies suggested that DOX might inhibit state 3 and state 4 respiration [15]. Although others have reported that DOX impedes state 3, which is phosphorylation-linked oxygen consumption, it is activated by the drug [13, 43]. Therefore, DOX triggers superoxide manufacturing. Also, this impact led to declining ATP synthesis [13]. The other mechanism for blocking the mitochondrial function is related to prevention of Mg-dependent F0F1-ATPase in muscle, including heart and skeletal muscle [15].

The ATP pool of cardiac tissue is reported to be 5 mmol/kg wet heart weight. When the demand for energy in the heart is increased, PCr (concentration around 10 mmol/kg wet heart weight) can compensate for the requirement. PCr can be transformed by CK, one of the energy reservoir regulators [34]. Interestingly, total ATP decline due to DOX treatment on cardiomyocytes vs. normal, healthy cardiomyocytes is reported to be ~30% [15]. Some compensating mechanism is recommended to modulate energy supply to maintain cellular function, e.g., CK or AMPK. Studies have shown that ATP and/or PCr decrease by using the drug. One μM DOX concentration has indicated a decline of ~50% ATP production within 24 h [43]. PCr is destroyed by DOX treatment due to the accumulation of ferrous iron by the drug. So, DOX declines both ATP and PCr. Children treated with DOX for 4 years have been reported to have decreased PCr/ATP ratios of around 20% [34]. Why the decline is vital to utilize around 90% ATP synthesized by mitochondria is because heart or tissue function is automatically affected by low energy supply when mitochondrial function is destroyed [43].

The other mechanism of energy dysfunction due to DOX treatment is AMPK destruction [87]. It is well known that the heart mainly utilizes fatty acid to generate energy by β-oxidation [43]. DOX inhibits fatty acid β-oxidation and myocardial function as well, but enhances glucose intake though AMPK phosphorylation [88]. AMPK inhibition means that DOX leads to a change in the metabolic activity of cells by declining fatty acid oxidant, particularly palmitate consumption. How the fatty acid oxidant decreases relates to enhancing acetyl-CoA carboxylase by AMPK inhibition, resulting in a decline in CPTI and/or its substrate L-carnitine by malonyl-CoA, eventually leading to a decrease in mitochondrial fatty acid oxidation [43]. Under physiological conditions, energy stress activates AMPK [43]. DOX elevates glycolysis as a compensatory response to a decline in fatty acid oxidation. However, some study results showed a decrease in both fatty acid and glucose oxidation by using cell line and rat models. Why glucose utilization is reduced after DOX treatment is explained by two theories. One is that DOX might minimize glucose supply. It is reported that DOX treatment initially increases glycolysis (~50%; within 1 h of exposure to the drug), but later causes it to depress sharply. The second explanation is that DOX leads to reduced PFK activity, one of the rate-limiting enzymes of glycolysis [43].

When energy disruption occurs such as CK dysfunction, AMPK is activated to regain energy balance. AMPK is one of the sensory energy proteins that compensates for shifting from ATP to ADP and/or AMP. It means AMPK is highly sensitive to a ratio of AMP/ATP and oxidative stress. Under energy stress, AMPK changes the metabolic activity of cells to increase ATP synthesis by elevation of fatty acid oxidation, glycolysis, and a decline in ATP utilization. All these processes are crucial to the surviving cell by maintaining proteins, lipids, and the manufacture of carbohydrate. It is reported that DOX inhibits AMPK, resulting in energy stress [43]. Another study noticed that AMPK can be inactivated with a 2 μM concentration of DOX. This explains how DOX can change substrate utilization to produce energy [24]. There is no clearly understood process as to how AMPK is inhibited. Therefore, further study is needed to evaluate the mechanism. However, it is suggested that DOX causes energy and oxidative stress in both reactive and nitrogen stress [43]. Kinase is also a crucial function in cardiolipin synthesis and remodeling. By AMPK, PGC-1α/β modulates cardiolipin synthesis as well [36]. Moreover, DOX could destroy desmin interaction with mitochondria, resulting in triggering apoptosis [89]. When our knowledge of AMPK, cardiolipin, DOX, and PGC1α/β are superimposed, it can easily be understood that DOX-induced cardiac mitochondrial toxicity is more complex and multifactorial. Metabolic dysfunction induced by DOX might also relate to gender [36].

One pathway of DOX's low-energy generation disrupts cell metabolism tissue. DOX destroys CK as an energy shuttle and storage system, AMPK as an energy-sensing and signaling system [24], and the channel of ATP and PCr from mitochondria to the cytosol. PCr and creatine can regulate the ATP/ADP ratio [14]. This is why the mechanism of DOX's mitochondrial energy dysfunction can be explained by DOX's cardiac cell metabolism CK system effects [43]. CK in the heart has two isoforms. One is located free at the cytosol (cytosolic CK (cCK)), and the other is bound to sarcoplasmic or mitochondrial membranes [14, 43]. cCK has two subtypes: muscle-type MCK and brain-type BCK. Also, MtCK has two subtypes known as sarcomeric MtCK (sMtCK) that exist only in the heart and skeletal muscles and ubiquitous MtCK (uMtCK) that is present in other organs and tissues, such as the brain, spermatozoa, and skin. Cardiac cCK has two forms as a homodimer (MMCK and/or BBCK) or heterodimer (MBCK), which is a cardiac-specific form [24]. According to this knowledge, it is said that MBCK can usually be determined as an indicator of a heart attack. sMtCK is the mainly octameric form [24] and places the outer intermembrane space and mitochondrial cristae between membranal protein ANT in the inner membrane and VDAC in the outer layer [24]). MtCK has high affinity to cardiolipin [14] and the outer surface of the inner mitochondrial membrane [24]. It must not be forgotten that DOX has a great relationship with cardiolipin. So, one of DOX's targets is MtCK. Moreover, DOX oxidizes MtCK at cysteine residues. Besides oxidation, DOX leads to inactivation of MtCK, resulting in enhanced embryonic CK isoform expression [14].

MtCK can efficiently produce PCr from creatine [24, 43]. Transformation of creatine to PCr firmly binds between energy generation and utilization. MtCK, an octameric, accompanies ANT, and VDAC (porin) [43]. ANT can transfer ADP to matrix space. Then, ADP resynthesizes ATP through oxidative phosphorylation. However, PCr can be sent to the cytosol via VDAC [24]. PCr is utilized by cCK to maintain the subcellular local ATP/ADP ratio [24].

Although DOX inactivates all CK, MtCK is especially destroyed [43] by the drug through dissociation of its structure from octamer to dimer [24, 43] or infusion of binding MtCK at mitochondrial membranes, such as cardiolipin [24]. Moreover, cardiac MtCK has been reported to be more sensitive to DOX than uMtCK, leading to selective toxicity in heart tissue. The inactivation of MtCK by DOX is linked to the drug's dosage. At a low dose below 100 μM, MtCK's inactivation occurs because of DOX's redox modification from its cysteine residues. Its high treatment, however, depresses MtCK due to ROS production. Furthermore, DOX and MtCK have been indicated to have a standard feature, they tend to attach an inner mitochondrial membrane, providing high DOX concentration around the MtCK. Additionally, when DOX is activated by peroxidase/H_2O_2, CK inhibition via DOX accelerates. The inhibition is linked to oxidative and nitrous stress, which means that CK is very vulnerable to the redox status of cells. Even a 2 μM DOX concentration has been reported to lead to dimerization of MtCK (ordinarily octameric), and augment the inhibition and dimerization at a 20 μM intensity. Also, it is indicated that total CK activity has been noticed to reduce (by nearly 20%) for DOX treatment concentrated at 20 μM. Under this circumstance, CK has still been maintaining its function due to a compensatory mechanism, which reduces MCK (a myofibrillar isoform) and high BCK (a fetal isoform) that is elevated by heart failure or cardiac hypertrophy. It is vital to know that CK shift is reported to be within 1 h at 2 μM of DOX. So, CK system dysfunction might probably participate in DOX-mediated heart failure. MtCK inhibition by dimerization not only causes energy transfer from mitochondria to the cytosol but also influences the mitochondrial respiratory chain. Moreover, this inhibition destroys the three-modal interaction between MtCK, ANT, and VDAC, which means that MtCK plays a role in MPT. So, damage to the modal interaction could first trigger apoptosis. Besides programmed cell death, myofibrillar CK functionally integrates with SERCA. When a CK defect occurs, cytosolic Ca^{2+} balance is destroyed, leading to defects in contraction and relaxation coupling due to Ca^{2+} accumulation. Ca^{2+}accumulation could also trigger apoptosis. This is why dysfunction of CK causes innate apoptosis in two ways [43].

http://dx.doi.org/10.5772/intechopen.80284

Besides the CK shuttle, the malate–aspartate shuttle (MAS) has a role in declining traffic equivalents between mitochondria and the cytosol. Moreover, TCA and MAS have demonstrated to be associated with each other physically. This interaction provides a direct reason for metabolic alternation of the mitochondrial matrix to the cytosol. MAS suppression in the heart has been proposed to reduce mitochondrial respiration before cardiac damage, thereby declining oxidative injury. A cancer cell produces energy by glycolysis known as the Warburg effect. So, it is suggested that MAS inhibition might be an excellent candidate for overt DOX toxicity, without affecting the anticancer drug's effects [29].

DOX directly affects oxidative phosphorylation enzymes, e.g., NADH dehydrogenase, Rieske iron sulfur protein, succinate dehydrogenase, cyclooxygenase, CK, carnitine palmitoyltransferase, fatty acid β-oxidation-related enzymes, as well as the translocation of phosphate and pyruvate to the mitochondrial matrix. DOX reduces fatty acid β-oxidation by blocking fatty acid transfer protein to mitochondria, resulting in an increase in the pyruvate dehydrogenase complex, which is a rate-limiting enzyme of glycolysis. The other effect of DOX metabolism is that the triosephosphate isomerase enzyme essential for glucose metabolism can be inhibited by the treatment [14]. The anthracyline causes mitochondrial dysfunction, e.g., displacing α-enolase from mitochondria [30]. ATP synthesis is decreased in both the cytosol and mitochondria by DOX [90].

7. Conclusion

It is impossible to ignore DOX therapy from cancer patients' treatment due to its inevitable chemotherapeutic efficiency on a variety of cancers. Unfortunately, there is limited knowledge available on DOX's cardiotoxicity, particularly mitochondriopathy. This is why the molecular clarifying mechanism of DOX's myocardial and mitochondrial toxicities will hopefully overcome the side effects and increase the survival rate of cancer patients as well. Therefore, further studies are needed to evaluate the detrimental effects of DOX on mitochondria to restore its limited utilization in cancer patients' therapy.

Author details

Celal Guven[1], Yusuf Sevgiler[2]* and Eylem Taskin[3]

*Address all correspondence to: ysevgiler@protonmail.com

1 Department of Biophysics, Faculty of Medicine, Omer Halisdemir University, Nigde, Turkey

2 Department of Biology, Faculty of Science and Letters, Adiyaman University, Adiyaman, Turkey

3 Department of Physiology, Faculty of Medicine, Omer Halisdemir University, Nigde, Turkey

References

[1] Fidler MM, Gupta S, Soerjomataram I, Ferlay J, Steliarova-Foucher E, Bray F. Cancer incidence and mortality among young adults aged 20-39 years worldwide in 2012: A population-based study. The Lancet Oncology. Dec 2017;**18**(12):1579-1589

[2] Tai X, Cai XB, Zhang Z, Wei R. In vitro and in vivo inhibition of tumor cell viability by combined dihydroartemisinin and doxorubicin treatment, and the underlying mechanism. Oncology Letters. Nov 2016;**12**(5):3701-3706

[3] Sorensen JC, Cheregi BD, Timpani CA, Nurgali K, Hayes A, Rybalka E. Mitochondria: Inadvertent targets in chemotherapy-induced skeletal muscle toxicity and wasting? Cancer Chemotherapy and Pharmacology. Oct 2016;**78**(4):673-683

[4] Bartlett JJ, Trivedi PC, Pulinilkunnil T. Autophagic dysregulation in doxorubicin cardiomyopathy. Journal of Molecular and Cellular Cardiology. Mar 2017;**104**:1-8

[5] Ludke A, Akolkar G, Ayyappan P, Sharma AK, Singal PK. Time course of changes in oxidative stress and stress-induced proteins in cardiomyocytes exposed to doxorubicin and prevention by vitamin C. PLoS One. 2017;**12**(7):e0179452

[6] Liu X, Zhu Y, Lin X, Fang L, Yan X. Mitral regurgitation after anthracycline-based chemotherapy in an adult patient with breast cancer: A case report. Medicine (Baltimore). Dec 2017;**96**(49):e9004

[7] Aramvash A, Rabbani Chadegani A, Lotfi S. Evaluation of apoptosis in multipotent hematopoietic cells of bone marrow by anthracycline antibiotics. Iranian Journal of Pharmaceutical Research. Summer 2017;**16**(3):1204-1213

[8] Manjanatha MG, Bishop ME, Pearce MG, Kulkarni R, Lyn-Cook LE, Ding W. Genotoxicity of doxorubicin in F344 rats by combining the comet assay, flow-cytometric peripheral blood micronucleus test, and pathway-focused gene expression profiling. Environmental and Molecular Mutagenesis. Jan 2014;**55**(1):24-34

[9] Shi J, Zhang L, Zhang YW, Surma M, Mark Payne R, Wei L. Downregulation of doxorubicin-induced myocardial apoptosis accompanies postnatal heart maturation. American Journal of Physiology. Heart and Circulatory Physiology. Apr 2012;**302**(8):H1603-H1613

[10] Conklin KA. Coenzyme q10 for prevention of anthracycline-induced cardiotoxicity. Integrative Cancer Therapies. Jun 2005;**4**(2):110-130

[11] Damiani RM, Moura DJ, Viau CM, Caceres RA, Henriques JA, Saffi J. Pathways of cardiac toxicity: Comparison between chemotherapeutic drugs doxorubicin and mitoxantrone. Archives of Toxicology. Sept 2016;**90**(9):2063-2076

[12] Yang F, Lei Q, Li L, et al. Delivery of epirubicin via slow infusion as a strategy to mitigate chemotherapy-induced cardiotoxicity. PLoS One. 2017;**12**(11):e0188025

[13] Berthiaume JM, Wallace KB. Adriamycin-induced oxidative mitochondrial cardiotoxicity. Cell Biology and Toxicology. Jan 2007;**23**(1):15-25

[14] Pereira GC, Silva AM, Diogo CV, Carvalho FS, Monteiro P, Oliveira PJ. Drug-induced cardiac mitochondrial toxicity and protection: From doxorubicin to carvedilol. Current Pharmaceutical Design. 2011;**17**(20):2113-2129

[15] Wallace KB. Adriamycin-induced interference with cardiac mitochondrial calcium homeostasis. Cardiovascular Toxicology. 2007;**7**(2):101-107

[16] Cui L, Guo J, Zhang Q, et al. Erythropoietin activates SIRT1 to protect human cardiomyocytes against doxorubicin-induced mitochondrial dysfunction and toxicity. Toxicology Letters. Jun 2017;**275**:28-38

[17] Carvalho FS, Burgeiro A, Garcia R, Moreno AJ, Carvalho RA, Oliveira PJ. Doxorubicin-induced cardiotoxicity: From bioenergetic failure and cell death to cardiomyopathy. Medicinal Research Reviews. Jan 2014;**34**(1):106-135

[18] Barenholz Y. Doxil(R)—The first FDA-approved nano-drug: Lessons learned. Journal of Controlled Release. Jun 2012;**160**(2):117-134

[19] Cortazar P, Justice R, Johnson J, Sridhara R, Keegan P, Pazdur R. US Food and Drug Administration approval overview in metastatic breast cancer. Journal of Clinical Oncology. May 2012;**30**(14):1705-1711

[20] Koleini N, Kardami E. Autophagy and mitophagy in the context of doxorubicin-induced cardiotoxicity. Oncotarget. Jul 2017;**8**(28):46663-46680

[21] Tang H, Tao A, Song J, Liu Q, Wang H, Rui T. Doxorubicin-induced cardiomyocyte apoptosis: Role of mitofusin 2. The International Journal of Biochemistry & Cell Biology. Jul 2017;**88**:55-59

[22] Meredith AM, Dass CR. Increasing role of the cancer chemotherapeutic doxorubicin in cellular metabolism. The Journal of Pharmacy and Pharmacology. Jun 2016;**68**(6):729-741

[23] Ascensao A, Oliveira PJ, Magalhaes J. Exercise as a beneficial adjunct therapy during doxorubicin treatment—Role of mitochondria in cardioprotection. International Journal of Cardiology. Apr 2012;**156**(1):4-10

[24] Tokarska-Schlattner M, Zaugg M, Zuppinger C, Wallimann T, Schlattner U. New insights into doxorubicin-induced cardiotoxicity: The critical role of cellular energetics. Journal of Molecular and Cellular Cardiology. Sept 2006;**41**(3):389-405

[25] Zhou F, Hao G, Zhang J, et al. Protective effect of 23-hydroxybetulinic acid on doxorubicin-induced cardiotoxicity: A correlation with the inhibition of carbonyl reductase-mediated metabolism. British Journal of Pharmacology. Dec 2015;**172**(23):5690-5703

[26] Lahoti TS, Patel D, Thekkemadom V, Beckett R, Ray SD. Doxorubicin-induced in vivo nephrotoxicity involves oxidative stress-mediated multiple pro- and anti-apoptotic signaling pathways. Current Neurovascular Research. Nov 2012;**9**(4):282-295

[27] Imstepf S, Pierroz V, Rubbiani R, et al. Organometallic rhenium complexes divert doxorubicin to the mitochondria. Angewandte Chemie (International Ed. in English). Feb 2016;**55**(8):2792-2795

[28] Varga ZV, Ferdinandy P, Liaudet L, Pacher P. Drug-induced mitochondrial dysfunction and cardiotoxicity. American Journal of Physiology. Heart and Circulatory Physiology. Nov 2015;**309**(9):H1453-H1467

[29] Liu Y, Asnani A, Zou L, et al. Visnagin protects against doxorubicin-induced cardiomyopathy through modulation of mitochondrial malate dehydrogenase. Science Translational Medicine. Dec 2014;**6**(266):266ra170

[30] Hsu HC, Chen CY, Chen MF. N-3 polyunsaturated fatty acids decrease levels of doxorubicin-induced reactive oxygen species in cardiomyocytes—Involvement of uncoupling protein UCP2. Journal of Biomedical Science. Nov 2014;**21**:101

[31] Xiong H, Du S, Ni J, Zhou J, Yao J. Mitochondria and nuclei dual-targeted heterogeneous hydroxyapatite nanoparticles for enhancing therapeutic efficacy of doxorubicin. Biomaterials. Jul 2016;**94**:70-83

[32] Jean SR, Tulumello DV, Riganti C, Liyanage SU, Schimmer AD, Kelley SO. Mitochondrial targeting of doxorubicin eliminates nuclear effects associated with cardiotoxicity. ACS Chemical Biology. Sep 2015;**10**(9):2007-2015

[33] Mendivil-Perez M, Velez-Pardo C, Jimenez-Del-Rio M. Doxorubicin induces apoptosis in Jurkat cells by mitochondria-dependent and mitochondria-independent mechanisms under normoxic and hypoxic conditions. Anti-Cancer Drugs. Jul 2015;**26**(6):583-598

[34] Govender J, Loos B, Marais E, Engelbrecht AM. Mitochondrial catastrophe during doxorubicin-induced cardiotoxicity: A review of the protective role of melatonin. Journal of Pineal Research. Nov 2014;**57**(4):367-380

[35] Dhingra R, Margulets V, Chowdhury SR, et al. Bnip3 mediates doxorubicin-induced cardiac myocyte necrosis and mortality through changes in mitochondrial signaling. Proceedings of the National Academy of Sciences of the United States of America. Dec 2014;**111**(51):E5537-E5544

[36] Moulin M, Piquereau J, Mateo P, et al. Sexual dimorphism of doxorubicin-mediated cardiotoxicity: Potential role of energy metabolism remodeling. Circulation. Heart Failure. Jan 2015;**8**(1):98-108

[37] Gonzalez Y, Pokrzywinski KL, Rosen ET, et al. Reproductive hormone levels and differential mitochondria-related oxidative gene expression as potential mechanisms for gender differences in cardiosensitivity to doxorubicin in tumor-bearing spontaneously hypertensive rats. Cancer Chemotherapy and Pharmacology. Sept 2015;**76**(3):447-459

[38] Yuan H, Zhang Q, Guo J, et al. A PGC-1alpha-mediated transcriptional network maintains mitochondrial redox and bioenergetic homeostasis against doxorubicin-induced

toxicity in human cardiomyocytes: Implementation of TT21C. Toxicological Sciences. Apr 2016;**150**(2):400-417

[39] Dirks-Naylor AJ, Kouzi SA, Bero JD, et al. Doxorubicin alters the mitochondrial dynamics machinery and mitophagy in the liver of treated animals. Fundamental & Clinical Pharmacology. Dec 2014;**28**(6):633-642

[40] Marques-Aleixo I, Santos-Alves E, Balca MM, et al. Physical exercise mitigates doxorubicin-induced brain cortex and cerebellum mitochondrial alterations and cellular quality control signaling. Mitochondrion. Jan 2016;**26**:43-57

[41] Zhu Q, Qi H, Long Z, et al. Extracellular control of intracellular drug release for enhanced safety of anti-cancer chemotherapy. Scientific Reports. Jun 2016;**6**:28596

[42] Singh P, Sharma R, McElhanon K, et al. Sulforaphane protects the heart from doxorubicin-induced toxicity. Free Radical Biology & Medicine. Sept 2015;**86**:90-101

[43] Tokarska-Schlattner M, Wallimann T, Schlattner U. Alterations in myocardial energy metabolism induced by the anti-cancer drug doxorubicin. Comptes Rendus Biologies. Sept 2006;**329**(9):657-668

[44] de Oliveira BL, Niederer S. A biophysical systems approach to identifying the pathways of acute and chronic doxorubicin mitochondrial cardiotoxicity. PLoS Computational Biology. Nov 2016;**12**(11):e1005214

[45] Qureshi R, Yildirim O, Gasser A, et al. FL3, a synthetic flavagline and ligand of prohibitins, protects cardiomyocytes via STAT3 from doxorubicin toxicity. PLoS One. 2015; **10**(11):e0141826

[46] Ahuja P, Sdek P, MacLellan WR. Cardiac myocyte cell cycle control in development, disease, and regeneration. Physiological Reviews. Apr 2007;**87**(2):521-544

[47] Valiente-Alandi I, Albo-Castellanos C, Herrero D, Sanchez I, Bernad A. Bmi1 (+) cardiac progenitor cells contribute to myocardial repair following acute injury. Stem Cell Research & Therapy. Jul 2016;**7**(1):100

[48] Jung K, Reszka R. Mitochondria as subcellular targets for clinically useful anthracyclines. Advanced Drug Delivery Reviews. Jul 2001;**49**(1-2):87-105

[49] Buondonno I, Gazzano E, Jean SR, et al. Mitochondria-targeted doxorubicin: A new therapeutic strategy against doxorubicin-resistant osteosarcoma. Molecular Cancer Therapeutics. Nov 2016;**15**(11):2640-2652

[50] Arola OJ, Saraste A, Pulkki K, Kallajoki M, Parvinen M, Voipio-Pulkki LM. Acute doxorubicin cardiotoxicity involves cardiomyocyte apoptosis. Cancer Research. Apr 2000; **60**(7):1789-1792

[51] Yapislar H, Taskin E, Ozdas S, Akin D, Sonmez E. Counteraction of apoptotic and inflammatory effects of adriamycin in the liver cell culture by clinopitolite. Biological Trace Element Research. Apr 2016;**170**(2):373-381

[52] Guven C, Taskin E, Akcakaya H. Melatonin prevents mitochondrial damage induced by doxorubicin in mouse fibroblasts through AMPK-PPAR gamma-dependent mechanisms. Medical Science Monitor. Feb 2016;**22**:438-446

[53] Taskin E, Dursun N. The protection of selenium on adriamycin-induced mitochondrial damage in rat. Biological Trace Element Research. Jun 2012;**147**(1-3):165-171

[54] Dursun N, Taskin E, Yerer Aycan MB, Sahin L. Selenium-mediated cardioprotection against adriamycin-induced mitochondrial damage. Drug and Chemical Toxicology. Apr 2011;**34**(2):199-207

[55] Ozdogan K, Taskin E, Dursun N. Protective effect of carnosine on adriamycin-induced oxidative heart damage in rats. Anadolu Kardiyoloji Dergisi. Feb 2011;**11**(1):3-10

[56] Dursun N, Taskin E, Ozturk F. Protection against adriamycin-induced cardiomyopathy by carnosine in rats: Role of endogenous antioxidants. Biological Trace Element Research. Oct 2011;**143**(1):412-424

[57] Guerriero E, Sorice A, Capone F, et al. Combining doxorubicin with a phenolic extract from flaxseed oil: Evaluation of the effect on two breast cancer cell lines. International Journal of Oncology. Feb 2017;**50**(2):468-476

[58] Zhang Y, Chen L, Li F, et al. Cryptotanshinone protects against adriamycin-induced mitochondrial dysfunction in cardiomyocytes. Pharmaceutical Biology. 2016;**54**(2):237-242

[59] Shakir DK, Rasul KI. Chemotherapy induced cardiomyopathy: Pathogenesis, monitoring and management. Journal of Clinical Medical Research. Apr 2009;**1**(1):8-12

[60] Ivanova M, Dovinova I, Okruhlicova L, et al. Chronic cardiotoxicity of doxorubicin involvesactivation of myocardial and circulating matrix metalloproteinases in rats. Acta Pharmacologica Sinica. Apr 2012;**33**(4):459-469

[61] Zhang YY, Meng C, Zhang XM, et al. Ophiopogonin D attenuates doxorubicin-induced autophagic cell death by relieving mitochondrial damage in vitro and in vivo. The Journal of Pharmacology and Experimental Therapeutics. Jan 2015;**352**(1):166-174

[62] Taskin E, Kindap EK, Ozdogan K, Aycan MB, Dursun N. Acute adriamycin-induced cardiotoxicity is exacerbated by angiotension II. Cytotechnology. Jan 2016;**68**(1):33-43

[63] Taskin E, Guven C, Sahin L, Dursun N. The cooperative effect of local angiotensin-II in liver with adriamycin hepatotoxicity on mitochondria. Medical Science Monitor. Mar 2016;**22**:1013-1021

[64] Sarosiek KA, Fraser C, Muthalagu N, et al. Developmental regulation of mitochondrial apoptosis by c-Myc Governs age- and tissue-specific sensitivity to cancer therapeutics. Cancer Cell. Jan 2017;**31**(1):142-156

[65] Amin KM, Syam YM, Anwar MM, Ali HI, Abdel-Ghani TM, Serry AM. Synthesis and molecular docking study of new benzofuran and furo[3,2-g]chromone-based cytotoxic

agents against breast cancer and p38alpha MAP kinase inhibitors. Bioorganic Chemistry. Jan 2018;**76**:487-500

[66] Chua CC, Liu X, Gao J, Hamdy RC, Chua BH. Multiple actions of pifithrin-alpha on doxorubicin-induced apoptosis in rat myoblastic H9c2 cells. American Journal of Physiology. Heart and Circulatory Physiology. Jun 2006;**290**(6):H2606-H2613

[67] Das J, Ghosh J, Manna P, Sil PC. Taurine protects rat testes against doxorubicin-induced oxidative stress as well as p53, Fas and caspase 12-mediated apoptosis. Amino Acids. May 2012;**42**(5):1839-1855

[68] Kazama K, Okada M, Yamawaki H. Adipocytokine, omentin inhibits doxorubicin-induced H9c2 cardiomyoblasts apoptosis through the inhibition of mitochondrial reactive oxygen species. Biochemical and Biophysical Research Communications. Feb 2015; **457**(4):602-607

[69] Bravo-Sagua R, Rodriguez AE, Kuzmicic J, et al. Cell death and survival through the endoplasmic reticulum-mitochondrial axis. Current Molecular Medicine. Feb 2013;**13**(2): 317-329

[70] Pecoraro M, Sorrentino R, Franceschelli S, Del Pizzo M, Pinto A, Popolo A. Doxorubicin-mediated cardiotoxicity: Role of mitochondrial connexin 43. Cardiovascular Toxicology. Oct 2015;**15**(4):366-376

[71] Xu C, Bailly-Maitre B, Reed JC. Endoplasmic reticulum stress: Cell life and death decisions. The Journal of Clinical Investigation. Oct 2005;**115**(10):2656-2664

[72] Nithipongvanitch R, Ittarat W, Cole MP, Tangpong J, Clair DK, Oberley TD. Mitochondrial and nuclear p53 localization in cardiomyocytes: Redox modulation by doxorubicin (Adriamycin)? Antioxidants & Redox Signaling. Jul 2007;**9**(7):1001-1008

[73] Hsu YN, Shyu HW, Hu TW, et al. Anti-proliferative activity of biochanin A in human osteosarcoma cells via mitochondrial-involved apoptosis. Food and Chemical Toxicology. Jan 2018;**112**:194-204

[74] Chen J, Chen B, Zou Z, et al. Costunolide enhances doxorubicin-induced apoptosis in prostate cancer cells via activated mitogen-activated protein kinases and generation of reactive oxygen species. Oncotarget. Dec 2017;**8**(64):107701-107715

[75] Yeung BH, Wong KY, Lin MC, et al. Chemosensitisation by manganese superoxide dismutase inhibition is caspase-9 dependent and involves extracellular signal-regulated kinase 1/2. British Journal of Cancer. Jul 2008;**99**(2):283-293

[76] Jablonska-Trypuc A, Kretowski R, Kalinowska M, Swiderski G, Cechowska-Pasko M, Lewandowski W. Possible mechanisms of the prevention of doxorubicin toxicity by cichoric acid-antioxidant nutrient. Nutrients. Jan 2018;**10**(1):44-65

[77] Moreira AC, Branco AF, Sampaio SF, et al. Mitochondrial apoptosis-inducing factor is involved in doxorubicin-induced toxicity on H9c2 cardiomyoblasts. Biochimica et Biophysica Acta. Dec 2014;**1842**(12 Pt A):2468-2478

[78] Alam SR, Wallrabe H, Svindrych Z, et al. Investigation of mitochondrial metabolic response to doxorubicin in prostate cancer cells: An NADH, FAD and tryptophan FLIM assay. Scientific Reports. Sept 2017;**7**(1):10451

[79] Kluza J, Marchetti P, Gallego MA, et al. Mitochondrial proliferation during apoptosis induced by anticancer agents: Effects of doxorubicin and mitoxantrone on cancer and cardiac cells. Oncogene. Sept 2004;**23**(42):7018-7030

[80] Ascensao A, Lumini-Oliveira J, Oliveira PJ, Magalhaes J. Mitochondria as a target for exercise-induced cardioprotection. Current Drug Targets. Jun 2011;**12**(6):860-871

[81] Guan N, Ren YL, Liu XY, et al. Protective role of cyclosporine A and minocycline on mitochondrial disequilibrium-related podocyte injury and proteinuria occurrence induced by adriamycin. Nephrology, Dialysis, Transplantation. Jun 2015;**30**(6):957-969

[82] Benard G, Karbowski M. Mitochondrial fusion and division: Regulation and role in cell viability. Seminars in Cell & Developmental Biology. May 2009;**20**(3):365-374

[83] Westermann B. Mitochondrial fusion and fission in cell life and death. Nature Reviews. Molecular Cell Biology. Dec 2010;**11**(12):872-884

[84] Arany Z, He H, Lin J, et al. Transcriptional coactivator PGC-1 alpha controls the energy state and contractile function of cardiac muscle. Cell Metabolism. Apr 2005;**1**(4):259-271

[85] Pillai VB, Kanwal A, Fang YH, et al. Honokiol, an activator of Sirtuin-3 (SIRT3) preserves mitochondria and protects the heart from doxorubicin-induced cardiomyopathy in mice. Oncotarget. May 2017;**8**(21):34082-34098

[86] Doktorova H, Hrabeta J, Khalil MA, Eckschlager T. Hypoxia-induced chemoresistance in cancer cells: The role of not only HIF-1. Biomedical Papers of the Medical Faculty of the University Palacky, Olomouc, Czech Republic. Jun 2015;**159**(2):166-177

[87] Deus CM, Zehowski C, Nordgren K, Wallace KB, Skildum A, Oliveira PJ. Stimulating basal mitochondrial respiration decreases doxorubicin apoptotic signaling in H9c2 cardiomyoblasts. Toxicology. Aug 2015;**334**:1-11

[88] Bauckneht M, Ferrarazzo G, Fiz F, et al. Doxorubicin effect on myocardial metabolism as a prerequisite for subsequent development of cardiac toxicity: A translational (18)F-FDG PET/CT observation. Journal of Nuclear Medicine. Oct 2017;**58**(10):1638-1645

[89] Finsterer J, Ohnsorge P. Influence of mitochondrion-toxic agents on the cardiovascular system. Regulatory Toxicology and Pharmacology. Dec 2013;**67**(3):434-445

[90] Yamada Y, Munechika R, Kawamura E, Sakurai Y, Sato Y, Harashima H. Mitochondrial delivery of doxorubicin using MITO-porter kills drug-resistant renal cancer cells via mitochondrial toxicity. Journal of Pharmaceutical Sciences. Sept 2017;**106**(9):2428-2437

Chapter 14

Ethanol Consumption Affects Neuronal Function: Role of the Mitochondria

Cheril Tapia-Rojas, María José Pérez, Claudia Jara,
Erick H. Vergara and Rodrigo A. Quintanilla

Additional information is available at the end of the chapter

http://dx.doi.org/10.5772/intechopen.71611

Abstract

Ethanol is a licit drug consumed by a large part of the population, from adolescence to adulthood. High ethanol consumption is a public health problem due to its addictiveness and the risk it produces of developing other diseases, including cardiovascular, hepatic, and mental pathologies. Different patterns of ethanol consumption and its toxic effects in the brain have been reported. Current studies suggest to mitochondria, one of the principal mediators for ethanol neurotoxicity. In this chapter, we will review the effects of ethanol on neurons in different scenarios of ethanol consumption and its relation with mitochondrial function. Finally, we will propose a mechanism of ethanol toxicity in which the mitochondria are the main mediator and in which the mitochondrial alterations correlate with the severity of ethanol consumption. Thus, improving mitochondrial health of brain cells could be considered as a potential therapeutic target to treat ethanol-associated disorders.

Keywords: ethanol, mitochondria, oxidative stress, neurodegeneration

1. Introduction

Ethanol is the most licit addictive drug worldwide, and its consumption in excess is the third leading cause of death in the world [1]. Global ethanol consumption is 6.2 L of pure ethanol per person, with 15 years or older, which corresponds to 13.5 g of pure ethanol per day [2, 3]. Ethanol abuse is a health concern, which can lead to problems associated with alcoholism and increases the risk factor for other diseases such as cardiovascular disease, cirrhosis, dementia, and depression [4]. Socially, ethanol abuse can trigger other problems as well as violence, low productivity at work, traffic accidents, and crime [5].

Excessive ethanol use results in brain intoxication, leading to motor and behavior alterations, and eventually to death as a consequence of the depressive effects on the central nervous system (CNS) [6]. These effects result in simultaneous alterations in neuronal circuits including the prefrontal cortex, which controls behavior [7]; the cerebellum, which regulates movement and coordination [8]; the frontal lobe, which controls emotions [9]; the reticular activating system, which determines the sleep-wake cycle [10]; the hippocampus, which mediates learning and memory [8]; and the medulla, which controls vital functions [6]. Ethanol intoxication induces cellular damage and neuronal death [11]. The precise mechanism participating in ethanol toxicity in the brain is unknown. However, at the cellular level, ethanol impairs the neurotransmitters signaling [12]. Also, ethanol promotes reactive oxygen species (ROS) production [13] and activates inflammatory processes [14]. Altogether these events could be responsible for ethanol-induced damage in the brain.

Mitochondria are dynamic organelles, which regulate the production of ATP, redox balance, and calcium homeostasis in the neuron [15]. Interestingly, many effectors described in ethanol toxicity are directly or indirectly related to mitochondria. Mitochondria are the main source of ROS in the brain, and they are mainly affected by the oxidative damage induced by ethanol intoxication [16]. Likewise, dysfunctional mitochondria play a role in inducing proinflammatory events [17]. Finally, during synaptic process, ATP production and calcium buffering capacity produced by mitochondria are critical [18, 19]; therefore, mitochondrial injury may have severe consequences on neuronal communication.

In fact, evidence suggests that ethanol produces catastrophic changes in the mitochondria of organs such as liver [20] and heart [21], and over the last decade, many studies have reported the toxicity of ethanol to the brain's mitochondria [22, 23]. Briefly, ethanol increases ROS production [23], alters mitochondrial respiration [23, 24], impairs ATP production [22, 25], and eventually induces cell death by opening the mitochondrial permeability transition pore (mPTP) [26], observed both *in vitro* and *in vivo* [27].

In this chapter, we will discuss the effects of ethanol toxicity in the brain, focusing on the mitochondria. We will describe the specific ethanol-induced alterations to mitochondrial integrity, dynamics, and bioenergetics in different scenarios of ethanol exposure including:

1. Acute ethanol toxicity, corresponding to the consumption of high ethanol concentrations for a short period, spanning over hours, and even days [26].

2. Hangover, a common term to describe the physical effects following excessive ethanol consumption. Veisalgia is the uncommonly used medical name for this condition [25].

3. Chronic ethanol consumption, a condition where ethanol intake lasts 3 months or more. High concentrations of ethanol consumed over time can trigger ethanol use disorder (AUD), commonly called alcoholism [23].

4. Ethanol withdrawal, a condition observed in individuals who have consumed a high amount of ethanol for a prolonged period followed by cessation in ethanol intake. Common symptoms are anxiety and shakiness, seizures, and eventually death [22].

5. Binge drinking ethanol consumption characterized by a short period of heavy ethanol consumption followed by a period of abstinence and by intermittent ethanol intake [28].

Finally, we will discuss evidence suggesting that mitochondrial dysfunction is a potential mechanism by which ethanol promotes neurotoxicity, placing ethanol intoxication as a mitochondrial disease.

2. Patterns of ethanol consumption: mitochondrial alterations

2.1. Acute ethanol consumption

Acute ethanol consumption refers to a high ingestion of ethanol at a rate faster than that at which the body can metabolize it. Acute ethanol intoxication leads to brain injury, resulting in significant alterations of brain structure and function, and induces neuronal apoptosis and neurodegeneration in mouse, rat, and cellular models [11, 29–33].

Although several studies have tried to explain how acute ethanol administration induces brain injury, data on pathophysiology and underlying molecular and cellular mechanisms are still insufficient [34]. One of the possible theories was shown *in vitro*. Acute ethanol exposure induces neuronal apoptosis and changes to the neuronal structure, which could be related to the development of mature synapses and lead to a deficit in brain development [35]. Another alternative is that ethanol triggers inflammatory processes by activating toll-like receptor (TLR4) signaling and down-regulating autophagy pathways that trigger cell death [36]. However, and most importantly, oxidative stress appears to be the main mechanism for explaining brain injury mediated by ethanol. Oxidative stress is significantly increased following ethanol administration in several animal and cellular models [32, 37–39].

Rats exposed to ethanol through gavage administration showed an increase in inflammatory and oxidative stress markers in the brain 1 h post ethanol exposure [38]. Also, pre-treatment for 3 days with 150 mg/kg of antioxidant vitamin E decreased inflammation, an effect that is not observed with other antioxidants such as *N*-acetylcysteine (NAC) or selenium [38]. Similarly, ethanol-related increases in ROS generation are a prime factor in ethanol neurotoxicity. Primary cortical neurons treated with 2.5 mg/mL ethanol for 24 h elicit a rapid onset of oxidative stress, which resulted in mitochondria-dependent apoptotic cell death both in cultured fetal rat cortical neurons and during embryonic development [32, 39]. Also, ethanol downregulates protective cellular antioxidant content in this neuronal model, thus seriously disturbing the cellular redox state [32]. Indeed, pretreatment with NAC increased cellular glutathione and prevented apoptosis, suggesting that oxidative stress precedes a cascade of events mediated by mitochondria. Prevention of apoptosis with NAC antioxidant supports the role of oxidative stress in neuronal death [32].

The mitochondria appear to be a major target of ethanol toxicity in the brain. Some studies suggest that disturbances of the integrity of the mitochondrial membrane are essential for ethanol-induced cell death in mitochondria isolated from ethanol-exposed fetal brains [40].

For example, ethanol treatment for 24 h decreased ATP production and apparently impaired mitochondrial function [41]. Also, ethanol treatment reduced peroxisome proliferator-activated receptor-gamma coactivator 1alpha (PGC-1α) promoter activity and expression. PCG-1α [41] is a transcriptional coactivator of peroxisome proliferator-activated gamma receptors (PPARγ) that regulates energy metabolism and mitochondrial biogenesis in the brain [42, 43]. These ethanol-mediated changes in PCG-1α could be involved in mitochondrial dysfunction and oxidative damage. In contrast, the overexpression of PCG-1α has shown protective effects against ethanol-induced neuronal death and toxicity [41].

Several reports indicate that acute ethanol induces neuronal death [44]. Bax is a proapoptotic protein that when it is activated, it is translocated to the mitochondrial membrane. In primary neuronal cultures, Bax dimerizes with protein inhibitors of apoptosis, such as Bcl-2 and Bcl-xL, in response to ethanol exposure, leading to cell death [44]. Ethanol exposure disrupts the mitochondrial membrane potential, increases ROS production, and finally induced apoptosis in cerebellar granule cells [45–48]. Interestingly, Bax could also interact with the mPTP [49], a high-conductance mitochondrial channel, involved in the mitochondrial permeability to ions and small solutes [50–52]. These result in a reduction in mitochondrial potential [53], dysregulated calcium homeostasis [54], increased ROS formation [55], decreased ATP production [56], and eventually lead to neuronal death [53].

Interestingly, ethanol treatment did not induce the mPTP opening in the isolated mitochondria from mice brain, suggesting that ethanol does not affect mitochondrial health directly in neurons [26]. Further studies showed that ethanol administration transiently decreased the oxygen consumption rate of the mouse brain, an effect that disappeared 24 h after the ethanol treatment ceased [26]. However, this impairment of mitochondrial respiratory function could contribute to spatial learning and memory impairment observed in young mice [57], and to the deficit in the nociceptive response, showed in infant mice [26]. Interestingly, mice treatment with mPTP inhibitors, such as cyclosporine A and nortriptyline, before the first ethanol injection improved the behavior of ethanol-exposed animals [26], highlighting the importance of mPTP opening in acute ethanol intoxication, despite that probably is an indirect effect.

All these evidences indicate that acute ethanol exposure induces an increase in the production of ROS that finally could lead to mitochondrial dysfunction through the opening of mPTP.

2.2. Hangover

In humans, a hangover is a physiological state that involves an unpleasant next day sensation following an evening of excessive ethanol consumption [58]. Hangover begins when ethanol is absent in plasma and is characterized by symptoms such as headaches, nausea, diarrhea, fatigue, tremor, combined with decreased functional, cognitive, or visual-spatial skill performance [59, 60]. This state has grave implications for activities such as job performance and driving [61, 62]. In different animal models, the hangover has been studied to provide insights into the physiological and behavioral changes that occur in this period [63, 64]. Some of these studies have reported decreased locomotor activity in adult rats [65].

Acetaldehyde, an ethanol metabolite, is the leading cause of hangover [66]. Acetaldehyde causes steatohepatitis, a condition characterized by inflammation of the liver with fat accumulation in this organ, hepatic cirrhosis, and downregulation of aldehyde dehydrogenase 2 (ALD2) expression due to mitochondrial dysfunction [67]. In the brain, an association between hangover and mitochondrial dysfunction has been proposed [68–70].

During the hangover state, alterations like the impairment in motor performance have been associated with mitochondrial dysfunction [68]. In mice studies using the ethanol hangover onset protocol, animals showed impaired motor performance that could be the result of disturbed motor control [68]. Because motor performance is associated with the cerebellar function, the effects of the hangover were evaluated in cerebellum. Mitochondria isolated from the cerebellum of AHO mice revealed that at the onset of ethanol hangover, malate-glutamate- and succinate-supported oxygen uptake is increased, accompanied by the decreased activity of mitochondrial I–III and IV respiratory complexes and reduced mitochondrial membrane potential [69]. Additionally, the opening of mPTP was reported [69]. Furthermore, the activity of antioxidant enzymes was also differentially affected; superoxide dismutase (SOD) and the monoamine oxidase (MAO) enzyme showed increased activity [69], whereas both catalase (CAT) and glutathione peroxidase (GPx) had decreased activity [69]. In this same context, neuronal nitric oxide synthase (nNOS) expression was reduced [69], indicating a specific effect of ethanol against oxidative defenses in hangover.

In the brain cortex, isolated mitochondria had increased hydrogen peroxide (H_2O_2) levels in ethanol hangover conditions [68]. Moreover, mitochondrial activity of I–III, II–III, and IV respiratory complexes and the membrane potential are reduced in hangover [68]. Also, in mitochondria from the brain cortex, NO production and NOS expression were decreased [68], and synaptic mitochondrial function was significantly affected [68]. Finally, mitochondria from the brain cortex of hangover mice are more prone to suffer damage, due to the opening of mPTP with dramatic consequences to neural cell survival [68].

Interestingly, hangover provokes an imbalance in cellular redox homeostasis in isolated mitochondria in AHO mice brain cortex [70]. Decreased activity of both CAT and SOD enzymes accompanied by increased MAO activity was reported in mitochondria from both nonsynaptic extracts and synaptosome, whereas the GSH/GSSG ratio was decreased only in synaptosome mitochondria, with a reduction in both GPx and glutathione reductase (GR) and an increase in glutathione S-transferase (GST) [70]. Also, H_2O_2 levels were higher in both mitochondrial pools [70], and treatment with diphenyl (a MAO inhibitor) prevented this increase in AHO in both non synaptic and synaptic mitochondria [70]. Altogether, these results show that ethanol hangover produces an imbalance in mitochondrial redox state, indicated by an overproduction of ROS and a decrease of antioxidant agents [70]. This evidence is consistent with previous studies that described oxidative stress as a key element of the hangover syndrome and suggests that antioxidants could suppress the toxicity caused by ethanol [71]. In fact, the importance of the antioxidant imbalance was confirmed by the administration of natural products to treat hangover mainly in liver and brain [72].

In line with the anterior, melatonin pretreatment prevented the impairment of motor performance and mitochondrial function during ethanol hangover [73]. Melatonin is a hormone mostly secreted by the pineal gland during the night in mammals [74]. Melatonin and its metabolites are endogenous free-radical scavengers and antioxidants [75–77]. The effects of melatonin pretreatment in AHO were evaluated, and it was reported that melatonin improved motor coordination [73] and partially prevent the decrease in malate-glutamate-dependent oxygen uptake [73]. Interestingly, decreased mitochondrial potential and overproduction of H_2O_2 and NO induced by ethanol hangover also were prevented by melatonin [73].

In summary, ethanol hangover affects ROS production and reduces the antioxidant activity in different brain regions. These events could lead to mitochondrial membrane depolarization and dysfunction of the respiratory activity, reducing the ATP production and favoring the opening of mPTP. ATP deficiency in the cortex and cerebellar synapses could be the cause of deterioration of motor coordination. More studies are necessary to understand the real implications of mitochondria on brain function during hangover state.

2.3. Chronic ethanol consumption

The chronic ethanol consumption severely affects mental and physical health, including the development of alcohol dependence and neurological, cardiovascular, and hepatic diseases, among others [24, 78–80]. This type of ethanol intake is characterized by the difficulty of controlling the ingestion of ethanol. In this condition, the person is highly dependent and consumes it whenever possible, ingesting highly dangerous levels despite the negative consequences [81–83]. High ethanol consumption can lead to serious health, mental, and social problems [84, 85]. Among these alterations, the alcohol use disorder (AUD) [78, 86] is defined by the diagnostic and statistical manual of mental disorders (DSM-V), as a pattern of habitual drinking of excessive amounts of ethanol over a prolonged period [78].

Chronic ethanol consumption or AUD produces neurobiological changes that lead to an increase in unsafe behaviors, impulsivity, and anxiety [78]. Researchers have shown that regular consumption of alcoholic beverages damages the CNS, affecting cerebral activity, motor coordination, and behavior and developing neurodegeneration and neurocognitive deficits through exacerbated oxidative stress and excitotoxicity [24, 87, 88].

At the cellular level, ethanol induces activation of inflammatory and degenerative processes in the brain [88, 89]. Ethanol affects neuronal communication by altering the synthesis, release, and signaling of neurotransmitters [90], including glutamate, dopamine, and GABA [88, 90, 91]. Studies performed in human alcoholics have demonstrated that alterations in dopamine signaling induced by chronic ethanol consumption produce alterations in the prefrontal cortex, resulting in deficits in executive functions. Altogether, these affect the quality of life and also increase the probability of relapse [91, 92].

Recent studies in rat brain have shown that common alterations due to chronic ethanol consumption, such as neuropathies and neurocognitive deficits, are associated with mitochondrial dysfunction [23, 24, 85]. Ethanol is toxic, and the most vulnerable organs are the liver and the brain [93]. Ethanol is metabolized to acetaldehyde by the enzyme alcohol dehydrogenase and cytochrome P450 2E1. Acetaldehyde is highly toxic to nerve cells as it promotes oxidative stress and apoptotic events [84, 93], and its generation and accumulation cause brain damage [23, 94]. In the brain, acetaldehyde is capable of interacting with neurotransmitters and generates an environment of oxidative stress, which affects cells, organelles, and biomolecules with the mitochondria being the first affected organelle [23, 94].

In rats, chronic ethanol consumption causes alterations in mitochondrial function in the brain, increasing the ROS and reactive nitrogen species (RNS) production through the activity of NADPH oxidase and NOS and altering the electron transport chain activity, which leads to decreased ATP production [23, 24, 84, 94, 95]. This leads to the peroxidation of fatty acids, resulting in increased oxidative damage [95]. The brain is the most vulnerable organ to oxidative injury, due to the high concentration of lipids in the neural membranes, especially the polyunsaturated fatty acids of the phospholipids [23, 94]. These can be converted into hyperperoxidized lipids, which are unstable and quickly decompose to form new free radicals [23, 94, 95]. Chronic ethanol exposure also results in decreased antioxidant capacity, by reducing SOD, CAT, GPx, and GR activities [90, 94, 95]. This altered redox state leads to alterations in Ca^{+2} homeostasis, increasing cytoplasmic Ca^{+2} levels and mitochondria uptake, which promotes ROS formation and destabilizes the electron transport chain [90].

Interestingly, mice treated chronically with ethanol for 7–8 weeks present an altered glucose metabolism and transport in the brain [24]. Ethanol causes hypoglycemia, limiting the availability of glucose for the ATP formation. Also, it produces alterations in the expression of carnitine palmitoyltransferase (cPT) 1 and 2, an internal and external membrane mitochondrial enzyme, respectively, that regulate β-oxidation and ATP production [24]. Furthermore, in a mouse model of chronic ethanol consumption treated with acetyl-L-carnitine (ALC), a cofactor of cPT1 and cPT2, mitochondria health was reestablished increasing the oxidative phosphorylation and improving ATP production in mitochondria isolated from the brain [24]. Complementary studies showed that chronic ethanol consumption decreased the expression of the mitochondrial complexes I and V (ATP synthase) [24]. Additionally, chronic ethanol intake significantly increased the release of cytochrome-c [24], suggesting that ethanol affects the physical properties and functions of the mitochondria.

Excessive ethanol consumption also represents a risk during the pregnancy, which can result in fetal alcohol syndrome (FAS) [96]. Brain of prenatal ethanol-exposed fetuses showed increased apoptosis, possibly as a consequence of impaired function of mitochondria [96], increased ROS [97–99], and reduced activity of electron respiratory chain, which lead to decreased ATP production [96]. This could contribute to the malformations and developmental abnormalities observed previously in the fetuses with FAS [100].

Altogether, these studies indicate that chronic ethanol intake affects the mitochondrial structure and function, promoting the ROS production, altering substrate transport through the mitochondrial membrane, expression of the electron transport chain complex I and V, and ATP synthesis [24]. In conclusion, excessive ethanol consumption affects cognitive function and damages brain cells by a mechanism that involves mitochondrial dysfunction.

2.4. Ethanol withdrawal

When ethanol consumption stops or is abruptly reduced after a prolonged period of elevated ingestion, a state of physical ethanol dependence characterized by the appearance of neurological manifestations is acquired [87, 101]. The symptoms include tremors, hallucinations, arrhythmias, seizures, and later delirium tremens [86, 87, 102]. The severity of symptoms is determined mainly by the degree of ethanol intake, time of ethanol consumption, and the previous history of ethanol withdrawal [101].

As it was described in the previous section, ethanol produces structural and molecular changes in the brain. It exerts a potent effect on synaptic plasticity and dendritic spine formation in specific brain regions, providing a neuroanatomical substrate for the pathophysiology of alcoholism [82]. Dendritic spines are specialized protrusions on neuronal dendrites, considered the postsynaptic region of the excitatory synapses [103]. These structural changes induced by ethanol could affect the organization and function of the neural network and could explain the behavioral and cognitive alterations in alcoholic individuals [82]. Several studies have shown that abstinence from chronic ethanol consumption, and especially repeated withdrawal, causes an abrupt decline in the number of dendritic spines in the amygdala and other important regions of the brain such as the prefrontal cortex, accompanied by an increase in behaviors similar to anxiety [82, 92].

In synapses, the synaptic mitochondria play a fundamental role in providing the ATP necessary for diverse functions including vesicle exocytosis and neurotransmitter release, restoration of membrane potential through active transport, and recycling of receptors and neurotransmitters [18, 104]. The alterations described in the mitochondria of the cerebellum are of particular interest because ethanol intoxication triggers altered movement of lower limbs and the lack of voluntary coordination of muscles [105].

Ethanol withdrawal generates an excitatory effect in neurons from the cerebellum [106]. Ethanol promotes the activation of inhibitory GABA neurotransmission [107]; however, when ethanol concentrations are completely reduced, the excitatory transmission is overactivated [108]. Excitatory activation is mediated by the overly release of glutamate, which in turn activates its receptors such as α-amino-3-hydroxy-5-methyl-4-isoxazolepropionic acid (AMPA) and *N*-methyl-D-aspartate (NMDA) [108]. The binding of glutamate to its receptors in neurons leads to a drastic increase of Ca^{2+} entry, inducing excitotoxicity that eventually leads to neuronal death [109]. In fact, the Ca^{2+}concentrations in a synaptosomal membrane fraction obtained from rat cerebellum were greater during ethanol withdrawal episodes compared with the period of ethanol consumption [110, 111].

The excessive uptake of Ca^{2+} by the neurons results in an increased in the Ca^{2+} uptake by the mitochondria, which in turn leads to overproduction of ROS and a decreased antioxidant response [22]. In a rat model of ethanol withdrawal, lipid peroxidation and mitochondrial protein oxidation is increased in the cortex, hippocampus and more drastically in the cerebellum [112]. During ethanol withdrawal, ATP production also is decreased in neurons from the cerebellum [113]; resulting in reduced cellular energy in this brain region. The high Ca^{2+} concentrations in the mitochondria can ultimately lead to prolonged opening of mPTP [114, 115]. Therefore, ethanol withdrawal toxicity is probably mediated by mitochondrial dysfunction, which implicates an imbalance in the redox state, decreased ATP production, and prolonged mPTP opening due to high Ca^{+2} overload in the mitochondria.

2.5. Binge drinking

Binge drinking is a recurrent pattern of ethanol consumption, characterized by a short period of heavy ethanol consumption followed by a period of abstinence, which continue with intermittent high ethanol consumption [116]. Binge drinking is common during adolescence [117] and relatively little is known about its effects and potential toxicity mechanisms. Binge drinking is described as the intake of four drinks in women and five drinks in men in a period less than 2 h [118]. It is of great interest to understand the damaging effects of binge drinking in the brain [119], mainly because the adolescent brain is more sensitive to ethanol toxicity than that of the adult brain [120, 121].

Rats trained to self-administration of binge-like ethanol is associated with the development of depression-like symptoms [122], which could be a result of decreased survival and differentiation of neural progenitor cells in the hippocampus, finally resulting in decreased adult neurogenesis [122]. Additionally, ethanol binge drinking induces neuroinflammation, such as indicated by the activation of innate immune receptors TLRs and by an increase in the expression of the inflammatory cytokines TNFα and IL-1β, and demyelination suggested by significantly reducing the levels of the myelin proteins myelin basic protein (MBP) and myelin oligodendrocyte glycoprotein (MOG) in the prefrontal cortex [123]. Also, adolescent binge-like ethanol consumption produced alterations to cognitive processes associated with the prefrontal cortex in adulthood [124]. Changes in executive functions, reduced anxiety, and disinhibition in the exploratory behavior were observed after ethanol exposure [124]. In addition, increase in the resistance to the extinction of ethanol-seeking behavior in adult rats trained to self-administer ethanol [124]. Studies in rats that simulate the adolescent binge drinking pattern also reported memory and motor alterations [125].

In other murine model of binge drinking, rats pups were exposed to ethanol consumption at postnatal day 25 (PND25) (3.0 g/kg), during 2 consecutive days, with gaps of 2 days without injections, during 2 weeks [28]. Then, 24 h or 20 days after the final ethanol administration, the animals were used to evaluate cognitive and motor functions. The results revealed that binge drinking treatment impaired conditional discrimination learning, motor learning, and recognition memory during adolescence and in the adult stage [28]. Additionally, binge drinking ethanol treatment increases cyclooxygenase (COX-2) and inducible NOS (iNOS) levels and cell death in the neocortex, hippocampus, and cerebellum 24 h after administration. These effects, as well as the cognitive alterations, were prevented by the administration of indomethacin, a COX-2 inhibitor [28]. Interestingly, new reports have showed that mitochondrial dysfunction promotes brain inflammatory response, which in turn could induce an additional mitochondrial damage in a positive feedback loop induced of toxicity induced by ethanol, which could be reverted by the indomethacin treatment [17].

Mitochondrial alterations associated with binge alcohol drinking has not being described. For example, binge ethanol exposure in early postnatal stage induced defects in insulin and IGF signaling, resulting in impaired motor abilities [126]. Most important, deficiencies in insulin/IGF-1 signaling are associated to oxidative stress, DNA injury, loss of mitochondrial function, and apoptosis [126]. In other studies, rats submitted to binge alcohol drinking protocol showed an increase in the ventricular volume of the brain; reduced levels of N-acetyl aspartate (NAA) and creatine and increased choline-containing compound in the dorsal hippocampus, effects that were recovered after 7 days of alcohol treatment [127]. These metabolic changes could suggest transient deficiencies of mitochondrial NAA production, resulting finally in an impaired energy production of the brain immediately after binge ethanol consumption [127].

Currently, the most complete study associated to mitochondrial alterations corresponds to our findings [128]. In our study, adolescent rats PND25, were exposed to binge-like ethanol consumption using the same protocol described previously [128]. The rats were euthanized at 1, 3, or 7 weeks after treatment. Our results show that binge ethanol pretreatment (BEP) triggers alterations in hippocampal cell structure and function [128]. We found increase in oxidized proteins at 1-week posttreatment, which was subsequently restored at 3 and 7 weeks post BEP [128]. Additionally, proteins participating in the regulation of mitochondrial dynamics were affected. Mitochondrial dynamics involves fission and fusion events [129]. Fusion is mediated by the dynamin-related GTPases mitofusins (Mfn1 and Mfn2) and optic atrophy 1 (OPA1), which induce fusion of mitochondrial membranes [130]. Fission is performed by dynamin-related protein 1 (Drp1), which is recruited by the Fis1 protein [129] to the mitochondrial membrane to constrict mitochondria inducing its division [130]. BEP altered Drp1, Fis1, Mfn1, Mfn2, and Opa1 proteins levels [128], suggesting that binge-like ethanol consumption favors an pro-fission state at 1–3 weeks post BEP, and imbalance between fusion and fission proteins was restored but animals with 7 weeks after ethanol treatment showed reduced both mitochondrial fusion and fission processes compared to saline treated animals [128].

Interestingly, a decrease in ATP production was also reported in our study at 3 and 7 weeks post BEP [128], indicating a specific bioenergetics mitochondrial failure induced by binge ethanol exposure that persists over time. Finally, we observed a delayed increase in the expression of inflammatory markers such as NF-κB, Iba1, and GFAP, 7 weeks post BEP [128], suggesting a late inflammatory response due to adolescent ethanol consumption. Despite the damage present in the hippocampus of BEP rats, we detected the activation of a mechanism that could possibly protect the brain. These mechanisms include decreased expression of proteins that are key to mPTP formation, such as voltage-dependent anion channel (VDAC) and cyclophilin D (Cyp-D) [128], and the increased levels of nuclear factor erythroid-2 related factor 2 (Nrf2) [128], a transcription factor that is activated under stress conditions regulating the expression of antioxidant, anti-inflammatory, and detoxification enzymes that prevent mitochondrial impairment [131]. The increased Nrf2 levels were mainly observed at 3 and 7 weeks [128] suggesting that this signaling pathway could be involved in restoring redox balance.

http://dx.doi.org/10.5772/intechopen.71611

In summary, our and others studies about adolescent ethanol consumption indicate that adolescent binge-like ethanol exposure results in severe structural and functional alterations in the brain that persist until the adult stage, affecting mainly to mitochondria. The mitochondria plays a key role in binge ethanol toxicity, since it alters the redox balance of the cell and reduces ATP availability to vital functions such as synaptic communication.

3. Mitochondrial impairment as a possible mechanism of ethanol toxicity in the brain

In the previous sections, we described the effects of ethanol on neuronal cells, focusing our attention on alterations to the mitochondria. In all patterns of ethanol consumption described above, we reported changes associated with mitochondrial injury [11, 27, 132], therefore strongly suggesting that mitochondria is an important mediator of ethanol neurotoxicity and could be considered as a potential therapeutic approaches for treating ethanol-associated disorders. In this section, we will summarize the effects of ethanol linked to mitochondrial function, and finally, we propose a mechanism in which mitochondrial impairment plays a central role in the neurotoxicity induced by ethanol.

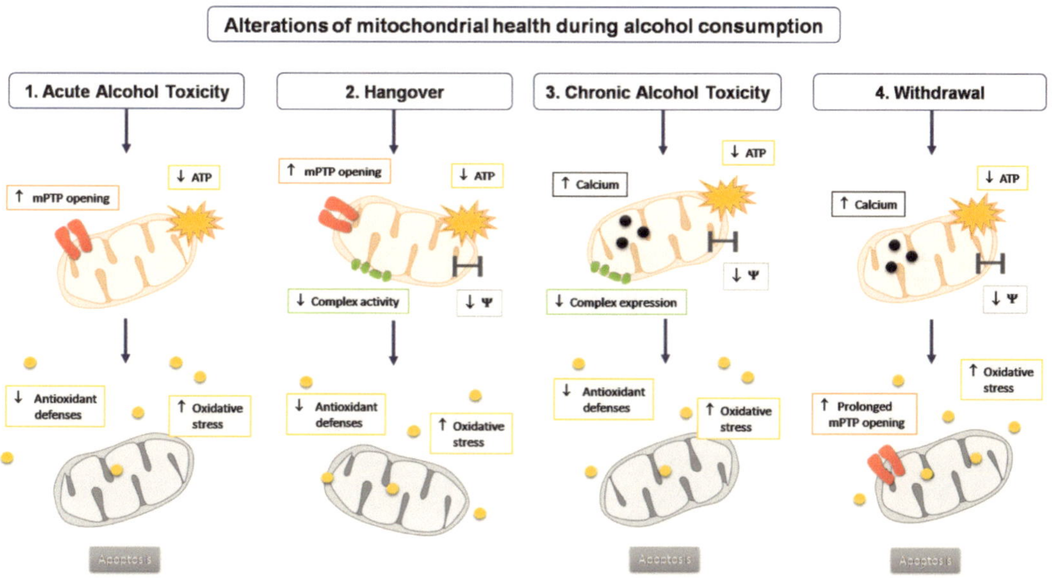

Figure 1. Alterations of mitochondrial health during ethanol consumption. A representative scheme is summarizing the mitochondrial alterations described in the different patterns of ethanol consumption. The severity of mitochondrial dysfunction is associated with the amount and time of ethanol exposure, starting with an imbalance in redox response, accompanied by decreased ATP production and the opening of the mPTP (1. Acute ethanol toxicity). Additionally, decreased activity of the electron transporter chain and the loss of mitochondrial membrane potential are observed (2. Hangover); following of high Ca^{+2} concentrations (3. Chronic ethanol toxicity) that lead finally to prolonged opening of mPTP that eventually triggers neuronal death (4. Withdrawal).

Figure 1 summarizes the mitochondrial alterations described after the different patterns of ethanol consumption (**Figure 1**). Acute ethanol exposure triggers mitochondrial toxicity, increasing ROS production and decreasing antioxidant defenses [38]. In turn, this leads to reduced ATP production [41] and finally to the opening of mPTP [26]. All these events could eventually lead to apoptotic neuronal death [32, 39] (**Figure 1.1**). After ethanol consumption, a hangover condition can be produced [58]. In this state, the mitochondrial alterations described in acute ethanol conditions are also accompanied by a period of reduced activity of the electron respiratory chain complexes [69] and a loss of mitochondrial membrane potential [69] that suggests a major state of mitochondrial dysfunction (**Figure 1.2**).

When ethanol consumption implicates the ingestion of a high amount of ethanol on repeated occasions and cannot be controlled, this is considered a pattern of chronic ethanol consumption [81–83]. This condition is pathological, and therefore the mitochondrial alterations are also more complex. In addition to redox imbalance [23, 94], deficiency in ATP generation and a loss of mitochondrial membrane potential can be detected by a reduction in the expression of respiratory complexes and increased levels of mitochondrial calcium [23, 94, 95]. Altogether, these events lead to severe loss of mitochondrial function (**Figure 1.3**). Chronic ethanol consumption implicates the development of addictive behaviors; therefore, in the absence of ethanol, those affected present ethanol withdrawal symptoms [87, 101]. In this state, the mitochondrial effects already described in chronic consumption are

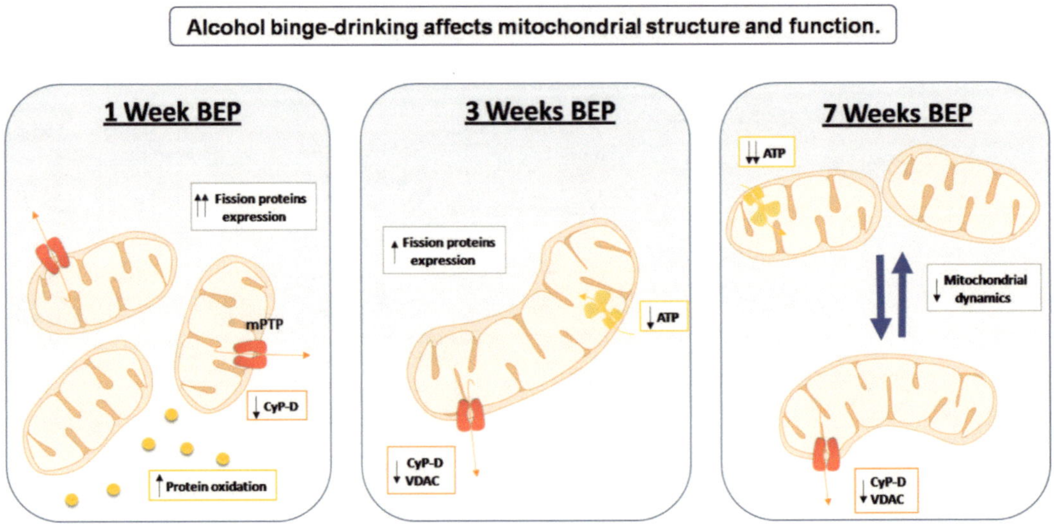

Figure 2. Ethanol binge-drinking affects mitochondrial structure and function. Binge-like ethanol consumption during the adolescence induces changes in the structure and function of the mitochondria that persist on time until adulthood. One week after binge ethanol pretreatment (BEP), rat hippocampus has increased expression of fission proteins and protein oxidation, accompanied by reduced expression of Cyp-D. Three weeks after BEP, addition is possibly observed decreased ATP production and reduced expression of VDAC. Finally, at adulthood (7 weeks post BEP), the levels of both fission and fusion proteins suggest decreased mitochondrial dynamics, and the deficiency in ATP production is more severe.

aggravated, mainly by the high amount of Ca^{+2} that enters to the mitochondria [110, 111], which leads to a prolonged opening of mPTP [114, 115] and neuronal death [22] (**Figure 1.4**). In summary, the mitochondrion plays a central role in all these patterns of ethanol consumption, and its alterations gradually increase according to the amount and time of ethanol exposure.

Binge drinking ethanol is associated with the adolescent population [116]. Diverse molecular alterations have been reported; however, the cellular mechanism involved in this process are unknown [11]. We recently indicated that adolescent binge ethanol consumption triggers cellular damage by a mechanism that probably involves the mitochondria [128]. Also, the mitochondrial alterations persist over time until adulthood [128]. **Figure 2** summarizes the mitochondrial changes induced by adolescent binge ethanol exposure. One week after BEP, the mitochondria showed increased protein oxidation, reduced expression of Cyp-D, and increased expression of proteins involved in mitochondrial fission, suggesting a mitochondrial pro-fission state [128]. Then, 3 weeks after BEP challenging the mitochondrial pro-fission state is less severe, indicated by a lower reduction in the expression of fission proteins; however, a decrease in VDAC protein, and a significant reduction of ATP, is also observed [128]. Finally, during adulthood, the balance in the fission/fusion state is restored, but the dynamics are decreased compared with the control condition. Also, the ATP deficiency persists and becomes even more drastic [128]. Nevertheless, the reduced expression of VDAC and Cyp-D suggests the activation of a protective mechanism that could prevent the opening of mPTP [128]. Altogether, these alterations indicate that mitochondria have an important role in the binge ethanol toxicity in the hippocampus of adolescent rats.

4. Future perspectives

We propose that the mitochondrion is the main mediator of ethanol neurotoxicity where mitochondrial alterations reveal the severity of ethanol toxicity. The initial effect of ethanol exposure implicates an imbalance in the cellular redox state, followed by changes in the respiratory complexes from the electron transport chain that leads to the reduction in ATP production and the opening of mPTP. Persistent ethanol consumption also induced the loss of mitochondrial membrane potential and increased Ca^{+2} entries into the mitochondria that provoke the prolonged opening of mPTP and finally promote neurodegeneration. Interestingly, these mitochondrial alterations ethanol-associated may could occur mainly in glial cells, inducing inflammation and interfering with the glial-neuronal communication in specific brain areas [119]. The hippotalamus, important to ethanol dependence, and the hippocampus, associated to learning and memory, are particularly vulnerable; possibly due to the downregulation of melanocortin system induced by ethanol [119]. Therefore, the description of all these events highlights the importance of maintaining the function of the mitochondria to prevent the harmful effects of ethanol consumption and propose a new potential treatment for the pathological condition related to ethanol use and abuse.

Acknowledgements

Work supported by FONDECYT: 1140968; 1170441, and Anillo ACT1411.

Author details

Cheril Tapia-Rojas[1,2], María José Pérez[1,2], Claudia Jara[1,2], Erick H. Vergara[1,2] and Rodrigo A. Quintanilla[1,2*]

*Address all correspondence to: rodrigo.quintanilla@uautonoma.cl

1 Centro de Investigación y Estudio del Consumo de Alcohol en Adolescentes (CIAA), Santiago, Chile

2 Laboratory of Neurodegenerative Diseases, Universidad Autónoma de Chile, Chile

References

[1] Koob GF, Le Moal M. Plasticity of reward neurocircuitry and the 'dark side' of drug addiction. Nature Neuroscience. 2005;**8**:1442-1444

[2] Dawson DA, Goldstein RB, Chou SP, Ruan WJ, Grant BF. Age at first drink and the first incidence of adult-onset DSM-IV alcohol use disorders. Alcoholism, Clinical and Experimental Research. 2008;**32**:2149-2160

[3] Kirby T, Barry AE. Alcohol as a gateway drug: A study of US 12th graders. The Journal of School Health. 2012;**82**:371-379

[4] Rehm J. The risks associated with alcohol use and alcoholism. Alcohol Research & Health. 2011;**34**:135-143

[5] Ali MM, Dwyer DS. Social network effects in alcohol consumption among adolescents. Addictive Behaviors. 2010;**35**:337-342

[6] Mukherjee S. Alcoholism and its effects on the central nervous system. Current Neurovascular Research. 2013;**10**:256-262

[7] Abernathy K, Chandler LJ, Woodward JJ. Alcohol and the prefrontal cortex. International Review of Neurobiology. 2010;**91**:289-320

[8] Oscar-Berman M, Marinkovic K. Alcohol: Effects on neurobehavioral functions and the brain. Neuropsychology Review. 2007;**17**:239-257

[9] Moselhy HF, Georgiou G, Kahn A. Frontal lobe changes in alcoholism: A review of the literature. Alcohol and Alcoholism. 2001;**36**:357-368

[10] Brower KJ. Alcohol's effects on sleep in alcoholics. Alcohol Research & Health. 2001; **25**:110-125

[11] Crews FT, Nixon K. Mechanisms of neurodegeneration and regeneration in alcoholism. Alcohol and Alcoholism. 2009;**44**:115-127

[12] McCool BA. Ethanol modulation of synaptic plasticity. Neuropharmacology. 2011;**61**: 1097-1108

[13] Albano E. Alcohol, oxidative stress and free radical damage. The Proceedings of the Nutrition Society. 2006;**65**:278-290

[14] Garcia-Valdecasas-Campelo E, Gonzalez-Reimers E, Santolaria-Fernandez F, De La Vega-Prieto MJ, Milena-Abril A, Sanchez-Perez MJ, Martinez-Riera A, Rodriguez-Rodriguez E. Brain atrophy in alcoholics: Relationship with alcohol intake; liver disease; nutritional status, and inflammation. Alcohol and Alcoholism. 2007;**42**:533-538

[15] Liesa M, Palacin M, Zorzano A. Mitochondrial dynamics in mammalian health and disease. Physiological Reviews. 2009;**89**:799-845

[16] Murphy MP. How mitochondria produce reactive oxygen species. The Biochemical Journal. 2009;**417**:1-13

[17] Tschopp J. Mitochondria: Sovereign of inflammation? European Journal of Immunology. 2011;**41**:1196-1202

[18] Cheng A, Hou Y, Mattson MP. Mitochondria and neuroplasticity. ASN Neuro. 2010; **2**:e00045

[19] Kann O, Kovacs R. Mitochondria and neuronal activity. American Journal of Physiology. Cell Physiology. 2007;**292**:C641-C657

[20] Garcia-Ruiz C, Kaplowitz N, Fernandez-Checa JC. Role of mitochondria in alcoholic liver disease. Current Pathobiology Reports. 2014;**1**:159-168

[21] Hajnoczky G, Buzas CJ, Pacher P, Hoek JB, Rubin E. Alcohol and mitochondria in cardiac apoptosis: Mechanisms and visualization. Alcoholism, Clinical and Experimental Research. 2005;**29**:693-701

[22] Jung ME. Alcohol withdrawal and cerebellar mitochondria. Cerebellum. 2015;**14**: 421-437

[23] Reddy VD, Padmavathi P, Kavitha G, Saradamma B, Varadacharyulu N. Alcohol-induced oxidative/nitrosative stress alters brain mitochondrial membrane properties. Molecular and Cellular Biochemistry. 2013;**375**:39-47

[24] Haorah J, Rump TJ, Xiong H. Reduction of brain mitochondrial beta-oxidation impairs complex I and V in chronic alcohol intake: The underlying mechanism for neurodegeneration. PLoS One. 2013;**8**:e70833

[25] Bustamante J, Karadayian AG, Lores-Arnaiz S, Cutrera RA. Alterations of motor performance and brain cortex mitochondrial function during ethanol hangover. Alcohol. 2011;**46**:473-479

[26] Lamarche F, Carcenac C, Gonthier B, Cottet-Rousselle C, Chauvin C, Barret L, Leverve X, Savasta M, Fontaine E. Mitochondrial permeability transition pore inhibitors prevent ethanol-induced neuronal death in mice. Chemical Research in Toxicology. 2013;**26**: 78-88

[27] Manzo-Avalos S, Saavedra-Molina A. Cellular and mitochondrial effects of alcohol consumption. International Journal of Environmental Research and Public Health. 2010;**7**:4281-4304

[28] Pascual M, Blanco AM, Cauli O, Minarro J, Guerri C. Intermittent ethanol exposure induces inflammatory brain damage and causes long-term behavioural alterations in adolescent rats. The European Journal of Neuroscience. 2007;**25**:541-550

[29] Dikranian K, Qin YQ, Labruyere J, Nemmers B, Olney JW. Ethanol-induced neuroapoptosis in the developing rodent cerebellum and related brain stem structures. Brain research. Developmental Brain Research. 2005;**155**:1-13

[30] Garic-Stankovic A, Hernandez MR, Chiang PJ, Debelak-Kragtorp KA, Flentke GR, Armant DR, Smith SM. Ethanol triggers neural crest apoptosis through the selective activation of a pertussis toxin-sensitive G protein and a phospholipase Cbeta-dependent Ca^{2+} transient. Alcoholism, Clinical and Experimental Research. 2005;**29**:1237-1246

[31] Olney JW, Wozniak DF, Jevtovic-Todorovic V, Farber NB, Bittigau P, Ikonomidou C. Drug-induced apoptotic neurodegeneration in the developing brain. Brain Pathology. 2002;**12**:488-498

[32] Ramachandran V, Watts LT, Maffi SK, Chen J, Schenker S, Henderson G. Ethanol-induced oxidative stress precedes mitochondrially mediated apoptotic death of cultured fetal cortical neurons. Journal of Neuroscience Research. 2003;**74**:577-588

[33] Heaton MB, Paiva M, Siler-Marsiglio K. Ethanol influences on Bax translocation, mitochondrial membrane potential, and reactive oxygen species generation are modulated by vitamin E and brain-derived neurotrophic factor. Alcoholism, Clinical and Experimental Research. 2011;**35**:1122-1133

[34] Adachi M, Ishii H. Role of mitochondria in alcoholic liver injury. Free Radical Biology & Medicine. 2002;**32**:487-491

[35] Guadagnoli T, Caltana L, Vacotto M, Gironacci MM, Brusco A. Direct effects of ethanol on neuronal differentiation: An in vitro analysis of viability and morphology. Brain Research Bulletin. 2016;**127**:177-186

[36] Pla A, Pascual M, Guerri C. Autophagy constitutes a protective mechanism against ethanol toxicity in mouse astrocytes and neurons. PLoS One. 2016;**11**:e0153097

[37] Schlorff EC, Husain K, Somani SM. Dose- and time-dependent effects of ethanol on plasma antioxidant system in rat. Alcohol. 1999;**17**:97-105

[38] Ozkol H, Bulut G, Balahoroglu R, Tuluce Y, Ozkol HU. Protective effects of selenium, N-acetylcysteine and vitamin E against acute ethanol intoxication in rats. Biological Trace Element Research. 2017;**175**:177-185

[39] Lee RD, An SM, Kim SS, Rhee GS, Kwack SJ, Seok JH, Chae SY, Park CH, Choi YW, Kim HS, et al. Neurotoxic effects of alcohol and acetaldehyde during embryonic development. Journal of Toxicology and Environmental Health Part A. 2005;**68**:2147-2162

[40] Ramachandran V, Perez A, Chen J, Senthil D, Schenker S, Henderson GI. In utero ethanol exposure causes mitochondrial dysfunction, which can result in apoptotic cell death in fetal brain: A potential role for 4-hydroxynonenal. Alcoholism, Clinical and Experimental Research. 2001;**25**:862-871

[41] Liu Z, Liu Y, Gao R, Li H, Dunn T, Wu P, Smith RG, Sarkar PS, Fang X. Ethanol suppresses PGC-1alpha expression by interfering with the cAMP-CREB pathway in neuronal cells. PLoS One. 2014;**9**:e104247

[42] Liang HL, Wong-Riley MT. Activity-dependent regulation of nuclear respiratory factor-1, nuclear respiratory factor-2, and peroxisome proliferator-activated receptor gamma coactivator-1 in neurons. Neuroreport. 2006;**17**:401-405

[43] St-Pierre J, Drori S, Uldry M, Silvaggi JM, Rhee J, Jager S, Handschin C, Zheng K, Lin J, Yang W, et al. Suppression of reactive oxygen species and neurodegeneration by the PGC-1 transcriptional coactivators. Cell. 2006;**127**:397-408

[44] Siler-Marsiglio KI, Pan Q, Paiva M, Madorsky I, Khurana NC, Heaton MB. Mitochondrially targeted vitamin E and vitamin E mitigate ethanol-mediated effects on cerebellar granule cell antioxidant defense systems. Brain Research. 2005;**1052**:202-211

[45] Heaton MB, Siler-Marsiglio K, Paiva M, Kotler A, Rogozinski J, Kubovec S, Coursen M, Madorsky V. Ethanol influences on Bax associations with mitochondrial membrane proteins in neonatal rat cerebellum. Developmental Neurobiology. 2013;**73**:127-141

[46] Hamre KM, West JR. The effects of the timing of ethanol exposure during the brain growth spurt on the number of cerebellar Purkinje and granule cell nuclear profiles. Alcoholism, Clinical and Experimental Research. 1993;**17**:610-622

[47] Bhave SV, Snell LD, Tabakoff B, Hoffman PL. Ethanol sensitivity of NMDA receptor function in developing cerebellar granule neurons. European Journal of Pharmacology. 1999;**369**:247-259

[48] Moore DB, Walker DW, Heaton MB. Neonatal ethanol exposure alters bcl-2 family mRNA levels in the rat cerebellar vermis. Alcoholism, Clinical and Experimental Research. 1999; **23**:1251-1261

[49] Marzo I, Brenner C, Zamzami N, Susin SA, Beutner G, Brdiczka D, Remy R, Xie ZH, Reed JC, Kroemer G. The permeability transition pore complex: A target for apoptosis regulation by caspases and bcl-2-related proteins. The Journal of Experimental Medicine. 1998;**187**:1261-1271

[50] Haworth RA, Hunter DR. The Ca^{2+}–induced membrane transition in mitochondria. II. Nature of the Ca^{2+} trigger site. Archives of Biochemistry and Biophysics. 1979;**195**: 460-467

[51] Hunter DR, Haworth RA. The Ca^{2+}–induced membrane transition in mitochondria. I. The protective mechanisms. Archives of Biochemistry and Biophysics. 1979;**195**:453-459

[52] Hunter DR, Haworth RA. The Ca^{2+}–induced membrane transition in mitochondria. III. Transitional Ca^{2+} release. Archives of Biochemistry and Biophysics. 1979;**195**:468-477

[53] Galluzzi L, Blomgren K, Kroemer G. Mitochondrial membrane permeabilization in neuronal injury. Nature Reviews Neuroscience. 2009;**10**:481-494

[54] Elrod JW, Wong R, Mishra S, Vagnozzi RJ, Sakthievel B, Goonasekera SA, Karch J, Gabel S, Farber J, Force T, et al. Cyclophilin D controls mitochondrial pore-dependent Ca(2+) exchange, metabolic flexibility, and propensity for heart failure in mice. The Journal of Clinical Investigation. 2010;**120**:3680-3687

[55] Hou Y, Ghosh P, Wan R, Ouyang X, Cheng H, Mattson MP, Cheng A. Permeability transition pore-mediated mitochondrial superoxide flashes mediate an early inhibitory effect of amyloid beta1-42 on neural progenitor cell proliferation. Neurobiology of Aging. 2014;**35**:975-989

[56] Budd SL, Nicholls DG. Mitochondria, calcium regulation, and acute glutamate excitotoxicity in cultured cerebellar granule cells. Journal of Neurochemistry. 1996;**67**: 2282-2291

[57] Wozniak DF, Hartman RE, Boyle MP, Vogt SK, Brooks AR, Tenkova T, Young C, Olney JW, Muglia LJ. Apoptotic neurodegeneration induced by ethanol in neonatal mice is associated with profound learning/memory deficits in juveniles followed by progressive functional recovery in adults. Neurobiology of Disease. 2004;**17**:403-414

[58] Verster JC. The "hair of the dog": A useful hangover remedy or a predictor of future problem drinking? Current Drug Abuse Reviews. 2009;**2**:1-4

[59] Kim DJ, Yoon SJ, Lee HP, Choi BM, Go HJ. The effects of alcohol hangover on cognitive functions in healthy subjects. The International Journal of Neuroscience. 2003;**113**: 581-594

[60] Wiese JG, Shlipak MG, Browner WS. The alcohol hangover. Annals of Internal Medicine. 2000;**132**:897-902

[61] Frone MR. Prevalence and distribution of alcohol use and impairment in the workplace: A U.S. national survey. Journal of Studies on Alcohol. 2006;**67**:147-156

[62] Verster JC, Penning R. Treatment and prevention of alcohol hangover. Current Drug Abuse Reviews. 2010;**3**:103-109

[63] Gauvin DV, Briscoe RJ, Baird TJ, Vallett M, Carl KL, Holloway FA. Cross-generalization of an EtOH "hangover" cue to endogenously and exogenously induced stimuli. Pharmacology, Biochemistry, and Behavior. 1997;**57**:199-206

[64] Gauvin DV, Cheng EY, Holloway FA. Recent developments in alcoholism: Biobehavioral correlates. Recent Developments in Alcoholism. 1993;**11**:281-304

[65] Lal H, Prather PL, Rezazadeh SM. Anxiogenic behavior in rats during acute and protracted ethanol withdrawal: Reversal by buspirone. Alcohol. 1991;**8**:467-471

[66] Penning R, van Nuland M, Fliervoet LA, Olivier B, Verster JC: The pathology of alcohol hangover. Current Drug Abuse Reviews. 2010;**3**:68-75

[67] Helander A, Tottmar O. Effect of acute ethanol administration on human blood aldehyde dehydrogenase activity. Alcoholism, Clinical and Experimental Research. 1988; **12**:643-646

[68] Bustamante J, Karadayian AG, Lores-Arnaiz S, Cutrera RA. Alterations of motor performance and brain cortex mitochondrial function during ethanol hangover. Alcohol. 2012;**46**:473-479

[69] Karadayian AG, Bustamante J, Czerniczyniec A, Lombardi P, Cutrera RA, Lores-Arnaiz S. Alcohol hangover induces mitochondrial dysfunction and free radical production in mouse cerebellum. Neuroscience. 2015;**304**:47-59

[70] Karadayian AG, Malanga G, Czerniczyniec A, Lombardi P, Bustamante J, Lores-Arnaiz S. Free radical production and antioxidant status in brain cortex non-synaptic mitochondria and synaptosomes at alcohol hangover onset. Free Radical Biology & Medicine. 2017;**108**:692-703

[71] Marino MD, Aksenov MY, Kelly SJ. Vitamin E protects against alcohol-induced cell loss and oxidative stress in the neonatal rat hippocampus. International Journal of Developmental Neuroscience. 2004;**22**:363-377

[72] Wang F, Li Y, Zhang YJ, Zhou Y, Li S, Li HB. Natural products for the prevention and treatment of hangover and alcohol use disorder. Molecules. 2016;**21**:64

[73] Karadayian AG, Bustamante J, Czerniczyniec A, Cutrera RA, Lores-Arnaiz S. Effect of melatonin on motor performance and brain cortex mitochondrial function during ethanol hangover. Neuroscience. 2014;**269**:281-289

[74] Cardinali DP, Pevet P. Basic aspects of melatonin action. Sleep Medicine Reviews. 1998;**2**: 175-190

[75] Tan DX, Manchester LC, Reiter RJ, Qi WB, Karbownik M, Calvo JR. Significance of melatonin in antioxidative defense system: Reactions and products. Biological Signals and Receptors. 2000;**9**:137-159

[76] Manda K, Ueno M, Anzai K. AFMK, a melatonin metabolite, attenuates X-ray-induced oxidative damage to DNA, proteins and lipids in mice. Journal of Pineal Research. 2007; **42**:386-393

[77] Reiter RJ, Paredes SD, Korkmaz A, Manchester LC, Tan DX. Melatonin in relation to the "strong" and "weak" versions of the free radical theory of aging. Advances in Medical Sciences. 2008;**53**:119-129

[78] Mehta AJ. Alcoholism and critical illness: A review. World Journal of Critical Care Medicine. 2016;**5**:27-35

[79] Wu D, Zhai Q, Shi X. Alcohol-induced oxidative stress and cell responses. Journal of Gastroenterology and Hepatology. 2006;**21**(Suppl 3):S26-S29

[80] Linhart K, Bartsch H, Seitz HK. The role of reactive oxygen species (ROS) and cytochrome P-450 2E1 in the generation of carcinogenic etheno-DNA adducts. Redox Biology. 2014;**3**:56-62

[81] Kyzar EJ, Floreani C, Teppen TL, Pandey SC. Adolescent alcohol exposure: Burden of epigenetic reprogramming, synaptic remodeling, and adult psychopathology. Frontiers in Neuroscience. 2016;**10**:222

[82] Kyzar EJ, Pandey SC. Molecular mechanisms of synaptic remodeling in alcoholism. Neuroscience Letters. 2015;**601**:11-19

[83] Vengeliene V, Celerier E, Chaskiel L, Penzo F, Spanagel R. Compulsive alcohol drinking in rodents. Addiction Biology. 2009;**14**:384-396

[84] Yan T, Zhao Y, Zhang X. Acetaldehyde induces cytotoxicity of SH-SY5Y cells via inhibition of Akt activation and induction of oxidative stress. Oxidative Medicine and Cellular Longevity. 2016;**2016**:4512309

[85] Almansa I, Fernandez A, Garcia-Ruiz C, Muriach M, Barcia JM, Miranda M, Fernandez-Checa JC, Romero FJ. Brain mitochondrial alterations after chronic alcohol consumption. Journal of Physiology and Biochemistry. 2009;**65**:305-312

[86] Walter NA, Denmark DL, Kozell LB, Buck KJ, Systems Approach A. Implicates a brain mitochondrial oxidative homeostasis co-expression network in genetic vulnerability to alcohol withdrawal. Frontiers in Genetics. 2016;**7**:218

[87] Spanagel R. Alcoholism: A systems approach from molecular physiology to addictive behavior. Physiological Reviews. 2009;**89**:649-705

[88] Fernandez GM, Lew BJ, Vedder LC, Savage LM. Chronic intermittent ethanol exposure leads to alterations in brain-derived neurotrophic factor within the frontal cortex and impaired behavioral flexibility in both adolescent and adult rats. Neuroscience. 2017;**348**:324-334

[89] Alfonso-Loeches S, Urena-Peralta J, Morillo-Bargues MJ, Gomez-Pinedo U, Guerri C. Ethanol-induced TLR4/NLRP3 neuroinflammatory response in microglial cells promotes leukocyte infiltration across the BBB. Neurochemical Research. 2016;**41**:193-209

[90] Ji C. Mechanisms of alcohol-induced endoplasmic reticulum stress and organ injuries. Biochemistry Research International. 2012;**2012**:216450

[91] Trantham-Davidson H, Chandler LJ. Alcohol-induced alterations in dopamine modulation of prefrontal activity. Alcohol. 2015;**49**:773-779

[92] Rando K, Hong KI, Bhagwagar Z, Li CS, Bergquist K, Guarnaccia J, Sinha R. Association of frontal and posterior cortical gray matter volume with time to alcohol relapse: A prospective study. The American Journal of Psychiatry. 2011;**168**:183-192

[93] Auta J, Zhang H, Pandey SC, Guidotti A. Chronic alcohol exposure differentially alters one-carbon metabolism in rat liver and brain. Alcoholism, Clinical and Experimental Research. 2017;**41**:1105-1111

[94] Casanas-Sanchez V, Perez JA, Quinto-Alemany D, Diaz M. Sub-toxic ethanol exposure modulates gene expression and enzyme activity of antioxidant systems to provide neuroprotection in hippocampal HT22 cells. Frontiers in Physiology. 2016;**7**:312

[95] Das SK, Vasudevan DM. Alcohol-induced oxidative stress. Life Sciences. 2007;**81**:177-187

[96] Xu Y, Liu P, Li Y. Impaired development of mitochondria plays a role in the central nervous system defects of fetal alcohol syndrome. Birth Defects Research. Part A, Clinical and Molecular Teratology. 2005;**73**:83-91

[97] Brocardo PS, Gil-Mohapel J, Christie BR. The role of oxidative stress in fetal alcohol spectrum disorders. Brain Research Reviews. 2011;**67**:209-225

[98] Khalighi M, Brzezinski MR, Chen H, Juchau MR. Inhibition of human prenatal biosynthesis of all-trans-retinoic acid by ethanol, ethanol metabolites, and products of lipid peroxidation reactions: A possible role for CYP2E1. Biochemical Pharmacology. 1999;**57**:811-821

[99] Person RE, Chen H, Fantel AG, Juchau MR. Enzymic catalysis of the accumulation of acetaldehyde from ethanol in human prenatal cephalic tissues: Evaluation of the relative contributions of CYP2E1, alcohol dehydrogenase, and catalase/peroxidases. Alcoholism, Clinical and Experimental Research. 2000;**24**:1433-1442

[100] Moren C, Hernandez S, Guitart-Mampel M, Garrabou G. Mitochondrial toxicity in human pregnancy: An update on clinical and experimental approaches in the last 10 years. International Journal of Environmental Research and Public Health. 2014;**11**: 9897-9918

[101] Bayard M, McIntyre J, Hill KR, Woodside J Jr. Alcohol withdrawal syndrome. American Family Physician. 2004;**69**:1443-1450

[102] Prakash J, Setlur R, Saini RK. Symptom triggered therapy in delirium tremens. Medical Journal Armed Forces India. 2010;**66**:180-181

[103] Lee KF, Soares C, Beique JC. Examining form and function of dendritic spines. Neural Plasticity. 2012;**2012**:704103

[104] Hollenbeck PJ. Mitochondria and neurotransmission: Evacuating the synapse. Neuron. 2005;**47**:331-333

[105] Bargiela D, Shanmugarajah P, Lo C, Blakely EL, Taylor RW, Horvath R, Wharton S, Chinnery PF, Hadjivassiliou M. Mitochondrial pathology in progressive cerebellar ataxia. Cerebellum Ataxias. 2015;**2**:16

[106] Hoffman PL. Glutamate receptors in alcohol withdrawal-induced neurotoxicity. Metabolic Brain Disease. 1995;**10**:73-79

[107] Carta M, Mameli M, Valenzuela CF. Alcohol enhances GABAergic transmission to cerebellar granule cells via an increase in Golgi cell excitability. The Journal of Neuroscience. 2004;**24**:3746-3751

[108] Li CY, Chin TY, Chueh SH. Rat cerebellar granule cells are protected from glutamate-induced excitotoxicity by S-nitrosoglutathione but not glutathione. American Journal of Physiology. Cell Physiology. 2004;**286**:C893-C904

[109] Nguyen D, Alavi MV, Kim KY, Kang T, Scott RT, Noh YH, Lindsey JD, Wissinger B, Ellisman MH, Weinreb RN, et al. A new vicious cycle involving glutamate excitotoxicity, oxidative stress and mitochondrial dynamics. Cell Death & Disease. 2011; **2**:e240

[110] Virmani M, Majchrowicz E, Swenberg CE, Gangola P, Pant HC. Alteration in calcium-binding activity in synaptosomal membranes from rat brains in association with physical dependence upon ethanol. Brain Research. 1985;**359**:371-374

[111] Netzeband JG, Schneeloch JR, Trotter C, Caguioa-Aquino JN, Gruol DL. Chronic ethanol treatment and withdrawal alter ACPD-evoked calcium signals in developing Purkinje neurons. Alcoholism, Clinical and Experimental Research. 2002;**26**:386-393

[112] Jung ME, Yan LJ, Forster MJ, Simpkins JW. Ethanol withdrawal provokes mitochondrial injury in an estrogen preventable manner. Journal of Bioenergetics and Biomembranes. 2008;**40**:35-44

[113] Follesa P, Mancuso L, Biggio F, Mostallino MC, Manca A, Mascia MP, Busonero F, Talani G, Sanna E, Biggio G. Gamma-hydroxybutyric acid and diazepam antagonize a rapid increase in GABA(a) receptors alpha(4) subunit mRNA abundance induced by ethanol withdrawal in cerebellar granule cells. Molecular Pharmacology. 2003;**63**: 896-907

[114] Friberg H, Wieloch T. Mitochondrial permeability transition in acute neurodegeneration. Biochimie. 2002;**84**:241-250

[115] Perez MJ, Quintanilla RA. Development or disease: Duality of the mitochondrial permeability transition pore. Developmental Biology. 2017;**426**:1-7

[116] SAMHSA: Substance Abuse and Mental Health Services Administration. National Survey on Drug Use and Health: National Findings. Rockville: SAMHSA; 2007

[117] Schulteis G, Archer C, Tapert SF, Frank LR. Intermittent binge alcohol exposure during the periadolescent period induces spatial working memory deficits in young adult rats. Alcohol. 2008;**42**:459-467

[118] Merrill JE, Carey KB. Drinking over the lifespan: Focus on college ages. Alcohol Research: Current Reviews. 2016;**38**:103-114

[119] Orellana JA, Cerpa W, Carvajal MF, Lerma-Cabrera JM, Karahanian E, Osorio-Fuentealba C, Quintanilla RA. New implications for the Melanocortin system in alcohol drinking behavior in adolescents: The glial dysfunction hypothesis. Frontiers in Cellular Neuroscience. 2017;**11**:90

[120] Slawecki CJ, Thorsell A, Ehlers CL. Long-term neurobehavioral effects of alcohol or nicotine exposure in adolescent animal models. Annals of the New York Academy of Sciences. 2004;**1021**:448-452

[121] Spear LP. Adolescent alcohol exposure: Are there separable vulnerable periods within adolescence? Physiology & Behavior. 2015;**148**:122-130

[122] Briones TL, Woods J. Chronic binge-like alcohol consumption in adolescence causes depression-like symptoms possibly mediated by the effects of BDNF on neurogenesis. Neuroscience. 2013;**254**:324-334

[123] Pascual M, Pla A, Minarro J, Guerri C. Neuroimmune activation and myelin changes in adolescent rats exposed to high-dose alcohol and associated cognitive dysfunction: A review with reference to human adolescent drinking. Alcohol and Alcoholism. 2014;**49**:187-192

[124] Gass JT, Glen WB, Jr., McGonigal JT, Trantham-Davidson H, Lopez MF, Randall PK, Yaxley R, Floresco SB, Chandler LJ: Adolescent alcohol exposure reduces behavioral flexibility, promotes disinhibition, and increases resistance to extinction of ethanol self-administration in adulthood. Neuropsychopharmacology. 2014;**39**:2570-2583

[125] Ledesma JC, Miquel M, Pascual M, Guerri C, Aragon CM. Induction of brain cytochrome P450 2E1 boosts the locomotor-stimulating effects of ethanol in mice. Neuropharmacology. 2014;**85**:36-44

[126] Ewenczyk A, Ziplow J, Tong M, Le T, de la Monte SM: Sustained impairments in brain insulin/IGF signaling in adolescent rats subjected to binge alcohol exposures during development. Journal of Clinical and Experimental Pathology. 2012;**2**

[127] Zahr NM, Mayer D, Rohlfing T, Hasak MP, Hsu O, Vinco S, Orduna J, Luong R, Sullivan EV, Pfefferbaum A. Brain injury and recovery following binge ethanol: Evidence from in vivo magnetic resonance spectroscopy. Biological Psychiatry. 2010;**67**:846-854

[128] Tapia-Rojas C, Carvajal FJ, Mira RG, Arce C, Lerma-Cabrera JM, Orellana JA, Cerpa W, Quintanilla RA. Adolescent binge alcohol exposure affects the brain function through mitochondrial impairment. Molecular Neurobiology. 2017:1-19

[129] Chen H, Chan DC. Mitochondrial dynamics – fusion, fission, movement, and mitophagy – in neurodegenerative diseases. Human Molecular Genetics. 2009;**18**:R169-R176

[130] Detmer SA, Chan DC. Functions and dysfunctions of mitochondrial dynamics. Nature Reviews. Molecular Cell Biology. 2007;**8**:870-879

[131] Dinkova-Kostova AT, Abramov AY. The emerging role of Nrf2 in mitochondrial function. Free Radical Biology & Medicine. 2015;**88**:179-188

[132] Guerri C, Pascual M. Mechanisms involved in the neurotoxic, cognitive, and neurobehavioral effects of alcohol consumption during adolescence. Alcohol. 2010;**44**:15-26

Chapter 15

Mitochondrial Oxidative Stress and Calcium-Dependent Permeability Transition are Key Players in the Mechanisms of Statins-Associated Side Effects

Estela N.B. Busanello, Ana C. Marques,
Estela Lorza-Gil, Helena C.F. de Oliveira and
Anibal E. Vercesi

Additional information is available at the end of the chapter

http://dx.doi.org/10.5772/intechopen.71610

Abstract

Statins are cholesterol-lowering medicines utilized worldwide and are associated with reduced risk of cardiovascular mortality and events. However, 0.5–10% of patients suffer from adverse effects especially on skeletal muscle. Recently, new onset of diabetes has been reported in subjects on statin therapy. Pro- and anti-oxidant effects of statins have been reported, thus fostering a debate. Previously reported data provide evidence that statins induce alterations in intracellular calcium homeostasis and mitochondrial dysfunctions that can be counteracted by antioxidants (e.g., CoQ10, creatine, and L-carnitine). Therefore, we have proposed that statin-induced inhibition of mitochondrial respiration leads to oxidative stress that opens a calcium-dependent permeability transition pore, an event that may lead to cell death. In addition, mitochondrial oxidative stress caused by statin treatment may be a signal for cellular antioxidant system responses such as catalase upregulation, possibly explaining the alleged statins' antioxidant properties. Muscle mitochondrial dysfunction induced by statin treatment may be associated with the peripheral insulin resistance and may explain statins-induced new onset of diabetes. Together, the data presented in this review suggest that the statins' detrimental effects can be prevented by co-administration of antioxidants.

Keywords: statins adverse effects, statins pleiotropic effects, reactive oxygen species (ROS), mitochondrial permeability transition, antioxidants

1. Introduction

Familial hypercholesterolemia (FH) is an autosomal dominant disorder characterized by the presence of very high levels of low-density lipoprotein cholesterol (LDLc) in the blood stream since birth. This cholesterol disorder was first described in the 1960s, and the existence of a mutated LDL receptor (LDLr) in FH patients was later discovered by Brown and Goldstein [1]. They observed that FH fibroblasts did not specifically bind and internalize LDL when compared with normal fibroblasts; that finding was the beginning of decades of work and discoveries concerning cholesterol metabolism regulation that led the pair to Nobel Prize award in 1985. Although the homozygous mutants for LDLr have an early cardiac death in the first or second decade of life, heterozygous FH patients usually do not present any early severe symptoms. The lack of diagnosis and treatment may have severe consequences considering the lifetime exposure to high LDLc concentrations. Increased LDLc levels are a well-established independent risk factor for cardiovascular diseases [2], and lowering LDL serum levels remains the primary treatment target in hypercholesterolemia [3, 4] that is undertaken in order to prevent and reduce cardiovascular and coronary heart diseases [5, 6].

Cholesterol is synthesized from acetyl-CoA by a 30-step pathway, in which 3-hydroxy-3-methylglutaryl coenzyme-A (HMG-CoA) reductase is the rate-limiting enzyme, converting HMG-CoA into mevalonate. However, besides being involved in cholesterol synthesis, mevalonate is also a precursor for isoprenoids farnesyl diphosphate. Geranyl- (GPP), farnesyl- (FPP) and geranylgeranyl-pyrophosphate (GGPP) are precursors of sterols, dolichols, CoQ10, isoprenoids, and carotenoids. These important metabolites are involved in membrane structures, protein glycosylation and prenylation, electron transport in mitochondrial respiratory chain, and scavenging of ROS [7].

The first cholesterol-lowering agent, citrinin, was discovered in the 1970s. It was derived from fungal cultures, but this product was discontinued due to its hepatotoxicity [8, 9]. After this, another fungal-derived compound called compactin was purified and tested in rats; however, it failed to reduce plasma cholesterol because it had the rebound effect of inducing HMG-CoA reductase activity a few hours after administration [10]. At the end of the 1970s, a very potent compound chemically similar to compactin was synthesized based on independent studies from Endo and Alberts [11, 12], and after several trials, this potent compound, lovastatin, was approved and commercially available in 1986 [13]. Presently, there are seven natural (fungal-derived) or synthetic statins that are commercially available; this group consists of three hydrophilic (pravastatin, rosuvastatin, and pitavastatin) and four lipophilic (lovastatin, simvastatin, fluvastatin, and atorvastatin) [14–16]. Cerivastatin was approved by the Food and Drug Administration in 1998, but it was removed from the market in 2001 after reports of fatal rhabdomyolysis [17].

Statins are one of the most successful drugs for reducing cardiovascular diseases. High-intensity statins treatment is associated with the greatest reduction in mortality [18]. In addition to lowering plasma cholesterol, various studies have reported that statins have pleiotropic effects such as antioxidant, anti-inflammatory, and anti-tumorigenesis. Regarding statins redox effects, some groups have demonstrated protective roles of these compounds against cell oxidative damage [19, 20], whereas others have reinforced their toxic effects [21, 22]. Despite these discrepancies in these results over the last decade, accumulated data have indicated that alterations in mitochondrial energy-linked functions such as respiration, oxidative phosphorylation, redox state,

Ca^{2+}-dependent permeability transition underlie statins toxicity. The impact on cell or tissue pathophysiology will depend on the intensity of statins' effects on mitochondria. In this chapter, we review the literature data on the statins effects on mitochondrial functions and consequent toxic tissue events.

1.1. Mitochondrial energy-linked functions and reactive oxygen generation

Mitochondria participation in the process of statin toxicity adds to the numerous roles of these organelles in cell pathophysiology [23, 24]. Considering that statin-mediated mitochondrial dysfunctions include many aspects of mitochondrial physiology such as inhibition of respiration, depletion of ubiquinone, redox imbalance, opening of the mitochondrial permeability transition pore (PTP) and disruption of energy conservation, we next outline some of these mitochondrial properties in the following sections.

During the last several decades, mitochondria have emerged as the center of attention in processes of cell signaling, cell injury, and cell death [25, 26]. According to the concept of coupling between respiration and oxidative phosphorylation through a transmembrane proton electrochemical potential that was introduced by Peter Mitchell [27], it is not difficult to understand that any condition that interferes with the ability to sustain the inner membrane proton potential leads to mitochondrial dysfunction [28]. In addition, the continuous oxygen reduction by the mitochondrial electron transport chain to build up the transmembrane proton gradient also generates a well-regulated amount of superoxide [23, 29]. Therefore, mitochondria have developed a complex antioxidant defense system composed of Mn-superoxide dismutase that converts the superoxide radical generated during respiration into hydrogen peroxide (H_2O_2). H_2O_2 is then reduced to water by glutathione and thioredoxin peroxidase or catalase [30]. Oxidized glutathione (GSSG) and thioredoxin (TSST) generated by peroxidases are converted to their reduced forms by glutathione and thioredoxin reductases, using NADPH as reducing power. NADH then reduces $NADP^+$, in a reaction catalyzed by NADP transhydrogenase that is present in the inner mitochondrial membrane [31–33]. Therefore mitochondria redox state is tightly regulated and connected with whole cell redox balance [34–36]. Furthermore, it is now generally accepted that superoxide as well as other forms of ROS can function as a signal for either adaptation or maladaptation to stress conditions [35]. In this regard, mitochondrial ROS generation leads to a nonlinear dose-response relationship called mitohormesis. In mitohormesis, high reactive oxygen concentrations exert devastating and irreversible effects on cell function and structures, whereas low concentrations may be associated with protective effects due to activation of cellular defense mechanisms [37, 38]. In fact, at progressively increasing physiological levels, ROS may successively regulate cellular processes such as proliferation and differentiation, activate adaptive programs such as transcriptional upregulation of antioxidant genes, and at higher levels, ROS may be a signal for senescence and regulated cell death [35]. In addition to the physiological processes, it seems that mitochondrial oxidative stress is responsible for the development and progression of a series of diseases such as cancer, diabetes, inflammatory diseases, hypertension, neurodegenerative and ischemia-related diseases, and aging [39–46]. Statin toxicity may also include the participation of mitochondrial generated ROS [47–49].

1.2. Mitochondrial Ca^{2+} transport and mitochondrial membrane permeability transition (MPT)

Ca^{2+} modulates several metabolic pathways through transient changes in its free concentrations in different cell compartments [50, 51]. In order to fulfill these physiological roles, Ca^{2+} movements across cell membranes are driven directly or indirectly by ATP hydrolysis. Therefore, defects in processes that supply cellular ATP may lead to deregulation in Ca^{2+} signaling that may compromise cell functioning, redox balance, and mitochondrial membrane permeability transition (MPT) [51, 52]. In this review, we briefly describe how mitochondrial Ca^{2+} load promotes MPT [53].

MPT is characterized by the opening of a high conductance, nonspecific proteinaceous pore, the PTP. It was first described by Hunter and collaborators [54] and then demonstrated by Vercesi's group to be dependent on redox imbalance promoted either by thiol oxidants or oxidative stress [55]. Matrix Ca^{2+} participates in at least two steps in the process of PTP opening: (a) stimulates superoxide generation by mitochondria and (b) binds to membrane sites exposing specific buried thiols to the oxidants (**Figure 1**) [55]. Accordingly, Ca^{2+} binding to cardiolipin alters mitochondria inner membrane lipid organization characterized by increased lipid packing and domain formation. As a consequence, the electron transfer along the respiratory complexes is impaired favoring superoxide generation [56].

Robust data has provided evidence that PTP opening is a main step in the mitochondrial pathway leading to cell death either by apoptosis or necrosis [57, 58], and is a major cause of cell death under a variety of pathophysiological conditions, including ischemia/reperfusion injury, traumatic brain injury, neurodegenerative diseases, metabolic diseases, muscular dystrophy, and drug toxicity [59–67].

Since mitochondrial Ca^{2+} overload stimulates superoxide generation and MPT, the mechanisms of Ca^{2+} transport by mitochondria will be outlined next. The inner mitochondrial membrane possesses three different carriers for Ca^{2+} influx and efflux [68]. A mitochondrial calcium uniporter (MCU) located in the inner membrane mediates the influx of Ca^{2+} down its electrochemical gradient without coupling Ca^{2+} transport to the flux of another ion. This mechanism was discovered in the 1960s [69, 70], but the molecular nature of the channel was only recently identified [71, 72]. Ca^{2+} release from mitochondria occurs via $Ca^{2+}/3Na^{+}$ or a $Ca^{2+}/2H^{+}$ exchangers [73–75] depending on the tissue [68, 76].

The high loads of matrix Ca^{2+} that stimulate ROS production in mitochondria [55] appear to be associated with either dysregulation of cellular Ca^{2+} homeostasis or regulated release from endo(sarco)plasmic reticulum [77–79] (**Figure 1**). Under both conditions, the opening of the PTP can occur allowing for the movements of molecules up to 1.5 KDa. The entry of solutes and water to the matrix causes large amplitude mitochondrial swelling. These conditions disrupt both the electrochemical proton potential and oxidative phosphorylation [23, 55]. When PTP opens in a large number of mitochondria, cell death occurs by necrosis due to the lack of ATP, and when PTP is limited to a small number of mitochondria, apoptosis is triggered by the release of cytochrome c [80]. Anti-apoptotic proteins (members of Bcl-2 family) or cyclosporine A inhibits the opening of PTP [81, 82]. Evidence has been provided that high intracellular Ca^{2+} levels and ROS have additive effects in the process of PTP opening [23, 53, 55, 83–88].

It is well recognized that mitochondrial Ca^{2+} is essential for PTP opening [54, 55, 89, 90], whereas oxidative modifications of inner membrane protein thiols, oxidative stress, presence

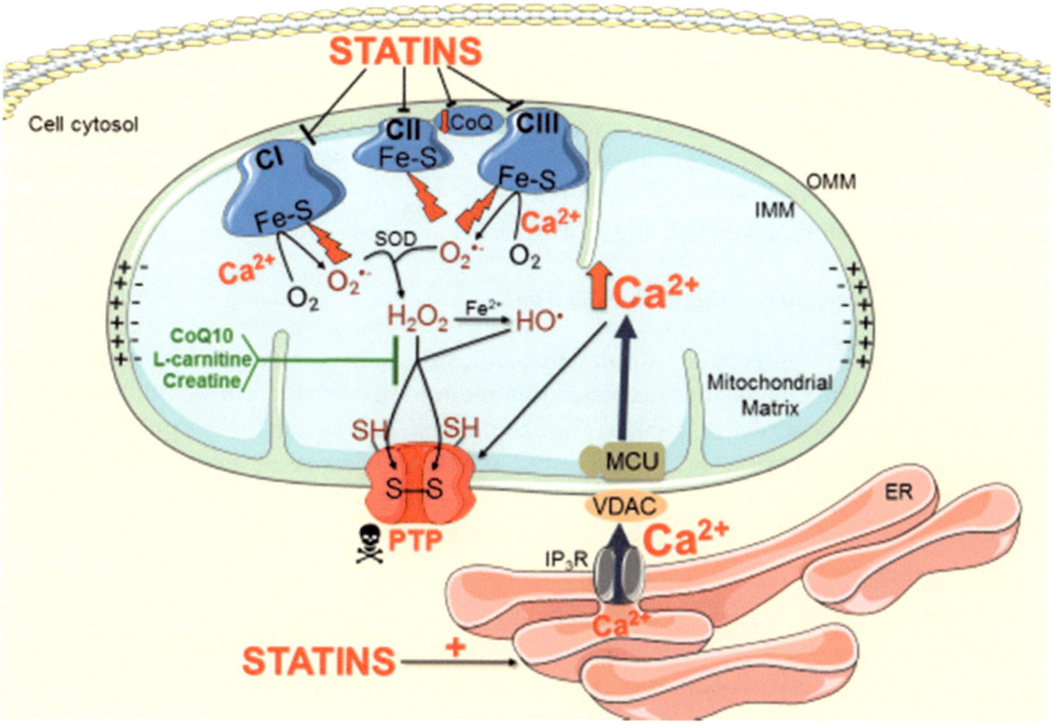

Figure 1. Statins triggers mitochondrial oxidative stress and calcium-dependent permeability transition. Statins diminishes the respiratory capacity at the level of complexes I, II and III of the respiratory chain, increasing superoxide generation ($O_2^{\cdot-}$). The Fe-S clusters present in these respiratory complexes are vulnerable to superoxide attack, thus inhibiting their activity and diminishing their resistance to Ca^{2+} induced MPT. Superoxide is dismutated in hydrogen peroxide (H_2O_2). When not metabolized by mitochondrial antioxidant systems, H_2O_2 can induce (directly or indirectly) membrane protein sulfhydryl-disulfide transitions, a process involved in PTP opening. Statins also impair cellular Ca^{2+} homeostasis, inducing Ca^{2+} release from the ER via IP_3R and increasing cytosolic Ca^{2+} levels. Thus, mitochondria uptake the excessive cytosolic Ca^{2+} via VDAC and MCU channels, leading to its accumulation in mitochondrial matrix. Ca^{2+} binds to membrane sites exposing specific buried thiols to the oxidants and also impairs mitochondrial respiration, increasing $O_2^{\cdot-}$ formation. The association of ROS and mitochondrial Ca^{2+} overload, PTP may open and trigger cell death. In addition, a decrease in the levels of CoQ10 that acts as an electron carrier and antioxidant also occurs due to inhibition of the mevalonate pathway by statins. The antioxidants CoQ10, L-carnitine and creatine prevent PTP opening induced by statins.

of inorganic phosphate [53, 55, 83, 85, 91], and Bcl-2 family proteins [81, 82] participate in PTP modulation. The close location of mitochondria and the endoplasmic reticulum (ER) [75] permits mitochondria to take up large amounts of Ca^{2+} that are released from the ER. This process seems to be controlled via a redox-regulated cross talk between mitochondria and ER that is mediated by NADPH oxidases [36]. Such redox interactions may link PTP opening to the induction of Ca^{2+} signals specifically for cell death [26]. Considering the understanding on how Ca^{2+} and ROS act synergistically in the mechanism of PTP opening, it should be emphasized that mitochondria are more susceptible to MPT when their antioxidant systems are exhausted, especially due to an oxidized state of NADPH and GSH [55]. Accordingly, mitochondria isolated from mice deficient in nicotinamide nucleotide transhydrogenase (NNT), which cannot sustain NADPH in the reduced state, present defective antioxidant capacity and increased susceptibility to MPT [92, 93]. Thus, MPT can be induced by pro-oxidants and prevented or even reversed by antioxidants [85, 86, 94, 95].

2. Statins pleiotropic effects

Statins are among the most commonly prescribed medicines worldwide. They are safe and well-tolerated and seem to present a range of cholesterol-independent protective actions called pleiotropic effects. Indeed, several studies claim that statins act as antioxidants [19, 96], anti-inflammatory agents [97], and can increase stability of the atherosclerotic plaque [98], improve endothelial function [99], and induce cancer cell death [100].

2.1. Antioxidant responses triggered by statins

Extensive literature reports have indicated that antioxidant effects can be attributed to statins. It has been postulated that statins decrease systemic or local oxidative stress and this appears to confer additional vascular protection. The first possible mechanism for this protective effect could be secondary to statins' main target effect, which is to decrease the concentration of the oxidizable substrate, LDLc. This decrease may lead to a reduction in oxidized-LDL, which constitutes a very early step involved in atherosclerosis development [101–103].

Another antioxidant mechanism frequently attributed to statins is the upregulation of cellular antioxidant defenses. For instance, atorvastatin treatment decreased the expression of essential NAD(P)H oxidase subunits and upregulated catalase expression in cultured rat vascular smooth muscle cells and in the vasculature of spontaneous hypertensive rats (SHR) [104]. Simvastatin treatment restored endothelial function in SHR by increasing superoxide dismutase and glutathione peroxidase activities [105].

Other studies have demonstrated a protective effect by statins against oxidative damage of biomolecules. In whole blood leukocytes of non-treated dyslipidemic diabetic type 2 patients, simvastatin treatment [19] protected against DNA oxidative damage. Similarly, rosuvastatin inhibited lipid peroxidation and attenuated the oxidative damage to DNA in treated rat liver [106]. Rosuvastatin-treated HL-60 cells exhibited a glutathione-dependent protective mechanism against DNA oxidation [107]. In addition, simvastatin or fluvastatin administration prevented lipid peroxidation, superoxide generation, cytokine production, and neutrophil accumulation in a rat colitis model [108].

With respect to statins' effects on specific mitochondrial redox homeostasis, literature reports are more controversial. It was shown that atorvastatin and simvastatin reduced oxidative stress triggered by Ca^{2+} and prevented MPT and cytochrome c release in rat liver mitochondria [96]. On the other hand, results from our group and others suggest that statins, when administered to mitochondria, muscle biopsies, or *in vivo* exert pro-oxidant activities (this will be discussed in more detail in the next section) [47, 49, 109]. Thus, our hypothesis for the alleged statin antioxidant effects is based on the mitohormesis concept [37, 38]: mild mitochondrial oxidative stress caused by statins may function as a signal that leads to a cellular adaptive response such as increasing the expression and activity of cellular antioxidant systems in order to overcome this stress.

2.2. Statins and cancer

Statins have been proposed as adjuvant in cancer therapy since the 1990s and, until then, several mechanisms have been proposed for this specific function depending on the type of cancer and statins lipophilicity [100, 110–112]. In this regard, literature reports suggest that the mevalonate pathway inhibition is associated with anti-proliferative, pro-apoptotic, and anti-metastatic statins effects [113]. In addition, statins may impair cell membrane function, due to the lowering of cholesterol levels and inhibition of the tumor cell cycle, and may lead to cell death by distinct pathways, including the mitochondrial pathway (for more details, see Ref. [114] and other reviews).

Prostate cancer is one of the most commonly diagnosed cancer in men and is a significant cause of male morbidity and mortality [115]. Literature reports have shown that statins protect against prostate cancer in human patients [116, 117], and some of these effects may be attributed to a decreased isoprenoid synthesis due to mevalonate pathway inhibition. As a consequence, Ras proteins that regulate signaling pathways of cell proliferation, angiogenesis, and metastasis are not able to be isoprenylated, thus reducing their function and triggering apoptosis [118]. Statins also stimulate the mitochondrial apoptosis pathway [119, 120] via an increase in pro- and decrease in anti-apoptotic Bcl-2 proteins [121], activation of caspases 3, 7, 8, and 9 [122–124], and decrease in the formation of lipid rafts, membrane microdomains involved in several regulatory functions, including cell survival [125, 126]. In addition, statins have a dose-dependent effect on cell death. For instance, simvastatin at concentrations below 10 μM induced PC3 prostate cancer cells apoptosis [21] via a mechanism sensitive to mevalonate but not to cyclosporin A (CysA), an MPT inhibitor. On the other hand, necrosis is stimulated by higher doses of simvastatin (≥60 μM) and is preceded by an increase in free cytosolic Ca^{2+} concentration and PTP opening, sensitive to CysA, but not to mevalonate [21]. Both MPT and necrosis induced by simvastatin (60 μM) are sensitive to L-carnitine (antioxidant) and piracetam (membrane stabilizer) in an additive manner. When combined, these compounds act at lower doses than when each compound is used separately [22]. These data provide evidence that statin toxicity to tumor cells is not only the result of HMG-CoA reductase inhibition but also is mediated by the increase in free cytosolic Ca^{2+} concentration, stimulation of ROS generation, and PTP opening [21, 22]. Although many studies show that statins which are efficient in inducing tumor cell death claim their potential use as adjuvant therapy, there are no robust data that non-tumor cells are less affected by statins' toxic effects than tumor cells. Therefore, it is still premature to conclude that statins are anti-tumorigenic agent.

3. Statins adverse effects

After decades of statins' use, some side effects have been consistently described in a minority of patients, particularly regarding muscle function. Adverse effects other than muscle symptoms such as headache, digestive problems, liver enzymes abnormalities, and neurological dysfunction may occur in some patients [127, 128]. The side effects are often the decisive factor for the noncompliance to statins treatment [129, 130] and its discontinuation usually makes the side effect symptoms disappear [131].

The precise mechanisms involved in statins toxicity and the reasons why only a few subjects are affected remain unclear. Several groups, including ours, have proposed that mitochondria are the main players in statin-induced toxicity.

3.1. Mitochondrial dysfunction caused by statins treatment

Mitochondrial redox imbalance is associated with aging, degenerative disorders, and drug-induced toxicity [26, 132]. Several reports concerning statin *in vitro* effects on isolated tissues or mitochondria from experimental models demonstrated that statins promote inhibition of mitochondrial respiration, mitochondrial oxidative stress, and cell death [47, 49, 109, 133]. It has been previously shown that lipophilic (cerivastatin, fluvastatin, atorvastatin, and simvastatin) and hydrophilic (pravastatin) statins-induced mitochondrial membrane potential decrease in rat skeletal muscle cell line (L6) [133]. The four lipophilic statins also induced mitochondrial swelling, cytochrome c release, and DNA fragmentation in these L6 cells. Mitochondrial β-oxidation enzymes activities were strongly impaired by all lipophilic statins, but in the case of pravastatin, it occurred only at high concentrations. In isolated rat skeletal muscle mitochondria, glutamate-supported state 3 respiration and respiratory control ratios were decreased by all lipophilic statins, but not by pravastatin [133]. According to the authors, this mitochondrial dysfunction caused by lipophilic statins in skeletal muscle might partially explain the muscle symptoms presented by some patients. Abdoli and coworkers demonstrated in isolated rat liver mitochondria that atorvastatin, simvastatin, and lovastatin increased ROS formation followed by lipid peroxidation, inner mitochondrial membrane depolarization, and a decreased GSH/GSSG ratio [47].

More recently, mitochondrial redox imbalance [67, 134] was observed in a genetic human familial hypercholesterolemia mouse model, the LDL receptor knockout mouse (*LDLr*$^{-/-}$) [135]. Mitochondria isolated from several tissues of these mice (liver, heart, and brain) and intact spleen mononuclear cells presented higher ROS production and higher susceptibility to MPT. In addition, these mitochondria showed lower capacity to sustain reduced NADPH [67, 134], which is the most important reducing power involved in reconstituting mitochondrial antioxidant systems [132]. As a consequence, H_2O_2 accumulates and PTP opens [67, 134]. Since cholesterol synthesis consumes a large amount of NADPH, we have proposed that the increased steroidogenesis observed in these mice would be partially responsible for the lower mitochondrial content of NADPH and Krebs cycle intermediates observed in their liver mitochondria [67, 134]. Therefore, we hypothesized that inhibition of cholesterol synthesis by statins treatment could prevent the decrease in NADPH oxidation in *LDLr*$^{-/-}$ mice mitochondria. Unexpectedly, liver mitochondria from wild type and *LDLr*$^{-/-}$ mice treated with lovastatin presented a higher susceptibility to PTP opening, and *in vitro* experiments revealed a drug dose- and class-dependence of this effect [109]. Statin induced PTP opening was shown to be Ca^{2+}-dependent and associated with oxidation of protein thiol groups. Thus, statins induced a direct oxidative damage in mitochondrial proteins [109].

3.2. Ca^{2+} and statins toxicity

It has been proposed by our group and others that statins impair cellular Ca^{2+} homeostasis, leading to mitochondrial dysfunction. Increased cytosolic Ca^{2+} levels were observed after simvastatin treatment of myoblasts culture [136], rat skeletal muscle [137], and human skeletal muscle fibers, and this was followed by mitochondrial Ca^{2+} accumulation [138]. Indeed, Hattori and coworkers [139] proposed that statins induced Ca^{2+} release from the endoplasmic reticulum to the cytosol in human CD19+ primary lymphocytes. As a consequence of high Ca^{2+} levels in the cytosol, Ca^{2+} enters the mitochondria and induces MPT as demonstrated by our group in PC3 cells after simvastatin treatment [21, 22].

3.3. Statins effects on respiratory chain complexes

It is well known that enzymes containing 4Fe-4S clusters are particularly vulnerable to damage by superoxide or peroxynitrite radicals [140–145]. Complexes I and II present six and one of these 4Fe-4S clusters, respectively, thus showing a high superoxide-sensitivity. Some studies have demonstrated that superoxide generation inhibits respiration at complex I and II levels as a result of 4Fe-4S clusters damage. These alterations diminish resistance to Ca^{2+}-induced MPT and induce necrotic cell death [65, 145]. As mentioned before, our group demonstrated that mitochondrial dysfunction caused by simvastatin incubation in permeabilized skeletal muscle was L-carnitine and CoQ10 sensitive [49]. L-carnitine did not protect against CoQ10 depletion, indicating that both CoQ10 and L-carnitine are protecting mitochondrial respiration due to its ROS scavenging properties. Since L-carnitine also binds Fe^{2+} [146], it is feasible that this antioxidant molecule interacts with 4Fe-4S clusters in complexes I and II of the respiratory chain, protecting these sites against superoxide attack. Simvastatin lowered the ADP-stimulated respiration supported by substrates of complexes I and II in primary human skeletal myotubes and increased susceptibility to MPT, mitochondrial oxidative stress, and apoptosis [48]. These results are in agreement with a decrease in complex I activity in muscle of patients undergoing statin treatment [147].

Another study performed in myoblasts culture (C2C12) incubated with several statins (atorvastatin, cerivastatin, fluvastatin, lovastatin, pitavastatin, pravastatin, rosuvastatin, and simvastatin) showed that the respiratory capacity is reduced not only at the levels of respiratory chain complexes I and II but also in complex III [148]. In this case, it was suggested that statins in the lactone form binds to Q_o site of complex III, inhibiting its activity. Similarly, complex III activity of muscle from patients presenting myopathies induced by statins was also reduced [148]. On the other hand, statins do not seem to affect the complex IV-supported respiration [49, 148].

4. Muscle sensitivity to statins

It is well known that about 10% of patients undergoing statin treatment develop mild myopathic symptoms such as weakness, muscle pain, exercise intolerance, and other symptoms that are usually with normal or minimally elevated creatine kinase (CK) serum levels [149, 150]. Moreover, myositis, defined as muscle symptoms associated with increased CK, is usually present [151, 152]. Rhabdomyolysis, the most severe adverse effect of statins, is a very rare condition affecting 1.6/100,000 patients-years. It may result in acute renal failure and disseminated intravascular coagulation, leading to death. This condition is frequently related to drug interactions and occurs with CK levels 10-fold higher than the normal limit and elevated levels of creatinine [153, 154]. Increased intracellular lipid stores, cytochrome oxidase-negative myofibers, ragged red fibers, and subsarcolemmal accumulation of mitochondria were found in patients with muscle symptoms during statin therapy [155, 156]. Schick and colleagues also observed reduced mitochondrial DNA levels in patients treated with simvastatin [157]. Muscle-associated statin toxicity seems to be more severe with increasing lipophilicity, whereas more hydrophilic statins exert only mild or no toxicity [133, 153]. The myotoxic effect is attributed to their ability to penetrate and accumulate in cell membranes and alter their structural conformation [158–160].

On the other hand, high statin sensitivity may also be related to genetic factors; for instance, the activity of specific liver transporters may be impaired, thus reducing statins hepatic uptake and increasing its plasma concentrations that may potentially affect muscles [161–163].

Skeletal muscles are highly heterogeneous and present distinct fiber types classified as I or II and their respective subtype spectrum as determined by the myosin heavy chain isoforms. Type I and II fibers present relatively distinct metabolic, contractile, and motor properties in addition to antioxidant defense capacity. Thus, type I fibers appear red due to high myoglobin content, extensive mitochondrial content, and oxidative capacity, whereas type II fibers have relatively low myoglobin and mitochondrial content that depends mostly on glycolytic activity [164, 165]. In this regard, our group observed that respiratory rates were inhibited in the presence of Ca^{2+} in permeabilized plantaris muscle (predominantly type II fibers) in $LDLr^{-/-}$ mice chronically treated with pravastatin and catalase activity increased. In contrast, no alterations were observed in soleus muscle (predominantly type I fibers) [166]. Similarly, previous studies reported a distinct sensitivity of different muscle fiber types to lovastatin [162]. After 10 days of lovastatin administration, rat gastrocnemius muscles showed organelle degeneration, microvacuolization, and 20–50% necrosis, whereas soleus muscle was spared, suggesting that type II fibers are more vulnerable to lovastatin-induced myopathy [167]. In line with this finding, Westwood and colleagues characterized time-dependent muscle necrosis triggered by simvastatin or cerivastatin in rats after 10 days of treatment. The authors demonstrated that glycolytic fibers were more prone to necrosis than oxidative fibers, which in turn were consistently spared even when myotoxicity was severe. Since these fibers present distinct metabolism and MPT may precede necrosis, it is conceivable that mitochondria exert a central role in this process. In fact, it was observed that the first subcellular alterations were found in mitochondria of type II fibers, characterized by vacuolization as well as myeloid and vesicular body accumulation in sarcolemma areas [168]. Later, the same group performed a similar study using rosuvastatin in rats. Although a much higher statin dose was required to achieve muscle necrosis in comparison to the earlier study, the same pattern of muscle damage was observed and the soleus muscle remained unaffected [169]. Specific soleus-insensitivity to statin toxicity has also been demonstrated by other groups. Schaefer and coworkers demonstrated necrosis and inflammation in muscles with predominance of type II fibers in rats after 15 days of cerivastatin administration. Sarcomere disruption and altered mitochondria was also found in degenerated fibers, while these alterations were not found in type I fibers [170]. Similarly, cerivastatin-induced degeneration was evident in several muscles but not in the soleus muscle of female rats after the same treatment time (15 days). After 15 days of treadmill exercises, the severity of muscle damage had increased, but the soleus remained unaltered. Degenerated mitochondria were also observed with no changes in contractile elements such as endoplasmic reticulum and other subcellular compartments [171]. Although the role of mitochondria in myotoxicity in type II fibers is well established, there is no consensus as to whether this involvement precedes myofiber degeneration, thus justifying further studies to clarify this matter [170, 171]. In addition, MPT is associated with apoptosis or necrosis in several diseases [172] and is probably an important statin-induced event in muscle necrosis.

5. Statins toxicity to liver

Although rare, the main liver injury studies have reported statins toxicity alone [173–176] or in combination with other drugs with variable patterns of injury [177–181]. Some cases exhibited autoimmune features [180, 182, 183] and a range of latencies to onset [184] and progression was also observed [182, 185]. Liver adverse symptoms are unspecific and most patients remain asymptomatic [186]. A 3-fold increase in serum aspartate (AST) and alanine (ALT) aminotransferases activities have been described in less than 1% of patients receiving starting and intermediate statins doses [187–191] and this alteration may be accompanied by bilirubin elevation [192]. Two factors are frequently related to the hepatotoxic effects of statins: (a) the lipophilicity of these medicines and (b) alterations in cytochrome P450 system [193–195]. Accordingly, lipophilic statins (atorvastatin and simvastatin) are associated with more than 130 cases of liver injury, and a few cases progress to liver transplantation and death [173, 174, 178]. Rare cases of portal inflammation or fibrosis and mild necrosis were also described in patients undergoing lovastatin treatment [196] or atorvastatin treatment [197]. On the other hand, hydrophilic statins are minimally metabolized by the cytochrome P450 pathway [193–195] and are generally less toxic [109, 198]. A multicenter report also showed that pravastatin was well-tolerated in patients with compensated chronic liver disease [199]. Our group also attributes statin-induced liver toxicity to mitochondrial dysfunction associated with oxidative stress and MPT [193].

6. Statins and new onset of diabetes

Recent studies suggest that chronic use of statins is associated with risk of developing type 2 diabetes [200–202]. Meta-analyses of large-scale statin trials support the concept of the diabetogenic effect of statins, but the precise mechanisms have not yet been identified [203, 204]. We have recently revealed diabetes-related mechanisms induced by statin treatment in a familial hypercholesterolemia animal model, the $LDLr^{-/-}$. We demonstrated that pravastatin-treated $LDLr^{-/-}$ mice exhibit marked reductions of insulinemia and of glucose-stimulated insulin secretion by isolated pancreatic islets. These effects were associated with increased oxidative stress and apoptosis [205] and were counteracted by co-treatment with CoQ10 (Lorza-Gil et al., unpublished data). Therefore, we have proposed that pancreatic toxic effects of pravastatin could be caused by statin inhibition of CoQ10 biosynthesis. On the other hand, we and others have hypothesized that insulin signaling in their target tissues (such as muscle) could also be impaired by chronic statin treatment. However, studies relating statins therapy and insulin sensitivity are controversial [206–208]. A meta-analysis by Baker and colleagues shows that while pravastatin improved insulin sensitivity, atorvastatin, simvastatin, and rosuvastatin worsened it [209]. Experimental studies suggest that atorvastatin leads to reduced expression of GLUT4 in adipocytes *in vivo* and *in vitro* [210] and that simvastatin decreases IGF-1 signaling (pAKT, pERK) in muscle cells [211]. Kain et al. [212] showed that myotubes treated with simvastatin and atorvastatin presented impaired insulin signaling pathway and glucose uptake. We have evidence that long-term pravastatin treatment of hypercholesterolemic mice also induces marked insulin resistance and increased muscle protein degradation (Lorza-Gil et al., unpublished data). Therefore, toxic effects on insulin secreting cells in conjunction with impaired muscle insulin signaling may explain the new onset of diabetes reported in statin-treated subjects.

7. Antioxidant supplement and statins toxicity

The cholesterol biosynthesis pathway generates several products including CoQ10 [213]. CoQ10 is an essential component of the electron transport chain where it acts as an electron carrier [214]. Ubiquinol, the reduced form of ubiquinone, when associated with proteins in the inner mitochondrial membrane, has an important function as a lipophilic antioxidant [215, 216]. CoQ10 also has additional functions such as regeneration of reduced intra- and extracellular forms of ascorbic acid and tocopherol (vitamin E) [217, 218], participation in redox processes associated with PTP opening [219], and regulation of muscle uncoupling proteins [220]. It is also known that the reduced form of ubiquinone occurs in all cellular membranes [221–223] as well as in serum lipoproteins and DNA, protecting them from oxidative damage [224]. CoQ10 content is larger in tissues such as cardiac and skeletal muscles that have high energy demand [223]. Therefore, decreased synthesis of ubiquinone may result in two harmful conditions: (a) insufficient rates of mitochondrial ATP synthesis [225] and (b) decreased mitochondrial antioxidant capacity [49].

Some studies have proposed that statin-induced mitotoxicity may be mediated by diminished CoQ10 content with consequent impairment of mitochondrial respiration [111, 226–234]. On the other hand, our group has provided evidence that under our experimental conditions, the reduction of mitochondrial respiration associated with CoQ10 depletion was mainly due to its free radical scavenging action rather than its electron carrier function. Indeed, it has been demonstrated that incubation of permeabilized rat soleus muscle with simvastatin inhibited both ADP and FCCP-stimulated oxygen consumption supported by complex I or II substrates. Additionally, ubiquinone content was diminished by 40% and the H_2O_2 content was significantly increased. Under these conditions, all of the following compounds, including mevalonate, CoQ10, or L-carnitine protected against H_2O_2 generation but only mevalonate prevented CoQ10 depletion. Thus, independent of CoQ10 levels, L-carnitine prevented the toxic effects of simvastatin. This allows for the conclusion that L-carnitine antioxidant action prevailed in the protection against simvastatin-induced respiratory inhibition [49]. Therefore, it can be concluded that CoQ10 also acted as a free radical scavenger in this mechanism. Accordingly, Kettawan and coworkers previously demonstrated that a decrease in ubiquinone levels in serum, liver, and heart in mice undergoing simvastatin treatment increased lipoperoxidation. Simvastatin also reduced NADPH-CoQ reductase activity, whereas the co-administration of CoQ10 and simvastatin to mice diminished these deleterious effects [235]. Another study revealed that simvastatin reduced mitochondrial CoQ10 levels associated with DNA oxidative damage and reduced ATP synthesis followed by cell death in hepatocytes (HepG2). All of these alterations were reversed by CoQ10 supplementation [236]. Furthermore, it was recently shown that CoQ10 supplementation improved respiratory control in liver mitochondria isolated from rats treated with high doses of atorvastatin and/or a cholesterol-rich diet [237]. Despite all data correlating CoQ10 depletion with statin toxicity, the efficacy of ubiquinone supplementation in patients with side effects is still under debate [231, 238–240].

Creatine is a guanidine compound synthesized endogenously [241] and widely and safely used as supplement by athletes to increase their performance [242]. The role of creatine on the maintenance of ATP/ADP ratio by activating CK is very well known, but it also exerts other actions. Creatine participates on a protein complex involved in MPT regulation [55, 243, 244] and was firstly mentioned as antioxidant in 1998 [245]. A few years later, Lawler and coworkers showed that this compound was capable of scavenging radicals such as superoxide and peroxynitrite [246]. In our recent work, we showed that diet supplementation with creatine protected *LDLr*$^{-/-}$ mice against pravastatin sensitization to Ca^{2+}-induced MPT [166].

L-carnitine stimulates β-oxidation by increasing carnitine palmitoyltransferase 1A mRNA expression. This action prevents mitochondrial oxidative stress induced by free fatty acids, increasing mitochondrial function [22, 247]. Another property of L-carnitine is to bind Fe^{2+} [248] that participates in the mitochondrial oxidative stress involved in MPT [249]. Thus, it is feasible to propose that L-carnitine protects complexes I and II of the respiratory chain against superoxide attack by interacting with 4Fe-4S clusters in these sites. In a previous work performed in PC3 prostate cancer, we showed that L-carnitine and piracetam (a membrane stabilizer) prevented MPT and necrosis induced by simvastatin (60 μM) [22].

Taken together, these experimental results suggest that ROS generation and mitochondrial oxidative stress play an important role on statins toxicity.

8. Conclusions

Cardiovascular benefits of statins therapy are undoubted and appear to be present across diverse demographic and clinical groups. However, the side effects may affect a minority of patients. In this review, we addressed the cellular and molecular mechanisms related to statin side effects. Mitochondrial oxidative stress seems to be the main cause of toxicity in statin sensitive tissues (**Figure 1**). The levels and consequences of mitochondrial oxidative stress seem to be more deleterious in skeletal muscle. This effect is secondary to: (a) inhibition of electrons flow at the levels of respiratory complexes I, II, and III, and (b) decrease in the levels of CoQ10 due to inhibition of the mevalonate pathway. In association with mitochondrial Ca^{2+} overload due to increased cytosolic free Ca^{2+} concentrations, the PTP may open and trigger cell death. *In vitro* experiments provide evidence that this can be blocked in a concerted manner by L-carnitine plus the membrane stabilizer piracetam. Experiments performed with muscle biopsies taken from hypercholesterolemic mice, chronically treated with pravastatin, show that either CoQ10 or creatine can protect against statin-induced mitochondrial muscle toxicity both *in vitro* and *in vivo*. Statin treatment may also result in pro- or antioxidant actions depending on statin class (lipophilicity), dose, and patient's background. We suggest that mitochondrial oxidative stress caused by statin treatment may be a signal for cellular antioxidant system response (such as catalase upregulation) possibly explaining the alleged statin antioxidant properties. Together, the experimental evidence presented in this review suggests that statins' detrimental effects could be prevented by antioxidants administration such as CoQ10, L-carnitine, and creatine.

Acknowledgements

We are grateful to the financial support of Fundação de Amparo à Pesquisa do Estado de São Paulo (FAPESP # 2011/50400-0 and # 2014/11261-2), Obesity and Co-morbidities Research Center (OCRC/Fapesp # 2013/07607-8), Conselho Nacional de Desenvolvimento Científico e Tecnológico (CNPq), and Coordenação de Aperfeiçoamento de Pessoal de Nível Superior (CAPES).

Conflict of interest statement

The authors declare no conflicts of interest.

Abbreviations

ALT	Alanine transaminase
AST	Aspartate transaminase
CK	Creatine kinase
CoQ10	Coenzyme Q10
Cys A	Cyclosporin A
ER	Endoplasmic reticulum
FCCP	Carbonyl cyanide 4-(trifluoromethoxy)phenylhydrazone
FH	Familial hypercholesterolemia
FPP	Farnesyl-pyrophosphate
GGPP	Geranylgeranyl-pyrophosphate
GPP	Geranyl-pyrophosphate
GSH	Glutathione
GSSG	Glutathione oxidized
HMG-CoA	3-Hydroxy-3-methylglutaryl coenzyme-A
IMM	Inner mitochondria membrane

IP_3R	Inositol 1,4,5-trisphosphate receptor
MCU	Mitochondrial calcium uniporter
MPT	Mitochondrial permeability transition
NNT	Nicotinamide nucleotide transhydrogenase
OMM	Outer mitochondria membrane
PTP	Permeability transition pore
ROS	Reactive oxygen species
SHR	Spontaneous hypertensive rats
TSST	Thioredoxin
VDAC	Voltage-dependent anion-selective channel

Author details

Estela N.B. Busanello[1], Ana C. Marques[1], Estela Lorza-Gil[2], Helena C.F. de Oliveira[2] and Anibal E. Vercesi[1]*

*Address all correspondence to: anibal@unicamp.br

1 Faculty of Medical Sciences, Department of Clinical Pathology, UNICAMP, SP, Brazil

2 Institute of Biology, Department of Structural and Functional Biology, UNICAMP, SP, Brazil

References

[1] Brown MS, Goldstein JL. Receptor-mediated endocytosis: Insights from the lipoprotein receptor system. Proceedings of the National Academy of Sciences of the United States of America. 1974;**71**:788-792

[2] Vogt A. The genetics of familial hypercholesterolemia and emerging therapies. The Application of Clinical Genetics. 2015;**8**:27-36. DOI: 10.2147/TACG.S44315

[3] Shepherd J, Cobbe SM, Ford I, Isles CG, Lorimer AR, MacFarlane PW, McKillop JH, Packard CJ. Prevention of coronary heart disease with pravastatin in men with hypercholesterolemia. West of Scotland Coronary Prevention Study Group. The New England Journal of Medicine. 1995;**333**:1301-1307. DOI: 10.1056/NEJM199511163332001

[4] Collins R, Armitage J, Parish S, Sleigh P, Peto R, HPSC Group. MRC/BHF Heart Protection Study of cholesterol-lowering with simvastatin in 5963 people with diabetes: A randomised placebo-controlled trial. Lancet. 2003;**361**:2005-2016. DOI: 10.1016/S0140-6736(03)13636-7

[5] Gazzerro P, Proto MC, Gangemi G, Malfitano AM, Ciaglia E, Pisanti S, Santoro A, Laezza C, Bifulco M. Pharmacological actions of statins: A critical appraisal in the management of cancer. Pharmacological Reviews. 2012;**64**:102-146. DOI: 10.1124/pr.111.004994

[6] Vaughan CJ, Gotto AM, Basson CT. The evolving role of statins in the management of atherosclerosis. Journal of the American College of Cardiology. 2000;**35**:1-10. DOI: 10.1016/S0735-1097(99)00525-2

[7] Goldstein JL, Brown MS. Regulation of the mevalonate pathway. Nature. 1990;**343**:425-430. DOI: 10.1038/343425a0

[8] Endo A, Kuroda M. Citrinin, an inhibitor of cholesterol synthesis. The Journal of Antibiotics. 1976;**29**:841-843. DOI: 10.7164/antibiotics. 29.841

[9] Tanzawa K, Kuroda M, Endo A. Time-dependent, irreversible inhibition of 3-hydroxy-3-methylglutaryl-coenzyme A reductase by the antibiotic citrinin. Biochimica et Biophysica Acta. 1977;**488**:97-101

[10] Endo A, Tsujita Y, Kuroda M, Tanzawa K. Effects of ML-236B on cholesterol metabolism in mice and rats: Lack of hypocholesterolemic activity in normal animals. Biochimica et Biophysica Acta. 1979;**575**:266-276

[11] Endo AJ. Monacolin K. A new hypercholesterolemic agent produced by a monascus species. Antibiotics. 1979;**32**:852-854. DOI: 10.7164/antibiotics.32.852

[12] Alberts AW, Chen J, Kuron G, Hunt V, Huff J, Hoffman C, Rothrock J, Lopez M, Joshua H, Harris E, Patchett A, Monaghan R, Currie S, Stapley E, Albers-Schonberg G, Hensens O, Hirshfield J, Hoogsteen K, Liesch J, Springer J. Mevinolin: A highly potent competitive inhibitor of hydroxymethylglutaryl-coenzyme A reductase and a cholesterol-lowering agent. Proceedings of the National Academy of Sciences of the United States of America. 1980;**77**:3957-3961

[13] Endo A. A historical perspective on the discovery of statins. Proceedings of the Japan Academy. Series B, Physical and Biological Sciences. 2010;**86**:484-493. DOI: 10.2183/pjab.86.484

[14] Endo A. The discovery and development of HMG-CoA reductase inhibitors. Journal of Lipid Research. 1992;**33**:1569-1582

[15] Tobert JA. Lovastatin and beyond: The history of the HMG-CoA reductase inhibitors. Nature Reviews. Drug Discovery. 2003;**2**:517-526. DOI: 10.1038/nrd1112: 10.1038/nrd1112

[16] Saito Y. Pitavastatin: An overview. Atherosclerosis. Supplements. 2011;**12**:271-276. DOI: 10.1016/S1567-5688(11)70886-8

[17] Psaty BM, Furberg CD, Ray WA, Weiss NS. Potential for conflict of interest in the evaluation of suspected adverse drug reactions: Use of cerivastatin and risk of rhabdomyolysis. Journal of the American Medical Association. 2004;**292**:2622-2263. DOI: 10.1001/jama.292.21.2622

[18] Wise J. High intensity statins are associated with greatest reduction in mortality. British Medical Journal. 2016;**355**:1-1. DOI: 10.1136/bmj.i6048

[19] Manfredini V, Biancini GB, Vanzin CS, Dal Vesco AM, Cipriani F, Biasi L, Treméa R, Deon M, Peralba MC, Wajner M, Vargas CR. Simvastatin treatment prevents oxidative damage to DNA in whole blood leukocytes of dyslipidemic type 2 diabetic patients. Cell Biochemistry and Function. 2010;**28**:360-366. DOI: 10.1002/cbf.1654

[20] Li J, Sun YM, Wang LF, Li ZQ, Pan W, Cao HY. Comparison of effects of simvastatin versus atorvastatin on oxidative stress in patients with coronary heart disease. Clinical Cardiology. 2010;**33**:222-227. DOI: 10.1002/clc.20724

[21] Oliveira KA, Zecchin KG, Alberici LC, Castilho RF, Vercesi AE. Simvastatin inducing PC3 prostate cancer cell necrosis mediated by calcineurin and mitochondrial dysfunction. Journal of Bioenergetics and Biomembranes. 2008;**40**:307-314. DOI: 10.1007/s10863-008-9155-9

[22] Costa RA, Fernandes MP, de Souza-Pinto NC, Vercesi AE. Protective effects of l-carnitine and piracetam against mitochondrial permeability transition and PC3 cell necrosis induced by simvastatin. European Journal of Pharmacology. 2013;**701**:82-86. DOI: 10.1016/j.ejphar.2013.01.001

[23] Vercesi AE, Kowaltowski AJ, Oliveira HC, Castilho RF. Mitochondrial Ca2+ transport, permeability transition and oxidative stress in cell death: Implications in cardiotoxicity, neurodegeneration and dyslipidemias. Frontiers in Bioscience. 2006;**11**:2554-2564. DOI: 10.2741/1990

[24] Kowaltowski AJ. Alternative mitochondrial functions in cell physiopathology: Beyond ATP production. Brazilian Journal of Medical and Biological Research. 2000;**33**:241-250. DOI: 10.1590/S0100-879X2000000200014

[25] Vercesi AE, Castilho RF, Kowaltowski AJ, Oliveira HC. Mitochondrial energy metabolism and redox state in dyslipidemias. IUBMB Life. 2007;**59**:263-268. DOI: 10.1080/15216540601178091

[26] Figueira TR, Barros MH, Camargo AA, Castilho RF, Ferreira JC, Kowaltowski AJ, Sluse FE, Souza-Pinto NC, Vercesi AE. Mitochondria as a source of reactive oxygen and nitrogen species: From molecular mechanisms to human health. Antioxidants & Redox Signaling. 2013;**18**:2029-2074. DOI: 10.1089/ars.2012.4729

[27] Mitchell P. Coupling of phosphorylation to electron and hydrogen transfer by a chemiosmotic type of mechanism. Nature. 1961;**191**:144-148

[28] Korshunov SS, Skulachev VP, Starkov AA. High protonic potential actuates a mechanism of production of reactive oxygen species in mitochondria. FEBS Letters. 1997;**416**:15-18. DOI: 10.1016/S0014-5793(97)01159-9

[29] Turrens JF. Mitochondrial formation of reactive oxygen species. The Journal of Physiology. 2003;**552**:335-344. DOI: 10.1113/jphysiol.2003.049478

[30] Radi R, Turrens JF, Chang LY, Bush KM, Crapo JD, Freeman BA. Detection of catalase in rat heart mitochondria. The Journal of Biological Chemistry. 1991;**266**:22028-22034

[31] Yin F, Sancheti H, Cadenas E. Silencing of nicotinamide nucleotide transhydrogenase impairs cellular redox homeostasis and energy metabolism in PC12 cell. Biochimica et Biophysica Acta. 2012;**1817**:401-409. DOI: 10.1016/j.bbabio.2011.12.004

[32] Rydström J. Mitochondrial NADPH, transhydrogenase and disease. Biochimica et Biophysica Acta. 2006;**1757**:721-726. DOI: 10.1016/j.bbabio.2006.03.010

[33] Jo SH, Son MK, Koh HJ, Lee SM, Song IH, Kim YO, Lee YS, Jeong KS, Kim WB, Park JW, Song BJ, Huh TL, Huhe TL. Control of mitochondrial redox balance and cellular defense against oxidative damage by mitochondrial NADP+-dependent isocitrate dehydrogenase. The Journal of Biological Chemistry. 2001;**276**:16168-16176. DOI: 10.1074/jbc.M010120200

[34] Toledo JC, Augusto O. Connecting the chemical and biological properties of nitric oxide. Chemical Research in Toxicology. 2012;**25**:975-989. DOI: 10.1021/tx300042g

[35] Hamanaka RB, Chandel NS. Mitochondrial reactive oxygen species regulate cellular signaling and dictate biological outcomes. Trends in Biochemical Sciences. 2010;**35**:505-513. DOI: 10.1016/j.tibs.2010.04.002

[36] Dikalov S. Cross talk between mitochondria and NADPH oxidases. Free Radical Biology & Medicine. 2011;**51**:1289-1301. DOI: 10.1016/j.freeradbiomed.2011.06.033

[37] Ristow M. Unraveling the truth about antioxidants: Mitohormesis explains ROS-induced health benefits. Nature Medicine. 2014;**20**:709-711. DOI: 10.1038/nm.3624

[38] Yun J, Finkel T. Mitohormesis. Cell Metabolism. 2014;**19**:757-766. DOI: 10.1016/j.cmet.2014.01.011

[39] Husain K, Hernandez W, Ansari RA, Ferder L. Inflammation, oxidative stress and renin angiotensin system in atherosclerosis. World Journal of Biological Chemistry. 2015;**6**:209-217. DOI: 10.4331/wjbc.v6.i3.209

[40] Liu J, Wang Z. Increased oxidative stress as a selective anticancer therapy. Oxidative Medicine and Cellular Longevity. 2015;**2015**:294-303. DOI: 10.1155/2015/294303

[41] Santilli F, D'Ardes D, Davì G. Oxidative stress in chronic vascular disease: From prediction to prevention. Vascular Pharmacology. 2015;**74**:23-37. DOI: 10.1016/j.vph.2015.09.003

[42] Bhat AH, Dar KB, Anees S, Zargar MA, Masood A, Sofi MA, Ganie SA. Oxidative stress, mitochondrial dysfunction and neurodegenerative diseases: A mechanistic insight. Biomedicine & Pharmacotherapy. 2015;**74**:101-110. DOI: 10.1016/j.biopha.2015.07.025

[43] Ferrari RS, Andrade CF. Oxidative stress and lung ischemia-reperfusion injury. Oxidative Medicine and Cellular Longevity. 2015;**2015**:590-987. DOI: 10.1155/2015/590987

[44] Jones DP. Redox theory of aging. Redox Biology. 2015;**5**:71-79. DOI: 10.1016/j.redox.2015.03.004

[45] Sinha N, Dabla PK. Oxidative stress and antioxidants in hypertension-a current review. Current Hypertension Reviews. 2015;**11**:132-142. DOI: 10.2174/1573402111666150529130922

[46] Maiese K. New insights for oxidative stress and diabetes mellitus. Oxidative Medicine and Cellular Longevity. 2015;**2015**:875-961. DOI: 10.1155/2015/875961

[47] Abdoli N, Heidari R, Azarmi Y, Eghbal MA. Mechanisms of the statins cytotoxicity in freshly isolated rat hepatocytes. Journal of Biochemical and Molecular Toxicology. 2013;**27**:287-294. DOI: 10.1002/jbt.21485

[48] Kwak HB, Thalacker-Mercer A, Anderson EJ, Lin CT, Kane DA, Lee NS, Cortright RN, Bamman MM, Neufer PD. Simvastatin impairs ADP-stimulated respiration and increases mitochondrial oxidative stress in primary human skeletal myotubes. Free Radical Biology & Medicine. 2012;**52**:198-207. DOI: 10.1016/j.freeradbiomed.2011.10.449

[49] La Guardia PG, Alberici LC, Ravagnani FG, Catharino RR, Vercesi AE. Protection of rat skeletal muscle fibers by either L-carnitine or coenzyme Q10 against statins toxicity mediated by mitochondrial reactive oxygen generation. Frontiers in Physiology. 2013;**4**:103. DOI: 10.3389/fphys.2013.00103

[50] Berridge MJ, Bootman MD, Roderick HL. Calcium signalling: Dynamics, homeostasis and remodelling. Nature Reviews. Molecular Cell Biology. 2003;**4**:517-529. DOI: 10.1038/nrm1155

[51] Lehninger AL, Vercesi A, Bababunmi EA. Regulation of Ca2+ release from mitochondria by the oxidation-reduction state of pyridine nucleotides. Proceedings of the National Academy of Sciences of the United States of America. 1978;**75**:1690-1694

[52] Bhosale G, Sharpe JA, Sundier SY, Duchen MR. Calcium signaling as a mediator of cell energy demand and a trigger to cell death. Annals of the New York Academy of Sciences. 2015;**1350**:107-116. DOI: 10.1111/nyas.12885

[53] Vercesi AE, Kowaltowski AJ, Grijalba MT, Meinicke AR, Castilho RF. The role of reactive oxygen species in mitochondrial permeability transition. Bioscience Reports. 1997;**17**:43-52. DOI: 10.1023/A:1027335217774

[54] Hunter DR, Haworth RA, Southard JH. Relationship between configuration, function, and permeability in calcium-treated mitochondria. The Journal of Biological Chemistry. 1976;**251**:5069-5077

[55] Kowaltowski AJ, Castilho RF, Vercesi AE. Mitochondrial permeability transition and oxidative stress. FEBS Letters. 2001;**495**:12-15. DOI: 10.1016/S0014-5793(01)02316-X

[56] Grijalba MT, Vercesi AE, Schreier S. Ca2+-induced increased lipid packing and domain formation in submitochondrial particles. A possible early step in the mechanism of Ca2+-stimulated generation of reactive oxygen species by the respiratory chain. Biochemistry. 1999;**38**:13279-13287. DOI: 10.1021/bi9828674

[57] Javadov S, Kuznetsov A. Mitochondrial permeability transition and cell death: The role of cyclophilin d. Frontiers in Physiology. 2013;**4**:76. DOI: 10.3389/fphys.2013.00076

[58] Lemasters JJ, Nieminen AL, Qian T, Trost LC, Elmore SP, Nishimura Y, Crowe RA, Cascio WE, Bradham CA, Brenner DA, Herman B. The mitochondrial permeability transition in cell death: A common mechanism in necrosis, apoptosis and autophagy. Biochimica et Biophysica Acta. 1998;**1366**:177-196. DOI: 10.1016/S0005-2728(98)00112-1

[59] Bernardi P, Krauskopf A, Basso E, Petronilli V, Blachly-Dyson E, Blalchy-Dyson E, Di Lisa F, Forte MA. The mitochondrial permeability transition from in vitro artifact to disease target. The FEBS Journal. 2006;**273**:2077-2099. DOI: 10.1111/j.1742-4658.2006.05213.x

[60] Halestrap AP, Pasdois P. The role of the mitochondrial permeability transition pore in heart disease. Biochimica et Biophysica Acta. 2009;**1787**:1402-1415. DOI: 10.1016/j.bbabio.2008.12.017

[61] Kroemer G, Galluzzi L, Brenner C. Mitochondrial membrane permeabilization in cell death. Physiological Reviews. 2007;**87**:99-163. DOI: 10.1152/physrev.00013.2006:

[62] Mbye LH, Singh IN, Carrico KM, Saatman KE, Hall ED. Comparative neuroprotective effects of cyclosporin A and NIM811, a nonimmunosuppressive cyclosporin A analog, following traumatic brain injury. Journal of Cerebral Blood Flow and Metabolism. 2009;**29**:87-97. DOI: 10.1038/jcbfm.2008.93

[63] Russmann S, Kullak-Ublick GA, Grattagliano I. Current concepts of mechanisms in drug-induced hepatotoxicity. Current Medicinal Chemistry. 2009;**16**:3041-3053. DOI: 10.2174/092986709788803097

[64] Starkov AA, Chinopoulos C, Fiskum G. Mitochondrial calcium and oxidative stress as mediators of ischemic brain injury. Cell Calcium. 2004;**36**:257-264. DOI: 10.1016/j.ceca.2004.02.012

[65] Vaseva AV, Marchenko ND, Ji K, Tsirka SE, Holzmann S, Moll UM. p53 opens the mitochondrial permeability transition pore to trigger necrosis. Cell. 2012;**149**:1536-1548. DOI: 10.1016/j.cell.2012.05.014

[66] Alberici LC, Oliveira HC, Patrício PR, Kowaltowski AJ, Vercesi AE. Hyperlipidemic mice present enhanced catabolism and higher mitochondrial ATP-sensitive K+ channel activity. Gastroenterology. 2006;**131**:1228-1234. DOI: 10.1053/j.gastro.2006.07.021

[67] Oliveira HC, Cosso RG, Alberici LC, Maciel EN, Salerno AG, Dorighello GG, Velho JA, de Faria EC, Vercesi AE. Oxidative stress in atherosclerosis-prone mouse is due to low antioxidant capacity of mitochondria. The FASEB Journal. 2005;**19**:278-280. DOI: 10.1096/fj.04-2095fje

[68] Gunter TE, Sheu SS. Characteristics and possible functions of mitochondrial Ca(2+) transport mechanisms. Biochimica et Biophysica Acta. 2009;**1787**:1291-1308. DOI: 10.1016/j.bbabio.2008.12.011

[69] Deluca HF, Engstom GW. Calcium uptake by rat kidney mitochondria. Proceedings of the National Academy of Sciences of the United States of America. 1961;**47**:1744-1750

[70] Vasington FD, Murphy JV. Ca ion uptake by rat kidney mitochondria and its dependence on respiration and phosphorylation. The Journal of Biological Chemistry. 1962; **237**:2670-2677

[71] Baughman JM, Perocchi F, Girgis HS, Plovanich M, Belcher-Timme CA, Sancak Y, Bao XR, Strittmatter L, Goldberger O, Bogorad RL, Koteliansky V, Mootha VK. Integrative genomics identifies MCU as an essential component of the mitochondrial calcium uniporter. Nature. 2011;**476**:341-345. DOI: 10.1038/nature10234

[72] De Stefani D, Raffaello A, Teardo E, Szabo I, Rizzuto R. A forty-kilodalton protein of the inner membrane is the mitochondrial calcium uniporter. Nature. 2011;**476**:336-340. DOI: 10.1038/nature10230

[73] Palty R, Silverman WF, Hershfinkel M, Caporale T, Sensi SL, Parnis J, Nolte C, Fishman D, Shoshan-Barmatz V, Herrmann S, Khananshvili D, Sekler I. NCLX is an essential component of mitochondrial Na+/Ca2+ exchange. Proceedings of the National Academy of Sciences of the United States of America. 2010;**107**:436-441. DOI: 10.1073/pnas.0908099107

[74] Kang TM, Hilgemann DW. Multiple transport modes of the cardiac Na+/Ca2+ exchanger. Nature. 2004;**427**:544-548. DOI: 10.1038/nature02271

[75] Hajnóczky G, Csordás G. Calcium signalling: Fishing out molecules of mitochondrial calcium transport. Current Biology. 2010;**20**:888-891. DOI: 10.1016/j.cub.2010.09.035

[76] Docampo R, Vercesi AE. Ca2+ transport by coupled Trypanosoma cruzi mitochondria in situ. The Journal of Biological Chemistry. 1989;**264**:108-111

[77] Rizzuto R, Brini M, Murgia M, Pozzan T. Microdomains with high Ca2+ close to IP3-sensitive channels that are sensed by neighboring mitochondria. Science. 1993;**262**:744-747. DOI: 10.1126/science.8235595

[78] Pozzan T, Rizzuto R, Volpe P, Meldolesi J. Molecular and cellular physiology of intracellular calcium stores. Physiological Reviews. 1994;**74**:595-636

[79] Rizzuto R, Pinton P, Carrington W, Fay FS, Fogarty KE, Lifshitz LM, Tuft RA, Pozzan T. Close contacts with the endoplasmic reticulum as determinants of mitochondrial Ca2+ responses. Science. 1998;**280**:1763-1766. DOI: 10.1126/science.280.5370.1763

[80] Bonfils C, Bec N, Larroque C, Del Rio M, Gongora C, Pugnière M, Martineau P. Cyclophilin A as negative regulator of apoptosis by sequestering cytochrome c. Biochemical and Biophysical Research Communications. 2010;**393**:325-330. DOI: 10.1016/j.bbrc.2010.01.135

[81] Kowaltowski AJ, Vercesi AE, Fiskum G. Bcl-2 prevents mitochondrial permeability transition and cytochrome c release via maintenance of reduced pyridine nucleotides. Cell Death and Differentiation 2000;**7**:903-910. DOI: 10.1038/sj.cdd.4400722

[82] Murphy AN, Bredesen DE, Cortopassi G, Wang E, Fiskum G. Bcl-2 potentiates the maximal calcium uptake capacity of neural cell mitochondria. Proceedings of the National Academy of Sciences of the United States of America. 1996;**93**:9893-9898

[83] Castilho RF, Kowaltowski AJ, Meinicke AR, Bechara EJ, Vercesi AE. Permeabilization of the inner mitochondrial membrane by Ca2+ ions is stimulated by t-butyl hydroperoxide and mediated by reactive oxygen species generated by mitochondria. Free Radical Biology & Medicine. 1995;**18**:479-486. DOI: 10.1016/0891-5849(94)00166-H

[84] Castilho RF, Kowaltowski AJ, Vercesi AE. The irreversibility of inner mitochondrial membrane permeabilization by Ca2+ plus prooxidants is determined by the extent of membrane protein thiol cross-linking. Journal of Bioenergetics and Biomembranes. 1996;**28**:523-529

[85] Fagian MM, Pereira-da-Silva L, Martins IS, Vercesi AE. Membrane protein thiol cross-linking associated with the permeabilization of the inner mitochondrial membrane by Ca2+ plus prooxidants. The Journal of Biological Chemistry. 1990;**265**:19955-19960

[86] Kowaltowski AJ, Netto LE, Vercesi AE. The thiol-specific antioxidant enzyme prevents mitochondrial permeability transition. Evidence for the participation of reactive oxygen species in this mechanism. The Journal of Biological Chemistry. 1998;**273**:12766-12769. DOI: 10.1074/jbc.273.21.12766

[87] Kowaltowski AJ, de Souza-Pinto NC, Castilho RF, Vercesi AE. Mitochondria and reactive oxygen species. Free Radical Biology & Medicine. 2009;**47**:333-343. DOI: 10.1016/j.freeradbiomed.2009.05.004

[88] Vercesi AE, Pereira-da-Silva L. NADP redox state and mitochondrial Ca2+ efflux: A controversial issue. Brazilian Journal of Medical and Biological Research. 1984;**17**:353-356

[89] Maciel EN, Kowaltowski AJ, Schwalm FD, Rodrigues JM, Souza DO, Vercesi AE, Wajner M, Castilho RF. NADP redox state and mitochondrial Ca2+ efflux: A controversial issue. Journal of Neurochemistry. 2004;**90**:1025-1035. DOI: 10.1111/j.1471-4159.2004.02565.x

[90] Kowaltowski AJ, Castilho RF. Ca2+ acting at the external side of the inner mitochondrial membrane can stimulate mitochondrial permeability transition induced by phenylarsine oxide. Biochimica et Biophysica Acta. 1997;**1322**:221-229. DOI: 10.1016/S0005-2728(97)00078-9

[91] Kowaltowski AJ, Castilho RF, Vercesi AE. Opening of the mitochondrial permeability transition pore by uncoupling or inorganic phosphate in the presence of Ca2+ is dependent on mitochondrial-generated reactive oxygen species. FEBS Letters. 1996;**378**:150-152. DOI: 10.1016/0014-5793(95)01449-7

[92] Ronchi JA, Figueira TR, Ravagnani FG, Oliveira HC, Vercesi AE, Castilho RF. A spontaneous mutation in the nicotinamide nucleotide transhydrogenase gene of C57BL/6J mice results in mitochondrial redox abnormalities. Free Radical Biology & Medicine. 2013;**63**:446-456. DOI: 10.1016/j.freeradbiomed.2013.05.049

[93] Ronchi JA, Francisco A, Passos LA, Figueira TR, Castilho RF. The contribution of nicotinamide nucleotide transhydrogenase to peroxide detoxification is dependent on the respiratory state and counterbalanced by other sources of NADPH in liver mitochondria. The Journal of Biological Chemistry. 2016;**291**:20173-20187. DOI: 10.1074/jbc.M116.730473

[94] Valle VG, Fagian MM, Parentoni LS, Meinicke AR, Vercesi AE. The participation of reactive oxygen species and protein thiols in the mechanism of mitochondrial inner membrane permeabilization by calcium plus prooxidants. Archives of Biochemistry and Biophysics. 1993;**307**:1-7. DOI: 10.1006/abbi.1993.1551

[95] Castilho RF, Kowaltowski AJ, Meinicke AR, Vercesi AE. Oxidative damage of mitochondria induced by Fe(II)citrate or t-butyl hydroperoxide in the presence of Ca^{2+}: Effect of coenzyme Q redox state. Free Radical Biology & Medicine. 1995;**18**:55-59

[96] Parihar A, Parihar MS, Zenebe WJ, Ghafourifar P. Statins lower calcium-induced oxidative stress in isolated mitochondria. Human & Experimental Toxicology. 2012;**31**:355-363. DOI: 10.1177/0960327111429141

[97] Futterman LG, Lemberg L. Statin pleiotropy: Fact or fiction? American Journal of Critical Care. 2004;**13**:244-249

[98] Du R, Zhao XQ, Cai J, Cui B, Wu HM, Ye P. Journal of Clinical Lipidology. 2016;**10**:587-593. DOI: 10.1016/j.jacl.2016.01.004

[99] Zhou Q, Liao JK. Changes in carotid plaque tissue composition in subjects who continued and discontinued statin therapy. Circulation Journal. 2010;**74**:818-826. DOI: 10.1253/circj.CJ-10-0110

[100] Demierre MF, Higgins PD, Gruber SB, Hawk E, Lippman SM. Statins and cancer prevention. Nature Reviews. Cancer. 2005;**5**:930-942. DOI: 10.1038/nrc1751

[101] Steinberg D. The LDL modification hypothesis of atherogenesis: An update. Journal of Lipid Research. 2009;**50**(Suppl):S376-S381. DOI: 10.1194/jlr

[102] Morel DW, DiCorleto PE, Chisolm GM. Endothelial and smooth muscle cells alter low density lipoprotein in vitro by free radical oxidation. Arteriosclerosis. 1984;**4**:357-364. DOI: 10.1161/01.ATV.4.4.357

[103] Lamb DJ, Wilkins GM, Leake DS. The oxidative modification of low density lipoprotein by human lymphocytes. Atherosclerosis. 1992;**92**:187-192. DOI: 10.1016/0021-9150(92)90277-N

[104] Wassmann S, Laufs U, Müller K, Konkol C, Ahlbory K, Bäumer AT, Linz W, Böhm M, Nickenig G. Cellular antioxidant effects of atorvastatin in vitro and in vivo. Arteriosclerosis, Thrombosis, and Vascular Biology. 2002;**22**:300-305

[105] Carneado J, Alvarez de Sotomayor M, Perez-Guerrero C, Jimenez L, Herrera MD, Pamies E, Martin-Sanz MD, Stiefel P, Miranda M, Bravo L, Marhuenda E. Simvastatin improves endothelial function in spontaneously hypertensive rats through a superoxide dismutase mediated antioxidant effect. Journal of Hypertension. 2002;**20**:429-437

[106] Ajith TA, Riji T, Anu V. In vitro anti-oxidant and DNA protective effects of the novel 3-hydroxy-3-methylglutaryl coenzyme A reductase inhibitor rosuvastatin. Clinical and Experimental Pharmacology and Physiology. 2008;**35**:625-629. DOI: 10.1111/j.1440-1681.2007.04853.x

[107] Schupp N, Schmid U, Heidland A, Stopper H. Rosuvastatin protects against oxidative stress and DNA damage in vitro via upregulation of glutathione synthesis. Atherosclerosis. 2008;**199**:278-287. DOI: 10.1016/j.atherosclerosis.2007.11.016

[108] Jahovic N, Gedik N, Ercan F, Sirvanci S, Yüksel M, Sener G, Alican I. Effects of statins on experimental colitis in normocholesterolemic rats. Scandinavian Journal of Gastroenterology. 2006;**41**:954-962. DOI: 10.1080/00365520600554444

[109] Velho JA, Okanobo H, Degasperi GR, Matsumoto MY, Alberici LC, Cosso RG, Oliveira HC, Vercesi AE. Statins induce calcium-dependent mitochondrial permeability transition. Toxicology. 2006;**219**:124-132. DOI: 10.1016/j.tox.2005.11.007

[110] Menter DG, Ramsauer VP, Harirforoosh S, Chakraborty K, Yang P, Hsi L, Newman RA, Krishnan K. Differential effects of pravastatin and simvastatin on the growth of tumor cells from different organ sites. PLoS One. 2011;**6**:28813. DOI: 10.1371/journal.pone.0028813

[111] Thibault A, Samid D, Tompkins AC, Figg WD, Cooper MR, Hohl RJ, Trepel J, Liang B, Patronas N, Venzon DJ, Reed E, Myers CE. Phase I study of lovastatin, an inhibitor of the mevalonate pathway, in patients with cancer. Clinical Cancer Research. 1996;**2**:483-491

[112] Larner J, Jane J, Laws E, Packer R, Myers C, Shaffrey M. A phase I-II trial of lovastatin for anaplastic astrocytoma and glioblastoma multiforme. American Journal of Clinical Oncology. 1998;**21**:579-583

[113] Hindler K, Cleeland CS, Rivera E, Collard CD. The role of statins in cancer therapy. The Oncologist. 2006;**11**:306-315. DOI: 10.1634/theoncologist.11-3-306

[114] Matusewicz L, Meissner J, Toporkiewicz M, Sikorski AF. The effect of statins on cancer cells–review. Tumour Biology. 2015;**36**:4889-4904. DOI: 10.1007/s13277-015-3551-7

[115] Ke Zhou C, Check DP, Lortet-Tieulent J, Laversanne M, Jemal A, Ferlay J, Bray F, Cook MB, Devesa SS. Prostate cancer incidence in 43 populations worldwide: An analysis of time trends overall and by age group. International Journal of Cancer. 2015;**6**:1388-1400. DOI: 10.1002/ijc.29894

[116] Marcella SW, David A, Ohman-Strickland PA, Carson J, Rhoads GG. Statin use and fatal prostate cancer: A matched case-control study. Cancer. 2012;**118**:4046-4052. DOI: 10.1002/cncr.26720

[117] Mondul AM, Weinstein SJ, Virtamo J, Albanes D. Serum total and HDL cholesterol and risk of prostate cancer. Cancer Causes & Control 2011;**22**:1545-1552. DOI: 10.1007/s10552-011-9831-7

[118] Konstantinopoulos PA, Karamouzis MV, Papavassiliou AG. Post-translational modifications and regulation of the RAS superfamily of GTPases as anticancer targets. Nature Reviews. Drug Discovery. 2007;**6**:541-555. DOI: 10.1038/nrd2221: 10.1038/nrd2221

[119] Park YH, Seo SY, Lee E, Ku JH, Kim HH, Kwak C. Simvastatin induces apoptosis in castrate resistant prostate cancer cells by deregulating nuclear factor-κB pathway. The Journal of Urology. 2013;**189**:1547-1552. DOI: 10.1016/j.juro.2012.10.030

[120] Ghosh PM, Ghosh-Choudhury N, Moyer ML, Mott GE, Thomas CA, Foster BA, Greenberg NM, Kreisberg JI. Role of RhoA activation in the growth and morphology of a murine prostate tumor cell line. Oncogene. 1999;**18**:4120-4130. DOI: 10.1038/sj.onc.1202792

[121] Peng X, Li W, Yuan L, Mehta RG, Kopelovich L, McCormick DL. Inhibition of proliferation and induction of autophagy by atorvastatin in PC3 prostate cancer cells correlate with downregulation of Bcl2 and upregulation of miR-182 and p21. PLoS One. 2013;**8**:e70442. DOI: 10.1371/journal.pone.0070442

[122] Marcelli M, Cunningham GR, Haidacher SJ, Padayatty SJ, Sturgis L, Kagan C, Denner L. Caspase-7 is activated during lovastatin-induced apoptosis of the prostate cancer cell line LNCaP. Cancer Research. 1998;**58**:76-83

[123] Goc A, Kochuparambil ST, Al-Husein B, Al-Azayzih A, Mohammad S, Somanath PR. Simultaneous modulation of the intrinsic and extrinsic pathways by simvastatin in mediating prostate cancer cell apoptosis. BMC Cancer. 2012;**12**:409. DOI: 10.1186/1471-2407-12-409

[124] Hoque A, Chen H, Xu XC. Statin induces apoptosis and cell growth arrest in prostate cancer cells. Cancer Epidemiology, Biomarkers & Prevention. 2008;**17**:88-94. DOI: 10.1158/1055-9965.EPI-07-0531

[125] Li YC, Park MJ, Ye SK, Kim CW, Kim YN. Elevated levels of cholesterol-rich lipid rafts in cancer cells are correlated with apoptosis sensitivity induced by cholesterol-depleting agents. The American Journal of Pathology. 2006;**168**:1107-1118. quiz 1404-1105. DOI: 10.2353/ajpath.2006.050959

[126] Zhuang L, Kim J, Adam RM, Solomon KR, Freeman MR. Cholesterol targeting alters lipid raft composition and cell survival in prostate cancer cells and xenografts. The Journal of Clinical Investigation. 2005;**115**:959-968. DOI: 10.1172/JCI19935

[127] Hu M, Cheung BM, Tomlinson B. Safety of statins: An update. Therapeutic Advances in Drug Safety. 2012;**3**:133-144. DOI: 10.1177/2042098612439884

[128] Evans M, Rees A. The myotoxicity of statins. Current Opinion in Lipidology. 2002;**13**:415-420

[129] Andrade SE, Walker AM, Gottlieb LK, Hollenberg NK, Testa MA, Saperia GM, Platt R. Discontinuation of antihyperlipidemic drugs–do rates reported in clinical trials reflect rates in primary care settings? The New England Journal of Medicine. 1995;**332**:1125-1131. DOI: 10.1056/NEJM199504273321703

[130] Sung JC, Nichol MB, Venturini F, Bailey KL, McCombs JS, Cody M. Factors affecting patient compliance with antihyperlipidemic medications in an HMO population. The American Journal of Managed Care. 1998;**4**:1421-1430

[131] Stojaković N, Igić R. Simvastatin-lnduced nocturnal leg pain disappears with pravastatin substitution. Srpski Arhiv za Celokupno Lekarstvo. 2013;**141**:387-389. DOI: 10.2298/SARH1306387S

[132] Kowaltowski AJ, Vercesi AE. Mitochondrial damage induced by conditions of oxidative stress. Free Radical Biology and Medicine. 1999;**26**:463-471. DOI: S0891-5849(98)00216-0

[133] Kaufmann P, Török M, Zahno A, Waldhauser KM, Brecht K, Krähenbühl S. Toxicity of statins on rat skeletal muscle mitochondria. Cellular and Molecular Life Sciences. 2006;**63**:2415-2425. DOI: 10.1007/s00018-006-6235-z

[134] Paim BA, Velho JA, Castilho RF, Oliveira HC, Vercesi AE. Oxidative stress in hypercholesterolemic LDL (low-density lipoprotein) receptor knockout mice is associated with low content of mitochondrial NADP-linked substrates and is partially reversed by citrate replacement. Free Radical Biology & Medicine. 2008;**44**:444-451. DOI: 10.1016/j.freeradbiomed.2007.10.005

[135] Ishibashi S, Brown MS, Goldstein JL, Gerard RD, Hammer RE, Herz J. Hypercholesterolemia in low density lipoprotein receptor knockout mice and its reversal by adenovirus-mediated gene delivery. The Journal of Clinical Investigation. 1993;**92**:883-893. DOI: 10.1172/JCI116663

[136] Nakahara K, Yada T, Kuriyama M, Osame M. Cytosolic Ca2+ increase and cell damage in L6 rat myoblasts by HMG-CoA reductase inhibitors. Biochemical and Biophysical Research Communications. 1994;**202**:1579-1585. DOI: 10.1006/bbrc.1994.2112

[137] Pierno S, De Luca A, Liantonio A, Camerino C, Conte Camerino D. Effects of HMG-CoA reductase inhibitors on excitation-contraction coupling of rat skeletal muscle. European Journal of Pharmacology. 1999;**364**:43-48. DOI: 10.1016/S0014-2999(98)00817-6

[138] Sirvent P, Mercier J, Vassort G, Lacampagne A. Simvastatin triggers mitochondria-induced Ca2+ signaling alteration in skeletal muscle. Biochemical and Biophysical Research Communications. 2005;**329**:1067-1075. DOI: 10.1016/j.bbrc.2005.02.070

[139] Hattori T, Saito K, Takemura M, Ito H, Ohta H, Wada H, Sei Y, Kawamura M, Seishima M. Statin-induced Ca(2+) release was increased in B lymphocytes in patients who showed elevated serum creatine kinase during statin treatment. Journal of Atherosclerosis and Thrombosis. 2009;**16**:870-877. DOI: 10.5551/jat.2048

[140] Flint DH, Tuminello JF, Emptage MH. The inactivation of Fe-S cluster containing hydro-lyases by superoxide. The Journal of Biological Chemistry. 1993;**268**:22369-22376

[141] Radi R, Rodriguez M, Castro L, Telleri R. Inhibition of mitochondrial electron transport by peroxynitrite. Archives of Biochemistry and Biophysics. 1994;**308**:89-95. DOI: 10.1006/abbi.1994.1013

[142] Fridovich I. Superoxide radical and superoxide dismutases. Annual Review of Biochemistry. 1995;**64**:97-112. DOI: 10.1146/annurev.bi.64.070195.000525

[143] Bouton C, Raveau M, Drapier JC. Modulation of iron regulatory protein functions. Further insights into the role of nitrogen- and oxygen-derived reactive species. The Journal of Biological Chemistry. 1996;**271**:2300-2306

[144] Demicheli V, Quijano C, Alvarez B, Radi R. Inactivation and nitration of human superoxide dismutase (SOD) by fluxes of nitric oxide and superoxide. Free Radical Biology & Medicine. 2007;**42**:1359-1368. DOI: 10.1016/j.freeradbiomed.2007.01.034

[145] Panov A, Dikalov S, Shalbuyeva N, Taylor G, Sherer T, Greenamyre JT. Rotenone model of Parkinson disease: Multiple brain mitochondria dysfunctions after short term systemic rotenone intoxication. The Journal of Biological Chemistry. 2005;**280**:42026-42035. DOI: 10.1074/jbc.M508628200

[146] Gülçin I. Antioxidant and antiradical activities of L-carnitine. Life Sciences. 2006;**78**:803-811. DOI: 10.1016/j.lfs.2005.05.103

[147] Sirvent P, Fabre O, Bordenave S, Hillaire-Buys D, Raynaud De Mauverger E, Lacampagne A, Mercier J. Muscle mitochondrial metabolism and calcium signaling impairment in patients treated with statins. Toxicology and Applied Pharmacology. 2012;**259**:263-268. DOI: 10.1016/j.taap.2012.01.008

[148] Schirris TJ, Renkema GH, Ritschel T, Voermans NC, Bilos A, van Engelen BG, Brandt U, Koopman WJ, Beyrath JD, Rodenburg RJ, Willems PH, Smeitink JA, Russel FG. Statin-induced myopathy is associated with mitochondrial complex III inhibition. Cell Metabolism. 2015;**22**:399-407. DOI: 10.1016/j.cmet.2015.08.002

[149] Bruckert E, Hayem G, Dejager S, Yau C, Bégaud B. Mild to moderate muscular symptoms with high-dosage statin therapy in hyperlipidemic patients–the PRIMO study. Cardiovascular Drugs and Therapy. 2005;**19**:403-414. DOI: 10.1007/s10557-005-5686-z

[150] Stroes ES, Thompson PD, Corsini A, Vladutiu GD, Raal FJ, Ray KK, Roden M, Stein E, Tokgözoğlu L, Nordestgaard BG, Bruckert E, De Backer G, Krauss RM, Laufs U, Santos RD, Hegele RA, Hovingh GK, Leiter LA, Mach F, März W, Newman CB, Wiklund O, Jacobson TA, Catapano AL, Chapman MJ, Ginsberg HN. Statin-associated muscle symptoms: Impact on statin therapy-European atherosclerosis society consensus panel statement on assessment, aetiology and management. EASC panel. European Heart Journal. 2015;**36**:1012-1022. DOI: 10.1093/eurheartj/ehv043

[151] Trøseid M, Henriksen OA, Lindal S. Statin-associated myopathy with normal creatine kinase levels. Case report from a Norwegian family. Acta Pathologica, Microbiologica et Immunologica Scandinavica. 2005;**113**:635-637. DOI: 10.1111/j.1600-0463.2005.apm_270.x

[152] Draeger A, Monastyrskaya K, Mohaupt M, Hoppeler H, Savolainen H, Allemann C, Babiychuk EB. Statin therapy induces ultrastructural damage in skeletal muscle in patients without myalgia. The Journal of Pathology. 2006;**210**:94-102. DOI: 10.1002/path.2018

[153] Taha DA, De Moor CH, Barrett DA, Gershkovich P. Translational insight into statin-induced muscle toxicity: From cell culture to clinical studies. Translational Research. 2014;**164**:85-109. DOI: 10.1016/j.trsl.2014.01.013

[154] Tomaszewski M, Stępień KM, Tomaszewska J, Czuczwar SJ. Statin-induced myopathies. Pharmacological Reports. 2011;**63**:859-866

[155] Phillips PS, Haas RH, Bannykh S, Hathaway S, Gray NL, Kimura BJ, Vladutiu GD, England JD. Statin-associated myopathy with normal creatine kinase levels. SMCR Center. Annals of Internal Medicine. 2002;**137**:581-585. DOI: 10.7326/0003-4819-137-7-200210010-00009

[156] Gambelli S, Dotti MT, Malandrini A, Mondelli M, Stromillo ML, Gaudiano C, Federico A. Mitochondrial alterations in muscle biopsies of patients on statin therapy. Journal of Submicroscopic Cytology and Pathology. 2004;**36**:85-89

[157] Schick BA, Laaksonen R, Frohlich JJ, Päivä H, Lehtimäki T, Humphries KH, Côté HC. Decreased skeletal muscle mitochondrial DNA in patients treated with high-dose simvastatin. Clinical Pharmacology and Therapeutics. 2007;**81**:650-653. DOI: 10.1038/sj.clpt.6100124

[158] Masters BA, Palmoski MJ, Flint OP, Gregg RE, Wang-Iverson D, Durham SK. In vitro myotoxicity of the 3-hydroxy-3-methylglutaryl coenzyme A reductase inhibitors, pravastatin, lovastatin, and simvastatin, using neonatal rat skeletal myocytes. Toxicology and Applied Pharmacology. 1995;**131**:163-174. DOI: 10.1006/taap.1995.1058

[159] Pierno S, Didonna MP, Cippone V, De Luca A, Pisoni M, Frigeri A, Nicchia GP, Svelto M, Chiesa G, Sirtori C, Scanziani E, Rizzo C, De Vito D, Conte Camerino D. Effects of chronic treatment with statins and fenofibrate on rat skeletal muscle: A biochemical, histological and electrophysiological study. British Journal of Pharmacology. 2006;**149**:909-919. DOI: 10.1038/sj.bjp.0706917

[160] Chatzizisis YS, Koskinas KC, Misirli G, Vaklavas C, Hatzitolios A, Giannoglou GD. Risk factors and drug interactions predisposing to statin-induced myopathy: Implications for risk assessment, prevention and treatment. Drug Safety. 2010;**33**:171-187. DOI: 10.2165/11319380-000000000-00000

[161] Generaux GT, Bonomo FM, Johnson M, Doan KM. Impact of SLCO1B1 (OATP1B1) and ABCG2 (BCRP) genetic polymorphisms and inhibition on LDL-C lowering and myopathy of statins. Xenobiotica. 2011;**41**:639-651. DOI: 10.3109/00498254.2011.562566

[162] Voora D, Shah SH, Spasojevic I, Ali S, Reed CR, Salisbury BA, Ginsburg GS. The SLCO1B1*5 genetic variant is associated with statin-induced side effects. Journal of the American College of Cardiology. 2009:**54**;1609-1616. DOI: 10.1016/j.jacc.2009.04.053

[163] Donnelly LA, Doney AS, Tavendale R, Lang CC, Pearson ER, Colhoun HM, McCarthy MI, Hattersley AT, Morris AD, Palmer CN. Common nonsynonymous substitutions in SLCO1B1 predispose to statin intolerance in routinely treated individuals with type 2 diabetes: A go-DARTS study. Clinical Pharmacology and Therapeutics. 2011; **89**:210-216. DOI: 10.1038/clpt.2010.255

[164] Cornachione AS, Benedini-Elias PC, Polizello JC, Carvalho LC, Mattiello-Sverzut AC. Characterization of fiber types in different muscles of the hindlimb in female weanling and adult Wistar rats. Acta Histochemica et Cytochemica. 2011;**44**:43-50. DOI: 10.1267/ahc.10031

[165] Ji LL, Fu R, Mitchell EW. Glutathione and antioxidant enzymes in skeletal muscle: Effects of fiber type and exercise intensity. Journal of Applied Physiology. 1992;**73**:1854-1859

[166] Busanello ENB, Marques AC, Lander N, de Oliveira DN, Catharino RR, Oliveira HCF, Vercesi AE. Pravastatin chronic treatment sensitizes hypercholesterolemic mice muscle

to mitochondrial permeability transition: Protection by creatine or coenzyme Q10. Frontiers in Pharmacology. 2017;**8**:185. DOI: 10.3389/fphar.2017.00185

[167] Waclawik AJ, Lindal S, Engel AG. Experimental lovastatin myopathy. Journal of Neuropathology and Experimental Neurology. 1993;**52**:542-549

[168] Westwood FR, Bigley A, Randall K, Marsden AM, Scott RC. Statin-induced muscle necrosis in the rat: Distribution, development, and fibre selectivity. Toxicologic Pathology. 2005; **33**:246-257. DOI: 10.1080/01926230590908213

[169] Westwood FR, Scott RC, Marsden AM, Bigley A, Randall K. Rosuvastatin: Characterization of induced myopathy in the rat. Toxicologic Pathology. 2008;**36**:345-352. DOI: 10.1177/0192623307311412

[170] Schaefer WH, Lawrence JW, Loughlin AF, Stoffregen DA, Mixson LA, Dean DC, Raab CE, NX Y, Lankas GR, Frederick CB. Evaluation of ubiquinone concentration and mitochondrial function relative to cerivastatin-induced skeletal myopathy in rats. Toxicology and Applied Pharmacology. 2004;**194**:10-23. DOI: 10.1016/j.taap.2003.08.013

[171] Seachrist JL, Loi CM, Evans MG, Criswell KA, Rothwell CE. Roles of exercise and pharmacokinetics in cerivastatin-induced skeletal muscle toxicity. Toxicological Sciences. 2005;**88**:551-561

[172] Rasola A, Sciacovelli M, Pantic B, Bernardi P. Signal transduction to the permeability transition pore. FEBS Letters. 2010;**584**:1989-1996. DOI: 10.1016/j.febslet.2010.02.022

[173] Björnsson E, Jacobsen EI, Kalaitzakis E. Hepatotoxicity associated with statins: Reports of idiosyncratic liver injury post-marketing. Journal of Hepatology. 2012;**56**:374-380. DOI: 10.1016/j.jhep.2011.07.023

[174] Perdices EV, Medina-Cáliz I, Hernando S, Ortega A, Martín-Ocaña F, Navarro JM, Peláez G, Castiella A, Hallal H, Romero-Gómez M, González-Jiménez A, Robles-Díaz M, Lucena MI, Andrade RJ. Hepatotoxicity associated with statin use: Analysis of the cases included in the Spanish Hepatotoxicity Registry. Revista Española de Enfermedades Digestivas. 2014;**106**:246-254

[175] Carrascosa MF, Salcines-Caviedes JR, Lucena MI, Andrade RJ. Acute liver failure following atorvastatin dose escalation: is there a threshold dose for idiosyncratic hepatotoxicity? Journal of Hepatology. 2015;**62**:751-752. DOI: 10.1016/j.jhep.2014.11.019

[176] Medina-Caliz I, Robles-Diaz M, Garcia-Muñoz B, Stephens C, Ortega-Alonso A, Garcia-Cortes M, González-Jimenez A, Sanabria-Cabrera JA, Moreno I, Fernandez MC, Romero-Gomez M, Navarro JM, Barriocanal AM, Montane E, Hallal H, Blanco S, Soriano G, Roman EM, Gómez-Dominguez E, Castiella A, Zapata EM, Jimenez-Perez M, Moreno JM, Aldea-Perona A, Hernández-Guerra M, Prieto M, Zoubek ME, Kaplowitz N, Lucena MI, Andrade RJ. Definition and risk factors for chronicity following acute idiosyncratic drug-induced liver injury. SD registry. Journal of Hepatology. 2016;**65**:532-542. DOI: 10.1016/j.jhep.2016.05.003

[177] Goldberg AC, Sapre A, Liu J, Capece R, Mitchel YB, Group ES. Efficacy and safety of ezetimibe coadministered with simvastatin in patients with primary hypercholesterolemia: a randomized, double-blind, placebo-controlled trial. Mayo Clinic Proceedings. 2004;**79**:620-629. DOI: 10.1016/S0025-6196(11)62283-0

[178] Björnsson ES. Hepatotoxicity of statins and other lipid-lowering agents. Liver International. 2017;**37**:173-178. DOI: 10.1111/liv.13308

[179] Andrade RJ, Lucena MI, Fernández MC, Pelaez G, Pachkoria K, García-Ruiz E, García-Muñoz B, González-Grande R, Pizarro A, Durán JA, Jiménez M, Rodrigo L, Romero-Gomez M, Navarro JM, Planas R, Costa J, Borras A, Soler A, Salmerón J, Martin-Vivaldi R. SGftSoD-IL disease. Drug-induced liver injury: An analysis of 461 incidences submitted to the Spanish registry over a 10-year period. Gastroenterology. 2005;**129**:512-521. DOI: 10.1016/j.gastro.2005.05.006

[180] van Heyningen C. Drug-induced acute autoimmune hepatitis during combination therapy with atorvastatin and ezetimibe. Annals of Clinical Biochemistry 2005;**42**:402-404. DOI: 10.1258/0004563054890105

[181] Chalasani N, Fontana RJ, Bonkovsky HL, Watkins PB, Davern T, Serrano J, Yang H, Rochon J. DILIN. Causes, clinical features, and outcomes from a prospective study of drug-induced liver injury in the United States. Gastroenterology. 2008;**135**:1924-1934. 1934.e1921-1924. DOI: 10.1053/j.gastro.2008.09.011

[182] Russo MW, Scobey M, Bonkovsky HL. Drug-induced liver injury associated with statins. Seminars in Liver Disease. 2009;**29**:412-422. DOI: 10.1055/s-0029-1240010

[183] Lucena MI, Kaplowitz N, Hallal H, Castiella A, García-Bengoechea M, Otazua P, Berenguer M, Fernandez MC, Planas R, Andrade RJ. Recurrent drug-induced liver injury (DILI) with different drugs in the Spanish Registry: The dilemma of the relationship to autoimmune hepatitis. Journal of Hepatology. 2011;**55**:820-827. DOI: 10.1016/j.jhep.2010.12.041

[184] Reuben A, Koch DG, Lee WM, ALFS Group. Drug-induced acute liver failure: results of a U.S. multicenter, prospective study. Hepatology. 2010;**52**:2065-2076. DOI: 10.1002/hep.23937

[185] Russo MW, Hoofnagle JH, Gu J, Fontana RJ, Barnhart H, Kleiner DE, Chalasani N, Bonkovsky HL. Spectrum of statin hepatotoxicity: Experience of the drug-induced liver injury network. Hepatology. 2014;**60**:679-686. DOI: 10.1002/hep.27157

[186] Tzefos M, Olin JL. 3-hydroxyl-3-methylglutaryl coenzyme A reductase inhibitor use in chronic liver disease: A therapeutic controversy. Journal of Clinical Lipidology. 2011;**5**:450-459. DOI: 10.1016/j.jacl.2011.06.013

[187] Tolman KG. Defining patient risks from expanded preventive therapies. The American Journal of Cardiology. 2000;**85**:15-19. DOI: 10.1016/S0002-9149(00)00946-2

[188] Chalasani N. Statins and hepatotoxicity: focus on patients with fatty liver. Hepatology. 2005;**41**:690-695. DOI: 10.1002/hep.20671

[189] Cohen DE, Anania FA, Chalasani N. NLASSTFLE panel. An assessment of statin safety by hepatologists. The American Journal of Cardiology. 2006;**97**:77C-81C. DOI: 10.1016/j.amjcard.2005.12.014

[190] McKenney JM. An assessment of statin safety. The American Journal of Managed Care. 2006;**12**:S310-S317

[191] Aguirre L, Hijona E, Macarulla MT, Gracia A, Larrechi I, Bujanda L, Hijona L, Portillo MP. Several statins increase body and liver fat accumulation in a model of metabolic syndrome. Journal of Physiology and Pharmacology. 2013;**64**:281-288

[192] Herrick C, Bahrainy S, Gill EA. Statins and the liver. Endocrinology and Metabolism Clinics of North America. 2016;**45**:117-128. DOI: 10.1016/j.ecl.2015.09.008

[193] Bhardwaj SS, Chalasani N. Lipid-lowering agents that cause drug-induced hepatotoxicity. Clinics in Liver Disease. 2007;**11**:597-613, vii. DOI: 10.1016/j.cld.2007.06.010

[194] Parra JL, Reddy KR. Hepatotoxicity of hypolipidemic drugs. Clinics in Liver Disease. 2003;**7**:415-433

[195] Souk K, Al-Badri M, Azar ST. The safety and benefit of statins in liver cirrhosis: A review. Experimental and Clinical Endocrinology & Diabetes. 2015;**123**:577-580. DOI: 10.1055/s-0035-1564093

[196] MacDonald JS, Gerson RJ, Kornbrust DJ, Kloss MW, Prahalada S, Berry PH, Alberts AW, Bokelman DL. Preclinical evaluation of lovastatin. The American Journal of Cardiology. 1988;**62**:16J-27J

[197] Nakad A, Bataille L, Hamoir V, Sempoux C, Horsmans Y. Atorvastatin-induced acute hepatitis with absence of cross-toxicity with simvastatin. Lancet. 1999;**353**:1763-1764. DOI: 10.1016/S0140-6736(99)00569-3

[198] Argo CK, Loria P, Caldwell SH, Lonardo A. Statins in liver disease: A molehill, an iceberg, or neither? Hepatology. 2008;**48**:662-669. DOI: 10.1002/hep.22402

[199] Lewis JH, Mortensen ME, Zweig S, Fusco MJ, Medoff JR, Belder R. PiCLDS investigators. Efficacy and safety of high-dose pravastatin in hypercholesterolemic patients with well-compensated chronic liver disease: Results of a prospective, randomized, double-blind, placebo-controlled, multicenter trial. Hepatology. 2007;**46**:1453-1463. DOI: 10.1002/hep.21848

[200] Sattar NA, Ginsberg H, Ray K, Chapman MJ, Arca M, Averna M, Betteridge DJ, Bhatnagar D, Bilianou E, Carmena R, Ceška R, Corsini A, Erbel R, Flynn PD, Garcia-Moll X, Gumprecht J, Ishibashi S, Jambart S, Kastelein JJ, Maher V, da Silva PM, Masana L, Odawara M, Pedersen TR, Rotella CM, Salti I, Teramoto T, Tokgozoglu L, Toth PP, Valensi P, Vergès B. The use of statins in people at risk of developing diabetes mellitus: evidence and guidance for clinical practice. Atherosclerosis. 2014;**15**(Suppl):1-15. DOI: 10.1016/j.atherosclerosissup.2014.04.001

[201] Cederberg H, Stančáková A, Yaluri N, Modi S, Kuusisto J, Laakso M. Increased risk of diabetes with statin treatment is associated with impaired insulin sensitivity and

insulin secretion: a 6 year follow-up study of the METSIM cohort. Diabetologia. 2015; **58**:1109-1117. DOI: 10.1007/s00125-015-3528-5

[202] Betteridge DJ, Carmena R. The diabetogenic action of statins–mechanisms and clinical implications. Nature Reviews. Endocrinology. 2016;**12**:99-110. DOI: 10.1038/nrendo.2015.194

[203] Chan DC, Pang J, Watts GF. Pathogenesis and management of the diabetogenic effect of statins: A role for adiponectin and coenzyme Q10? Current Atherosclerosis Reports. 2015;**17**:472. DOI: 10.1007/s11883-014-0472-7

[204] Thakker D, Nair S, Pagada A, Jamdade V, Malik A. Statin use and the risk of developing diabetes: A network meta-analysis. Pharmacoepidemiology and Drug Safety. 2016; **25**:1131-1149. DOI: 10.1002/pds.4020

[205] Lorza-Gil E, Salerno AG, Wanschel AC, Vettorazzi JF, Ferreira MS, Rentz T, Catharino RR, Oliveira HC. Chronic use of pravastatin reduces insulin exocytosis and increases β-cell death in hypercholesterolemic mice. Toxicology. 2016;**344-346**:42-52. DOI: 10.1016/j.tox.2015.12.007

[206] Koh KK, Quon MJ, Han SH, Lee Y, Kim SJ, Park JB, Shin EK. Differential metabolic effects of pravastatin and simvastatin in hypercholesterolemic patients. Atherosclerosis. 2009;**204**:483-490. DOI: 10.1016/j.atherosclerosis.2008.09.021

[207] Muscogiuri G, Sarno G, Gastaldelli A, Savastano S, Ascione A, Colao A, Orio F. The good and bad effects of statins on insulin sensitivity and secretion. Endocrine Research. 2014;**39**:137-143. DOI: 10.3109/07435800.2014.952018

[208] Benes LB, Bassi NS, Davidson MH. The risk of hepatotoxicity, new onset diabetes and rhabdomyolysis in the era of high-intensity statin therapy: Does statin type matter? Progress in Cardiovascular Diseases. 2016;**59**:145-152. DOI: 10.1016/j.pcad.2016.08.001

[209] Baker WL, Talati R, White CM, Coleman CI. Differing effect of statins on insulin sensitivity in non-diabetics: a systematic review and meta-analysis. Diabetes Research and Clinical Practice. 2010;**87**:98-107. DOI: 10.1016/j.diabres.2009.10.008

[210] Nakata M, Nagasaka S, Kusaka I, Matsuoka H, Ishibashi S, Yada T. Effects of statins on the adipocyte maturation and expression of glucose transporter 4 (SLC2A4): Implications in glycaemic control. Diabetologia. 2006;**49**:1881-1892. DOI: 10.1007/s00125-006-0269-5

[211] Ogura T, Tanaka Y, Nakata T, Namikawa T, Kataoka H, Ohtsubo YJ. Simvastatin reduces insulin-like growth factor-1 signaling in differentiating C2C12 mouse myoblast cells in an HMG-CoA reductase inhibition-independent manner. Toxicological Sciences. 2007;**32**:57-67. DOI: 10.2131/jts.32.57

[212] Kain V, Kapadia B, Misra P, Saxena U. Simvastatin may induce insulin resistance through a novel fatty acid mediated cholesterol independent mechanism. Scientific Reports. 2015;**5**:13823. DOI: 10.1038/srep13823

[213] Löw P, Andersson M, Edlund C, Dallner G. Effects of mevinolin treatment on tissue dolichol and ubiquinone levels in the rat. Biochimica et Biophysica Acta. 1992;**1165**: 102-109

[214] Ernster L, Dallner G. Biochemical, physiological and medical aspects of ubiquinone function. Biochimica et Biophysica Acta. 1995;**1271**:195-204

[215] James AM, Smith RA, Murphy MP. Antioxidant and prooxidant properties of mitochondrial coenzyme Q. Archives of Biochemistry and Biophysics. 2004;**423**:47-56

[216] Crane FL, Navas P. The diversity of coenzyme Q function. Molecular Aspects of Medicine. 1997;**18**(Suppl):S1-S6

[217] Arroyo A, Navarro F, Gómez-Díaz C, Crane FL, Alcaín FJ, Navas P, Villalba JM. Interactions between ascorbyl free radical and coenzyme Q at the plasma membrane. Journal of Bioenergetics and Biomembranes. 2000;**32**:199-210

[218] Constantinescu A, Maguire JJ, Packer L. Interactions between ubiquinones and vitamins in membranes and cells. Molecular Aspects of Medicine. 1994;**15**(Suppl):s57-s65

[219] Kowaltowski AJ, Castilho RF, Vercesi AE. Ca(2+)-induced mitochondrial membrane permeabilization: Role of coenzyme Q redox state. The American Journal of Physiology. 1995; **269**:C141-C147

[220] Jarmuszkiewicz W, Navet R, Alberici LC, Douette P, Sluse-Goffart CM, Sluse FE, Vercesi AE. Redox state of endogenous coenzyme q modulates the inhibition of linoleic acid-induced uncoupling by guanosine triphosphate in isolated skeletal muscle mitochondria. Journal of Bioenergetics and Biomembranes. 2004;**36**:493-502. DOI: 10.1023/B:JOB B.0000047331.25248.7a

[221] Marcoff L, Thompson PD. The role of coenzyme Q10 in statin-associated myopathy: A systematic review. Journal of the American College of Cardiology. 2007;**49**:2231-2237. DOI: 10.1016/j.jacc.2007.02.049

[222] Miles L, Miles MV, Tang PH, Horn PS, Wong BL, DeGrauw TJ, Morehart PJ, Bove KE. Muscle coenzyme Q: A potential test for mitochondrial activity and redox status. Pediatric Neurology. 2005;**32**:318-324. DOI: 10.1016/j.pediatrneurol.2005.01.009

[223] Turunen M, Olsson J, Dallner G. Metabolism and function of coenzyme Q. Biochimica et Biophysica Acta. 2004;**1660**:171-199. DOI: 10.1016/j.bbamem.2003.11.012

[224] Littarru GP, Tiano L. Bioenergetic and antioxidant properties of coenzyme Q10: Recent developments. Molecular Biotechnology. 2007;**37**:31-37

[225] Laaksonen R, Jokelainen K, Sahi T, Tikkanen MJ, Himberg JJ. Decreases in serum ubiquinone concentrations do not result in reduced levels in muscle tissue during short-term simvastatin treatment in humans. Clinical Pharmacology and Therapeutics. 1995;**57**:62-66. DOI: 10.1016/0009-9236(95)90266-X

[226] Ghirlanda G, Oradei A, Manto A, Lippa S, Uccioli L, Caputo S, Greco AV, Littarru GP. Evidence of plasma CoQ10-lowering effect by HMG-CoA reductase inhibitors: A double-blind, placebo-controlled study. Journal of Clinical Pharmacology. 1993;**33**:226-229. DOI: 10.1002/j.1552-4604.1993.tb03948.x

[227] Miyake Y, Shouzu A, Nishikawa M, Yonemoto T, Shimizu H, Omoto S, Hayakawa T, Inada M. Effect of treatment with 3-hydroxy-3-methylglutaryl coenzyme A reductase

inhibitors on serum coenzyme Q10 in diabetic patients. Arzneimittel-Forschung. 1999;**49**:324-329. DOI: 10.1055/s-0031-1300422

[228] Rundek T, Naini A, Sacco R, Coates K, DiMauro S. Atorvastatin decreases the coenzyme Q10 level in the blood of patients at risk for cardiovascular disease and stroke. Archives of Neurology. 2004;**61**:889-892. DOI: 10.1001/archneur.61.6.889

[229] Päivä H, Thelen KM, Van Coster R, Smet J, De Paepe B, Mattila KM, Laakso J, Lehtimäki T, von Bergmann K, Lütjohann D, Laaksonen R. High-dose statins and skeletal muscle metabolism in humans: A randomized, controlled trial. Clinical Pharmacology and Therapeutics 2005;78:60-68. DOI: 10.1016/j.clpt.2005.03.006

[230] Littarru GP, Langsjoen P. Coenzyme Q10 and statins: Biochemical and clinical implications. Mitochondrion. 2007;**7**(Suppl):S168-S174. DOI: 10.1016/j.mito.2007.03.002

[231] Mabuchi H, Nohara A, Kobayashi J, Kawashiri MA, Katsuda S, Inazu A, Koizumi J, HLR Group. Effects of CoQ10 supplementation on plasma lipoprotein lipid, CoQ10 and liver and muscle enzyme levels in hypercholesterolemic patients treated with atorvastatin: A randomized double-blind study. Atherosclerosis. 2007;**195**:e182-e189. DOI: 10.1016/j.atherosclerosis.2007.06.010

[232] Young JM, Molyneux SL, Reinheimer AM, Florkowski CM, Frampton CM, Scott RS, George PM. Relationship between plasma coenzyme Q10, asymmetric dimethylarginine and arterial stiffness in patients with phenotypic or genotypic familial hypercholesterolemia on long-term statin therapy. Atherosclerosis. 2011;**218**:188-193. DOI: 10.1016/j.atherosclerosis.2011.04.034

[233] Bookstaver DA, Burkhalter NA, Hatzigeorgiou C. Effect of coenzyme Q10 supplementation on statin-induced myalgias. The American Journal of Cardiology. 2012;**110**:526-529. DOI: 10.1016/j.amjcard.2012.04.026

[234] Vaughan RA, Garcia-Smith R, Bisoffi M, Conn CA, Trujillo KA. Ubiquinol rescues simvastatin-suppression of mitochondrial content, function and metabolism: implications for statin-induced rhabdomyolysis. European Journal of Pharmacology. 2013;**711**:1-9. DOI: 10.1016/j.ejphar.2013.04.009

[235] Kettawan A, Takahashi T, Kongkachuichai R, Charoenkiatkul S, Kishi T, Okamoto T. Protective effects of coenzyme q(10) on decreased oxidative stress resistance induced by simvastatin. Journal of Clinical Biochemistry and Nutrition. 2007;**40**:194-202. DOI: 10.3164/jcbn.40.194

[236] Tavintharan S, Ong CN, Jeyaseelan K, Sivakumar M, Lim SC, Sum CF. Reduced mitochondrial coenzyme Q10 levels in HepG2 cells treated with high-dose simvastatin: A possible role in statin-induced hepatotoxicity? Toxicology and Applied Pharmacology. 2007;**223**:173-179. DOI: 10.1016/j.taap.2007.05.013

[237] Jiménez-Santos MA, Juárez-Rojop IE, Tovilla-Zárate CA, Espinosa-García MT, Juárez-Oropeza MA, Ramón-Frías T, Bermúdez-Ocaña DY, Díaz-Zagoya JC. Coenzyme Q10 supplementation improves metabolic parameters, liver function and mitochondrial respiration in rats with high doses of atorvastatin and a cholesterol-rich diet. Lipids in Health and Disease. 2014;**13**:22. DOI: 10.1186/1476-511X-13-22

[238] Caso G, Kelly P, McNurlan MA, Lawson WE. Effect of coenzyme q10 on myopathic symptoms in patients treated with statins. The American Journal of Cardiology. 2007;**99**:1409-1412. DOI: 10.1016/j.amjcard.2006.12.063

[239] Young JM, Florkowski CM, Molyneux SL, McEwan RG, Frampton CM, George PM, Scott RS. Effect of coenzyme Q(10) supplementation on simvastatin-induced myalgia. The American Journal of Cardiology. 2007;**100**:1400-1403. DOI: 10.1016/j.amjcard.2007.06.030

[240] Levy HB, Kohlhaas HK. Considerations for supplementing with coenzyme Q10 during statin therapy. The Annals of Pharmacotherapy. 2006;**40**:290-294. DOI: 10.1345/aph.1G409

[241] Wyss M, Kaddurah-Daouk R. Creatine and creatinine metabolism. Physics Review. 2000; **80**:1107-1213

[242] Volek JS, Duncan ND, Mazzetti SA, Staron RS, Putukian M, Gómez AL, Pearson DR, Fink WJ, Kraemer WJ. Performance and muscle fiber adaptations to creatine supplementation and heavy resistance training. Medicine and Science in Sports and Exercise. 1999;**31**:1147-1156

[243] Dolder M, Walzel B, Speer O, Schlattner U, Wallimann T. Inhibition of the mitochondrial permeability transition by creatine kinase substrates. Requirement for microcompartmentation. The Journal of Biological Chemistry. 2003;**278**:17760-17766. DOI: 10.1074/jbc.M208705200

[244] Meyer LE, Machado LB, Santiago AP, da-Silva WS, De Felice FG, Holub O, Oliveira MF, Galina A. Mitochondrial creatine kinase activity prevents reactive oxygen species generation: Antioxidant role of mitochondrial kinase-dependent ADP re-cycling activity. Journal of Biological Chemistry. 2006;**281**:37361-37371. DOI: 10.1074/jbc.M604123200

[245] Matthews RT, Yang L, Jenkins BG, Ferrante RJ, Rosen BR, Kaddurah-Daouk R, Beal MF. Neuroprotective effects of creatine and cyclocreatine in animal models of Huntington's disease. The Journal of Neuroscience. 1998;**18**:156-163

[246] Lawler JM, Barnes WS, Wu G, Song W, Demaree S. Direct antioxidant properties of creatine. Biochemical and Biophysical Research Communications. 2002;**290**:47-52. DOI: 10.1006/bbrc.2001.6164

[247] Jun DW, Cho WK, Jun JH, Kwon HJ, Jang KS, Kim HJ, Jeon HJ, Lee KN, Lee HL, Lee OY, Yoon BC, Choi HS, Hahm JS, Lee MH. Prevention of free fatty acid-induced hepatic lipotoxicity by carnitine via reversal of mitochondrial dysfunction. Liver International. 2011;**31**:1315-1324. DOI: 10.1111/j.1478-3231.2011.02602.x

[248] Gulcin I. Antioxidant and antiradical activities of L-carnitine. Life Sciences. 2006;**78**:803-811. DOI: 10.1016/j.lfs.2005.05.103

[249] Castilho RF, Kowaltowski AJ, Meinicke AR, Vercesi AE. Oxidative damage of mitochondria induced by Fe(II)citrate or t-butyl hydroperoxide in the presence of Ca2+: Effect of coenzyme Q redox state. Free rad. Biologie et Médecine. 1995;**18**:55-59. DOI: 10.1016/0891-5849(94)00098-5

Chapter 16

Ketamine Induces Neuroapoptosis in Stem Cell–Derived Developing Human Neurons Possibly through Intracellular Calcium/Mitochondria/microRNA Signaling Pathway

Danielle Twaroski, Yasheng Yan, Congshan Jiang, Sarah Logan, Zeljko J. Bosnjak and Xiaowen Bai

Additional information is available at the end of the chapter

http://dx.doi.org/10.5772/intechopen.72939

Abstract

Ketamine, one of the commonly used agents in pediatric anesthesia, has been linked to neurodegeneration and cognitive dysfunction in developing animal models. Previous studies on developing neurons derived from human embryonic stem cells (hESCs) indicate that ketamine induces neuroapoptosis and the mechanisms remain largely unknown. This study aims to investigate the effect of ketamine on intracellular calcium, mitochondrial signaling, and microRNA profiles in hESCs-derived 2-week-old neurons. The neurons were exposed to ketamine for 6 or 24 hours. Neuroapoptosis was assessed by TUNEL staining. Intracellular calcium level was analyzed using Fluo-4 AM staining. The mitochondria-related neuroapoptosis pathway including mitochondrial membrane potential, cytochrome c release from mitochondria to cytosol, and mitochondrial fission was also investigated. miScript miRNA arrays were used in microRNA target identification studies. The results showed that ketamine exposure induced neuroapoptosis and alterations in intracellular calcium levels. In addition, ketamine decreased mitochondrial membrane potential, resulted in cytochrome c release from mitochondria into cytosol, and increased mitochondrial fission. Among 88 microRNAs investigated, let-7a/e, miR-21, miR-23b, miR-28-5p, and miR-423-5p were found downregulated, while miR-96 was upregulated in the neurons treated with ketamine. Collectively, our findings indicate that ketamine induces neuroapoptosis possibly through the dysregulated intracellular calcium, mitochondria, and microRNA pathway.

Keywords: ketamine, calcium, mitochondria, microRNAs, neuroapoptosis

1. Introduction

Studies performed in a variety of animal models including mice and rhesus monkeys have found that prolonged exposure of developing animals to most inhalational and intravenous anesthetic agents including sevoflurane, isoflurane, ketamine, propofol and anesthetic combinations induce neuroapoptosis [1–3]. The period of rapid synaptogenesis has been linked to the time of greatest vulnerability in developing brains to anesthetic-induced neurotoxicity [4–6]. The period of rapid brain growth in mice peaks at roughly 7 days after birth while this time frame in humans ranges from late in pregnancy until the 2nd or 3rd year of life [7, 8]. The neuroapoptosis observed in the growing brains of the young animals was also found to be coupled to long-term memory and learning deficits. For example, Shen and colleagues noted significant deficiencies in both memory and spatial learning in postnatal day 3 Sprague–Dawley rats following exposure to 1% sevoflurane. Their studies relied on the Morris water maze test to assess spatial learning/memory in the animals. Additionally, they found that these effects were both exposure number and dose dependent. They also observed that 7-week-old (adult) rats were insensitive to sevoflurane exposure with both the control and sevoflurane exposed animals displaying comparable results in the Water maze test [3]. The results of this study confirm that vulnerability to anesthetics is confined to an early period in development.

The many animal studies have raised concerns regarding the applicability of the models to humans. Of particular concern are the many rodent studies in which hemodynamic properties were not properly controlled. While extensive studies in rhesus macaques, a non-human primate model have been performed [9–14], a suitable human model in the study of anesthetic-induced neurotoxicity is currently lacking and exposure of young children to anesthetics for study purposes would be unethical. Several human epidemiologic studies have been performed and many have suggested a link between anesthetic exposure in young children and learning and behavioral abnormalities when compared to their unexposed counterparts [15–17]. However, the human epidemiologic studies face many confounding variables that are often difficult to properly account for, leaving the results of these studies uncertain. While many of these studies are still ongoing, it is imperative to develop a proper human model to assess the effects of anesthetics in young children. Our study aimed to identify an appropriate human model to assess the effects of anesthetics on the developing human brain and also to dissect out the mechanisms behind the toxicity.

Human embryonic stem cells (hESCs) are derived from the inner cell mass of a human blastocyst. In 1998 James Thompson and colleagues at the University of Wisconsin-Madison developed a technique to isolate and culture hESCs *in vitro* [18]. The formative work of this group opened up the possibility for mechanistic-based studies using a human cell line, effectively eliminating the potential concerns regarding the relevancy of studies using animal models to humans. hESCs are immature, divide indefinitely and are capable of generating cells from all three germ layers which makes these cells an ideal model of early human neurons once differentiated. Using hESC-derived neurons has provided us with a reasonable human model by which to study anesthetic-induced developmental neurotoxicity.

While many anesthetic agents are used clinically in the pediatric population, we choose to study the effects of the widely used anesthetic ketamine on our model of hESC-derived neurons. Ketamine is an N-methyl-D-aspartate-receptor antagonist and provides pain relief and sedation in children undergoing a variety of procedures. Additionally, ketamine is a drug that is often abused and abuse of ketamine during pregnancy is of concern for the developing brain of the fetus [19]. Despite the many studies implicating the negative effects of anesthetic agents on developing brains, the mechanisms behind the toxicity remain largely unknown. Possible roles of neuroinflammation, reactive oxygen species production, epigenetic changes, and calcium signaling in the mechanism of anesthetic-induced neurotoxicity have all been suggested [20–23]. However, considerable work remains to fully elucidate the mechanisms behind the neuronal toxicity. In this study, we investigated the effect of ketamine on the cell viability, intracellular calcium level, mitochondrial signaling, and microRNA profile using the hESC-derived developing human neuron model.

Proper maintenance of intracellular calcium levels is critical for nearly every cellular process. In neurons, calcium is involved in the regulation of electrical activity, cell growth, metabolic activity, and many other processes [24]. Several studies have suggested that aberrant intracellular calcium level in neurons plays a critical role in the neuronal degeneration observed in many different neurological disorders [25]. The dysregulated intracellular calcium might induce the neurotoxicity through mitochondrial signaling. Mitochondria are highly dynamic organelles that undergo continuous cycles of fusion and fission in order to maintain cellular homeostasis. Mitochondrial fusion and fission result in a change in mitochondrial shape: either elongated, tubular, interconnected mitochondrial networks, or fragmented and discontinuous mitochondria, respectively. Unbalanced fission-fusion can lead to various pathological processes including neurodegeneration [26–29]. Shifting the balance towards fission has been associated with neuronal death in age-related neurodegenerative disease and brain injury [30, 31]. Inhibition of mitochondrial fission attenuated glutamate-induced neuronal death [31], translating to an increase in cell survival in the presence of oxidative stress [32]. Recent studies from Dr. Jevtovic's groups have shown that mitochondrial fission plays an important role in anesthetic neurotoxicity. The increased mitochondrial fission was found in neonatal rat brains after a sedative dose of midazolam followed by combined nitrous oxide and isoflurane anesthesia for 6 h [33].

MicroRNAs are small, non-coding RNAs that function as negative regulators of gene expression. MicroRNAs are transcribed in hairpin structures in the nucleus by RNA polymerase II and the pri-miRNA produced is processed by the enzyme Drosha to cleave off a single hairpin loop. This forms the pre-miRNA which is exported to the cytoplasm. Once in the cytoplasm, the pre-miRNA is further processed to remove the hairpin loop and forms the mature microRNA strand. The mature microRNA strand then incorporates into an RNA-induced silencing complex where it can act to promote silencing of its target genes [34, 35]. Over 1000 microRNAs have been discovered in humans and they have been shown to play an important role in nearly every cellular process. Dysregulation of microRNAs has also been linked to several diseases including certain cancers [36]. The role of microRNAs in anesthetic-induced neurotoxicity is just beginning to be studied.

This chapter will outline: (1) the use of hESCs as a model system to study anesthetic-induced neurotoxicity in the developing human brain, (2) the protocols involved in dissecting the mechanisms behind anesthetic-induced developmental neurotoxicity. We have focused on the role of deregulated intracellular calcium, mitochondrial signaling (e.g., mitochondrial membrane potential, cytochrome c release from mitochondria into cytosol, and mitochondrial fission), and microRNAs, and (3) a brief discussion on the possible role of intracellular calcium levels, mitochondrial signaling, and altered microRNA profiles in ketamine-induced developmental neurotoxicity.

2. Materials and methods

2.1. Stem cell culture and neuronal differentiation

hESCs (H1 cell line, WiCell Research Institute Inc., Madison, WI) were cultured on a feeder layer of mouse embryonic fibroblasts (MEFs) that were mitotically inactivated using mitomycin C (Sigma-Aldrich, St. Louis, MO) in hESC media containing DMEM/F12 supplemented with, 1% nonessential amino acids, 20% Knockout serum (Gibco), 1 mM L-glutamine, 4 ng/mL human recombinant basic fibroblast growth factor (bFGF, Invitrogen), 1% penicillin–streptomycin (Invitrogen) and 0.1 mM β-mercaptoethanol (Sigma-Aldrich). The media was changed daily and the cells were mechanically passaged every 5–6 days. For the studies described in this chapter, hESCs at passage 55–70 were used. To generate neurons, the hESCs were taken through a four-step differentiation protocol. The hESCs were dissociated using the protease Dispase (1.5 unit/mL, Invitrogen). The hESCs were then cultured in ultra-low attachment six-well plates (Corning Inc., Corning, NY) in a normoxic incubator (20% O_2/5% CO_2, 37°C). The media was changed once per day and spherical embryoid bodies (EBs) were present 24 h after dispase digestion. Five days after digestion, EBs were moved to neural induction media containing DMEM/F12 supplemented with 1% N_2 (Invitrogen), 1% nonessential amino acids, 1 mg/mL heparin (Sigma) and 5 ng/mL bFGF. On day 9, the EBs were plated to matrigel-coated 35-mm dishes. Rosette-like structures were present within 5 days of the EBs plating down. The rosettes were manually separated from the surrounding cells using a serological pipette approximately 2 days after the morphology was clearly visible. The rosette cells were then transferred to matrigel-coated culture dishes and cultured in neural expansion media containing DMEM/F12 supplemented with 2% B27 without vitamin A, 1% N_2 (Invitrogen), 1% nonessential amino acids, 20 ng/mL bFGF and 1 mg/mL heparin. The neural stem cells (NSCs) were passaged enzymatically every 5 days. NSCs were cultured in 60-mm matrigel-coated dishes (500,000 cells/dish) in neuron differentiation media containing neurobasal media (Gibco) supplemented with 2% B27, 100 ng/mL ascorbic acid (Sigma-Aldrich), 0.1 μM cyclic adenosine monophosphate, 10 ng/mL brain-derived neurotrophic factor, 10 ng/mL insulin-like growth factor 1 (PeproTech Inc., Rocky Hill, NJ) and 10 ng/mL glial cell-derived neurotrophic factor. The media was changed every other day. Following 2 weeks of culture, the cells displayed clear neuronal morphology and were used for the studies.

2.2. Neuronal characterization by immunofluorescence staining

hESC-derived neurons cultured on matrigel-coated, glass coverslips for 2 weeks were fixed for 30 min in 1% paraformaldehyde at room temperature. The cells were then washed with phosphate-buffered saline (PBS). Next, the cells were incubated for 15 min in 0.5% Triton X-100 (Sigma-Aldrich) in PBS. The cells were washed once again with PBS and blocked for 20 min with 10% donkey serum at room temperature. The cells were then incubated with the primary antibodies [microtubule-associated protein 2 (MAP2), β-tubulin III or doublecortin (Abcam, Cambridge, MA)] for 1 h in a humidified, 37°C incubator. The cells were washed with PBS and incubated for 45 min with Alexa Fluor 488 or 594 donkey anti-mouse or rabbit immunoglobulin G (Invitrogen) secondary antibodies at 37°C. The cell nuclei were stained with Hoechst 33342 (Invitrogen). The coverslips were then mounted onto glass slides and imaged using a laser-scanning confocal microscope (Nikon Eclipse TE2000-U, Nikon Inc., Melville, NY).

2.3. Ketamine exposure

While the brain concentration of ketamine in humans during the induction and maintenance of anesthesia is not well understood, reports have found that the peak blood levels of ketamine could be as high as 103 μM. The levels required to maintain anesthesia are typically in the range of 10–20 μM. hESC-derived neurons were exposed to 6 h of 20 μM ketamine or neurobasal media as a vehicle-control in a 5% CO_2 incubator with normoxic conditions only for the microRNA studies. For all remaining studies, the cells were exposed to 24 h of 20 or 100 μM ketamine or neurobasal media as the vehicle control in the same incubator.

2.4. Assessment of cell death by TUNEL staining

Apoptosis of the hESC-derived neurons was assessed using a cell death detection kit (Roche Applied Bio Sciences, Indianapolis, IN) based on terminal deoxynucleotidyl transferase-mediated deoxyuridine triphosphate in situ nick end labeling (TUNEL) following directions provided by the manufacturer. This kit identifies single or double-stranded DNA breaks by labeling the free 3′-OH termini with altered nucleotides in a reaction with terminal deoxynucleotidyl transferase (TdT). Cells cultured on glass coverslips were exposed to ketamine or control conditions, rinsed and fixed with 1% paraformaldehyde. DNA fragmentation was analyzed using TdT, which incorporates into sites of DNA breaks. The nuclei were stained with Hoechst 33342 and the cells were imaged using the confocal microscope. Apoptosis/necrosis was quantified by assessing the ratio of TUNEL-positive nuclei to total cell nuclei in a field.

2.5. Calcium imaging

Neurons were plated on matrigel-coated glass coverslips for the calcium imaging studies. Intracellular calcium was assayed using Fluo-4AM (Thermo Fisher Scientific). Neurons were loaded with 2 μM Fluo-4AM for 30 min in the presence/absence of ketamine at 37°C followed by a 20-min washout deesterification. The coverslips were placed in a polycarbonate recording chamber (Warner Instruments) on the stage of a laser-scanning confocal microscope. Fluo-4AM fluorescence ($\lambda_{ex}/\lambda_{em}$ = 485/520 nm) was visualized using the confocal microscope and the studies were completed in under 8 min to ensure minimal confounding stress to the cells. Fluorescent intensity was then quantified using ImageJ software 1.41 (Wayne Rasband; National Institutes of Health).

2.6. Mitochondrial membrane potential ($\Delta\Psi_m$) assay

hESC-derived neurons cultured on glass coverslips were incubated with 50 nM tetramethylrhodamine ethyl ester (TMRE) (Thermo Fisher Scientific) for 20 min at room temperature. TMRE fluorescent intensity representing $\Delta\Psi_m$ was recorded using the confocal microscope (Nikon). Images were obtained from six random fields per coverslip. The data were analyzed using ImageJ software.

2.7. Analysis of release of cytochrome c from mitochondria into cytosol

NSCs were cultured in neuronal differentiation medium. Ten days later, the differentiated neurons were transduced with the virus CellLight™ mitochondria-green fluorescence protein (GFP) (Thermo Fisher Scientific) for 24 h to label mitochondria. This fluorescent protein-based reagent contains the leader sequence of E1-*α* pyruvate dehydrogenase fused to emerald GFP. The transduced neurons expressed GFP within mitochondria. Four days later, the labeled neurons were used for analysis of the effect of ketamine on the cytochrome c translocation. Virus transduction efficiency was calculated as the ratio between GFP-positive cells and total cells. GFP expression in mitochondria was confirmed by the colocalization of GFP and TMRE fluorescence signals within cells. The distribution of cytochrome c in the neurons was analyzed using immunofluorescence staining with antibody against cytochrome c (Abcam).

2.8. Assessment of mitochondrial shape by electron microscopy

hESC-derived neurons were cultured on matrigel-coated plastic coverslips and were exposed to either 20 μM or 100 μM ketamine or control conditions for 24 h. The cells were fixed at 4°C with 2% glutaraldehyde in 0.1 M sodium cacodylate buffer and postfixed for 1 h on ice with 1% osmium tetroxide. The cells were rinsed with distilled water and dehydrated using acetonitrile and graded methanol (50%, 20 min; 70%, 20 min; 95%, 20 min; 100% 3×, 20 min). The cells were embedded in epoxy resin (EMbed-812, Electron Microscopy Sciences, Hatfield, PA) and polymerized at 70°C overnight. Thin (60 nm) sections were cut and the sections were stained with lead citrate and uranyl acetate. The samples were imaged using a Hitachi H600 Electron Microscope.

2.9. RNA extraction and cDNA preparation

Following exposure to ketamine or control conditions, total RNA was extracted using an RNeasy mini kit (Qiagen, Valencia, CA). Briefly, the cells were rinsed with PBS and lysed with QIAzol lysis reagent (Qiagen). Chloroform was added and the lysates were centrifuged. The upper phase was removed and RNA was precipitated from it with 100% ethanol. The RNA was collected using the RNeasy spin columns (Qiagen). The samples were rinsed with buffer RPE. To elute the RNA from the column, 30 μL of RNase-free water (Qiagen) was added. An Epoch nanodrop spectrophotometer (BioTek Instruments Inc., Winooski, VT) was used to assess the quantity and quality of the RNA in each sample. Each RNA sample was then diluted to 100 ng/μL in RNase-free water. The RNA was reverse transcribed to cDNA using the miScript II RT kit (Qiagen) following the manufacturer's directions. Briefly, a mixture containing 1 μg of RNA, RNase-free water, 10× miScript nucleics mix, reverse transcriptase mix and 5× HiSpec buffer (Qiagen) was prepared. The RT reaction mixture was incubated for 1 h at 37°C and for 5 min at 95°C to stop the reaction. The RT product was diluted in 200 μL in RNase-free water which yielded a final RNA concentration of 4.5 ng/μL in each sample.

2.10. Quantitative reverse transcription-PCR (qRT-PCR) analysis of MicroRNAs

To screen for potential microRNAs contributing to the ketamine-induced neurotoxicity, we used human miFinder miRNA PCR arrays (Qiagen) which screen 84 microRNAs. For the arrays, a master mix (25 μL/well) containing the template cDNA (4.5 ng/well), RNase-free water, universal primer and miScript SYBR Green (Qiagen) was prepared according to the manufacturer's instructions. The primers for each microRNAs to be analyzed come lyophilized in the wells of the array plates. To confirm the array results, validation assays were performed in which the three cDNA samples used for the arrays were each run in triplicate on the same PCR run. The PCR was run using a BioRad iCycler for 15 min at 95°C followed by 40 cycles of: denaturation (15 s at 94°C), annealing (30 s at 55°C) and extension (30 s at 70°C). Melt curve and reverse transcriptase controls were run to ensure sample purity and primer specificity, respectively. The epoch nanodrop spectrophotometer was also used to assess RNA quality using the A260:A280 ratio. To be considered pure, the A260:A280 for an RNA sample must fall between 1.8 and 2.2. Samples with an A260:A280 ratio outside of this accepted range were not used for the studies. MicroRNAs that displayed a 1.3 fold change in expression between the ketamine and control treated cells were considered to be of interest.

2.11. Statistical analysis

The data presented in this chapter was all collected from at least 3 independent neuronal differentiations. Values were reported as means ± the standard deviation with normal distributions. Statistical analysis was completed using the Student's t-test when comparing 2 groups. All statistical analysis was performed using the SigmaStat 3.5 software (Systat Software, Inc., San Jose, CA).

3. Results and discussion

3.1. Neuronal differentiation and characterization

To generate neurons from the hESCs, the cells were taken through a four-step differentiation protocol as outlined in **Figure 1A** and described previously [20, 37, 38]. The neurons

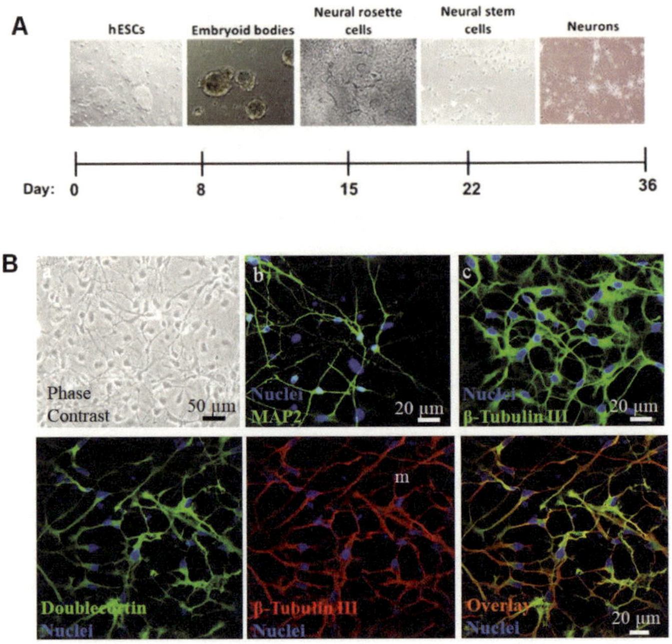

Figure 1. Differentiation protocol and confocal images of immunolabeled human embryonic stem cell (hESC)-derived neurons. (A) Neurons were derived from hESCs through a four step differentiation protocol. (B) Neurons were stained with antibodies against the neuron-specific proteins, microtubule-associated protein 2 (MAP2) and β-tubulin III to assess the differentiation efficiency, and doublecortin to confirm the immaturity of the neurons [37].

exhibited a characteristic neuronal morphology with small cell bodies and long projections. The neurons also formed extensive, interconnected networks over time. The cells displayed a very distinct morphology at each stage of the differentiation protocol. The hESCs formed tight colonies when cultured on a feeder layer and the EBs formed three-dimensional aggregates when suspended in culture media. At the neural rosette stage, the NSCs formed tightly packed arrangements with a characteristic design and were bordered by several additional cell types. Once mechanically separated from the surrounding non-NSCs and digested, the NSCs separated from one another and spread out on the matrigel-coated dishes. At this point, the cells proliferated extensively.

The neurons were immunostained after 2 weeks in differentiation media and expressed the neuron-specific markers MAP2 and β-tubulin III and formed synapses as assessed by the positive staining of Synapsin I. Based upon the immunostaining, the differentiation protocol was 90–95% efficient in the generation of neurons. In an attempt to better gauge the maturity level of the hESC-derived neurons, the cells were also immunostained for doublecortin, a marker of immature/migrating neurons. In assessing the staining results, most of the neurons in culture (90–95%) were positive for this marker of immature neurons (**Figure 1B**) which suggests that this model system is a valuable representation of developing human neurons.

3.2. Ketamine-induced apoptosis

TUNEL staining was used to assess cell death in hESC-derived neurons following ketamine exposure by labeling breaks in the DNA. The cells were exposed to 100 μM ketamine or control conditions for 24 h. The number of TUNEL-positive cells was significantly increased when compared to control treated cells following ketamine exposure (**Figure 2**). These findings confirm many of the previously published animal studies which have shown increased neuronal cell death following exposure of the developing brain to ketamine [39]. We focused on the investigation of the effect of ketamine on the intracellular calcium level, mitochondrial signaling, and microRNA expression in order to understand the mechanisms governing ketamine-induced cell death.

3.3. Alterations in intracellular calcium levels

Following exposure of 2-week-old hESC-derived neurons to 100 μM ketamine or control conditions for 24 h, the intracellular calcium levels in the cells were assessed using Fluo-4AM fluorescence. The intracellular calcium levels were significantly elevated in the ketamine-treated cells when compared to control treatment (**Figure 3**). Calcium is a critical ion in the body and is fundamental in proper neuronal functioning. In neurons, calcium is crucial in synaptic activity and plasticity, cell signaling, neurotransmitter release and is involved in nearly every aspect of the cell cycle [24]. The careful balance of intracellular calcium levels is crucial to cell survival. Calcium homeostasis dysregulation, in particular calcium overload in the cell, has been linked to many different neurodegenerative diseases [25]. The findings from this study suggest that disrupted intracellular calcium homeostasis may also be linked to ketamine-induced cell death in developing neurons which could prove to be a novel therapeutic target.

3.4. Ketamine induces neuronal apoptosis via mitochondrial pathway

The mitochondria are extremely important organelles involved in many cellular processes including energy production, cell signaling, and apoptosis [40–46]. Given that ketamine may

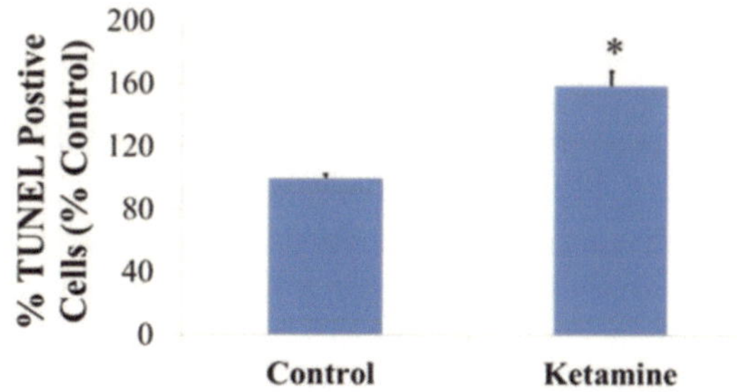

Figure 2. Exposure to 100 μM ketamine for 24 h induced significant cell death in the hESC-derived neurons. Ketamine induced an increase in the number of TUNEL-positive cells indicating significant cell death when compared to control-treated cells. *P < 0.05 vs. control. n = 3 for each group.

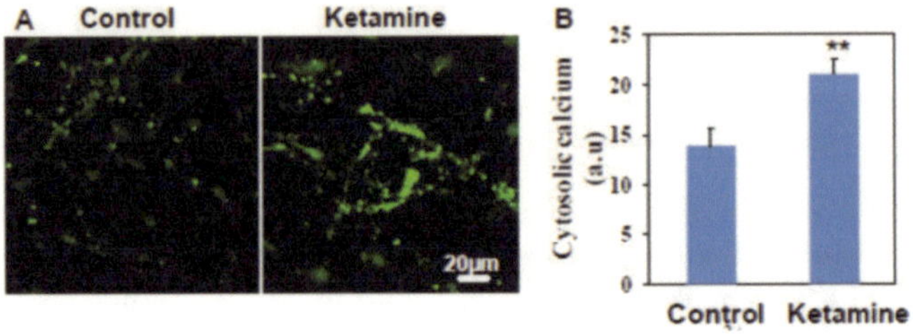

Figure 3. Ketamine exposure for 24 h induced elevated cytosolic Ca^{2+} [$(Ca^{2+})_c$] of neurons. (A) Ketamine increased $(Ca^{2+})_c$. Neurons were loaded with the Ca^{2+} indicator Fluo-4AM. The fluorescence images of free cytosolic Ca^{2+} in the 2-week-old differentiated neurons are shown. (B) Ketamine (100 μM, 24 h) significantly increased $(Ca^{2+})_c$ (**$P < 0.01$, $n = 3$).

cause mitochondrial damage, we measured $\Delta\Psi_m$ and distribution of cytochrome c in the cells. Treatment of hESC-derived neurons with 100 μM ketamine for 24 h significantly decreased $\Delta\Psi_m$ (**Figure 4A**). In order to investigate the distribution of cytochrome c within the cells, the neurons were transduced with the virus CellLight™ mitochondria-GFP (green). GFP and TMRE signals were colocalized in the cells (**Figure 4B**), confirming that successfully labeling of mitochondria with GFP. GFP-positive cells reached 40% (**Figure 4C**). The distribution of cytochrome c in mitochondria and cytosol was examined using immunofluorescence staining. The results showed that cytochrome c was located within mitochondria in the control culture (**Figure 4D**). However, in the ketamine-treated cells, cytochrome c was released from the mitochondria into cytosol.

Neuroapoptosis is a commonly recognized harmful effect by anesthetics with mechanisms that are not fully understood. Apoptosis is a programmed cell death. Cytochrome c release from mitochondria precededing the loss of $\Delta\Psi_m$ is a key event in initiating mitochondria-involved apoptosis [47], eventually leading to the typical alterations related to apoptosis such as DNA fragmentation in cell nuclei [48, 49]. In this study, following ketamine exposure, there was a significantly increase in the TUNEL-positive apoptotic cells (**Figure 2**). Ketamine-induced cell death was accompanied by the significant decrease in $\Delta\Psi_m$ and the increased cytochrome c release from mitochondria into cytosol (**Figure 4**). These data were in agreement with those previously reported by others [48, 50–52], suggesting that ketamine induces human neuron to undergo mitochondria-mediated apoptosis pathway.

To maintain proper cellular function, the mitochondria continuously undergo cycles of fusion and fission. Unbalanced fusion/fission, particularly excessive fission/fragmentation can lead to various pathological conditions including neurodegeneration [53]. To assess mitochondrial fission shape in the hESC-derived neurons following exposure to ketamine, electron microscopy was used. The neurons were exposed to either 20 μM or 100 μM ketamine or control conditions for 24 h. The cells were then prepared and imaged on an electron microscope. The mitochondria appeared considerably fragmented in the ketamine- treated neurons when compared to control cells (**Figure 5**). Increased mitochondrial fission has been linked to the propofol-induced cell death in hESC-derived neurons as previously published by our group [54]. Our findings suggest that ketamine exposure results in an increase of mitochondrial fission within the developing neurons, which may contribute to the increased cell death observed in the ketamine-treated group.

http://dx.doi.org/10.5772/intechopen.72939

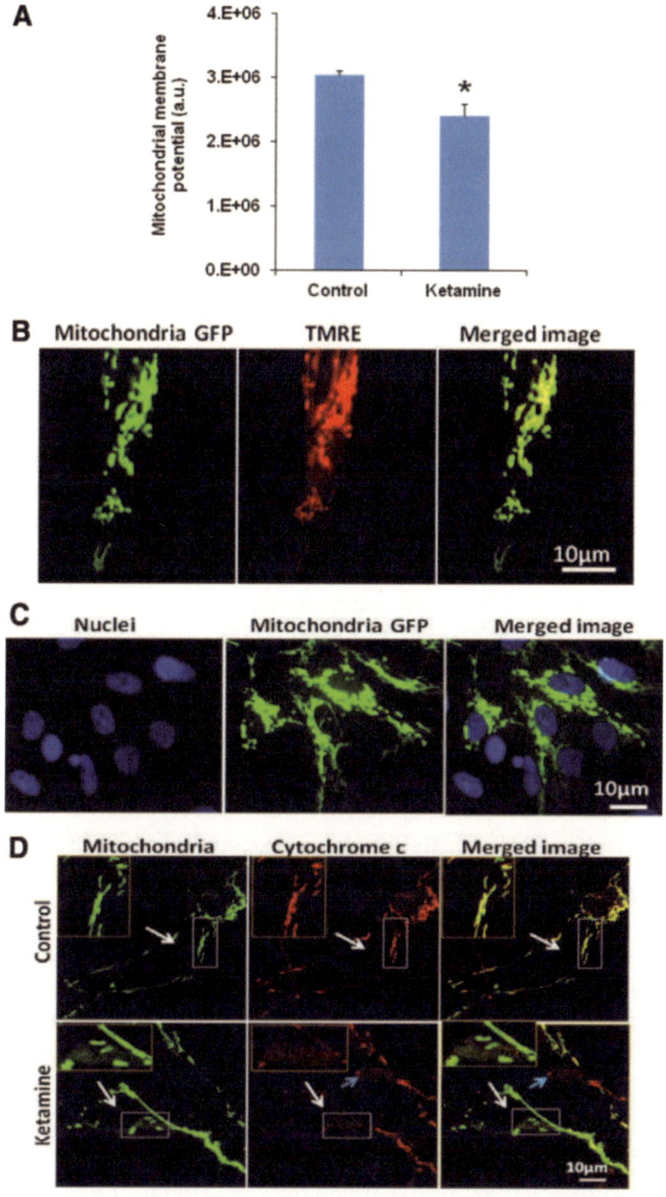

Figure 4. Ketamine decreases mitochondrial membrane potential ($\Delta\Psi_m$) and increases cytochrome c release from mitochondria into cytosol. (A) $\Delta\Psi_m$ assay. Ketamine (100 Mm) treatment for 24 h decreased $\Delta\Psi_m$ (*P < 0.05 vs. control, n = 3). (B) Labeling mitochondria of neurons with CellLight™ mitochondria-green fluorescence protein (GFP) reagent. The GFP-positive cells were loaded with TMRE. GFP expression in mitochondria was confirmed by the colocalization of tetramethylrhodamine ethyl ester (TMRE/mitochondrial probe) and GFP signals within the cells. (C) Representative fluorescent images of the neurons transduced with CellLight™ mitochondria-GFP reagent. Blue are cell nuclei. 40% cells were GFP positive. (D) the effect of ketamine on the distribution of cytochrome c in neurons. Cells were labeled with CellLight™ mitochondria-GFP reagent expressed GFP in mitochondria and then treated with ketamine (100 μM, 24 h). The distribution of cytochrome c in cells was analyzed by immunofluorescence staining. Column 1 is the image of mitochondria; column 2 is the image of cytochrome c; and column 3 is the merged image. The inset in the top corner of each image is the magnified box indicated by white arrows. The orange signals in the merged images indicate the existence of cytochrome c inside the mitochondria, and the signals in the merged images indicate the existence of cytochrome c outside the mitochondria. Ketamine treatment (100 μM, 24 h) increased cytochrome c release from mitochondria into cytosol. *Note: The cytochrome c signals (indicated by blue arrows) that do not overlap with GFP florescence were from non-transduced cells.* Scale bar = 10 μm [20].

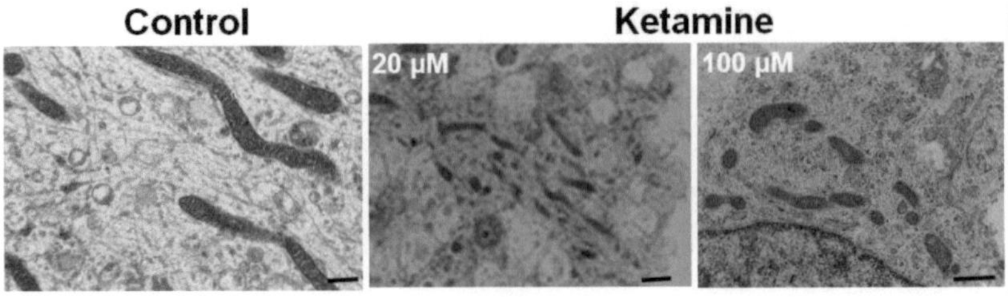

Figure 5. Ketamine increases mitochondrial fission as evidenced by the electron microscope images of differentiated neurons treated with the indicated concentrations (20 and 100 μM) of ketamine for 24 h. Scale bars = 500 nm.

3.5. qRT-PCR analysis of microRNA expression

Our lab was the first to show the role of microRNAs, specifically miR-21 in propofol-induced neurotoxicity in hESC-derived neurons [37]. Using a similar approach, we have identified several microRNAs with altered expression profiles in ketamine-treated hESC-derived neurons when compared to control-treated cells suggesting a role of microRNAs in ketamine-induced neurotoxicity. A total of 84 of the most abundantly expressed microRNAs were analyzed using the miFinder miRNA PCR arrays. A fold change of 1.3 between the control and ketamine-treated cells was considered significant. The data are expressed as percent of control with the control group set to 100%. The expression of seven microRNAs was found to be significantly altered following exposure to 6 h of ketamine when compared to control-treated cells. Of these seven, only miR-96 was found to be significantly upregulated with ketamine treatment. The remaining microRNAs (miRs-Let 7A, Let 7E, 21, 23b, 28-5p, 423-5p) were significantly downregulated with ketamine exposure compared to control-treated cells (**Figure 6**). Of these microRNAs, the downregulation of miR-21 was of particular interest since miR-21 is protective against ischemic injuries [55]. Downregulation of a protective microRNA may provide a mechanism by which ketamine is inducing neuronal toxicity in the hESC-derived neurons. Interestingly, we also reported a significant downregulation of miR-21 in hESC-derived neurons following exposure to the anesthetic propofol and went on to confirm a functional role of this expression change in the propofol-induced neurotoxicity [37]. This research suggests that the mechanism of anesthetic-induced neurotoxicity among multiple anesthetic agents might converge on altered expression of microRNAs such as miR-21. While the other 6 microRNAs identified through these array studies have not been implicated previously in neuronal diseases, this approach has the potential to uncover novel roles of these microRNAs in ketamine-induced neurotoxicity. An aim of future studies will include functional studies to further elucidate the role of these microRNAs and the signaling components connecting these altered microRNAs and attenuated mitochondrial function in ketamine-induced neurotoxicity. Additionally, the current microRNA studies were done using a different time point (6 h) than the cell death and mitochondrial studies previously mentioned which used a time point of 24 h. This was done to ensure any potentially transient changes in microRNA expression were observed. Future studies will include the addition of microRNA

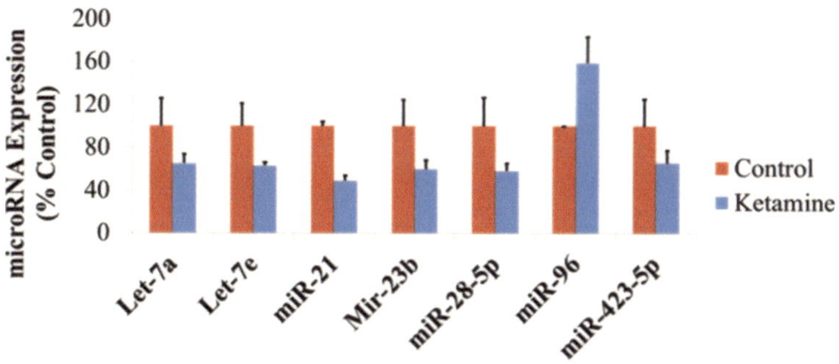

Figure 6. The expression of several microRNAs was significantly altered following exposure to ketamine. Among 88 microRNAs investigated, exposure to ketamine decreased the expression of six microRNAs and increased the expression of one microRNA. n = 3–4 for each group.

expression changes following exposure to 24 h of ketamine along with additional cell death and mitochondrial signaling assays following 6 h of exposure to ketamine which will allow for proper interpretation of the results.

3.6. Summary

The mechanisms governing anesthetic-induced neurotoxicity in the developing brain are currently not well understood and this research has been limited by the lack of an appropriate human model. Collectively, the findings from this study indicate that (1) hESC-derived neurons represent a promising model to investigate the effects of anesthetic exposure in the developing human brain, (2) ketamine induces neuroapoptosis via mitochondrial pathway, and (3) dysregulation of intracellular calcium, increased mitochondrial fission, and altered microRNA expression might play important roles in ketamine-induced neuroapoptosis. The role of microRNAs in anesthetic-induced neurotoxicity is just beginning to be understood. Functional studies including knockdown and overexpression of microRNAs of interest will further establish their role in the ketamine-induced neurotoxicity. Additionally, much work remains to establish a functional link between dysregulation of intracellular calcium, increased mitochondrial fission, decreased mitochondrial membrane potential, altered microRNA expression, and the observed neuroapoptosis. These studies are very promising and may reveal novel mechanisms of ketamine-induced developmental neurotoxicity.

Acknowledgements

The following grants supported this work: R01GM112696 from the NIH (to Dr. Xiaowen Bai) and P01GM066730 from the NIH (to Dr. Zeljko J. Bosnjak).

Author details

Danielle Twaroski[2], Yasheng Yan[1], Congshan Jiang[1], Sarah Logan[2], Zeljko J. Bosnjak[1,2] and Xiaowen Bai[1,2*]

*Address all correspondence to: xibai@mcw.edu

1 Department of Anesthesiology, Medical College of Wisconsin, Milwaukee, WI, United States

2 Department of Physiology, Medical College of Wisconsin, Milwaukee, WI, United States

References

[1] Jevtovic-Todorovic V, Hartman RE, Izumi Y, Benshoff ND, Dikranian K, Zorumski CF, Olney JW, Wozniak DF. Early exposure to common anesthetic agents causes widespread neurodegeneration in the developing rat brain and persistent learning deficits. The Journal of Neuroscience. 2003;**23**(3):876-882. PubMed PMID: 12574416

[2] Kahraman S, Zup SL, McCarthy MM, Fiskum G. GABAergic mechanism of propofol toxicity in immature neurons. Journal of Neurosurgical Anesthesiology. 2008;**20**(4):233-240. DOI: 10.1097/ANA.0b013e31817ec34d. PubMed PMID: 18812886; PMCID: PMC2730603

[3] Shen X, Liu Y, Xu S, Zhao Q, Guo X, Shen R, Wang F. Early life exposure to sevoflurane impairs adulthood spatial memory in the rat. Neurotoxicology. 2013;**39**:45-56. DOI: 10.1016/j.neuro.2013.08.007. PubMed PMID: 23994303

[4] Jevtovic-Todorovic V. Developmental synaptogenesis and general anesthesia: A kiss of death? Current Pharmaceutical Design. 2012;**18**(38):6225-6231. PubMed PMID: 22762476

[5] Jevtovic-Todorovic V. General anesthetics and the developing brain: Friends or foes? Journal of Neurosurgical Anesthesiology. 2005;**17**(4):204-206. PubMed PMID: 16184065

[6] Lunardi N, Ori C, Erisir A, Jevtovic-Todorovic V. General anesthesia causes long-lasting disturbances in the ultrastructural properties of developing synapses in young rats. Neurotoxicity Research. 2010;**17**(2):179-188. DOI: 10.1007/s12640-009-9088-z. PubMed PMID: 19626389; PMCID: PMC3629551

[7] Dobbing J, Sands J. Comparative aspects of the brain growth spurt. Early Human Development. 1979;**3**(1):79-83. PubMed PMID: 118862

[8] Dekaban AS. Changes in brain weights during the span of human life: Relation of brain weights to body heights and body weights. Annals of Neurology. 1978;**4**(4):345-356. DOI: 10.1002/ana.410040410. PubMed PMID: 727739

[9] Brambrink AM, Evers AS, Avidan MS, Farber NB, Smith DJ, Martin LD, Dissen GA, Creeley CE, Olney JW. Ketamine-induced neuroapoptosis in the fetal and neonatal rhesus macaque brain. Anesthesiology. 2012;**116**(2):372-384. DOI: 10.1097/ALN.0b013e318242b2cd. PubMed PMID: 22222480; PMCID: PMC3433282

[10] Brambrink AM, Evers AS, Avidan MS, Farber NB, Smith DJ, Zhang X, Dissen GA, Creeley CE, Olney JW. Isoflurane-induced neuroapoptosis in the neonatal rhesus macaque brain. Anesthesiology. 2010;**112**(4):834-841. DOI: 10.1097/ALN.0b013e3181d049cd. PubMed PMID: 20234312; PMCID: PMC3962067

[11] Creeley C, Dikranian K, Dissen G, Martin L, Olney J, Brambrink A. Propofol-induced apoptosis of neurones and oligodendrocytes in fetal and neonatal rhesus macaque brain. British Journal of Anaesthesia. 2013;**110**(Suppl 1):i29-i38. DOI: 10.1093/bja/aet173. PubMed PMID: 23722059; PMCID: PMC3667347

[12] Paule MG, Li M, Allen RR, Liu F, Zou X, Hotchkiss C, Hanig JP, Patterson TA, Slikker W Jr, Wang C. Ketamine anesthesia during the first week of life can cause long-lasting cognitive deficits in rhesus monkeys. Neurotoxicology and Teratology. 2011;**33**(2):220-230. DOI: 10.1016/j.ntt.2011.01.001. PubMed PMID: 21241795; PMCID: PMC3071878

[13] Slikker W Jr, Zou X, Hotchkiss CE, Divine RL, Sadovova N, Twaddle NC, Doerge DR, Scallet AC, Patterson TA, Hanig JP, Paule MG, Wang C. Ketamine-induced neuronal cell death in the perinatal rhesus monkey. Toxicological Sciences. 2007;**98**(1):145-158. DOI: 10.1093/toxsci/kfm084. PubMed PMID: 17426105

[14] Zou X, Patterson TA, Divine RL, Sadovova N, Zhang X, Hanig JP, Paule MG, Slikker W, Jr., Wang C. Prolonged exposure to ketamine increases neurodegeneration in the developing monkey brain. International Journal of Developmental Neuroscience 2009;**27**(7): 727-731. DOI: 10.1016/j.ijdevneu.2009.06.010. PubMed PMID: 19580862

[15] DiMaggio C, Sun LS, Kakavouli A, Byrne MW, Li GA. Retrospective cohort study of the association of anesthesia and hernia repair surgery with behavioral and developmental disorders in young children. Journal of Neurosurgical Anesthesiology. 2009;**21**(4):286-291. DOI: 10.1097/ANA.0b013e3181a71f11. PubMed PMID: 19955889; PMCID: PMC2789336

[16] Wilder RT, Flick RP, Sprung J, Katusic SK, Barbaresi WJ, Mickelson C, Gleich SJ, Schroeder DR, Weaver AL, Warner DO. Early exposure to anesthesia and learning disabilities in a population-based birth cohort. Anesthesiology. 2009;**110**(4):796-804. DOI: 10.1097/01.anes.0000344728.34332.5d. PubMed PMID: 19293700; PMCID: PMC2729550

[17] Ing C, DiMaggio C, Whitehouse A, Hegarty MK, Brady J, von Ungern-Sternberg BS, Davidson A, Wood AJ, Li G, Sun LS. Long-term differences in language and cognitive function after childhood exposure to anesthesia. Pediatrics. 2012;**130**(3):e476-e485. DOI: 10.1542/peds.2011-3822. PubMed PMID: 22908104

[18] Thomson JA, Itskovitz-Eldor J, Shapiro SS, Waknitz MA, Swiergiel JJ, Marshall VS, Jones JM. Embryonic stem cell lines derived from human blastocysts. Science. 1998;**282**(5391): 1145-1147. PubMed PMID: 9804556

[19] Zhao T, Li C, Wei W, Zhang H, Ma D, Song X, Zhou L. Prenatal ketamine exposure causes abnormal development of prefrontal cortex in rat. Scientific Reports. 2016;**6**:26865. DOI: 10.1038/srep26865. PubMed PMID: 27226073; PMCID: PMC4881038

[20] Bai X, Yan Y, Canfield S, Muravyeva MY, Kikuchi C, Zaja I, Corbett JA, Bosnjak ZJ. Ketamine enhances human neural stem cell proliferation and induces neuronal apoptosis

via reactive oxygen species-mediated mitochondrial pathway. Anesthesia and Analgesia. 2013;**116**(4):869-880. DOI: 10.1213/ANE.0b013e3182860fc9. PubMed PMID: 23460563; PMCID: PMC3606677

[21] Han XD, Li M, Zhang XG, Xue ZG, Cang J. Single sevoflurane exposure increases methyl-CpG island binding protein 2 phosphorylation in the hippocampus of developing mice. Molecular Medicine Reports. 2015;**11**(1):226-230. DOI: 10.3892/mmr.2014.2751. PubMed PMID: 25338822

[22] Cui Y, Ling-Shan G, Yi L, Xing-Qi W, Xue-Mei Z, Xiao-Xing Y. Repeated administration of propofol upregulated the expression of c-Fos and cleaved-caspase-3 proteins in the developing mouse brain. Indian J Pharmacol. 2011;**43**(6):648-651. DOI: 10.4103/0253-7613.89819. PubMed PMID: 22144767; PMCID: PMC3229778

[23] Wei H. The role of calcium dysregulation in anesthetic-mediated neurotoxicity. Anesthesia and Analgesia. 2011;**113**(5):972-974. DOI: 10.1213/ANE.0b013e3182323261. PubMed PMID: 22021793; PMCID: PMC3201768

[24] Toth AB, Shum AK, Prakriya M. Regulation of neurogenesis by calcium signaling. Cell Calcium. 2016;**59**(2-3):124-134. DOI: 10.1016/j.ceca.2016.02.011. PubMed PMID: 27020657; PMCID: PMC5228525

[25] Bezprozvanny I. Calcium signaling and neurodegenerative diseases. Trends in Molecular Medicine. 2009;**15**(3):89-100. DOI: 10.1016/j.molmed.2009.01.001. PubMed PMID: 19230774; PMCID: PMC3226745

[26] Perfettini JL, Roumier T, Kroemer G. Mitochondrial fusion and fission in the control of apoptosis. Trends in Cell Biology. 2005;**15**(4):179-183. Epub 2005/04/09. DOI: 10.1016/j.tcb.2005.02.005. PubMed PMID: 15817372. S0962-8924(05)00049-8 [pii]

[27] Youle RJ, Karbowski M. Mitochondrial fission in apoptosis. Nature reviews Molecular cell biology. 2005;**6**(8):657-663. Epub 2005/07/19. DOI: nrm1697 [pii]10.1038/nrm1697. PubMed PMID: 16025099

[28] Batlevi Y, La Spada AR. Mitochondrial autophagy in neural function, neurodegenerative disease, neuron cell death, and aging. Neurobiology of Disease. 2011;**43**(1):46-51. Epub 2010/10/05. DOI: 10.1016/j.nbd.2010.09.009. PubMed PMID: 20887789; PMCID: 3096708

[29] Rambold AS, Lippincott-Schwartz J. Mechanisms of mitochondria and autophagy crosstalk. Cell Cycle. 2011;**10**(23):4032-4038. Epub 2011/11/22. DOI: 10.4161/cc.10.23.18384. PubMed PMID: 22101267; PMCID: 3272286

[30] Benard G, Bellance N, James D, Parrone P, Fernandez H, Letellier T, Rossignol R. Mitochondrial bioenergetics and structural network organization. Journal of Cell Science. 2007;**120**(Pt 5):838-848. Epub 2007/02/15. DOI: 10.1242/jcs.03381. PubMed PMID: 17298981

[31] Grohm J, Kim SW, Mamrak U, Tobaben S, Cassidy-Stone A, Nunnari J, Plesnila N, Culmsee C. Inhibition of Drp1 provides neuroprotection in vitro and in vivo. Cell Death and Differentiation. 2012;**19**(9):1446-1458. Epub 2012/03/06. DOI: 10.1038/cdd.2012.18. PubMed PMID: 22388349; PMCID: 3422469

[32] Ong SB, Subrayan S, Lim SY, Yellon DM, Davidson SM, Hausenloy DJ. Inhibiting mitochondrial fission protects the heart against ischemia/reperfusion injury. Circulation. 2010;**121**(18):2012-2022. DOI: 10.1161/CIRCULATIONAHA.109.906610 Epub 2010/04/28. PubMed PMID: 20421521 CIRCULATIONAHA.109.906610 [pii]

[33] Boscolo A, Milanovic D, Starr JA, Sanchez V, Oklopcic A, Moy L, Ori CC, Erisir A, Jevtovic-Todorovic V. Early exposure to general anesthesia disturbs mitochondrial fission and fusion in the developing rat brain. Anesthesiology. 2013;**118**(5):1086-1097. DOI: 10.1097/ALN.0b013e318289bc9b. Epub 2013/02/16. PubMed PMID: 23411726

[34] Bartel DP. MicroRNAs: Genomics, biogenesis, mechanism, and function. Cell. 2004; **116**(2):281-297. PubMed PMID: 14744438

[35] Shukla GC, Singh J, Barik S. MicroRNAs: Processing, Maturation, Target Recognition and Regulatory Functions. Mol Cell Pharmacol. 2011;**3**(3):83-92. PubMed PMID: 22468167; PMCID: PMC3315687

[36] Zhang LF, Jiang S, Liu MF. MicroRNA regulation and analytical methods in cancer cell metabolism. Cellular and Molecular Life Sciences. 2017. DOI: 10.1007/s00018-017-2508-y. PubMed PMID: 28321489

[37] Twaroski DM, Yan Y, Olson JM, Bosnjak ZJ, Bai X. Down-regulation of microRNA-21 is involved in the propofol-induced neurotoxicity observed in human stem cell-derived neurons. Anesthesiology. 2014;**121**(4):786-800. DOI: 10.1097/ALN.0000000000000345. PubMed PMID: 24950164; PMCID: PMC4174986

[38] Bosnjak ZJ, Yan Y, Canfield S, Muravyeva MY, Kikuchi C, Wells CW, Corbett JA, Bai X. Ketamine induces toxicity in human neurons differentiated from embryonic stem cells via mitochondrial apoptosis pathway. Curr Drug Saf. 2012;**7**(2):106-119. PubMed PMID: 22873495; PMCID: PMC3684944

[39] Liu F, Paule MG, Ali S, Wang C. Ketamine-induced neurotoxicity and changes in gene expression in the developing rat brain. Current Neuropharmacology. 2011;**9**(1):256-261. DOI: 10.2174/157015911795017155. PubMed PMID: 21886601; PMCID: PMC3137194

[40] Tait SW, Green DR. Mitochondria and cell signalling. Journal of Cell Science. 2012;**125**(Pt 4): 807-815. DOI: 10.1242/jcs.099234. PubMed PMID: 22448037; PMCID: PMC3311926

[41] Wang W, Wang R, Zhang Q, Mor G, Zhang H. Benzo(a)pyren-7,8-dihydrodiol-9,10-epoxide induces human trophoblast Swan 71 cell dysfunctions due to cell apoptosis through disorder of mitochondrial fission/fusion. Environmental Pollution. 2017;**233**:820-832. DOI: 10.1016/j.envpol.2017.11.022. PubMed PMID: 29144987

[42] Yu Y, Xu L, Qi L, Wang C, Xu N, Liu S, Li S, Tian H, Liu W, Xu Y, Li Z. ABT737 induces mitochondrial pathway apoptosis and mitophagy by regulating DRP1-dependent mitochondrial fission in human ovarian cancer cells. Biomedicine & Pharmacotherapy. 2017;**96**:22-29. DOI: 10.1016/j.biopha.2017.09.111. PubMed PMID: 28963947

[43] Li S, Zhao H, Wang Y, Shao Y, Li J, Liu J, Xing M. The inflammatory responses in Cu-mediated elemental imbalance is associated with mitochondrial fission and intrinsic

apoptosis in Gallus gallus heart. Chemosphere. 2017;**189**:489-497. DOI: 10.1016/j.chemosphere.2017.09.099. PubMed PMID: 28957766

[44] Cui J, Li Z, Zhuang S, Qi S, Li L, Zhou J, Zhang W, Zhao Y. Melatonin alleviates inflammation-induced apoptosis in human umbilical vein endothelial cells via suppression of Ca^{2+}-XO-ROS-Drp1-mitochondrial fission axis by activation of AMPK/SERCA2a pathway. Cell Stress & Chaperones. 2017. DOI: 10.1007/s12192-017-0841-6. PubMed PMID: 28889229

[45] Zhao G, Cao K, Xu C, Sun A, Lu W, Zheng Y, Li H, Hong G, Wu B, Qiu Q, Crosstalk LZ. Between mitochondrial fission and oxidative stress in Paraquat-induced apoptosis in mouse alveolar type II cells. International Journal of Biological Sciences. 2017;**13**(7):888-900. DOI: 10.7150/ijbs.18468. PubMed PMID: 28808421; PMCID: PMC5555106

[46] Gou H, Zhao M, Xu H, Yuan J, He W, Zhu M, Ding H, Yi L, Chen JCSFV. Induced mitochondrial fission and mitophagy to inhibit apoptosis. Oncotarget. 2017;**8**(24):39382-39400. DOI: 10.18632/oncotarget.17030. PubMed PMID: 28455958; PMCID: PMC5503620

[47] Budd SL, Tenneti L, Lishnak T, Lipton SA. Mitochondrial and extramitochondrial apoptotic signaling pathways in cerebrocortical neurons. Proceedings of the National Academy of Sciences of the United States of America. 2000;**97**(11):6161-6166. Epub 2000/05/17. DOI: 10.1073/pnas.100121097100121097 [pii]. PubMed PMID: 10811898; PMCID: 18575

[48] Braun S, Gaza N, Werdehausen R, Hermanns H, Bauer I, Durieux ME, Hollmann MW, Stevens MF. Ketamine induces apoptosis via the mitochondrial pathway in human lymphocytes and neuronal cells. British Journal of Anaesthesia. 2010;**105**(3):347-354. Epub 2010/07/28. DOI: aeq169 [pii]10.1093/bja/aeq169. PubMed PMID: 20659914

[49] Zhang Y, Dong Y, Wu X, Lu Y, Xu Z, Knapp A, Yue Y, Xu T, Xie Z. The mitochondrial pathway of anesthetic isoflurane-induced apoptosis. Journal of Biological Chemistry. 2010;**285**(6):4025-4037. Epub 2009/12/17. DOI: M109.065664 [pii] 10.1074/jbc.M109.065664. PubMed PMID: 20007710; PMCID: 2823544

[50] Takadera T, Ishida A, Ohyashiki T. Ketamine-induced apoptosis in cultured rat cortical neurons. Toxicology and Applied Pharmacology. 2006;**210**(1-2):100-107. Epub 2005/11/26. DOI: S0041-008X(05)00599-5 [pii]10.1016/j.taap.2005.10.005. PubMed PMID: 16307766

[51] Zou X, Patterson TA, Sadovova N, Twaddle NC, Doerge DR, Zhang X, Fu X, Hanig JP, Paule MG, Slikker W, Wang C. Potential neurotoxicity of ketamine in the developing rat brain. Toxicological Sciences. 2009;**108**(1):149-158. Epub 2009/01/08. DOI: kfn270 [pii]10.1093/toxsci/kfn270. PubMed PMID: 19126600; PMCID: 2721655

[52] Soriano SG, Liu Q, Li J, Liu JR, Han XH, Kanter JL, Bajic D, Ibla JC. Ketamine activates cell cycle signaling and apoptosis in the neonatal rat brain. Anesthesiology. 2010;**112**(5):1155-1163. Epub 2010/04/27. DOI: 10.1097/ALN.0b013e3181d3e0c200000542-201005000-00021 [pii]. PubMed PMID: 20418696

[53] Reddy PH. Role of mitochondria in neurodegenerative diseases: mitochondria as a therapeutic target in Alzheimer's disease. CNS Spectrums. 2009;**14**(8 Suppl 7):8-13; discussion 6-8. PubMed PMID: 19890241; PMCID: PMC3056539

[54] Twaroski DM, Yan Y, Zaja I, Clark E, Bosnjak ZJ, Bai X. Altered mitochondrial dynamics contributes to Propofol-induced cell death in human stem cell-derived neurons. Anesthesiology. 2015;**123**(5):1067-1083. DOI: 10.1097/ALN.0000000000000857. PubMed PMID: 26352374; PMCID: PMC4632973

[55] Sathyan P, Golden HB, Miranda RC. Competing interactions between micro-RNAs determine neural progenitor survival and proliferation after ethanol exposure: Evidence from an ex vivo model of the fetal cerebral cortical neuroepithelium. The Journal of Neuroscience. 2007;**27**(32):8546-8557. DOI: 10.1523/JNEUROSCI.1269-07.2007. PubMed PMID: 17687032; PMCID: PMC2915840

Section 6

Viruses as Mitochondrial Modulators

Chapter 17

Modulation of Mitochondria During Viral Infections

Latif Reshi, Hao-Ven Wang and Jiann-Ruey Hong

Additional information is available at the end of the chapter

http://dx.doi.org/10.5772/intechopen.73036

Abstract

Mitochondria are organelles critical for cell survival because they produce ATP and modulate programmed cell death (PCD) pathways. PCD pathways are important in many clinical disorders, such as ischemia/reperfusion injuries, trauma, and toxic/metabolic syndromes, as well as in chronic neurodegenerative conditions, such as amyotrophic lateral sclerosis, Alzheimer's disease, Parkinson's disease, and Huntington's disease. Moreover, many viruses and other pathogens target the mitochondria. Viruses induce the production of various proteins in their hosts that have proapoptotic and anti-apoptotic activities, depending on the cellular environment. More specifically, many viruses that target mitochondria regulate the balance between the anti- and proapoptotic Bcl-2 family proteins and thereby increase their own survival within the host cell. Recent studies indicated that mitochondria centralize several critical innate immune responses based on the presence of several important signaling proteins within the mitochondria: mitochondrial antiviral signaling (MAVS), stimulation of interferon genes (STING), and NLR family member X1. Therefore, mitochondria are not only vital because they regulate cell survival and death but also they have broad roles in the control of cell functions following pathogen invasion. This chapter highlights the tight interplay between viral infection and mitochondria.

Keywords: virus, apoptosis, mitochondria, mitochondrial membrane potential (MMP), diseases, Bcl-2 family, viral death genes

1. Introduction

1.1. Viruses and hosts

Viral diseases are becoming increasingly common worldwide, so it is important to identify the causative species and examine the underlying pathogenesis to prevent future epidemics and reduce the spread of new diseases. Although many host responses can contribute to the pathogenesis of viral diseases, little is known about the role of mitochondria in viral pathogenesis.

Mitochondria are suitable targets for infectious microorganisms, such as viruses, because they act as powerhouses of the cell and have various other important functions. Therefore, "hijacking" the mitochondria disrupts overall cell function and makes it easy for a virus to control the cell and propagate. The host, in turn, has several responses that it uses to protect itself from viral invasions. One defense mechanism is based on the immune system, and another is based on cell autonomy, in which cells undergo certain physiological changes upon the onset of infection, such as unscheduled activation of the cell cycle following induction by certain viral proteins. When an infected cell undergoes programmed cell death (PCD), which includes apoptosis, autophagy, and necroptosis, this can prevent the spread of the virus infection to neighboring cells. A further complication is that viruses often promote apoptosis, but they can also block apoptosis by interacting with different signaling molecules of the host cell. Many viruses, especially human viruses, can perform either function, depending on the underlying conditions. Recent studies have shown that most viruses force cells to undergo apoptosis. However, from the perspective of the virus, apoptosis of the host seems to provide no benefit, so this is a topic of the current research. Therefore, additional studies that elucidate the mechanisms underlying the induction of the virus-induced PCD and cell lysis may help to identify new drug targets for the treatment of viral infections.

1.2. Intrinsic and extrinsic pathways of apoptosis in viral infections

Programmed cell death has a key role in the pathogenesis of many conditions including viral diseases, cancer, inflammation, and neurodegenerative diseases. Apoptosis is a highly complex process that is controlled by numerous cell signaling pathways [1]. The common event at the end point is activation of a set of cysteine-aspartic proteases (caspases) [2, 3]. Apoptosis may benefit host cells by limiting the production and dissemination of viruses [4]. However, apoptosis may benefit viruses if it allows them to increase production and dissemination of progeny [5, 6]. The PCD induced by a virus infection is often described as "typical apoptosis" [7]. However, recent studies reported that nonapoptotic forms of PCD are important for the pathogenesis of certain RNA viruses, including the JC virus, hepatitis C virus (HCV), coxsackievirus B3, enterovirus, and dengue virus [8]. The mechanism of DNA virus-induced nonapoptotic cell death is not well understood. Although not all signaling pathways that induce apoptosis are fully understood, the fate of a cell undergoing apoptosis mainly depends on the balance between the Bcl-2 family sensor proteins, which can promote and inhibit apoptosis (**Figure 1**) [9–11]. Recent studies have shown viral pathogenesis that involves oxidative damage and apoptosis.

1.3. Role of ROS in viral diseases

Recent studies have shown that mitochondria are the targets of the reactive oxygen species (ROS) that are produced inside a cell during viral infections, and that mtDNA is a major target of these ROS [11]. Mitochondrial ATP generation requires proteins from the nuclear and mitochondrial genomes. ROS disrupt the oxidative production of ATP, which is required for normal cellular function, because damage of mtDNA disrupts the normal synthesis of proteins needed for mitochondria function and making them suitable targets for attack by ROS produced during infections by viruses and other microorganisms, although ROS also have other

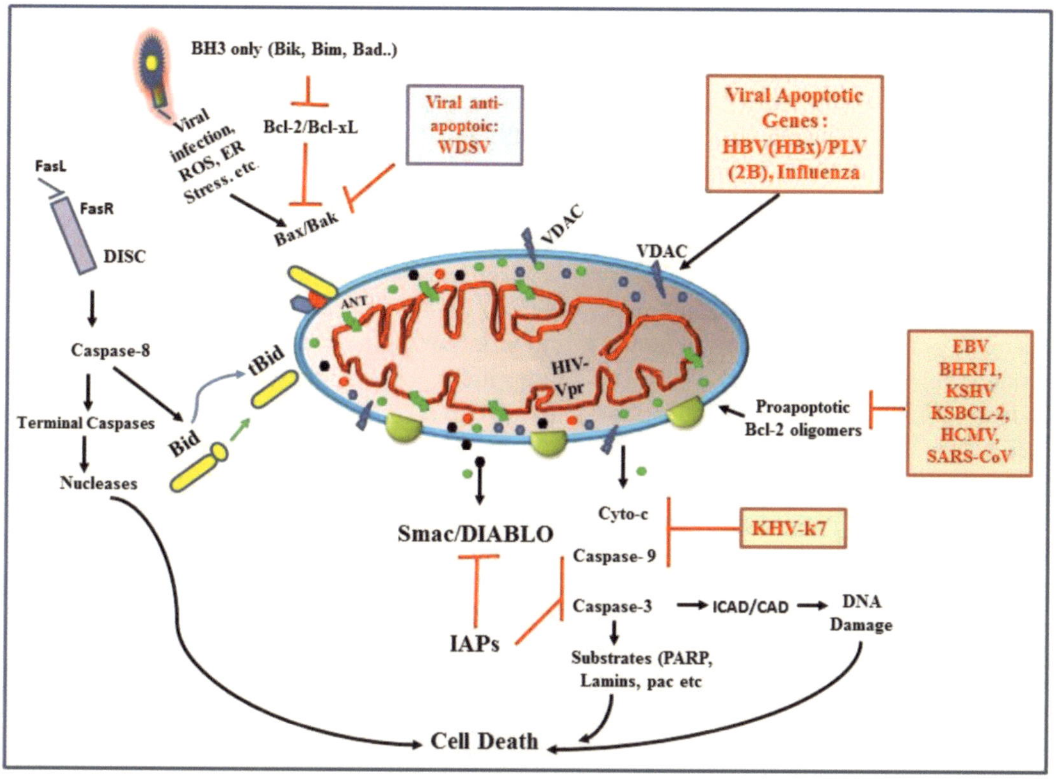

Figure 1. Modulation of cell death pathways in mitochondria by different viral infections or different viral proteins. In the extrinsic apoptosis pathway (middle left) [2], is activation of Fas death receptors at the cell surface by its ligand for activating the caspase-8 for either cleaved Bid to tBid for targeting into mitochondria [24] or activates the ROS/RIP3-mediated necroptosis via a nonmitochondria-mediated cell death process [2, 85]. In the intrinsic apoptosis pathway (top left), some death factors trigger death signals on disrupting mitochondrial function via loss of MMP and release the cytochrome c and activate the downstream caspase-3 for further triggering apoptotic cell death, but these mitochondria-mediated death signaling also regulated by anti-apoptotic family members such as Bcl-2 and Bcl-xL for rescuing host cells [8, 10, 11, 87]. On the other hand, IAP can inhibit the caspase-3 activation [88] but it is suppressed by the Smac/DIABLO molecule, which is released from mitochondria [24]. Finally, if viruses entering or expressing, they can also trigger proapoptotic signaling (indicated by black lines) or block anti-apoptotic signaling (indicated by red lines) via whole virus or viral gene productions in mammalian viruses, which is associated with activation of caspase-dependent [9] and caspase-independent executioner mechanisms [2], leads to cell death by viral genes from RNA and DNA viruses, respectively for inducing some damaged or human diseases [4, 27].

cellular targets. In HIV and hepatitis C virus infections, oxidative stress (OS) always plays a dominant pathogenic role. Peterhen and other researchers showed that almost all viruses (DNA/RNA viruses) cause cell death by generating oxidative stress in infected cells [12–14]. The OS generated during chronic hepatitis is associated with hepatic damage, a decrease in reduced glutathione (GSH) and decrease in plasma and hepatic zinc concentration [15, 16]. In case of influenza virus infection, the activated phagocytes release not only produces ROS but also cytokine and TNF. The pro-antioxidant effect of TNF may be relevant to influenza virus as shown by children with Rey's syndrome [17]. OS ultimately results in decrease in the functioning of the immune system.

2. Mitochondrial functions

Mitochondria are multifunctional organelles that are covered by an outer membrane (OM), within which lie the intermembrane space (IMS) and the inner membrane (IM). The IM is folded into special structures called cristae, so its surface area is much greater than that of the OM. The cristae function as matrices for protein complexes required for the electron transport chain (ETC), and they contain many integral membrane proteins, including adenine nucleotide translocator (ANT) and ATP synthase. The IM remains almost entirely impermeable under normal physiological conditions, thereby allowing the respiratory chain to create an electrochemical gradient. This electric potential is important for maintaining the mitochondrial membrane potential (MMP, $\Delta\psi m$) of the IM. The pumping of protons by the ETC out of the IM activates ATP synthase, which phosphorylates ADP to ATP. The ATP generated on the matrix side of the IM is then exported by ANT in exchange for ADP. The OM has many voltage-dependent anion channels (VDACs), which maintains permeability of solutes up to 5000 Da in size under normal physiological conditions. The IMS is chemically equivalent to the cytosol in terms of low molecular weight solutes and has its own special set of proteins. The human mitochondrial genome (about 16,500 bp), which is in the matrix (within the IM), only codes for 13 subunits of the respiratory chain. More than 99% of mitochondrial proteins are encoded by the nuclear genome and then selectively imported into one of the mitochondrial compartments. Thus, the mitochondrial OM, IM, IMS, and matrix have highly unique protein compositions.

Mitochondria act "powerhouse" of the cell and have several other important functions. The numerous functions of mitochondria make them indispensable to the cell, so when a virus "hijacks" mitochondrial function, it allows it to control the whole cell. Mitochondria have important roles in several signal transduction pathways [18, 19], the process of aging [20], regulation of different biochemical pathways related to cell metabolism [21, 22], PCD [23, 24], development [25, 26], the pathogenesis of numerous diseases immune responses [19], and cell cycle control [19, 27]. The circular mitochondrial genome encodes 13 polypeptides, 2 rRNAs, and 22 tRNAs. All of these mtDNA products are essential for function of the ETC and the generation of ATP by oxidative phosphorylation [9, 27], although many proteins from the nuclear genome are also required. Thus, any injury to mtDNA can affect the whole cell. The mtDNA is more susceptible to damage from ROS because it lacks protective histones, the mitochondrion has more limited DNA repair enzymes, and it is close to ETC, the main center of ATP and ROS production. The matrix of IMS, which contains cytochrome c oxidase (Cyt C, encoded by mtDNA), SMAC/DIABLO (encoded by nuclear DNA), and endonuclease G (encoded by nuclear DNA), acts as a buffer zone between the IM and OM. This matrix region contains many of the enzymes needed for aerobic respiration, dissolved oxygen, water, carbon dioxide, and recyclable intermediates that serve as energy shuttles and have other functions.

2.1. Loss of mitochondrial membrane potential

A loss of the MMP ($\Delta\psi m$) leads to imbalances in the membrane potentials of the IM and OM, and then to arrest of normal cellular biosynthetic function and bioenergetics, and finally to a "crisis" within the cell. A loss of the MMP ($\Delta\psi m$) also leads to release of several proapoptotic proteins from the IMS, such as Cyt C and Smac/DIABLO, as well as caspase independent death effectors, such as apoptosis-inducing factor (AIF) and endonuclease G (EndoG) [9], which have important roles in caspase-independent and caspase-dependent cell death [9]. The MMP (Δψm) transition occurs during the pathogenesis of exogenous factors (e.g., viral proteins, toxins, and prooxidants [9, 10]). A prolonged loss of the MMP (Δψm) leads to serious cell damage, from which the cell cannot recover. Therefore, in the intrinsic pathway of apoptosis, any viral factor that influences the MMP (Δψm) has a major impact on cell fate, either by inducing or by blocking cell death [9].

In recent years, there has been an increasing focus on the role of the MMP (Δψm) in disease and health. Thus, several recent models based on *in vivo* and *in vitro* studies explain the mechanisms underlying the maintenance and loss of the MMP. A loss of the MMP by any mechanism leads to functional and structural collapse of the mitochondria and cell death [27]. A recent study for first time has shown that dengue virus (DV) infection of human hepatoma cell line (HepG2) leads alteration in the bioenergetic function of mitochondrial morphology leading to MMP loss [28]. The alteration in respiratory properties of HepG2 cells in DV infection results due to decrease in respiratory control ratio (PCR) and ADP/O ratio, which suggest significant alteration in mitochondrial morphology. Another additional feature observed by an increase in proton leak termed mitochondrial uncoupling which occurs by leaking of protons through F_oF_1 ATP synthase from inner membrane into matrix resulting in decrease in MMP loss. Thus, creating an imbalance in ATP synthesis ultimately affects the bioenergetic functions of cell. The biochemical mitochondrial damage induced in cell infected with HCV showed that E1 Protein together with core and NS3 are responsible for ROS production. Core and NS3 induce NO production which causes MMP loss by opening of transition pore [29]. NO could also interact with another free radical superoxide (O_2^-) to form strong peroxynitrite anion (ONOO–), which irreversibly inhibits multiple respiratory complexes (complexes I, II and IV) and aconitase, and activate proton leak and permeability transition pore [30, 31]. Therefore, interfering with energy metabolism by disrupting the ATP synthesis of cell results in modulation of mitochondrial function.

2.2. Effects of viral infections on mitochondrial processes

Mitochondria undergo a number of processes, such as fusion and fission, in normally functioning healthy cells. However, when mitochondria develop abnormalities, the cell can destroy it by the process of mitophagy [32]. Cells typically eliminate unhealthy mitochondria by mitochondrial fission; they typically use mitochondrial fusion to recycle matrix metabolites, including mtDNA and mitochondrial membranes, for the assembly of new and healthy mitochondria. Therefore, these three processes—mitophagy, fission, and fusion—are interlinked, and they all play prominent roles in maintaining healthy cells [33]. Mitophagy plays an important role in maintaining mitochondrial homeostasis, but can also eliminate healthy mitochondria in cases such as cell starvation, viral invasion, and erythroid cell differentiation [34, 35]. The mitochondrial fusion and fission are highly dynamic. Viruses interfere with these processes to distort mitochondrial dynamic to facilitate their proliferation. Thus, interfering with these processes promotes the interference of different cellular signaling pathways [36–38]. New castal virus

(NDV) uses strategy that interferes with P62-mediated mitophagy to promote viral propagation [39]. The severe acute respiratory syndrome coronovirus (SARS-CoV) escapes the innate immune response by translocating its ORF-9b to mitochondria and promotes proteosomal degradation of dynamin-like protein (Drp1) leading to mitochondrial fission [40]. However, still more studies are needed to explain the exact role of mitophagy in the viral disease pathogenesis, which regulates the cell death process [41].

2.3. Role of mitochondria in host immune response

During the coevolution of viruses and hosts, some viruses have evolved proteins that mimic the activity of host proteins, thereby allowing the virus to complete its life cycle without inducing an immune response in the host. For example, Mimivirus, a genus with a single species in the newly created Mimiviridae, has genes for many proteins, including a viral mitochondrial carrier protein (VMC-I) [42], which mimics the host cell's mitochondrial carrier protein, allowing it to control mitochondrial transport in infected cells. Therefore, this virus takes control of the host cell's transportation of ADP, dADP, TTP, dTTP, and UTP in exchange for dATP, which the virus uses as an energy source for genome replication and production of progeny [27].

2.4. Viruses target mitochondrial DNA and disable host cells

Numerous viruses appear to have adopted a "strategy" of damaging the host cell mitochondrial DNA to control the whole cell. For example, the herpes simplex virus (HSV) causes productive and latent infections in human hosts by disruption of mitochondrial function. The HSV-1UL12 gene encodes two distinct yet similar proteins, UL12 and UL12.5. UL12 is an alkaline nuclease, and UL12.5 is an N terminally truncated 500-aa polypeptide that lacks the first 126 residues of UL12. UL12 plays a crucial role in viral genome replication and processing; UL12.5 also has nuclease and strand-exchange activities but does not accumulate in the host cell nucleus. Instead, UL12.5 localizes predominantly to the mitochondria, where it triggers massive degradation of mitochondrial DNA during early HSV replication. In particular, UL12.5 occurs directly within the mitochondrial matrix, and its nuclease activity degrades mtDNA [43]. HIV and hepatitis C virus infections cause metabolic stress due to mtDNA depletion in coinfected patients [44]. The Zta protein encoded by Ebola virus (EBV) genome translocates into mitochondria and interacts with mitochondrial single-strand protein, which ultimately affects mtDNA replication [45]. The OS generated during HCV infection also interferes with mtDNA [31].

3. Human viruses in mitochondria-mediated diseases

3.1. Epstein: Barr virus

The Epstein–Barr virus (EBV) is an oncovirus that is associated with breast cancer, gastric cancer, and numerous other cancers. Recent studies showed that EBV-encoded latent membrane protein 2A (LMP2A) leads to increased mitochondrial fission [46]. Further, molecular studies showed that LMP2A activates the NOTCH pathway, which alters the expression of Drp1 and then increases mitochondrial fission. Although increased Drp expression does not directly increase mitochondrial fission, the recruitment of Drp by mitochondria and activation of GTPase leads to mitochondrial fission. Therefore, the EBV-induced changes in mitochondrial function, due to the LMP2A protein, may play a major role in the pathogenesis of several cancers [47].

3.2. Herpes simplex virus (alphaherpesvirus)

Infections by the herpes simplex virus type 1 (HSV-1) and pseudorabies virus (PRV) lead to imbalances in the calcium homeostasis of host cells. A study on rodents indicated that this calcium imbalance leads to disruption of mitochondrial function in the cervical ganglion neurons [48]. An imbalance in the cellular calcium pool affects the Miro protein (a calcium-binding protein), altering its interaction with kinesin-1. Therefore, HSV-1 and PRV "hijack" host cell proteins, and this disrupts mitochondrial dynamics, thereby allowing the viruses to replicate and spread to neighboring cells.

3.3. Influenza A virus

3.3.1. Influenza A virus induces oxidative stress in mitochondria

Reactive oxygen species have important roles in the overall function of normal cells and play a vital role in the host adaptive immune response [49, 50]. For example, production of $O_2^{\cdot-}$ is an important defense against microbial infections. However, a large increase in the production of $O_2^{\cdot-}$during influenza A virus infection leads to damage of lung parenchyma cells [51]. Further studies that OS increased lung injuries caused by the influenza virus and viral replication, irrespective of the viral strain [52, 53]. Excessive and nonspecific knockdown of stress-related enzymes, such as superoxide dismutase 2 (SOD2), led to T-cell apoptosis and many developmental defects, resulting in overall weakening of the adaptive immune system and an increased susceptibility to influenza A virus subtype H1N1 [54, 55].

3.3.2. Influenza A virus-encoded protein PB1-F2 targets mitochondria

Influenza A viruses encode the proapoptotic protein PB1-F2, which localizes to the mitochondria due to a target sequence on its C terminal domain. PB1-F2 is conserved within the influenza family [56]. After PB1-F2 binds to mitochondria, it interacts with two important mitochondrial proteins, VDAC1 on the OM and ANT3 on the IM [57, 58]. This leads to alterations in mitochondria morphology, release of proapoptotic proteins, loss of MMP, and then cell death.

3.4. HCV virus

3.4.1. HCV induces oxidative stress that damages mitochondria

HCV infection typically leads to generation of ROS, which interferes with the calcium signaling pathways of the cell [9]. This disruption of calcium homeostasis alters the structure of the endoplasmic reticulum, and increased calcium is taken up by the mitochondria, leading to disruption of the MMP. Recent molecular studies have shown that many other HCV proteins, such as E2 [59], and NS4B [60], are important in generating oxidative stress. In addition, the nonstructural HCV protein NS5A is an integral membrane protein that is important for viral replication, apoptosis, immune responses (such as interferon resistance), and changes in cellular calcium [61]. The proteins NS5Aand NS3 have roles in increasing calcium uptake and in the oxidation of glutathione (GSH) to glutathione disulfide (GSSG) in mitochondria, which ultimately leads to oxidative stress [61–63]. The imbalance of ROS created in the mitochondria leads to activation and translocation of NF-κB and STAT3 to the nucleus, as part of disease progression. Antioxidants block the NS5A-mediated activation of NF-κB and STAT3 [64]. NS4B also promotes translocation of NF-κB to the nucleus in a PTK-mediated pathway. The resulting production of ROS and nitric oxide (NO) causes oxidative damage and inhibits DNA repair [60] and leads to apoptosis. ROS-mediated disruption of mitochondria is believed to be the sole cause of liver inflammation in HCV infections [9].

3.4.2. HCV-encoded proteins target mitochondria

HCV remains persistent in its host because it lowers the host cell immune response. The HCV protein NS3/4A is a serine protease that inhibits interferon beta production by the retinoic acid-inducible gene I (RIG-I) pathway. Studies of the NS3/4A protein show that this protease cleaves MAVS at Cys-508, a few residues before its mitochondrial targeting domain. Cleavage of MAVS inactivates this protein because its soluble form is not functional. NS3/4A has a mitochondrial localizing signal, so it can directly cleave MAVS in the mitochondria [65, 66]. Substitution of Cys-508 with arginine prevents cleavage of MAVS. Cleavage of MAVS is thus an important mechanism by which HCV reduces host cell defenses [66].

3.5. Hepatitis B virus targets mitochondria

Hepatitis B virus x protein (HBx) is potentially essential for viral replication, and it has oncogenic properties in animal models [67]. HBx sensitizes hepatocytes to apoptosis induced by stimuli such TNF-α [68]. Studies of the overexpression of HBx showed that this protein causes apoptosis by causing a perinuclear clustering of mitochondria and a loss of the MMP [69]. Studies of HBx mutants identified that certain hydrophobic residues (a mitochondrial targeting sequence, MTS) are important for its induction of mitochondrial localization, loss of MMP, and cell death [70]. The HBx protein usually interacts with at least two mitochondrial proteins, heat shock protein 60 (HSP60) [71] and HVDAC3 [72]. The interaction of HBx with these two proteins (which are important in maintaining mitochondrial integrity) ultimately disrupts mitochondrial function in infected cells. These two mitochondrial proteins play major roles in chronic liver disease and carcinogenesis. Therefore, HBx plays a major role in the pathogenesis of HBV infection due to its alteration of host cell mitochondria.

4. Control strategies

4.1. RNA interference treatment of viral diseases that target mitochondria

Despite the many advances in molecular biology and in treatment of viral diseases, the prevention and control of viral infections remains a challenge. Alteration of the interaction of the virus and host is one general strategy. Therefore, a complete understanding of the interactions of the host and virus at the molecular level is needed to develop new antiviral drugs and vaccines. There is an urgent need to find more effective therapeutic agents for the treatment of viral infections. Researchers have recently started testing treatments based on RNA interference (RNAi), using either microRNA (miRNA) or small interfering RNA (siRNA). Although this approach is still in its infancy, there has been some success in silencing the viral genes responsible for virulence [73, 74].

RNAi is an endogenous defense that cells use as a defense against harmful nucleic acids, either generated by the cell itself or from external environment (such as a viral invasions) [75]. RNAi is successful against many virus infections, but the delivery and stability of RNAi molecules within the cell are major concerns. The stability of RNAi is affected by its charge and biochemical activity within a cell, so these two parameters must be considered when designing RNAi-based therapies. In addition, the effectiveness of RNAi-based therapies depends on the delivery route [76], target gene [77, 78], target pathogen [75, 78], and target tissue [75]. The adverse effects of using RNAi-based treatment on the environment and treatment costs must also be considered, and we must have a deeper understanding of RNAi at the molecular level. The growing interest of molecular virologists in the use of RNAi suggests that this is one of the most exciting new therapeutic approaches for treatment of viral diseases [75].

4.2. Host antioxidant defense system fights viral invasion

The increased generation of ROS and reactive nitrogen species (RNS) is a key part of the pathogenesis of many virus infections. OS induces loss of the MMP, so mitochondria are become more susceptible to ROS damage. However, cells also have defenses against ROS, such as reduced glutathione (GSH),which acts as an antioxidant during the oxidative production of ATP in healthy cells [9, 79–81]. An imbalance between the generation of ROS and ROS quenching by the cell's endogenous antioxidant defense system usually leads to a disease and is common during viral invasion. In recent years, due to the unavailability of antiviral drugs, researchers have proposed a number of new strategies to protect against free radical-induced OS. These strategies may be characterized as repair and protection. Protection is achieved by enzymes and by nonenzymatic compounds, such as carotenoids, vitamin C, vitamin E, GSH, and flavonoids [82]. Recent studies have shown the importance of both classes of these molecules in defense against oxidative stress [9, 83–86].

5. Concluding remarks

Identifying the main cause of a new epidemic is the most important factor in controlling disease outbreak. Many host responses appear to contribute to the pathogenesis of viral infections, and recent cellular and molecular studies have shown that many viruses specifically target mitochondria. Several different host responses and viral proteins directly or indirectly act on the mitochondria and lead to loss of the MMP. Mitochondria play important roles in cell survival and cell death, so a better understanding how different viruses use mitochondrial responses to control cells may provide a foundation for the development of new treatments for different viral diseases. More specifically, clarification of the roles of viruses and viral proteins in host mitochondria may help to develop methods that protect against pathogenic viruses. Therefore, molecular examination of the exact roles of viruses and viral proteins on mitochondria may help to guide the discovery of novel therapeutic strategies and provide important insights into different mitochondrial viral diseases. However, there are major unanswered questions regarding the mechanism of virus- and protein-induced loss of the MMP. Answering these questions may lead to the discovery of key molecules or pathways involved in loss of MMP, a common feature in the pathogenesis of many viral diseases. The research summarized in this review clearly shows that mitochondria are the main target of invading viruses, and that disruption of mitochondrial function is a major part of the pathogenesis of viral diseases. Although the prevention and treatment of viral diseases is challenging, molecular pathogenesis studies examining virus-host interactions will help in the design of new drugs and therapeutic strategies against different viral diseases.

Acknowledgements

This work was supported by a grant (NSC 98-2313-B-006-004-MY3 and NSC 101-3011-P-006-006) awarded to Dr. Jainn-Ruey Hong from the National Science Council, Taiwan, Republic of China.

Conflict of interest

The authors declare no conflicts of interest in terms of funding or authorship.

Abbreviations

DISC	death-inducing signaling complex
ER	endoplasmic reticulum
HCV	hepatitis C virus
HBV	hepatitis B virus
PLV	poliovirus
KPSV	Kaposi sarcoma virus
Bid	BH3 interacting-domain death agonist
WDSV	walleye dermal saecoma virus
HCMV	human cytomegalovirus
EBV	Epstein–Barr virus
SARS-CoV	severe acute respiratory syndrome coronovirus

VDAC	voltage-dependent anion channel
HIV	human immunodeficiency virus
IAPs	inhibitor of apoptosis proteins.

Author details

Latif Reshi[1,2], Hao-Ven Wang[2] and Jiann-Ruey Hong[1,3]*

*Address all correspondence to: jrhong@mail.ncku.edu.tw

1 Lab of Molecular Virology and Biotechnology, Institute of Biotechnology, College of Bioscience and Biotechnology, National Cheng Kung University, Tainan City, Taiwan, ROC

2 Department of Life Sciences, College of Bioscience and Biotechnology, National Cheng Kung University, Tainan City, Taiwan, ROC

3 Department of Biotechnology and Bioindustry Sciences, National Cheng Kung University, Tainan City, Taiwan, ROC

References

[1] Liu J, Chen I, Kwang J. Characterization of a previously unidentified viral protein in porcine circovirus type 2-infected cells and its role in virus-induced apoptosis. Journal of Virology. 2005;**79**:8262-8274

[2] Ashkenazi A, Dixit VM. Death receptors: Signaling and modulation. Science. 1998;**281**: 1305-1308

[3] Münz C. Viral evasion of autophagy. Cell Host & Microbe. 2007;**1**:9-11

[4] Benedict CA, Norris PS, Ware CF. To kill or be killed: Viral evasion of apoptosis. Nature Immunology. 2002;**3**:1013-1018

[5] Wong J, Zhang J, Si X, Gao G, Mao I, et al. Autophagosome supports coxsackie virus B3 replication in host cells. Journal of Virology. 2008;**82**:9143-9153

[6] Lee YR, Lei HY, Liu MT, Wang JR, Chen SH, et al. Autophagic machinery activated by dengue virus enhances virus replication. Virology. 2008;**374**:240-248

[7] Levine AJ. The cellular gatekeeper for growth and division. Cell. 1997;**1997**(88):323-331

[8] Rao L, White E. Bcl-2 and the ICE family of apoptotic regulators: Making a connection. Current Opinion in Genetics & Development. 1997;**7**:52-58

[9] Reshi L, Su YC, Hong JR. RNA viruses: ROS-mediated cell death. International Journal of Cell Biology. 2014;**2014**:467-452

[10] Reshi L, Wu JL, Wang HV, Hong JR. Aquatic viruses induce host cell death pathways and its application. Virus Research. 2016;**211**:133-144

[11] Reshi L, Wang HV, Hui CF, Su YC, Hong JR. Anti-apoptotic genes Bcl-2 and Bcl-xL overexpression can block iridovirus serine/threonine kinase-induced Bax/mitochondria-mediated cell death in GF-1 cells. Fish & Shellfish Immunology. 2017;**61**:120-129

[12] Peterhans E, Grob M, Urge TB, Zanoni R. Virus-induced formation of reactive oxygen intermediates in phagocytic cells. Free Radical Research Communications. 1987;**3**(1-5):39-46

[13] Vierucci A, DeMartino M, Graziani E. A mechanism for liver cell injury in viral hepatitis: Effects of hepatitis B virus on neutrophil function in vitro and in children with chronic active hepatitis. Pediatric Research. 1983;**17**(10):814-820

[14] Muller F. Reactive oxygen intermediates and human immunodeficiency virus (HIV) infection. Free Radical Biology and Medicine. 1992;**13**(6):651-657

[15] Boya P, Peña AD, Beloquietal O. Antioxidant status and glutathione metabolism in peripheral blood mononuclear cells from patients with chronic hepatitis C. Journal of Hepatology. 1999;**31**(5):808-814

[16] Bianchi GP, Marchesini G, Brizietal M. Nutritional effects of oral zinc supplementation in cirrhosis. Nutrition Research. 2000;**20**(8):1079-1089

[17] Cooperstock MS, Tucker RP, Baublis JV. Possible pathogenic role of endotoxin in Reye's syndrome. The Lancet. 1975;**1**(7919):1272-1274

[18] Bossy-Wetzel E, Barsoum MJ, Godzik A, Schwarzenbacher R, Lipton SA. Mitochondrial fission in apoptosis, neurodegeneration and aging. Current Opinion in Cell Biology. 2003;**15**: 706-716

[19] Wallace DC. A mitochondrial paradigm of metabolic and degenerative diseases, aging and cancer: A dawn for evolutionary medicine. Annual Review of Genetics. 2005;**39**:359-407

[20] Chan DC. Mitochondria: Dynamic organelles in disease, aging and development. Cell. 2006;**125**:1241-1252

[21] Hackenbrock CR. Ultrastructural bases for metabolically linked mechanical activity in mitochondria. I. Reversible ultrastructural changes with change in metabolic steady state in isolated liver mitochondria. Journal of Cell Biology. 1966;**30**:269-297

[22] Mannella CA, Pfeiffer DR, Bradshaw PC, Moraru II, Slepchenko B, et al. Topology of the mitochondrial inner membrane: Dynamics and bioenergetics implications. IUBMB Life. 2001;**52**:93-100

[23] McBride HM, Neuspiel M, Wasiak S. Mitochondria: More than just a powerhouse. Current Biology. 2006;**16**:R551-R560

[24] Kroemer G, Galluzzi L, Brenner C. Mitochondrial membrane permeabilization in cell death. Physiological Reviews. 2007;**87**:99-163

[25] Mandal S, Guptan P, Owusu-Ansah E, Banerjee U. Mitochondrial regulation of cell cycle progression during development as revealed by the tenured mutation in drosophila. Developmental Cell. 2005;**9**:843-854

[26] Honda S, Hirose S. Stage-specific enhanced expression of mitochondrial fusion and fission factors during spermatogenesis in rat testis. Biochemical and Biophysical Research Communications. 2003;**311**:424-432

[27] Reshi L, Hong JR. Mitochondria as a favourite organelle for invading viruses. Molecular Biology. 2017;**6**:181

[28] El-Bacha T et al. Mitochondrial and bioenergetic dysfunction in human hepatic cells infected with dengue 2 virus. Biochimica et Biophysica Acta (BBA)—Molecular Basis of Disease. 2007;**1772**(10):1158-1166

[29] Machida K et al. Hepatitis C virus infection activates the immunologic (type II) isoform of nitric oxide synthase and thereby enhances DNA damage and mutations of cellular genes. Journal of Virology. 2004;**78**(16):8835-8843

[30] Hortelano S et al. Nitric oxide induces apoptosis via triggering mitochondrial permeability transition. FEBS Letters. 1997;**410**(2-3):373-377

[31] Machida K et al. Hepatitis C virus triggers mitochondrial permeability transition with production of reactive oxygen species, leading to DNA damage and STAT3 activation. Journal of Virology. 2006;**80**(14):7199-7207

[32] Twig G, Shirihai OS. The interplay between mitochondrial dynamics and mitophagy. Antioxidants & Redox Signaling. 2011;**14**:1939-1951

[33] Chen H, Chan DC. Mitochondrial dynamics—Fusion, fission, movement, and mitophagy—in neurodegenerative diseases. Human Molecular Genetics. 2009;**18**:R169-R176

[34] Shitara H, Kaneda H, Sato A, Inoue K, Ogura A, Yonekawa H, Hayashi JL. Selective and continuous elimination of mitochondria microinjected into mouse eggs from spermatids, but not from liver cells, occurs throughout embryogenesis. Genetics. 2000;**156**:1277-1284

[35] Ebato C, Uchida T, Arakawa M, Komatsu M, Ueno T, Komiya K, et al. Autophagy is important in islet homeostasis and compensatory increase of beta cell mass in response to high-fat diet. Cell Metabolism. 2008;**8**:325-332

[36] Seth RB et al. Identification and characterization of MAVS, a mitochondrial antiviral signaling protein that activates NF-κB and IRF3. Cell. 2005;**122**(5):669-682

[37] Castanier C et al. Mitochondrial dynamics regulate the RIG-I-like receptor antiviral pathway. EMBO Reports. 2010;**11**(2):133-138

[38] West AP, Shadel GS, Ghosh S. Mitochondria in innate immune responses. Nature Reviews Immunology. 2011;**11**(6):389

[39] Meng G, Xia M, Wang D, Chen A, Wang Y, Wang H, Yu D, Wei J. Mitophagy promotes replication of oncolytic Newcastle disease virus by blocking intrinsic apoptosis in lung cancer cells. Oncotarget. 2014;**5**(15):6365-6374

[40] Shi C-S et al. SARS-coronavirus open reading frame-9b suppresses innate immunity by targeting mitochondria and the MAVS/TRAF3/TRAF6 signalosome. The Journal of Immunology. 2014;**193**(6):3080-3089

[41] Xia M, Meng G, Jiang A, et al. Mitophagy switches cell death from apoptosis to necrosis in NSCLC cells treated with oncolytic measles virus. Oncotarget. 2014;**5**(11):3907

[42] Monn'e M, Robinson AJ, Boes C, Harbour ME, Fearnley IM, et al. The mimivirus genome encodes a mitochondrial carrier that transports dATP and dTTP. Journal of Virology. 2007;**81**:3181-3186

[43] Martinez R, Shao L, Bronstein JC, Weber PC, Weller SK. The product of a 1.9-kb mRNA which overlaps the HSV-1 alkaline nuclease gene (UL12) cannot relieve the growth defects of a null mutant. Virology. 1996;**215**:152-164

[44] de Mendoza C, Sánchez-Conde M, Timmermans E, et al. Mitochondrial DNA depletion in HIV-infected patients with chronic hepatitis C and effect of pegylated interferon plus ribavirin therapy. AIDS .2007;**21**(5): 583-588

[45] Wiedmer A, Wang P, Zhou J, et al. Epstein-Barr virus immediate-early protein Zta co-opts mitochondrial single-stranded DNA binding protein to promote viral and inhibit mitochondrial DNA replication. Journal of Virology. 2008;**82**(9):4647-4655

[46] Young LS, Rickinson AB. Epstein–Barr virus: 40 years on. Nature Reviews. Cancer. 2004;**4**: 757-768

[47] Pal AD, Basak NP, Banerjee AS, Banerjee S. Epstein–Barr virus latent membrane protein-2A alters mitochondrial dynamics promoting cellular migration mediated by Notch signaling pathway. Carcinogenesis. 2014;**35**:1592-1601

[48] Kramer T, Enquist LW. Alphaherpesvirus infection disrupts mitochondrial transport in neurons. Cell Host & Microbe. 2012;**11**:504-514

[49] Rott R, Klenk HD, Nagai Y, Tashiro M. Influenza viruses, cell enzymes, and pathogenicity. American Journal of Respiratory and Critical Care Medicine. 1995;**152**(4):S16-S19

[50] Kido H, Sakai K, Kishino Y, Tashiro M. Pulmonary surfactant is a potential endogenous inhibitor of proteolytic activation of Sendai virus and influenza A virus. FEBS Letters. 1993;**322**(2):115-119

[51] Hennet T, Peterhans E, Stocker R. Alterations in antioxidant defences in lung and liver of mice infected with influenza A virus. Journal of General Virology. 1992;**3**:39-46

[52] Geiler J, Michaelis M, Naczk P, et al. N-acetyl-l-cysteine (NAC) inhibits virus replication and expression of proinflammatory molecules in A549 cells infected with highly pathogenic H5N1 influenza A virus. Biochemical Pharmacology. 2010;**79**(3):413-420

[53] Vlahos R, Selemidis S. NADPH oxidases as novel pharmacologic targets against influenza A virus infection. Molecular Pharmacology. 2014;**86**(6):747-759

[54] Case AJ, McGill JL, Tygrett LT, Shirasawa T, Spitz DR, Waldschmidt TJ, Legge KL, Domann FE. Elevated mitochondrial superoxide disrupts normal T cell development, impairing adaptive immune responses to an influenza challenge. Free Radical Biology & Medicine. 2011;**50**(3):448-458

[55] Allen RG, Balin AK. Oxidative influence on development and differentiation: An overview of a free radical theory of development. Free Radical Biology and Medicine. 1989;**6**(6): 631-661

[56] Bruns K, Studtrucker N, Sharma A, Fossen T, Mitzner D, et al. Structural characterization and oligomerization of PB1-F2, a proapoptotic influenza A virus protein. The Journal of Biological Chemistry. 2007;**282**:353-363

[57] Gibbs JS, Malide D, Hornung F, Bennink JR, Yewdell JW. The influenza A virus PB1-F2 protein targets the inner mitochondrial membrane via a predicted basic amphipathic helix that disrupts mitochondrial function. Journal of Virology. 2003;**77**:7214-7224

[58] Zamarin D, Garcia-Sastre A, Xiao X, Wang R, Palese P. Influenza virus PB1-F2 protein induces cell death through mitochondrial ANT3 and VDAC1. PLoS Pathogens. 2005;**1**:4

[59] Hsieh MJ, Hsieh YS, Chen TY, Chiou HL. Hepatitis C virus E2 protein induce reactive oxygen species (ROS)-related fibrogenesis in the HSC-T6 hepatic stellate cell line. Journal of Cellular Biochemistry. 2011;**112**(1):233-243

[60] Li S, Ye Y, Yu X, et al. Hepatitis C virus NS4B induces unfolded protein response and endoplasmic reticulum overload response-dependent NF-κB activation. Virology. 2009;**391**:257-264

[61] Liang Y, Ye H, Cong BK, HoS Y. Domain 2 of nonstructural protein 5A (NS5A) of hepatitis C virus is natively unfolded. Biochemistry. 2007;**46**:11550-11558

[62] Thoren F, Romero A, Lindh M, Dahlgren C, Hellstrand K. A hepatitis C virus-encoded, nonstructural protein (NS3) triggers dysfunction and apoptosis in lymphocytes: Role of NADPH oxidase-derived oxygen radicals. Journal of Leukocyte Biology. 2004;**76**(6):1180-1186

[63] García-Monzón C, Majano PL, Zubia I, Sanz P, Apolinario A, Moreno-Otero R. Intrahepatic accumulation of nitrotyrosine in chronic viral hepatitis is associated with histological severity of liver disease. Journal of Hepatology. 2000;**32**(2):331-338

[64] Gong G, Waris G, Tanveer R, Siddiqui A. Human hepatitis C virus NS5A protein alters intracellular calcium levels, induces oxidative stress, and activates STAT-3 and NF-κB. Proceedings of the National Academy of Sciences of the United States of America. 2001;**98**(17):9599-9604

[65] Meylan E, Curran J, Hofmann K, Moradpour D, Binder M, et al. Cardif is an adaptor protein in the RIG-I antiviral pathway and is targeted by hepatitis C virus. Nature. 2005;**437**: 1167-1172

[66] Li XD, Sun L, Seth RB, Pineda G, Chen ZJ. Hepatitis C virus protease NS3/4A cleaves mitochondrial antiviral signaling protein off the mitochondria to evade innate immunity. Proceedings of the National Academy of Sciences of the United States of America. 2005;**102**:17717-17722

[67] Wang Y, Lau SH, Sham JST, Wu MC, Wang T, et al. Characterization of HBV integrants in 14 hepatocellular carcinomas: Association of truncated X gene and hepatocellular carcinogenesis. Oncogene. 2004;**23**:142-148

[68] Su F, Schneider RJ. Hepatitis B virus HBx protein sensitizes cells to apoptotic killing by tumor necrosis factor alpha. Proceedings of the National Academy of Sciences of the United States of America. 1997;**94**:8744-8749

[69] Takada S, Shirakata Y, Kaneniwa N, Koike K. Association of hepatitis B virus X protein with mitochondria causes mitochondrial aggregation at the nuclear periphery, leading to cell death. Oncogene. 1999;**18**:6965-6973

[70] Henkler F, Hoare J, Waseem N, Goldin RD, McGarvey MJ, et al. Intracellular localization of the hepatitis B virus HBx protein. The Journal of General Virology. 2001;**82**:871-882

[71] Rahmani Z, Huh KW, Lasher R, Siddiqui A. Hepatitis B virus X protein colocalizes to mitochondria with a human voltage-dependent anion channel, HVDAC3, and alters its transmembrane potential. Journal of Virology. 2000;**74**:2840-2846

[72] Tanaka Y, Kanai F, Kawakami T, Tateishi K, Ijichi H, et al. Interaction of the hepatitis B virus X protein (HBx) with heat shock protein 60 enhances HBx-mediated apoptosis. Biochemical and Biophysical Research Communications. 2004;**318**:461-469

[73] Buchon N, Vaury C. RNAi: A defensive RNA-silencing against viruses and transposable elements. Heredity. 2006;**96**:195-202

[74] Rijiravanich E, Berezikov E. Small RNAs and the control of transposons and viruses in Drosophila. Trends in Microbiology. 2009;**17**:163-171

[75] Reshi ML, Wu JL, Wang HV, Hong JR. RNA interference technology used for the study of aquatic virus infections. Fish & Shellfish Immunology. 2014;**40**(1):14-23

[76] Attasart P, Kaewkhaw R, Chimwai C, Kongphom U, Namramoon O, Panyim S. Inhibition of white spot syndrome virus replication in *Penaeus monodon* by combined silencing of viral rr2 and shrimp PmRab7. Virus Research. 2009;**145**:127-133

[77] Shockey JE, O'Leary NA, de la Vega E, Browdy CL, Baatz JE, Gross PS. The role of crustins in *Litopenaeus vannamei* in response to infection with shrimp pathogens: An in vivo approach. Developmental and Comparative Immunology. 2009;**33**:668-673

[78] Han-Ching Wang K, Tseng CW, Lin HY, Chen IT, Chen YH, Chen YM, et al. RNAi knock-down of the *Litopenaeus vannamei* Toll gene (LvToll) significantly increases mortality and reduces bacterial clearance after challenge with Vibrioharveyi. Developmental and Comparative Immunology. 2010;**34**:49-58

[79] Stout AK, Raphael HM, Kanterewicz BI, Klann E, Reynolds IJ. Glutamate-induced neuron death requires mitochondrial calcium uptake. Nature Neuroscience. 1998;**1**(5):366-373

[80] White E, Shannon JS, Patterson RE. Relationship between vitamin and calcium supplement use and colon cancer. Cancer Epidemiology Biomarkers and Prevention. 1997;**6**(10):769-774

[81] Smith AR, Shenvi SV, Widlansky M, Suh JH, Hagen TM. Lipoic acid as a potential therapy for chronic diseases associated with oxidative stress. Current Medicinal Chemistry. 2004;**11**(9):1135-1146

[82] Sharoni Y, Danilenko M, Dubi N, Ben-Dor A, Levy J. Carotenoids and transcription. Archives of Biochemistry and Biophysics. 2004;**430**(1):89-96

[83] Schrauzer GN. Interactive effects of selenium and chromium on mammary tumor development and growth in MMTV infected female mice and their relevance to human cancer. Biological Trace Element Research. 2006;**109**(3):281-292

[84] Packer L, Suzuki YJ. Vitamin E and alpha-lipoate: Role in antioxidant recycling and activation of the NF-κB transcription factor. Molecular Aspects of Medicine. 1993;**4**(3):229-239

[85] Reshi ML, Hong JR. Role of oxidative stress in RNA virus–induced cell death. In: Shamimi A, editor. Reactive Oxygen Species in Biology and Human Health. New York: Taylor & Francis group; 2016. pp. 471-485

[86] Pryor WA. Vitamin E and heart disease: Basic science to clinical intervention trials. Free Radical Biology and Medicine. 2000;**28**(1):141-164

[87] Ferri KF, Kroemer G. Organelle-specific initiation of cell death pathways. Nature Cell Biology. 2001;**3**:E255-E263

[88] Clem RJ, Duckett CS. The IAP genes: Unique arbitrators of cell death. Trends in Cell Biology. 1997;**7**:337-339

Section 7

Regulation of Structure and Function of Mitochondrion by Estrogen

Chapter 18

Estrogen and Mitochondrial Function in Disease

Ved P. Mooga, C. Roger White and
Samantha Giordano-Mooga

Additional information is available at the end of the chapter

http://dx.doi.org/10.5772/intechopen.73015

Abstract

Anecdotal and scientific evidence suggest that the sex hormone estrogen provides significant health benefits in women. Women have higher estrogen levels than men. Circulating estrogen reaches its highest level during the reproductive period and steadily declines with the onset of menopause. The role of estrogen and estrogen receptors in both cellular physiology and pathophysiology has been controversial. Estrogen has anti-inflammatory and anti-oxidant effects, which preserve cell viability during cardiovascular incidents, but it enhances disease progression in the context of breast cancer. Estrogen mediates these responses *via* activation of estrogen receptor subtypes located in the cell membrane, nucleus, and mitochondrion. Further, transcription of nuclear and mitochondrial genes by estrogen yields products that play an important role in regulating mitochondrial function. Mitochondria are part of a highly dynamic network and undergo fission and fusion, produce cellular energy, adenosine 5′ triphosphate (ATP), and regulate cell death. Herein, we review the cell and receptor specific effects of estrogen on mitochondrial structure, function, and cell death under normal physiological conditions and in the context of cardiovascular disease, inflammation, neurodegeneration, and cancer. Further research is needed to elucidate the specific role of estrogenic control of mitochondria in health and disease.

Keywords: estrogen, mitochondria, aging, menopause, estrogen receptors

1. Introduction

The term estrogen refers to a family of chemically similar steroid hormones that include estrone, estradiol, and estriol. Estrogens are synthesized primarily by the ovarian follicles [1]. An important rate limiting step in steroid hormone synthesis is the production of pregnenolone in follicular granulosa cells. Cholesterol is transported from the outer to the inner mitochondrial membrane by the steroidogenic acute regulatory (StAR) protein, followed by conversion to pregnenolone by cytochrome P450 side chain cleavage (CYP11A1). Pregnenolone then diffuses to the theca cells where it is converted to androstenedione and then re-routed to the granulosa cells for the aromatase-mediated conversion to estrogen. Androstenedione can also be converted to testosterone. Thus, mitochondria play an important role in estrogen biosynthesis.

Estrogen serves a major role in determining female secondary sex characteristics during development and in regulating the estrous cycle. During puberty and throughout the female reproductive cycle, estrogen levels fluctuate, and as women age, sex steroid production decreases [1]. Estrogen levels oscillate during the estrous cycle. They are lowest during menstruation, steadily rise during the follicular stage and reach a maximal level during ovulation. If a woman becomes pregnant, estrogen levels will remain high, but if fertilization does not occur, hormone levels decline during the luteal phase. Following the luteal phase, menstruation occurs, and the cycle resumes. As estrogen levels fluctuate during the estrous cycle, mitochondria alter the production of pregnenolone accordingly.

Estrogen is a pleiotropic hormone that exerts its effects *via* both transcriptional and non-genomic mechanisms. In addition to regulating reproductive function, estrogen exerts numerous cytoprotective effects. With respect to atherosclerosis, estrogen regulates levels of circulating lipids by stimulating the formation of high density lipoprotein (HDL) and decreasing expression of low density lipoprotein (LDL) [2]. It exerts antioxidant and anti-inflammatory effects by preventing the oxidation of LDL, inhibiting the expression of endothelial cell adhesion molecules and stimulating nitric oxide formation [3]. As discussed in this chapter, differential responses to estrogen are due to activation of different receptor subtypes. Recent studies also suggest that many of the protective responses to estrogen are related to the ability of the hormone to maintain normal mitochondrial function. Mitochondrial localization of estrogen receptors has been shown to regulate mitochondrial gene expression. In this manner, estrogen plays an important role in the supporting mitochondrial respiration and adenosine 5′ triphosphate (ATP) production, reducing reactive oxygen species (ROS) formation and inhibiting activation of mitochondrial cell death pathways. The goal of this chapter is to discuss mechanisms by which estrogen regulates mitochondrial signaling and function under normal physiological conditions and in the context of disease.

2. Estrogen receptor types

Estrogen modulates cellular function *via* activation of one of four receptor subtypes: estrogen receptor alpha (ERα), estrogen receptor beta (ERβ), G-protein coupled estrogen receptor (GPER), and ER-X. ERα was first described in the 1950s as a ligand-activated receptor for estrogen, while ERβ was discovered more recently in 1996 [4]. ERs are located throughout the cell [5]. Two distinct genes encode ligand-activated ERα and ERβ. These genes and their products are subject to epigenetic modifications and alternative RNA splicing [6–11]. Nuclear ERα and ERβ can modulate gene transcription, while localization of these receptors on the cell membrane results in the rapid activation of signaling cascades *via* non-genomic mechanisms.

Studies utilizing ERα and ERβ knockout (KO) mice have provided insight into the function of each receptor type. Male and female ERα KO mice are infertile, while ERβ KO mice are fertile but produce small litters [12–14]. These studies highlight the importance of estrogen in the development of reproductive systems of both sexes [14, 15].

ERα and ERβ are also found on the membranes of cellular organelles, including the endoplasmic reticulum and the mitochondrion, where they mediate various cellular functions. Localization to mitochondria was first confirmed using radioligand binding methods in mitochondria isolated from rat uterus and later by immunocytochemistry in rat pancreatic acinar cells [16]. MALDI-TOF mass spectrometry studies have shown that mitochondrial ERs are identical to ERs located in the nucleus [17]. ERβ is the predominant mitochondrial receptor in most tissues: for example ovary, uterus, spermatocytes, cerebral and hippocampal neurons, cardiomyocytes, and endothelial cells [17, 18]. In contrast, the identification of mitochondrial ERα has been limited to the uterus, ovary, and the MCF-7 breast cancer cell line [18]. The presence of ERs on mitochondria and estrogen responsive elements on the mitochondrial DNA suggests a role for estrogen in regulating the structure and/or function of the organelle [19].

Estrogen also binds to a GPER on the plasma membrane. GPER specifically binds to estradiol and mediates numerous responses including cell proliferation, vasodilation, and regulation of glucose metabolism by non-genomic mechanisms [20]. GPER has also been localized to intracellular sites. In the endoplasmic reticulum, GPER activation induces calcium release and activation of the phosphoinositide 3-kinase (PI3K)-*Akt* pathway, which induces cell proliferation [21, 22]. While GPER is not associated with the mitochondria, its regulation of cellular calcium handling indirectly impacts mitochondrial function and mitochondrial-induced cell death [22, 23]. Calcium uptake by mitochondria results in the opening of the mitochondrial permeability transition pore (mPTP) and induction of the intrinsic cell death pathway. GPER-specific agonist G1 binding to GPER has been shown to attenuate these responses in a rodent model of ischemia/reperfusion (I/R) by preventing endoplasmic reticulum calcium release [23]. ER-X is an additional estrogen receptor type that is associated with the cell membrane. This novel receptor shares sequence homology with ERα and ERβ, which is expressed primarily in the brain during development and becomes re-expressed in response to ischemic brain injury [24]. While little is known regarding the function of ER-X, some data suggest that it exerts a cytoprotective role in the brain [24].

3. Mitochondrial function

The mitochondria are classically described as the powerhouse of the cell by virtue of its ability to generate ATP. Physiological processes underlying mitochondrial bioenergetics and respiration have been previously reviewed [25]. Under aerobic conditions, mitochondria utilize electron transport and a protomotive force to produce ~36 ATP molecules for every glucose molecule. Reducing equivalents produced by the Krebs cycle (NADH and $FADH_2$) are accepted by the respiratory chain at Complex I (NADH Dehydrogenase) and Complex

II (Succinate Dehydrogenase), respectively. Electrons are shuttled through the complexes with oxygen acting as the final electron acceptor at Complex IV. Concurrently, hydrogen ions are pumped from the electronegative mitochondrial matrix into the more positively charged inner membrane space by Complexes I, III (cytochrome C reductase), and IV (cytochrome C oxidase). The protomotive force thus generated allows hydrogen ions to flow down their concentration gradient at Complex V (ATP Synthase), resulting in the formation of ATP. This chemiosmotic process is tightly regulated and highly efficient. Although ATP is the primary (and often most studied) product of cellular respiration, ROS and thermal energy/heat are also generated by mitochondria. ROS include chemical species produced by the incomplete reduction of O_2. These molecules include superoxide anion ($O_2^{\bullet -}$), hydrogen peroxide (H_2O_2), and hydroxyl radical ($^{\bullet}OH$). Mitochondrial ROS are thought to perform a variety of cell signaling functions under normal physiological conditions.

Mitochondria are highly dynamic organelles that are components of a constantly changing, dynamic mitochondrial network. Damaged or old mitochondria can be cleared from the cell by autophagy/mitophagy or bulk clearance and degraded by lysosomal enzymes [26]. Furthermore, mitochondria can also undergo fission and fusion. Fission is the process by which mitochondria bud off from the mitochondrial network. This is regulated by the proteins DRP-1 and FIZZ1. Fusion represents the incorporation of mitochondria in the mitochondrial network and is regulated by mitofusin1 (Mfn1), mitofusin2 (Mfn2), or optic atrophy 1 (OPA1) [27]. These regulatory proteins help to maintain the balance between fission and fusion that is required to preserve cell viability. In different disease states, however, this balance can be disrupted causing mitochondrial dysfunction and cell death.

4. Mitochondria, cell injury, and apoptosis

Manganese superoxide dismutase (MnSOD) and glutathione represent endogenous molecules that minimize mitochondrial-derived ROS. Mitochondrial injury occurs, however, when ROS formation exceeds the capacity for their removal by these antioxidant mechanisms. ROS biochemically modify other molecules to produce cytotoxic species that induce cellular injury [28]. For example, ROS induce the formation of 4-hydroxynonenal (HNE), a reactive lipid species that is associated with neuronal damage in brains of Parkinson's disease patients [29, 30]. ROS production also leads to cell death *via* the induction of apoptosis. Activation of the intrinsic apoptotic pathway occurs in response to a decrease in mitochondrial membrane potential, opening of the mPTP and release of cytochrome C [23]. Cytochrome C initiates the pro-apoptotic cascade by activating the initiator caspase 9, which in turn cleaves the final effector caspase 3. There are also a number of proteins that regulate apoptosis, including anti-apoptotic Bcl-2, and pro-apoptotic *Bax* and *Bad* proteins [31]. When cytosolic *Bax* binds to the outer mitochondrial membrane, it induces apoptosis by stimulating cytochrome C release. Further, the binding of *Bax* to Bcl-2 inhibits the anti-apoptotic effects of Bcl-2, resulting in cell death. The dimerization and localization of this group of proteins modulate apoptosis under both basal and pathological conditions and can be modified by the cellular microenvironment.

5. Mitochondrial responses to estrogen

Both nuclear and mitochondrial genes are subject to regulation by estrogen [32]. Nuclear DNA encodes proteins that are incorporated in mitochondria and influence their function. For example, the binding of estrogen to nuclear ERα induces the expression of peroxisome proliferator-activated receptor gamma coactivator 1-alpha (PGC1α) [33]. This protein plays an important role in mitochondrial biogenesis, a process by which new mitochondria are formed. The mitochondrion also contains its own maternally inherited DNA, which encodes 37 genes [25]. A recent study in MCF-7 cells showed that estrogen regulates mitochondrial RNA production under serum starvation conditions [34]. Subsequent to estrogen treatment, ERα translocated to the mitochondria and increased expression of mitochondrial tRNAs used to translate mitochondrial proteins. In GH4C1 pituitary cells, treatment with estrogen increases expression of mitochondrial-encoded RNA for subunit II of cytochrome C oxidase [35]. In female rats, levels of mitochondrial-encoded 16S RNA, a housekeeping gene used as a marker for mitochondrial number, are four times higher than males of the same age [36, 37]. Ovariectomy (OVX) in rats is characterized by an increase in liver and brain peroxide production and formation of 8-oxo-2'deoxyguanosine, a marker of mitochondrial DNA damage. These changes were associated with a reduction in the antioxidant protein GSH and MnSOD [36]. Estrogen treatment in OVX rats reversed these responses [36]. Collectively, these data suggest that increased estrogen levels regulate mitochondrial and nuclear anti-oxidant protein expression.

Estrogen plays an important role in the regulation of apoptosis by stimulating Bcl-2 protein expression and translocation to the mitochondria. This is achieved *via* the Ca^{2+} regulated ERK pathway [38]. The regulation of both Bcl-2 and *Bax* expression by estrogen has been reported in THP-1 macrophages and human monocyte-derived macrophages. Pre-treatment with estrogen increased the Bcl-2: *Bax* ratio, thus increasing cell viability in the presence of pro-apoptotic stimuli. Estrogen treatment of cortical neurons has also been shown to inhibit glutamate toxicity and improve cell viability by upregulating Bcl-2 expression [39]. In SH-SY5Y neuroblastoma cells over-expressing ERβ, the receptor has been shown to interact with the pro-apoptotic protein *Bad* and prevent its binding to *Bax*, thereby inhibiting apoptosis [40]. These data suggest that both estrogen and ERs *per se* are anti-apoptotic and modulate disease pathogenesis. Estrogen also preserves cell viability by altering mitochondrial dynamics. In the myocardium of ischemia reperfusion injury rodents, OVX rodents display an increase in mitochondrial fusion after injury, which is reversed by estrogen treatment [41] Work in isolated cortical astrocytes from male and female postnatal day 1 mice shows that estrogen regulates fission and fusion genes in a gender-specific manner [42]. Further, estrogen stimulated mitochondrial biogenesis in skeletal muscle and adipocytes [43, 44]. These data suggest that estrogen can strengthen the mitochondrial network by increasing mitochondrial fusion, thus preserving mitochondrial function and cell viability.

Estrogen effects on mitochondrial function vary in different cell types. For example, estrogen binds specifically to the oligomycin-sensitivity conferring protein of ATP-synthase (Complex V) in brain mitochondria and inhibits ATP production [45]. In contrast, another study showed that the enzymatic activity of F0F1-ATPase, a Complex V subunit, is higher in mitochondria isolated from the heart than other tissues. Estrogen induced a further increase in cardiac ATPase activity implying a direct link between estrogen stimulation and ATP production [45, 46]. Estrogen can therefore exert different effects on mitochondria from different cell types. These differential responses may impact disease pathogenesis.

6. Estrogen, mitochondria, and cardiovascular disease

Cardiovascular disease (CVD) is the leading cause of death in men and women, and American Heart Association statistics reveal a significant increase in CVD mortality in women compared to men [47]. Mitochondrial dysfunction has been implicated as a causative factor in CVD, with mitochondrial DNA damage being significantly increased in the heart and aorta of patients with CVD compared to healthy controls [25, 48–50]. Women do not generally present with CVD until the seventh decade, while the incidence of death due to CVD is high in men throughout life. This age-dependent increase in CVD in women has been linked to the onset of menopause and a reduction in circulating estrogen levels. The "Free Radical Theory of Aging" proposes that, with increased age, an increase in free radical formation initiates a vicious cycle of ROS formation that causes progressive cell injury [51]. Data suggest that loss of the antioxidant and anti-inflammatory effects of estrogen after menopause contributes to the development of mitochondrial injury [52, 53]. Thus, maintaining high levels of estrogen may increase lifespan and/or health in postmenopausal women.

Studies using experimental animal models of CVD show that OVX increases vascular inflammation/injury in a manner that is prevented by estrogen treatment [54, 55]. Analysis of mitochondria isolated from hearts of OVX rats reveals increased levels of apoptotic markers compared to mitochondria of intact animals. Administration of estrogen to these animals significantly attenuated apoptosis [56]. Since mitochondrial damage and apoptosis can be mediated by ROS, it has been hypothesized that the estrogen can decrease ROS by activating the antioxidant pathway. Treatment of human aortic endothelial cells (HAECs) with estradiol upregulates the mitochondrial antioxidant MnSOD by an ERα-dependent mechanism. The ability of estrogen to increase MnSOD levels is ablated in ERα KO mice but not in ERβ KO mice. Interestingly, while ERβ does not regulate MnSOD expression, it was shown to be essential for preventing atherosclerotic progression *in vivo* [57, 58]. These data show that ERs modulate mitochondrial antioxidant production and have distinctive vasoprotective mechanisms.

Gender differences have been identified in mitochondrial genes isolated from rat hearts [59]. Whole genome microarray analysis showed that expression of genes associated with mitochondrial apoptosis pathways is significantly elevated in male mice compared to females. In contrast, genes associated with fatty acid and glucose metabolism were upregulated in females. Female rats also displayed higher transcription levels for mitochondrial Complexes I and IV. These data suggest that genes related to cellular metabolism, including mitochondrial respiration, are upregulated in cardiac mitochondria from female rats while genes associated with mitochondrial apoptosis are increased in males. Whether this difference is directly related to the circulating levels of estrogen *in vivo* is unclear.

Mitochondrial structure in the heart is influenced by estrogen. The hearts of OVX rats that underwent I/R injury had lower levels of mitochondrial respiratory function and increased myocardial cell death compared to intact animals. Transmission electron microscopy showed that the mitochondria in cardiomyocytes from OVX rats were more disordered within the cell and structurally damaged compared to mitochondria from intact animals [41]. Interestingly, even male ERα KO mice that underwent cardiac I/R injury display lower coronary blood flow rates, increased calcium accumulation, and reduced nitrite production compared to non-ischemic hearts. Further, electron microscopic analysis revealed that the mitochondria from ERα KO mice were abnormally shaped [60]. These studies suggest that estrogen signaling plays a role in regulating mitochondrial structure in both females and males. In another model of I/R injury, female wild-type mouse hearts were shown to have better functional recovery and an attenuated inflammatory response compared to female ERα KO mice and wild-type male mice [61]. These data further suggest the importance of ER signaling as a cardioprotective mechanism in females.

Effects of estrogen on mitochondrial function have been tested in a genetic model of hypertrophic cardiomyopathy (cTnT-Q92). Estrogen treatment improved ATP production, the mitochondrial respiratory ratio, and diastolic function in OVX cTnT-Q92 mice compared to untreated OVX mice [62]. OVX in cTnT-Q92 mice attenuated the expression of the mitochondrial biogenesis genes PGC1α, peroxisome proliferator-activated receptor alpha (PPARα), mitochondrial transcription factor A (tFAM), and the antioxidant protein nuclear respiratory factor 1 (NRF-1). Estrogen treatment improved cardiac mitochondrial organization and cristae structure and increased mitochondrial biogenesis. These data directly show that estrogen exerts cytoprotective effects at the level of the mitochondrion that translate into an improvement in cardiac function.

7. Estrogen, mitochondria, and inflammation

Macrophages contribute to the chronic inflammation associated with many diseases including CVD and neurodegeneration. Macrophages display plasticity in that they may adopt various phenotypes. The differentiation of these cells is highly dependent on the local microenvironment in which they are situated. M1 macrophages are pro-inflammatory and are induced by cytokines and lipopolysaccharide (LPS). M2 macrophages are anti-inflammatory, play a role in wound healing, and are induced by IL-4 and IL-13 [63, 64]. The metabolic characteristics of M1 and M2 macrophages are different. M1 macrophages rely on glycolysis for ATP formation while M2 macrophages are dependent on mitochondrial oxidative phosphorylation for energy [63, 64]. Damage to mitochondria induced by inflammatory stimuli can exacerbate cellular injury [65]. It was shown that both ERα knockout and mitochondrial dysfunction inhibit the IL-4 mediated conversion to macrophages from an M1 to an M2 phenotype [64, 66].

Treatment of macrophages with LPS/interferon-γ (IFN-γ) favors an increase in the M1 phenotype. In macrophages isolated from premenopausal women, estrogen treatment was shown to reduce the M1/M2 ratio in cells exposed to LPS/IFN-γ to a greater extent than macrophages isolated from postmenopausal women [67]. Recent studies from our group have shown that there is a significant decrease in ERα expression in macrophages from postmenopausal women compared to premenopausal women while estrogen therapy was able to preserve ERα expression [68]. These data imply that estrogen and ER levels play a crucial role in macrophage polarization, but the role of estrogen on the mitochondrial function in these groups is still unknown. Determining the role of estrogen on the mitochondria and how it affects macrophage phenotype can help us to better understand the anti-inflammatory roles of estrogen.

8. Estrogen, mitochondria, and neurodegeneration

Neurodegenerative disorders such as Alzheimer's disease (AD) and Parkinson's disease (PD) are characterized by the progressive deterioration and death of specific neuron types in the brain [69]. It is well known that mitochondrial dysfunction plays a pathogenic role in neurodegeneration [69]. AD is characterized by atrophy of the cortex and hippocampus. Additionally, increases in glucose metabolism and a reduction in the activities of mitochondrial Complexes I, III, and IV in the brain have been reported [69, 70]. Plaques containing amyloid beta and tau protein can become incorporated in the remaining brain cells [69]. These inclusions are known to increase oxidative stress and mitochondrial dysfunction.

In PD, the loss of dopaminergic neurons in the substantia nigra contributes to the development of motor disturbances. The protein alpha synuclein becomes entangled with these neurons, resulting in ROS production, mitochondrial dysfunction, and neuronal cell death [71]. A decrease in mitochondrial Complex I activity has been observed in postmortem brains of PD patients that is linked to a reduction in oxidative phosphorylation [72]. *In vivo* and *in vitro* models of PD utilize Complex I inhibitors, such as rotenone, to induce PD-like systems to study disease mechanisms [73, 74]. Most PD cases are of unknown etiology; however, data suggest that defects in the expression of the mitochondrial clearance genes parkin, pink1, and DJ-1 may be an underlying mechanism [69].

Gender differences have been identified in the pathology of both AD and PD [75, 76]. These include alterations in brain weight, regional atrophy, distribution of white and gray matter, cerebral blood flow, expression of neurotransmitter transporters and receptors, and age of onset [77]. In the case of PD, there is also an increased incidence of the disease in men compared to women [78, 79]. The gender difference in neurodegenerative phenotypes has led to the hypothesis that estrogen exerts neuroprotective effects and that these effects are mediated at the level of the mitochondrion [80]. In mouse spinal cord neurons, estrogen treatment increased mRNA levels of nuclear-encoded mitochondrial electron transport chain genes ND1, CytB, Cox2, and ATP6 [80]. ERα has been identified in the mitochondria of endothelial cells in the brain and forebrain. In these cells, estrogen increased expression of cytochrome C and reduced ROS formation [81]. ERβ has been localized to hippocampal mitochondria [17, 81, 82]. Hippocampal cells isolated from ERβ KO mice had lower mitochondrial membrane potential and were more resistant to oxidative stress compared to control mice [83]. Taken together, these data suggest opposing effects of ERα and ERβ in the brain. More cell-type specific studies are needed to better understand the role of these ERs in the brain and to help clarify these opposing views.

Estrogen also interacts with mitochondrial proteins in a non-genomic manner. Under *in vitro* conditions, estrogen had no effect on sodium dependent calcium influx from mitochondria isolated from synaptosomes and increased mitochondrial calcium efflux [84]. Thus, estrogen prevented mitochondrial calcium overload. Higher levels of cytoplasmic calcium increase mitochondrial ATP production and cause neuron-specific changes in cellular signaling. In aged, post-reproductive rodents, loss of estrogen is associated with a decrease in brain weight and a concomitant increase in the utilization of ketone bodies and fatty acids [85]. This was associated with a decrease in metabolic substrates for mitochondrial ATP production that was further decreased in an AD mouse model [85]. Taken together, we and others propose that reductions in estrogen levels that cause decreased mitochondrial function during the postmenopausal period may explain the increased incidence of AD in women at this stage.

Estrogen preserves mitochondrial structure/function by upregulating the mitochondrial anti-oxidant enzyme MnSOD in the brain of female rodents [37, 86, 87]. In SK-N-SH neuroblastoma cells, estrogen inhibits the effects of the mitochondrial Complex II inhibitor, 3-nitroprionic acid (3-NPA), by preserving mitochondrial ATP production and inhibiting the 3-NPA induced hydrogen peroxide and peroxynitrite formation [88]. These data suggest that estrogen also plays an anti-oxidant role in the brain. This has led many to hypothesize that the anti-oxidant effects of estrogen may play a role in slowing disease pathogenesis.

Estrogen also regulates mitochondrial dynamics in astrocytes in a gender-dependent manner. It reduces expression of the fusion protein Mfn1 in astrocytes isolated from male rodents but has no effect on astrocytes obtained from females [80]. Treatment of cortical primary astrocytes with estrogen increases the expression of fission (Dyn 1 and Fis 1) and fusion (Mfn2) proteins to a greater extent in female mice than males. The upregulation of both fission and fusion proteins suggests that mitochondrial network is more dynamic in females than males. Although the exact mechanisms and reasons for the differences in fission and fusion regulation between male and female rodents are unknown, these responses may explain the sexual dimorphism seen in neurodegenerative diseases and other pathologies.

9. Estrogen, mitochondria, and cancer

Cancer is the second leading cause of death in the United States, and, among all cancers, breast cancer is the second most commonly diagnosed cancer in women. Breast tumor cells that express estrogen receptors are classified as ER-positive and account for 80% of all breast cancers [89]. Further, the Women's Health Initiative Study showed that menopausal hormone therapy (MHT) increases the incidence of breast cancer in women compared to controls [90]. Modern day cancer treatment principally focuses on identifying estrogen signatures in breast cancers, and suppression of estrogen receptor function is a routine therapeutic strategy.

Estrogen is known to regulate mitochondrial function in the context of breast cancer by several mechanisms. First, it has been shown to alter mitochondrial morphology. Administration of physiologically relevant doses of estrogen to MCF-7 breast cancer cell lines results in enlargement of mitochondria [91]. Mitochondrial cristae adopt an abnormal structure that is reminiscent of mitochondria that are oxygen-deprived and rely on glycolysis for ATP formation. This change in structure was associated with a 2.5-fold increase in the mitochondrial content of ERα and ERβ and an increase in the mitochondrial expression of cytochrome C oxidase subunits I and II. Alternatively, activation of cell membrane estrogen receptors is reported to induce changes in the cytoskeleton that indirectly influences mitochondrial structure [92]. Alteration in mitochondrial structure not only affects the capacity of the energy production but also influences other crucial functions such as calcium signaling, ROS production, or biosynthetic processes.

Second, estrogen induces cellular ROS production in cancer cells by three main pathways: (1) direct inhibition of respiratory chain complexes; (2) accumulation of calcium within mitochondria; and (3) inhibition of the antioxidant response element (ARE) [92]. The increase in ROS generation by the mitochondria and the decrease in antioxidant capacity cause a cellular shift to high ROS production that plays an important role in cancer cell proliferation and cell damage. Estrogen also promotes ROS formation in breast cancer cells by inducing cyclin D1 gene expression [93]. NRF-1 regulates the expression of several nuclear-encoded mitochondrial genes [94] that encode respiratory protein subunits, mtDNA transcription/replication machinery, components of heme biosynthesis, and mitochondrial protein import [95]. Cyclin D1 phosphorylates NRF-1, resulting in repression of its activity. This inactivation of NRF-1 reduces mitochondrial activity and shift glucose metabolism toward glycolysis [96]. The reduction in mitochondrial ATP production, in part, increases mitochondrial ROS production.

Another characteristic of cancer cells is that they highjack apoptotic pathways in order to evade cell death. When normal cells are exposed to UV radiation, the generation of mitochondrial ROS activates c-jun N-terminal kinase (JNK) and protein kinase C (PKC)-δ. These signaling molecules trigger the translocation of *Bax* to the mitochondria and induce apoptosis. In breast cancer cells exposed to UV radiation, estrogen attenuates cytochrome C release, preserves mitochondrial membrane potential, and inhibits apoptotic cell death [97]. Other data show that addition of estrogen to MCF-7 breast cancer cells induced apoptotic signaling through the extrinsic cell death *Fas* ligand pathway. This response was accompanied by an increase in the expression of anti-apoptotic Bcl-2 [98].

The role of estrogen receptors in breast cancer development has been known for almost over 30 years. Subsequent studies strongly suggested that ER status is the single most important predictive and prognostic biomarker in breast cancer. Clinicians use several strategies to battle estrogen-sensitive breast cancer, which affect not only estrogen levels but also mitochondrial function. One approach is to block ovarian function. Ovarian ablation can either be performed surgically to remove the ovaries (oophorectomy) or by radiation. An alternative approach is to temporarily suppress the ovarian function pharmacologically using gonadotropin-releasing hormone (GnRH) agonists. GnRH interferes with signals that are produced by the pituitary gland that stimulate the ovaries to produce estrogen. GnRH agonists also act by inducing mitochondrial depolarization, thereby decreasing mitochondrial oxidative capacity. Aromatase inhibitors represent another pharmacological approach to inhibit estrogen synthesis. Addition of aromatase inhibitors to MCF-7 cells was shown to induce caspase 9 expression [99]. Thus, activation of the intrinsic cell death pathway may be an alternative mechanism by which aromatase inhibitors decrease cancer progression. Selective estrogen receptor modulators (SERMs) are another class of drugs that are used for treatment of breast cancers. The SERM tamoxifen blocks the ability of estrogen to stimulate the growth of breast cancer cells. Tamoxifen has also been shown to induce mitochondrial ROS and apoptosis by increasing mitochondrial nitric oxide synthase (mtNOS) [100]. Tamoxifen decreases cellular respiration, increases mitochondrial cytochrome C release, and increases mitochondrial lipid peroxide formation. These data suggest that tamoxifen induces the mitochondrial cell death pathway. While current breast cancer therapeutics inhibit both estrogen signaling and mitochondrial function, the development of next generation drugs that can more efficiently inhibit these processes is required.

10. Conclusions

Estrogen is a multi-functional hormone that exerts its effects by both transcriptional and non-genomic mechanisms. Nuclear transcriptional responses are classically induced by binding of estrogen to ERα and ERβ. Estrogen-dependent gene transcription plays an important role in the development of female reproductive structures and regulation of the estrous cycle. The local production of estrogen is now also thought to regulate physiological responses in males. Non-genomic responses to estrogen are more rapid and include induction of signaling pathways that promote cell proliferation. The differential expression of ERs in different cell types and cellular loci dictates their specific function.

Studies in recent years have defined a role for estrogen in the regulation of mitochondrial structure and function. Estrogen increases expression of respiratory complexes, antioxidant molecules, and anti-apoptotic factors that directly impact mitochondrial structure and function. Aging in women is associated with a reduction in estrogen formation and the development of mitochondrial dysfunction. An increase in free radical damage in cells also occurs with aging. Damaged mitochondria are more likely to produce additional ROS, thus initiating a vicious cycle that progressively degrades cellular function. This includes estrogen biosynthesis. Transgenic mice with a mutation in the inner mitochondrial membrane peptidase-2 (IMMP-2) had hyperpolarized mitochondria, which produced increased levels of superoxide and ATP and resulted in impaired ovulation and reduced fertility [101]. Other data show that defective mitochondrial DNA polymerase activity induces mitochondrial dysfunction and infertility in mice [102]. It follows that cytoprotective responses to estrogen at the level of the mitochondrion are ablated. Thus, a reciprocal relationship exists between estrogen and mitochondrial function. Under normal physiological conditions, mitochondria are critical mediators of estrogen biosynthesis and are also targets for estrogen action.

Strong evidence suggests that estrogen plays a major role in promoting the proliferation of both normal and the neoplastic breast cancer cells. However, cancer represents a unique scenario in which estrogen exerts tumorigenic responses in susceptible cells. Prolonged exposure to high levels of estrogen is associated with an increased incidence of breast cancer, which supports models of estrogen-induced carcinogenesis. In breast cancer cells, estrogen is shown to not only stimulate the cell proliferation but also inhibit apoptotic pathways, which can therefore lead to uncontrolled tumor growth. Estrogen increases mitochondrial ROS production that can also promote cancer progression. Further research is needed to expand our understanding of how estrogen induces carcinogenesis.

Estrogen and ER signaling in the mitochondria play an important role in health and disease. We have shown that estrogen effects are cell type and receptor type specific, which explains the varied effects of estrogen treatment described in this review. We also understand that despite the protective role of estrogen in inflammation, cardiovascular disease, and neurodegeneration, it promotes breast cancer through both nuclear and mitochondrial regulation. Further research is needed to understand the specific mechanisms of estrogen-induced mitochondrial changes in health and disease.

Acknowledgements

This work was supported by grants from the National Institutes of Health (GM115367 and DK108836).

Author details

Ved P. Mooga[1], C. Roger White[2] and Samantha Giordano-Mooga[3*]

*Address all correspondence to: sgiordan@uab.edu

1 GenScript USA Inc., Piscataway, New Jersey, United States

2 Vascular Biology and Hypertension Program, Department of Medicine, University of Alabama at Birmingham, Birmingham, Alabama, United States

3 Clinical and Diagnostic Sciences, School of Health Professions, University of Alabama at Birmingham, Birmingham, Alabama, United States

References

[1] Velarde MC. Mitochondrial and sex steroid hormone crosstalk during aging. Longevity & Healthspan. 2014;**3**(1):2

[2] Fåhraeus L. The effects of estradiol on blood lipids and lipoproteins in postmenopausal women. Obstetrics and Gynecology. 1988;**72**(5 Suppl):18S-22S

[3] Nathan L, Chaudhuri G. Estrogens and atherosclerosis. Annual Review of Pharmacology and Toxicology. 1997;**37**:477-515

[4] Dahlman-Wright K, Cavailles V, Fuqua SA, Jordan VC, Katzenellenbogen JA, Korach KS, et al. International Union of Pharmacology. LXIV. Estrogen receptors. Pharmacological Reviews. 2006;**58**(4):773-781

[5] Levin ER. Integration of the extranuclear and nuclear actions of estrogen. Molecular Endocrinology. 2005;**19**(8):1951-1959

[6] Zhou J, Cidlowski JA. The human glucocorticoid receptor: One gene, multiple proteins and diverse responses. Steroids. 2005;**70**(5-7):407-417

[7] Hirata S, Shoda T, Kato J, Hoshi K. Isoform/variant mRNAs for sex steroid hormone receptors in humans. Trends in Endocrinology and Metabolism. 2003;**14**(3):124-129

[8] Hirata S, Shoda T, Kato J, Hoshi K. Novel isoforms of the mRNA for human female sex steroid hormone receptors. The Journal of Steroid Biochemistry and Molecular Biology. 2002;**83**(1-5):25-30

[9] Lewandowski S, Kalita K, Kaczmarek L. Estrogen receptor beta. Potential functional significance of a variety of mRNA isoforms. FEBS Letters. 2002;**524**(1-3):1-5

[10] Post WS, Goldschmidt-Clermont PJ, Wilhide CC, Heldman AW, Sussman MS, Ouyang P, et al. Methylation of the estrogen receptor gene is associated with aging and atherosclerosis in the cardiovascular system. Cardiovascular Research. 1999;**43**(4):985-991

[11] Ying AK, Hassanain HH, Roos CM, Smiraglia DJ, Issa JJ, Michler RE, et al. Methylation of the estrogen receptor-alpha gene promoter is selectively increased in proliferating human aortic smooth muscle cells. Cardiovascular Research. 2000;**46**(1):172-179

[12] Couse JF, Korach KS. Estrogen receptor null mice: What have we learned and where will they lead us? Endocrine Reviews. 1999;**20**(3):358-417

[13] Dupont S, Krust A, Gansmuller A, Dierich A, Chambon P, Mark M. Effect of single and compound knockouts of estrogen receptors alpha (ERalpha) and beta (ERbeta) on mouse reproductive phenotypes. Development. 2000;**127**(19):4277-4291

[14] Krege JH, Hodgin JB, Couse JF, Enmark E, Warner M, Mahler JF, et al. Generation and reproductive phenotypes of mice lacking estrogen receptor beta. Proceedings of the National Academy of Sciences of the United States of America. 1998;**95**(26):15677-15682

[15] Luconi M, Forti G, Baldi E. Genomic and nongenomic effects of estrogens: Molecular mechanisms of action and clinical implications for male reproduction. The Journal of Steroid Biochemistry and Molecular Biology. 2002;**80**(4-5):369-381

[16] Noteboom WD, Gorski J. Stereospecific binding of estrogens in the rat uterus. Archives of Biochemistry and Biophysics. 1965;**111**(3):559-568

[17] Yang SH, Liu R, Perez EJ, Wen Y, Stevens SM, Valencia T, et al. Mitochondrial localization of estrogen receptor beta. Proceedings of the National Academy of Sciences of the United States of America. 2004;**101**(12):4130-4135

[18] Psarra AM, Sekeris CE. Steroid and thyroid hormone receptors in mitochondria. IUBMB Life. 2008;**60**(4):210-223

[19] Chen JQ, Eshete M, Alworth WL, Yager JD. Binding of MCF-7 cell mitochondrial proteins and recombinant human estrogen receptors alpha and beta to human mitochondrial DNA estrogen response elements. Journal of Cellular Biochemistry. 2004;**93**(2):358-373

[20] Sharma G, Mauvais-Jarvis F, Prossnitz ER. Roles of G protein-coupled estrogen receptor GPER in metabolic regulation. The Journal of Steroid Biochemistry and Molecular Biology. 2018;**176**(1879-1220):31-37

[21] Revankar CM, Cimino DF, Sklar LA, Arterburn JB, Prossnitz ER. A transmembrane intracellular estrogen receptor mediates rapid cell signaling. Science. 2005;**307**(5715):1625-1630

[22] Prossnitz ER, Barton M. The G-protein-coupled estrogen receptor GPER in health and disease. Nature Reviews. Endocrinology. 2011;**7**(12):715-726

[23] Bopassa JC, Eghbali M, Toro L, Stefani E. A novel estrogen receptor GPER inhibits mitochondria permeability transition pore opening and protects the heart against ischemia-reperfusion injury. American Journal of Physiology. Heart and Circulatory Physiology. 2010;**298**(1):H16-H23

[24] Toran-Allerand CD, Guan X, MacLusky NJ, Horvath TL, Diano S, Singh M, et al. ER-X: A novel, plasma membrane-associated, putative estrogen receptor that is regulated during development and after ischemic brain injury. The Journal of Neuroscience. 2002;**22**(19):8391-8401

[25] Ballinger SW. Mitochondrial dysfunction in cardiovascular disease. Free Radical Biology & Medicine. 2005;**38**(10):1278-1295

[26] Zhang J. Autophagy and mitophagy in cellular damage control. Redox Biology. 2013; **1**(1):19-23

[27] Archer SL. Mitochondrial dynamics – mitochondrial fission and fusion in human diseases. The New England Journal of Medicine. 2013;**369**(23):2236-2251

[28] D'Autréaux B, Toledano MB. ROS as signalling molecules: Mechanisms that generate specificity in ROS homeostasis. Nature Reviews. Molecular Cell Biology. 2007; **8**(10):813-824

[29] Yoritaka A, Hattori N, Uchida K, Tanaka M, Stadtman ER, Mizuno Y. Immunohistochemical detection of 4-hydroxynonenal protein adducts in Parkinson disease. Proceedings of the National Academy of Sciences of the United States of America. 1996;**93**(7):2696-2701

[30] Perluigi M, Coccia R, Butterfield A. HNE a reactive product of lipid peroxidation and neurodegenerative diseases: A toxic combination illuminated by Redox proteomics studies. Antioxidants & Redox Signaling 2012;**11**(1557-7716):1590-609

[31] Czabotar PE, Lessene G, Strasser A, Adams JM. Control of apoptosis by the BCL-2 protein family: Implications for physiology and therapy. Nature Reviews. Molecular Cell Biology. 2014;**15**(1):49-63

[32] Demonacos C, Djordjevic-Markovic R, Tsawdaroglou N, Sekeris CE. The mitochondrion as a primary site of action of glucocorticoids: The interaction of the glucocorticoid receptor with mitochondrial DNA sequences showing partial similarity to the nuclear glucocorticoid responsive elements. The Journal of Steroid Biochemistry and Molecular Biology. 1995;**55**(1):43-55

[33] Schreiber SN, Emter R, Hock MB, Knutti D, Cardenas J, Podvinec M, et al. The estrogen-related receptor alpha (ERRalpha) functions in PPARgamma coactivator 1alpha (PGC-1alpha)-induced mitochondrial biogenesis. Proceedings of the National Academy of Sciences of the United States of America. 2004;**101**(17):6472-6477

[34] Sanchez MI, Shearwood AM, Chia T, Davies SM, Rackham O, Filipovska A. Estrogen-mediated regulation of mitochondrial gene expression. Molecular Endocrinology. 2015; **29**(1):14-27

[35] Van Itallie CM, Dannies PS. Estrogen induces accumulation of the mitochondrial ribonucleic acid for subunit II of cytochrome oxidase in pituitary tumor cells. Molecular Endocrinology. 1988;**2**(4):332-337

[36] Borrás C, Sastre J, García-Sala D, Lloret A, Pallardó FV, Viña J. Mitochondria from females exhibit higher antioxidant gene expression and lower oxidative damage than males. Free Radical Biology & Medicine. 2003;**34**(5):546-552

[37] Borrás C, Gambini J, Gómez-Cabrera MC, Sastre J, Pallardó FV, Mann GE, et al. 17beta-oestradiol up-regulates longevity-related, antioxidant enzyme expression via the ERK1 and ERK2[MAPK]/NFkappaB cascade. Aging Cell. 2005;**4**(3):113-118

[38] Subramanian M, Shaha C. Up-regulation of Bcl-2 through ERK phosphorylation is associated with human macrophage survival in an estrogen microenvironment. Journal of Immunology. 2007;**179**(4):2330-2338

[39] Nilsen J, Diaz Brinton R. Mechanism of estrogen-mediated neuroprotection: Regulation of mitochondrial calcium and Bcl-2 expression. Proceedings of the National Academy of Sciences of the United States of America. 2003;**100**(5):2842-2847

[40] Liang J, Xie Q, Li P, Zhong X, Chen Y. Mitochondrial estrogen receptor β inhibits cell apoptosis via interaction with bad in a ligand-independent manner. Molecular and Cellular Biochemistry. 2015;**401**(1-2):71-86

[41] Zhai P, Eurell TE, Cotthaus R, Jeffery EH, Bahr JM, Gross DR. Effect of estrogen on global myocardial ischemia-reperfusion injury in female rats. American Journal of Physiology. Heart and Circulatory Physiology. 2000;**279**(6):H2766-H2775

[42] Arnold S, de Araújo GW, Beyer C. Gender-specific regulation of mitochondrial fusion and fission gene transcription and viability of cortical astrocytes by steroid hormones. Journal of Molecular Endocrinology. 2008;**41**(5):289-300

[43] Capllonch-Amer G, Sbert-Roig M, Galmés-Pascual BM, Proenza AM, Lladó I, Gianotti M, et al. Estradiol stimulates mitochondrial biogenesis and adiponectin expression in skeletal muscle. The Journal of Endocrinology. 2014;**221**(3):391-403

[44] Capllonch-Amer G, Lladó I, Proenza AM, García-Palmer FJ, Gianotti M. Opposite effects of 17-β estradiol and testosterone on mitochondrial biogenesis and adiponectin synthesis in white adipocytes. Journal of Molecular Endocrinology. 2014;**52**(2):203-214

[45] Zheng J, Ramirez VD. Purification and identification of an estrogen binding protein from rat brain: Oligomycin sensitivity-conferring protein (OSCP), a subunit of mitochondrial F0F1-ATP synthase/ATPase. The Journal of Steroid Biochemistry and Molecular Biology. 1999;**68**(1-2):65-75

[46] Kipp JL, Ramirez VD. Effect of estradiol, diethylstilbestrol, and resveratrol on F0F1-ATPase activity from mitochondrial preparations of rat heart, liver, and brain. Endocrine. 2001;**15**(2):165-175

[47] Benjamin EJ, Blaha MJ, Chiuve SE, Cushman M, Das SR, Deo R, et al. Heart disease and stroke Statistics-2017 update: A report from the American Heart Association. Circulation. 2017;**135**(10):e146-e603

[48] Corral-Debrinski M, Shoffner JM, Lott MT, Wallace DC. Association of mitochondrial DNA damage with aging and coronary atherosclerotic heart disease. Mutation Research. 1992;**275**(3-6):169-180

[49] Corral-Debrinski M, Stepien G, Shoffner JM, Lott MT, Kanter K, Wallace DC. Hypoxemia is associated with mitochondrial DNA damage and gene induction. Implications for cardiac disease. Journal of the American Medical Association. 1991;**266**(13):1812-1816

[50] Ballinger SW, Patterson C, Knight-Lozano CA, Burow DL, Conklin CA, Hu Z, et al. Mitochondrial integrity and function in atherogenesis. Circulation. 2002;**106**(5):544-549

[51] Harman D. Aging: A theory based on free radical and radiation chemistry. Journal of Gerontology. 1956;**11**(3):298-300

[52] Klinge CM. Estrogenic control of mitochondrial function and biogenesis. Journal of Cellular Biochemistry. 2008;**105**(6):1342-1351

[53] Klinge CM. Estrogens regulate life and death in mitochondria. Journal of Bioenergetics and Biomembranes. 2017;**49**(4):307-324

[54] Bowling MR, Xing D, Kapadia A, Chen YF, Szalai AJ, Oparil S, et al. Estrogen effects on vascular inflammation are age dependent: Role of estrogen receptors. Arteriosclerosis, Thrombosis, and Vascular Biology. 2014;**34**(7):1477-1485

[55] Xing D, Nozell S, Chen YF, Hage F, Oparil S. Estrogen and mechanisms of vascular protection. Arteriosclerosis, Thrombosis, and Vascular Biology. 2009;**29**(3):289-295

[56] Liou CM, Yang AL, Kuo CH, Tin H, Huang CY, Lee SD. Effects of 17beta-estradiol on cardiac apoptosis in ovariectomized rats. Cell Biochemistry and Function. 2010;**28**(6):521-528

[57] Liu Z, Gou Y, Zhang H, Zuo H, Yao D. Estradiol improves cardiovascular function through up-regulation of SOD2 on vascular wall. Redox Biology. 2014;**3**:88-99

[58] Zhao C, Dahlman-Wright K, Gustafsson J. Estrogen signaling via estrogen receptor {beta}. The Journal of Biological Chemistry. 2010;**285**(51):39575-39579

[59] Vijay V, Han T, Moland CL, Kwekel JC, Fuscoe JC, Desai VG. Sexual dimorphism in the expression of mitochondria-related genes in rat heart at different ages. PLoS One. 2015;**10**(1):e0117047

[60] Zhai P, Eurell TE, Cooke PS, Lubahn DB, Gross DR. Myocardial ischemia-reperfusion injury in estrogen receptor-alpha knockout and wild-type mice. American Journal of Physiology. Heart and Circulatory Physiology. 2000;**278**(5):H1640-H1647

[61] Wang M, Crisostomo P, Wairiuko GM, Meldrum DR. Estrogen receptor-alpha mediates acute myocardial protection in females. American Journal of Physiology. Heart and Circulatory Physiology. 2006;**290**(6):H2204-H2209

[62] Chen Y, Zhang Z, Hu F, Yang W, Yuan J, Cui J, et al. 17β-estradiol prevents cardiac diastolic dysfunction by stimulating mitochondrial function: A preclinical study in a mouse model of a human hypertrophic cardiomyopathy mutation. The Journal of Steroid Biochemistry and Molecular Biology. 2015;**147**:92-102

[63] Odegaard JI, Chawla A. Alternative macrophage activation and metabolism. Annual Review of Pathology. 2011;**6**:275-297

[64] Bolego C, Cignarella A, Staels B, Chinetti-Gbaguidi G. Macrophage function and polarization in cardiovascular disease: A role of estrogen signaling? Arteriosclerosis, Thrombosis, and Vascular Biology. 2013;**33**(6):1127-1134

[65] López-Armada MJ, Riveiro-Naveira RR, Vaamonde-García C, Valcárcel-Ares MN. Mitochondrial dysfunction and the inflammatory response. Mitochondrion. 2013; **13**(2):106-118

[66] Van den Bossche J, Neele AE, Hoeksema MA, de Winther MP. Macrophage polarization: The epigenetic point of view. Current Opinion in Lipidology. 2014;**25**(5):367-373

[67] Toniolo A, Fadini GP, Tedesco S, Cappellari R, Vegeto E, Maggi A, et al. Alternative activation of human macrophages is rescued by estrogen treatment in vitro and impaired by menopausal status. The Journal of Clinical Endocrinology and Metabolism. 2015;**100**(1):E50-E58

[68] Hage FG, Xing D, Guo Y, Colon C, Szalai AJ, Chen YF, Oparil S. Abstract 14875: Estrogen-induced vasoprotection is preserved after prolonged estrogen deprivation. Circulation. 2014;**130**:A14875

[69] Johri A, Beal MF. Mitochondrial dysfunction in neurodegenerative diseases. The Journal of Pharmacology and Experimental Therapeutics. 2012;**342**(3):619-630

[70] Trimmer PA, Swerdlow RH, Parks JK, Keeney P, Bennett JP, Miller SW, et al. Abnormal mitochondrial morphology in sporadic Parkinson's and Alzheimer's disease cybrid cell lines. Experimental Neurology. 2000;**162**(1):37-50

[71] Schapira AH, Gegg M. Mitochondrial contribution to Parkinson's disease pathogenesis. Parkinson's Disease. 2011;**2011**:159160

[72] Parker WD, Parks JK, Swerdlow RH. Complex I deficiency in Parkinson's disease frontal cortex. Brain Research. 2008;**1189**:215-218

[73] Giordano S, Lee J, Darley-Usmar VM, Zhang J. Distinct effects of rotenone, 1-methyl-4-phenylpyridinium and 6-hydroxydopamine on cellular bioenergetics and cell death. PLoS One. 2012;**7**(9):e44610

[74] Greenamyre JT, Cannon JR, Drolet R, Mastroberardino PG. Lessons from the rotenone model of Parkinson's disease. Trends in Pharmacological Sciences. 2010;**31**(4):141-142 author reply 2-3

[75] Mazure CM, Swendsen J. Sex differences in Alzheimer's disease and other dementias. Lancet Neurology. 2016;**15**(5):451-452

[76] Gillies GE, Pienaar IS, Vohra S, Qamhawi Z. Sex differences in Parkinson's disease. Frontiers in Neuroendocrinology. 2014;**35**(3):370-384

[77] Cosgrove KP, Mazure CM, Staley JK. Evolving knowledge of sex differences in brain structure, function, and chemistry. Biological Psychiatry. 2007;**62**(8):847-855

[78] Swerdlow RH, Parker WD, Currie LJ, Bennett JP, Harrison MB, Trugman JM, et al. Gender ratio differences between Parkinson's disease patients and their affected relatives. Parkinsonism & Related Disorders. 2001;**7**(2):129-133

[79] Taylor KS, Cook JA, Counsell CE. Heterogeneity in male to female risk for Parkinson's disease. Journal of Neurology, Neurosurgery, and Psychiatry. 2007;**78**(8):905-906

[80] Arnold S, Victor MB, Beyer C. Estrogen and the regulation of mitochondrial structure and function in the brain. The Journal of Steroid Biochemistry and Molecular Biology. 2012;**131**(1-2):2-9

[81] Razmara A, Sunday L, Stirone C, Wang XB, Krause DN, Duckles SP, et al. Mitochondrial effects of estrogen are mediated by estrogen receptor alpha in brain endothelial cells. The Journal of Pharmacology and Experimental Therapeutics. 2008;**325**(3):782-790

[82] Alvarez-Delgado C, Mendoza-Rodríguez CA, Picazo O, Cerbón M. Different expression of alpha and beta mitochondrial estrogen receptors in the aging rat brain: Interaction with respiratory complex V. Experimental Gerontology. 2010;**45**(7-8):580-585

[83] Yang SH, Sarkar SN, Liu R, Perez EJ, Wang X, Wen Y, et al. Estrogen receptor beta as a mitochondrial vulnerability factor. The Journal of Biological Chemistry. 2009; **284**(14):9540-9548

[84] Horvat A, Petrović S, Nedeljković N, Martinović JV, Nikezić G. Estradiol affect Na-dependent Ca^{2+} efflux from synaptosomal mitochondria. General Physiology and Biophysics. 2000;**19**(1):59-71

[85] Yao J, Hamilton RT, Cadenas E, Brinton RD. Decline in mitochondrial bioenergetics and shift to ketogenic profile in brain during reproductive senescence. Biochimica et Biophysica Acta. 2010;**1800**(10):1121-1126

[86] Simpkins JW, Yi KD, Yang SH, Dykens JA. Mitochondrial mechanisms of estrogen neuroprotection. Biochimica et Biophysica Acta. 2010;**1800**(10):1113-1120

[87] Razmara A, Duckles SP, Krause DN, Procaccio V. Estrogen suppresses brain mitochondrial oxidative stress in female and male rats. Brain Research. 2007;**1176**:71-81

[88] Wang J, Green PS, Simpkins JW. Estradiol protects against ATP depletion, mitochondrial membrane potential decline and the generation of reactive oxygen species induced by 3-nitroproprionic acid in SK-N-SH human neuroblastoma cells. Journal of Neurochemistry. 2001;**77**(3):804-811

[89] Kohler BA, Sherman RL, Howlader N, Jemal A, Ryerson AB, Henry KA, et al. Annual report to the nation on the status of cancer, 1975-2011, featuring incidence of breast cancer subtypes by race/ethnicity, poverty, and state. Journal of the National Cancer Institute. 2015;**107**(6):djv048

[90] Anderson GL, Limacher M, Assaf AR, Bassford T, Beresford SA, Black H, et al. Effects of conjugated equine estrogen in postmenopausal women with hysterectomy: The Women's Health Initiative randomized controlled trial. Journal of the American Medical Association. 2004;**291**(14):1701-1712

[91] Vic P, Vignon F, Derocq D, Rochefort H. Effect of estradiol on the ultrastructure of the MCF7 human breast cancer cells in culture. Cancer Research. 1982;**42**(2):667-673

[92] Felty Q, Roy D. Estrogen, mitochondria, and growth of cancer and non-cancer cells. Journal of Carcinogenesis. 2005;**4**(1):1

[93] Castro-Rivera E, Samudio I, Safe S. Estrogen regulation of cyclin D1 gene expression in ZR-75 breast cancer cells involves multiple enhancer elements. The Journal of Biological Chemistry. 2001;**276**(33):30853-30861

[94] Scarpulla RC. Nuclear control of respiratory gene expression in mammalian cells. Journal of Cellular Biochemistry. 2006;**97**(4):673-683

[95] Cam H, Balciunaite E, Blais A, Spektor A, Scarpulla RC, Young R, et al. A common set of gene regulatory networks links metabolism and growth inhibition. Molecular Cell. 2004;**16**(3):399-411

[96] Cuezva JM, Krajewska M, de Heredia ML, Krajewski S, Santamaría G, Kim H, et al. The bioenergetic signature of cancer: A marker of tumor progression. Cancer Research. 2002;**62**(22):6674-6681

[97] Pedram A, Razandi M, Wallace DC, Levin ER. Functional estrogen receptors in the mitochondria of breast cancer cells. Molecular Biology of the Cell. 2006;**17**(5):2125-2137

[98] Song RX, Zhang Z, Mor G, Santen RJ. Down-regulation of Bcl-2 enhances estrogen apoptotic action in long-term estradiol-depleted ER(+) breast cancer cells. Apoptosis. 2005; **10**(3):667-678

[99] Amaral C, Borges M, Melo S, da Silva ET, Correia-da-Silva G, Teixeira N. Apoptosis and autophagy in breast cancer cells following exemestane treatment. PLoS One. 2012; **7**(8):e42398

[100] Nazarewicz RR, Zenebe WJ, Parihar A, Larson SK, Alidema E, Choi J, et al. Tamoxifen induces oxidative stress and mitochondrial apoptosis via stimulating mitochondrial nitric oxide synthase. Cancer Research. 2007;**67**(3):1282-1290

[101] Lu B, Poirier C, Gaspar T, Gratzke C, Harrison W, Busija D, et al. A mutation in the inner mitochondrial membrane peptidase 2-like gene (Immp2l) affects mitochondrial function and impairs fertility in mice. Biology of Reproduction. 2008;**78**(4):601-610

[102] Trifunovic A, Wredenberg A, Falkenberg M, Spelbrink JN, Rovio AT, Bruder CE, et al. Premature ageing in mice expressing defective mitochondrial DNA polymerase. Nature. 2004;**429**(6990):417-423